LEARN. PRACTICE. APPLY.

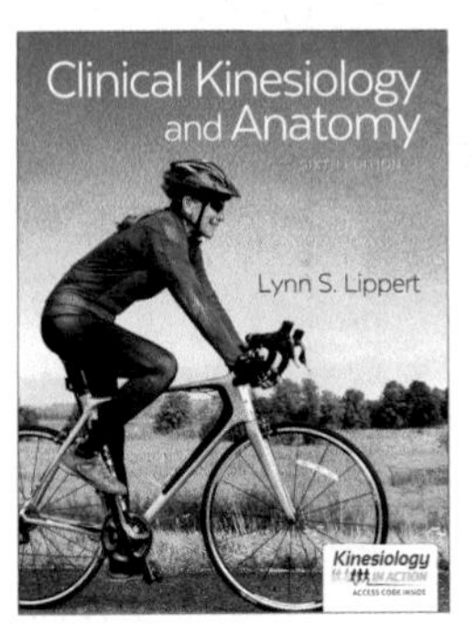

+

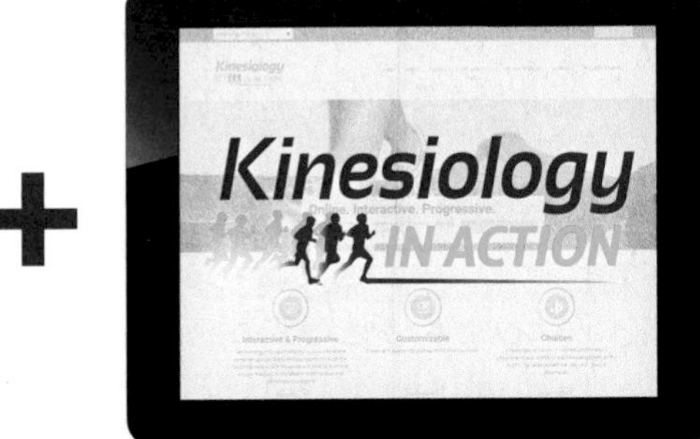

= KINESIOLOGY SUCCESS

STUDY SMARTER... NOT HARDER.

Clinical Kinesiology and Anatomy and **KinesiologyinAction.com** work together to create an immersive, multimedia experience that tracks your progress until you've mastered the concepts and techniques and are ready to apply them in class, lab, and clinic.

LEARN

Turn to your book for...

- Reviewing anatomy and how the various anatomical systems are related
- Developing foundational knowledge and critical-thinking skills
- Understanding the connection between anatomy and how the body moves.

PRACTICE & APPLY

Turn to the Kinesiology in Action for...

- Progressing through knowledge and skill-building activities and exercises
- Seeing how to apply what you're learning in practice

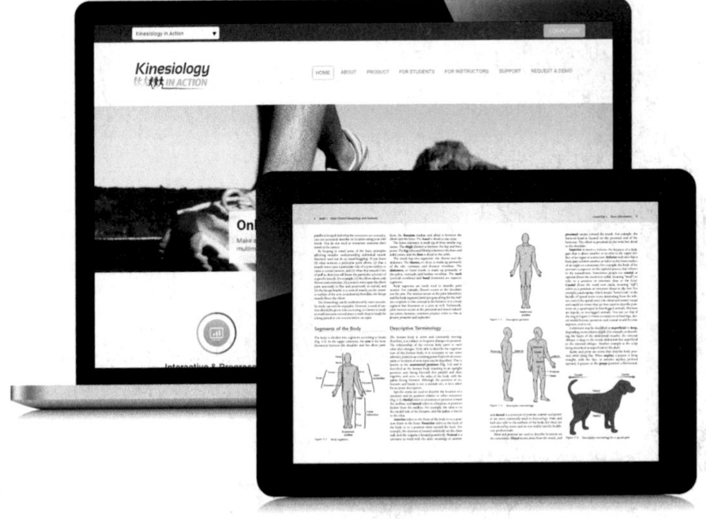

Study anytime, anywhere.

Desktop, laptop, or mobile phone.

An ebook version of your text and online access to Kinesiology in Action lets you study wherever there's an internet connection.

Kinesiology In Action

Experience the power of KinesiologyinAction.com

PRACTICE & APPLY

Kinesiology in Action is the online program that works with your text to make this challenging, must-know content easier to master. Ten online modules guide you step by step through the basic theory of joint structure and muscle action to provide the foundation you need to understand both normal and pathologic function.

PRACTICE

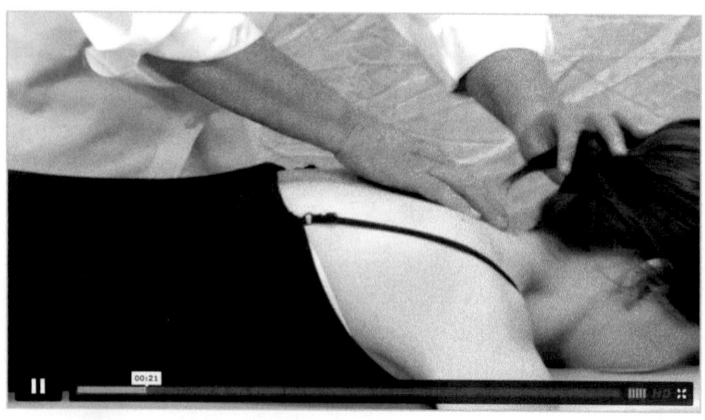

Build your confidence.

The Video Library not only offers full-color, narrated clips, but also animations that illustrate biomechanics, functional anatomy/kinesiology, posture and gait.

Practice. Practice. And more practice.

Interactive exercises, activities, and flashcards provide the know-how you need to master the content.

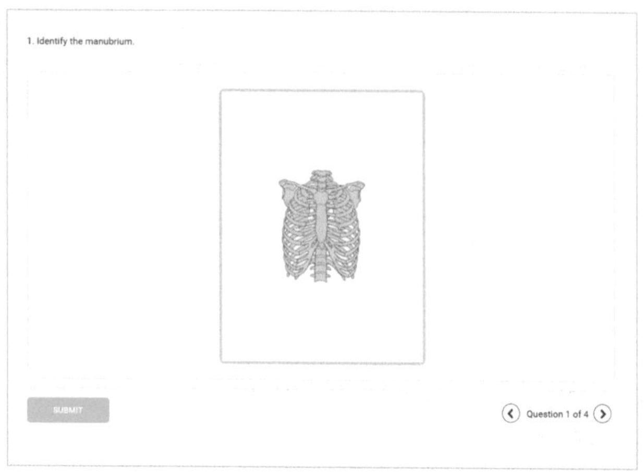

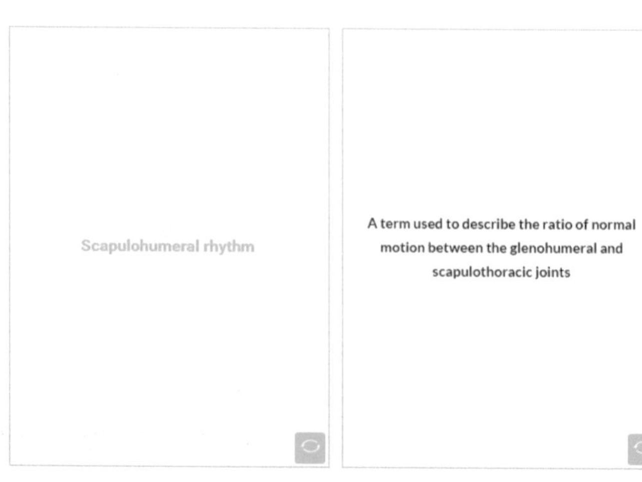

APPLY

Assess your knowledge.

Pre- and post-tests for each module evaluate your mastery of the content and how well you are able to apply your knowledge in practice.

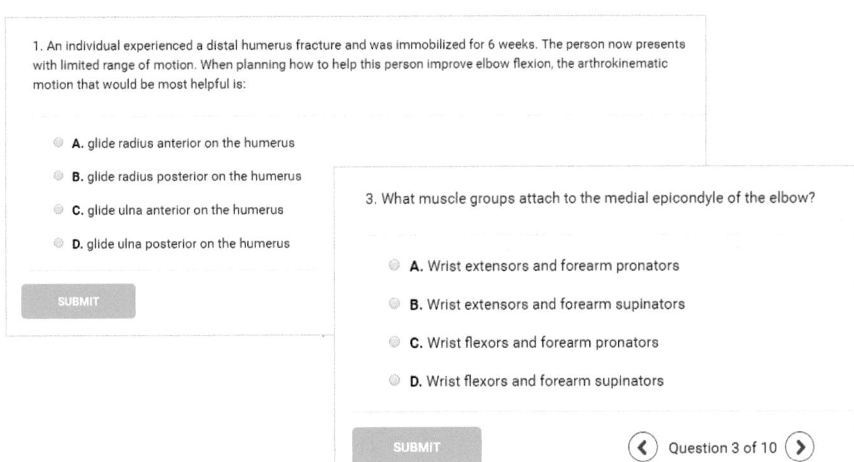

1. An individual experienced a distal humerus fracture and was immobilized for 6 weeks. The person now presents with limited range of motion. When planning how to help this person improve elbow flexion, the arthrokinematic motion that would be most helpful is:
A. glide radius anterior on the humerus
B. glide radius posterior on the humerus
C. glide ulna anterior on the humerus
D. glide ulna posterior on the humerus
SUBMIT
3. What muscle groups attach to the medial epicondyle of the elbow?
A. Wrist extensors and forearm pronators
B. Wrist extensors and forearm supinators
C. Wrist flexors and forearm pronators
D. Wrist flexors and forearm supinators
SUBMIT
Question 3 of 10

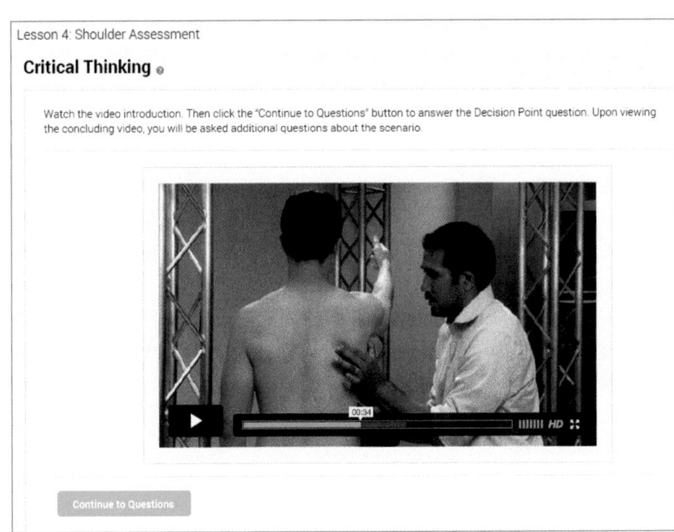

Lesson 4: Shoulder Assessment
Critical Thinking
Watch the video introduction. Then click the "Continue to Questions" button to answer the Decision Point question. Upon viewing the concluding video, you will be asked additional questions about the scenario.
Continue to Questions

Challenge yourself.

Critical-thinking exercises enhance your decision-making skills in real-world situations.

Assess your progress.

The **Gradebook** tracks your progress through each activity and each module and identifies the areas in which more study is needed.

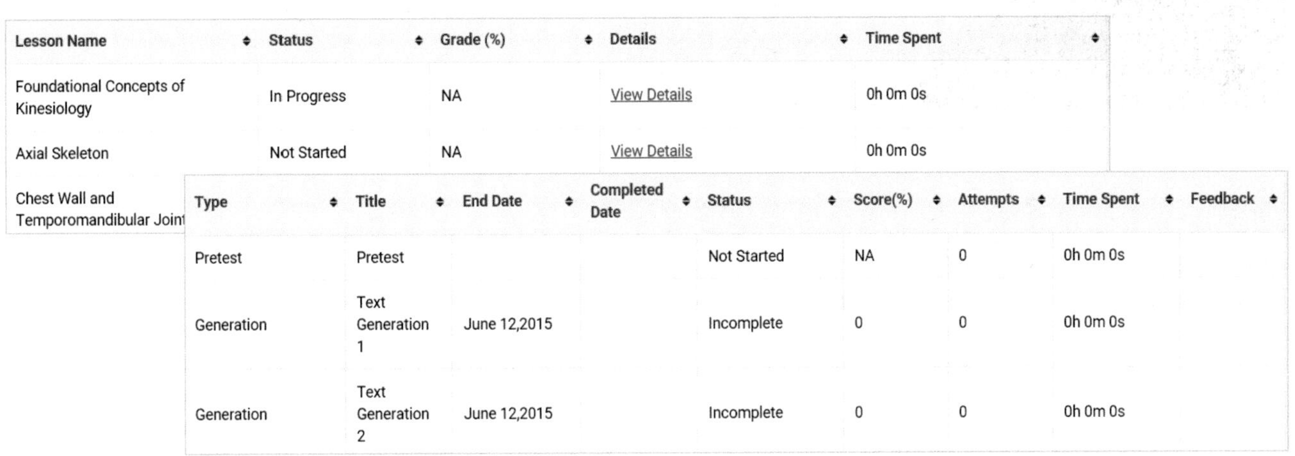

Lesson Name	Status	Grade (%)	Details	Time Spent
Foundational Concepts of Kinesiology	In Progress	NA	View Details	0h 0m 0s
Axial Skeleton	Not Started	NA	View Details	0h 0m 0s
Chest Wall and Temporomandibular Joint				

Type	Title	End Date	Completed Date	Status	Score(%)	Attempts	Time Spent	Feedback
Pretest	Pretest			Not Started	NA	0	0h 0m 0s	
Generation	Text Generation 1	June 12,2015		Incomplete	0	0	0h 0m 0s	
Generation	Text Generation 2	June 12,2015		Incomplete	0	0	0h 0m 0s	

Put Kinesiology in Action to work today!

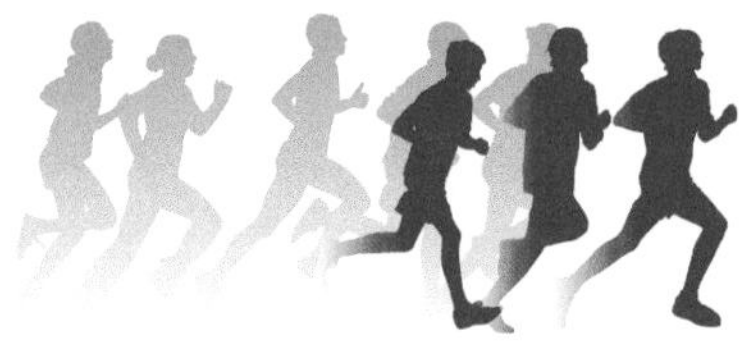

www.KinesiologyinAction.com

Follow the instructions on the inside front cover to use the access code to unlock Kinesiology in Action.

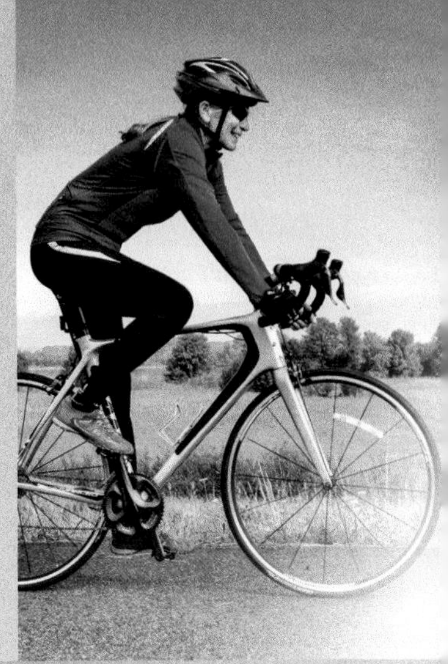

Clinical Kinesiology and Anatomy

SIXTH EDITION

Lynn S. Lippert, PT, MS
Program Director, Retired
Physical Therapist Assistant Program
Mount Hood Community College
Gresham, Oregon

With contributions from:

Jennifer Hurrell, PT, MS
Associate Professor/Rehab Health
Fieldwork Coordinator
Community College of Rhode Island
Warwick, Rhode Island

F.A. Davis Company • Philadelphia

F. A. Davis Company
1915 Arch Street
Philadelphia, PA 19103

Printed in the United States of America

Last digit indicates print number: 10 9 8 7 6 5

Senior Acquisitions Editor: Melissa A. Duffield
Manager of Content Development: George W. Lang
Developmental Editors: Lisa Consoli, Jennifer A. Pine
Art and Design Manager: Carolyn O'Brien

Library of Congress Cataloging-in-Publication Data

Names: Lippert, Lynn, 1942- author.
Title: Clinical kinesiology and anatomy / Lynn S. Lippert.
Description: Sixth edition. | Philadelphia, PA : F. A. Davis Company, [2017]
| Includes bibliographical references and index.
Identifiers: LCCN 2016057814 | ISBN 9780803658233 (pbk.)
Subjects: | MESH: Kinesiology, Applied | Movement | Musculoskeletal
System—anatomy & histology | Physical Therapy Modalities
Classification: LCC QP303 | NLM WE 103 | DDC 612.7/6—dc23
LC record available at https://lccn.loc.gov/2016057814

To Sal Jepson, who for over 27 years and six editions has provided invaluable support, advice, and wisdom. Your contribution is immeasurable. Thank you from the bottom of my heart.

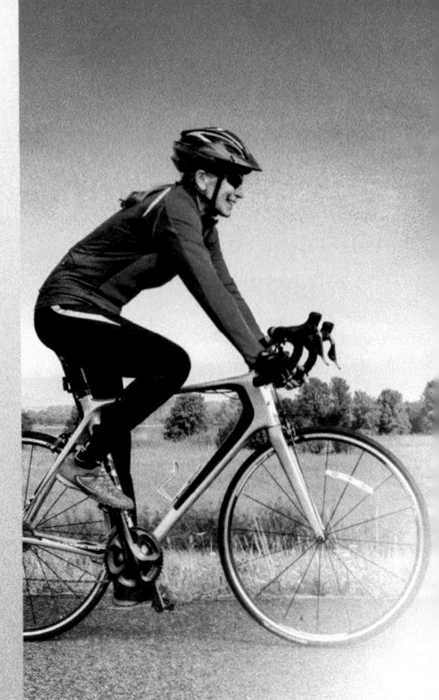

Acknowledgments

As Hillary Clinton made us so aptly aware that it takes a village to raise a child, the same can be said of the creation or revision of a book. My village includes so many individuals. Sal Jepson, who drew the original art for the first edition, and whose influence continues through to this edition, also donned Lycra and smiled while riding her bicycle for the cover shot. Mark Fitzgerald, with his knowledge of photography and helpful, easy-to-work-with style allowed the photo shoot for the cover to be accomplished to everyone's satisfaction. Don Davis has continued to make my explanations of physics simple, yet accurate. Shelby Clayson again has applied her eagle eyes to proofreading so I might accomplish my dream of an error-proof edition. Jennifer Hurrell somehow found enough time and energy while teaching full time, going to graduate school, and raising two teenage daughters to contribute some writing in this edition.

My appreciation goes out to Rob Craven, President, and the many individuals at F.A. Davis for their commitment to making this textbook one that will continue to make us all proud. Melissa Duffield, Senior Acquisitions Editor has maintained her support of this text, while juggling more projects than seemingly possible, and still kept her sense of humor. Margaret Biblis, publisher, has maintained her long history with, and support of, me and this book. Jennifer Pine, Senior Developmental Editor, whose expertise, wonderful communication skills, and calm demeanor has made the project move quite smoothly. Carolyn O'Brien, Design Manager, used her artistic eye and expertise in the creation of the book cover, and provided suggestions for improvement to the inside art.

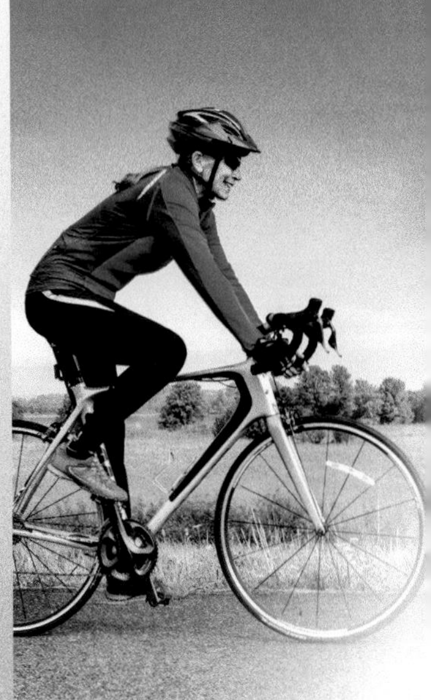

Preface to the Sixth Edition

For over 25 years *Clinical Kinesiology and Anatomy* has provided a fundamental understanding of kinesiology and anatomy from a clinical perspective. The sixth edition continues to provide this basic information. Simple, easy-to-follow explanations continue to be the hallmark of this book.

As with previous editions, the book is written so that instructors can omit information not needed for their particular discipline without putting the student at a disadvantage in terms of understanding other subject matter. For example, some disciplines may not need to study arthrokinematics, the temporomandibular joint, or gait. The joint-specific chapters are essentially self-standing, so the order in which they are read can be easily changed. Instead of beginning with joints of the upper extremity, one could begin with the lower extremity or axial skeleton, and not lose understanding.

Emphasis remains on basic understanding. To make the arthrokinematics chapter more clinically relevant, steps have been provided to perform a motion analysis.

A brief explanation at the cellular level has been provided for greater understanding of how force is produced during muscle contraction.

To provide a greater link between foundational knowledge and clinical application, several box features have been added throughout the joint-specific chapters. Many illustrations have been updated to provide uniformity and consistency across the text. To enhance clarity, consistent color-coding has been applied to several illustrations.

Lynn S. Lippert

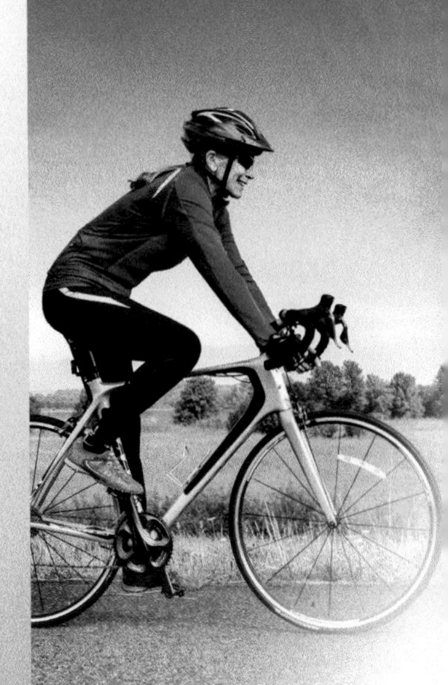

Contents in Brief

Part I
Basic Clinical Kinesiology and Anatomy

CHAPTER 1 Basic Information 3
CHAPTER 2 Skeletal System 13
CHAPTER 3 Articular System 21
CHAPTER 4 Arthrokinematics 31
CHAPTER 5 Muscular System 41
CHAPTER 6 Nervous System 63
CHAPTER 7 Circulatory System 85
CHAPTER 8 Basic Biomechanics 103

Part II
Clinical Kinesiology and Anatomy of the Upper Extremities

CHAPTER 9 Shoulder Girdle 127
CHAPTER 10 Shoulder Joint 145
CHAPTER 11 Elbow Joint 163
CHAPTER 12 Wrist Joint 181
CHAPTER 13 Hand 195

Part III
Clinical Kinesiology and Anatomy of the Trunk

CHAPTER 14 Temporomandibular Joint 223
CHAPTER 15 Neck and Trunk 239
CHAPTER 16 Respiratory System 267
CHAPTER 17 Pelvic Girdle 281

Part IV
Clinical Kinesiology and Anatomy of the Lower Extremities

CHAPTER 18 Hip Joint 297
CHAPTER 19 Knee Joint 323
CHAPTER 20 Ankle Joint and Foot 343

Part V
Clinical Kinesiology and Anatomy of the Body

CHAPTER 21 Posture 371
CHAPTER 22 Gait 381

Bibliography *399*
Answers to Review Questions *403*
Index *423*

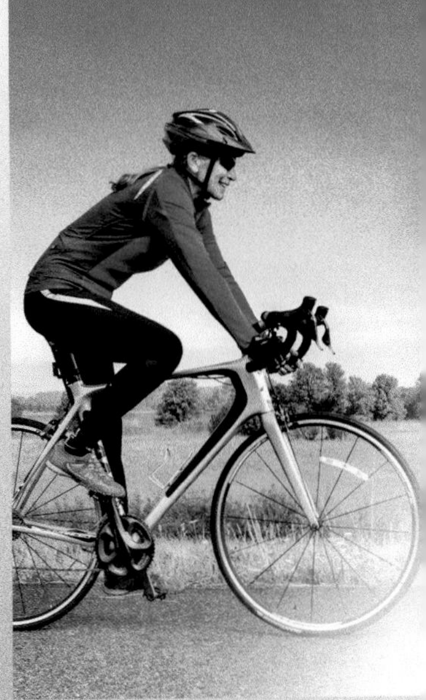

Table of Contents

Part I
Basic Clinical Kinesiology and Anatomy

CHAPTER 1 **Basic Information** 3
- Segments of the Body 4
- Descriptive Terminology 4
- Types of Motion 6
- Joint Movements (Osteokinematics) 7
- Review Questions 11

CHAPTER 2 **Skeletal System** 13
- Functions of the Skeleton 13
- Types of Skeletons 13
- Composition of Bone 13
- Structure of Bone 14
- Types of Bones 16
- Common Skeletal Pathologies 17
- Review Questions 19

CHAPTER 3 **Articular System** 21
- Types of Joints 21
- Joint Structure 25
- Planes and Axes 26
- Degrees of Freedom 28
- Common Pathological Terms 28
- Review Questions 29

CHAPTER 4 **Arthrokinematics** 31
- Osteokinematic Motion 31
  - *End Feel* 31
- Arthrokinematic Motion 32
  - *Accessory Motion Terminology* 32
  - *Joint Mobilization* 33
  - *Joint Surface Shape* 34
  - *Types of Arthrokinematic Motion* 34
  - *Convex-Concave Rule* 35
  - *Joint Surface Positions (Joint Congruency)* 36
- Review Questions 39

CHAPTER 5 **Muscular System** 41
- Muscle Attachments 41
- Muscle Names 42
- Muscle Fiber Arrangement 43
- Functional Characteristics of Muscle Tissue 45
- Sliding Filament Theory 45
- Length-Tension Relationship in Muscle Tissue 45
  - *Optimal Length* 47
  - *Active and Passive Insufficiency* 49
  - *Adaptive Shortening & Lengthening of Muscle Tissue* 51
  - *Stretching* 52
  - *Tendon Action of a Muscle (Tenodesis)* 53
- Types of Muscle Contraction 53
- Roles of Muscles 57
- Line of Pull 57
- Kinetic Chains 58
- Common Muscle Pathologies 59
- Review Questions 60

CHAPTER 6 **Nervous System** 63
- Introduction 63
- Nervous Tissue (Neurons) 64
  - *The Central Nervous System* 65
  - *Brain* 65
  - *Spinal Cord* 68

The Peripheral Nervous System 70
Functional Significance of Spinal Cord Level 72
Plexus Formation 74
Common Pathologies of the Central and Peripheral Nervous Systems 81
Common Pathologies of the Central Nervous System 81
Common Pathologies of Peripheral Nerves 82
Review Questions 83

CHAPTER 7 Circulatory System 85
Cardiovascular System 85
Heart 86
Blood Vessels 89
Lymphatic System 97
Functions 98
Drainage Patterns 99
Common Pathologies 101
Review Questions 102
Cardiovascular System 102
Lymphatic System 102

CHAPTER 8 Basic Biomechanics 103
Laws of Motion 104
Force 105
Torque 107
Stability 109
Simple Machines 113
Levers 113
Pulleys 118
Wheel and Axle 119
Inclined Plane 120
Review Questions 121

Part II
Clinical Kinesiology and Anatomy of the Upper Extremities

CHAPTER 9 Shoulder Girdle 127
Clarification of Terms 127
Bones and Landmarks 128
Important Bony Landmarks of the Scapula 128
Important Bony Landmarks of the Clavicle 129
Important Bony Landmarks of the Sternum 130
Joints and Ligaments 130
Sternoclavicular Joint 130
Acromioclavicular Joint 130
Scapulothoracic Articulation 131
Joint Motions 131
Companion Motions of the Shoulder Joint and Shoulder Girdle 133
Scapulohumeral Rhythm 133
Muscles of The Shoulder Girdle 133
Muscle Descriptions 134
Anatomical Relationships 138
Force Couples 139
Reverse Muscle Action 139
Summary of Muscle Innervation 141
Common Shoulder Girdle Pathologies 141
Review Questions 142
General Anatomy Questions 142
Functional Activity Questions 142
Clinical Exercise Questions 142

CHAPTER 10 Shoulder Joint 145
Joint Motions 145
Bones and Landmarks 147
Important Bony Landmarks of the Scapula 147
Important Bony Landmarks of the Humerus 148
Ligaments and Other Structures 148
Muscles of the Shoulder Joint 150
Anatomical Relationships 156
Glenohumeral Movement 157
Summary of Muscle Action 158
Summary of Muscle Innervation 158
Common Shoulder Pathologies 159
Review Questions 160
General Anatomy Questions 160
Functional Activity Questions 160
Clinical Exercise Questions 161

CHAPTER 11 **Elbow Joint** 163
Joint Structure and Motions 163
Carrying Angle 165
End Feel 165
Bones and Landmarks 165
Important Bony Landmarks of the Scapula 166
Important Bony Landmarks of the Humerus 166
Important Bony Landmarks of the Ulna 166
Important Bony Landmarks of the Radius 167
Ligaments and Other Structures 167
Muscles of the Elbow and Forearm 168
Anatomical Relationships 174
Summary of Muscle Action 175
Summary of Muscle Innervation 175
Common Elbow Pathologies 175
Review Questions 177
General Anatomy Questions 177
Functional Activity Questions 178
Clinical Exercise Questions 178

CHAPTER 12 **Wrist Joint** 181
Joint Structure 181
Joint Motions 182
Bones and Landmarks 183
Ligaments and Other Structures 184
Muscles of the Wrist 184
Anatomical Relationships 188
Common Wrist Pathologies 189
Summary of Muscle Action 190
Summary of Muscle Innervation 191
Review Questions 192
General Anatomy Questions 192
Functional Activity Questions 193
Clinical Exercise Questions 194

CHAPTER 13 **Hand** 195
Joint Structure and Motions of the Thumb 195
The Carpometacarpal Joint 195
The Metacarpophalangeal and Interphalangeal Joints 197
Joint Structure and Motions of the Fingers 197
The Carpometacarpal Joints 197
The Metacarpophalangeal Joints 198
The Interphalangeal Joints 198
Bones and Landmarks 199
Landmark of the Forearm 199
Ligaments and Other Structures 199
Muscles of the Thumb and Fingers 201
Extrinsic Muscles 201
Intrinsic Muscles 206
Anatomical Relationships 210
Common Wrist and Hand Pathologies 211
Summary of Muscle Actions 212
Summary of Muscle Innervation 213
Hand Function 213
Grasps 214
Review Questions 218
General Anatomy Questions 218
Functional Activity Questions 219
Clinical Exercise Questions 219

Part III
Clinical Kinesiology and Anatomy of the Trunk

CHAPTER 14 **Temporomandibular Joint** 223
Joint Structure and Motions 223
Bones and Landmarks 224
Important Landmarks of the Mandible 224
Important Landmarks of the Temporal Bone 225
Important Landmarks of the Sphenoid Bone 226
Important Landmarks of the Zygomatic Bone 227
Important Landmark of the Maxilla 227

Ligaments and Other Structures 227
Mechanics of Movement 228
Muscles of the TMJ 229
Anatomical Relationships 234
Summary of Muscle Action 235
Summary of Muscle Innervation 235
Pathological Conditions 236
Review Questions 237
General Anatomy Questions 237
Functional Activity Questions 237
Clinical Exercise Questions 237

CHAPTER 15 Neck and Trunk 239
Vertebral Curves 239
Clarification of Terms 239
Joint Motions 240
Bones and Landmarks 241
Important Bony Landmarks of the Skull 241
Important Bony Landmarks of the Vertebrae 242
Vertebrae with Unique Bony Landmarks 243
Joints and Ligaments 244
Atypical Vertebral Articulations 244
Typical Vertebral Articulations 244
Other Soft Tissue Structures 247
Muscles of the Neck and Trunk 248
Muscles of the Cervical Spine 248
Muscles of the Trunk 251
Anatomical Relationships 258
Summary of Muscle Actions 260
Summary of Muscle Innervation 260
Common Vertebral Column Pathologies 260
Review Questions 263
General Anatomy Questions 263
Functional Activity Questions 263
Clinical Exercise Questions 264

CHAPTER 16 Respiratory System 267
The Thoracic Cage 267
Bones and Landmarks 267
Bony Landmarks of the Ribs 268
Bony Landmarks of the Sternum 268
Bony Landmarks of the Thoracic Vertebra 268
Joints of the Thorax 269
Movements of the Thorax 269
Structures of Respiration 270
Mechanics of Respiration 271
Phases of Respiration 272
Muscles of Respiration 272
Diaphragm Muscle 272
Intercostal Muscles 273
Accessory Inspiratory Muscles 274
Accessory Expiratory Muscles 275
Anatomical Relationships 275
Diaphragmatic Versus Chest Breathing 276
Summary of Innervation of the Muscles of Respiration 277
Common Respiratory Conditions or Pathologies 278
Review Questions 279
General Anatomy Questions 279
Functional Activity Questions 279
Clinical Exercise Questions 280

CHAPTER 17 Pelvic Girdle 281
Structure and Function 281
False and True Pelvis 282
Sacroiliac Joint 283
Bones and Landmarks 283
Important Bony Landmarks of the Sacrum 283
Important Bony Landmarks of the Ilium 284
Important Bony Landmarks of the Ischium 285
Pubic Symphysis 286
Important Bony Landmarks of the Pubis 286
Lumbosacral Joint 287
Pelvic Girdle Motions 288
Muscle Control 291
Review Questions 293
General Anatomy Questions 293
Functional Activity Questions 294
Clinical Exercise Questions 294

Part IV
Clinical Kinesiology and Anatomy of the Lower Extremities

CHAPTER 18 Hip Joint 297
- Joint Structure and Motions 297
  - *Arthrokinematics* 298
- Bones and Landmarks 299
  - *Important Bony Landmarks of the Ilium* 299
  - *Important Bony Landmarks of the Ischium* 300
  - *Important Bony Landmarks of the Pubis* 300
  - *Important Bony Landmarks of the Femur* 301
  - *Important Bony Landmark of the Tibia* 301
- Ligaments and Other Structures 302
  - *Adductor Hiatus* 303
- Muscles of the Hip 303
  - *Anatomical Relationships* 311
  - *Common Hip Pathologies* 312
  - *Summary of Muscle Action* 315
  - *Summary of Muscle Innervation* 316
- Review Questions 317
  - *General Anatomy Questions* 317
  - *Functional Activity Questions* 318
  - *Clinical Exercise Questions* 320

CHAPTER 19 Knee Joint 323
- Joint Structure and Motions 323
  - *Arthrokinematics* 324
- Bones and Landmarks 325
  - *Important Bony Landmarks of the Femur* 327
  - *Important Bony Landmarks of the Tibia* 328
- Ligaments and Other Structures 328
- Muscles of the Knee 330
  - *Anterior Muscles* 331
  - *Posterior Muscles* 333
  - *Anatomical Relationships* 335
  - *Summary of Muscle Action* 335
  - *Summary of Muscle Innervation* 335
  - *Common Knee Pathologies* 336
- Review Questions 338
  - *General Anatomy Questions* 338
  - *Functional Activity Questions* 339
  - *Clinical Exercise Questions* 340

CHAPTER 20 Ankle Joint and Foot 343
- Bones and Landmarks 344
  - *Important Bony Landmarks of the Tibia and Fibula* 344
  - *Important Bony Landmarks of the Tarsal Bones* 344
  - *Important Bony Landmarks of the Metatarsals* 345
  - *Functional Aspects of the Foot* 345
- Joints and Motions 346
  - *Terminology* 346
  - *Ankle Joints* 347
  - *Motion at the Ankle Joint* 348
  - *Foot Joints* 350
- Ligaments and Other Structures 350
  - *Arches* 351
- Muscles of the Ankle and Foot 353
  - *Extrinsic Muscles* 353
  - *Intrinsic Muscles* 360
  - *Anatomical Relationships* 360
  - *Summary of Muscle Innervation* 363
  - *Common Ankle Pathologies* 364
- Review Questions 367
  - *General Anatomy Questions* 367
  - *Functional Activity Questions* 367
  - *Clinical Exercise Questions* 367

Part V
Clinical Kinesiology and Anatomy of the Body

CHAPTER 21 Posture 371
- Vertebral Alignment 371
  - *Development of Postural Curves* 372
- Standing Posture 374
  - *Lateral View* 374
  - *Anterior View* 375
  - *Posterior View* 376
- Sitting Posture 376
- Supine Posture 378

Common Postural Deviations 378
Review Questions 379
General Anatomy Questions 379
Functional Activity Questions 379
Clinical Exercise Questions 380

CHAPTER 22 Gait 381
Definitions 381
Analysis of Stance Phase 386
Analysis of Swing Phase 387
Additional Determinants of Gait 388
Age-Related Gait Patterns 390
Abnormal (Atypical) Gait 390
Review Questions 397
General Anatomy Questions 397
Functional Activity Questions 397
Clinical Exercise Questions 397

Bibliography ***399***
Answers to Review Questions ***403***
Index ***423***

PART I

Basic Clinical Kinesiology and Anatomy

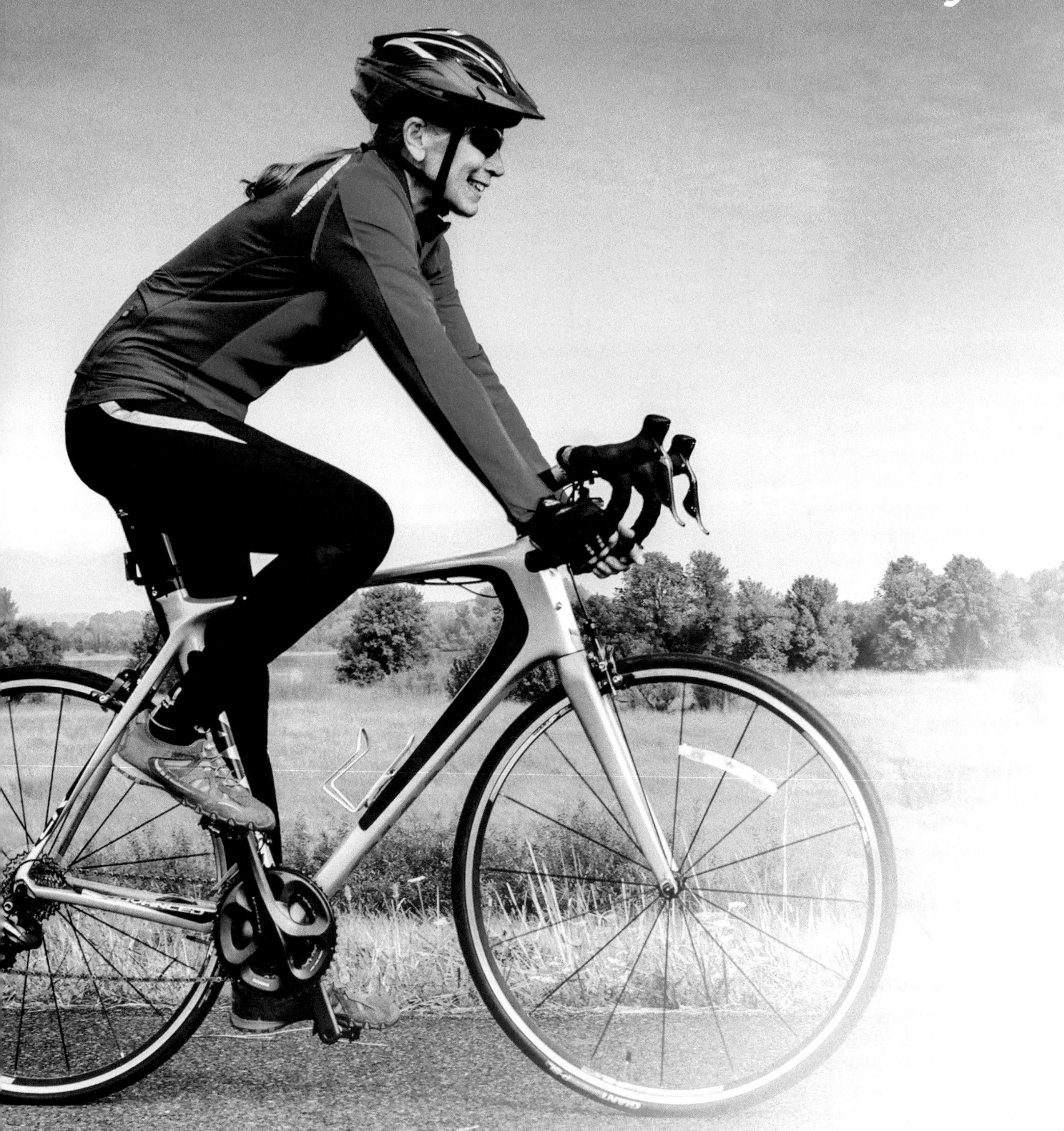

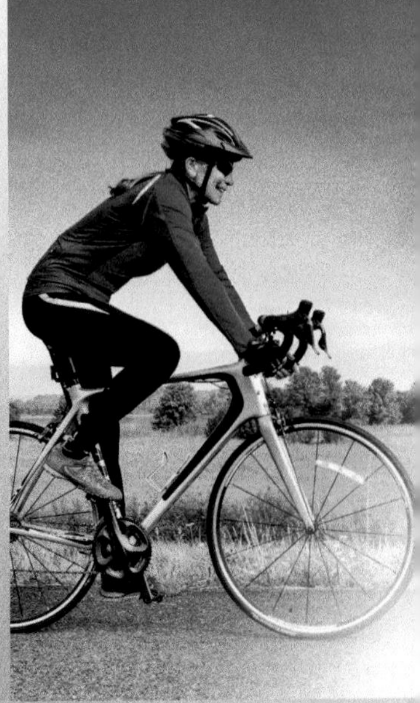

CHAPTER 1
Basic Information

Segments of the Body
Descriptive Terminology
Types of Motion
Joint Movements (Osteokinematics)
Review Questions

Kinesiology IN ACTION For additional practice activities and videos, please visit www.kinesiologyinaction.com

By definition, **kinesiology** is the study of movement. However, this definition is too general to be of much use. Kinesiology brings together the fields of anatomy, physiology, physics, and geometry and relates them to human movement. Thus, kinesiology utilizes principles of mechanics, musculoskeletal anatomy, and neuromuscular physiology.

Mechanical principles that relate directly to the human body are used in the study of **biomechanics.** Because we may use a ball, racket, crutch, prosthesis, or some other implement, we must consider our biomechanical interaction with them as well. This may involve looking at the *static* (nonmoving) and/or *dynamic* (moving) *systems* associated with various activities. Dynamic systems can be divided into kinetics and kinematics. **Kinetics** are those forces causing movement, whereas **kinematics** is the time, space, and mass aspects of a moving system. These and other basic biomechanical concepts will be discussed in Chapter 8.

This text will give most emphasis to the musculoskeletal anatomy components, which are considered the key to understanding and being able to apply the other components. Many students have negative thoughts at the mere mention of the word *kinesiology.* Their eyes glaze over and their brains freeze. Perhaps, based on past experience with anatomy, they feel that their only hope is mass memorization. However, this may prove to be an overwhelming task with no long-term memory gain.

As you proceed through this text, keep in mind a few simple concepts. First, the human body is arranged in a very logical way. Like all aspects of life, there are exceptions. Sometimes the logic of these exceptions is apparent, and sometimes the logic may be apparent only to some higher being. Whichever is the case, you should note the exception and move on. Second, if you have a good grasp of descriptive terminology and can visualize the concept or feature, strict memorization is not necessary. For example, if you know generally where the patella is located and what the structures are around it, you can accurately describe its location using your own words. You do not need to memorize someone else's words to be correct.

By keeping in mind some of the basic principles affecting muscles, understanding individual muscle function need not be so mind-boggling. If you know (1) what motions a particular joint allows, (2) that a muscle must span a particular side of a joint surface to cause a certain motion, and (3) what that muscle's line of pull is, then you will know the particular action(s) of a specific muscle. For example, (1) the elbow allows only flexion and extension, (2) a muscle must span the elbow joint anteriorly to flex and posteriorly to extend, and (3) the biceps brachii is a vertical muscle on the anterior surface of the arm; (conclusion) therefore, the biceps muscle flexes the elbow.

Yes, kinesiology *can* be understood by mere mortals. Its study can even be enjoyable. However, a word of caution should be given: Like exercising, it is better to study in small amounts several times a week than to study for a long period in one session before an exam.

Segments of the Body

The body is divided into segments according to bones (Fig. 1-1). In the upper extremity, the **arm** is the bone (humerus) between the shoulder and the elbow joint.

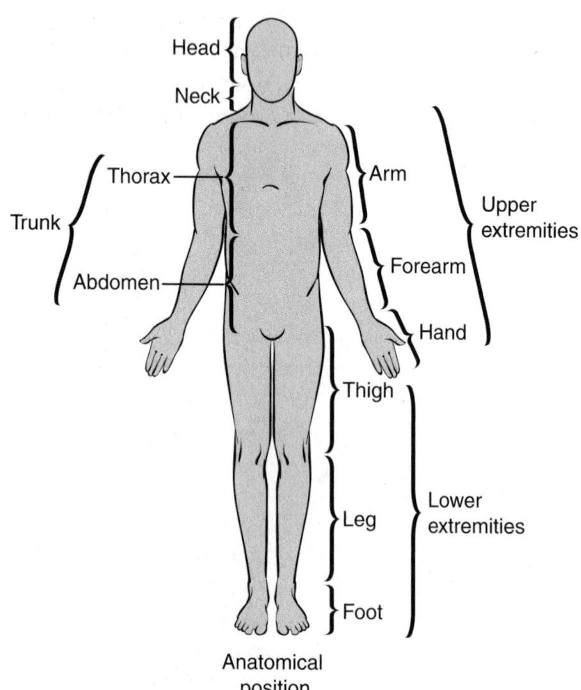

Figure 1-1. Body segments.

Next, the **forearm** (radius and ulna) is between the elbow and the wrist. The **hand** is distal to the wrist.

The lower extremity is made up of three similar segments. The **thigh** (femur) is between the hip and knee joints. The **leg** (tibia and fibula) is between the knee and ankle joints, and the **foot** is distal to the ankle.

The trunk has two segments: the thorax and the abdomen. The **thorax,** or chest, is made up primarily of the ribs, sternum, and thoracic vertebrae. The **abdomen,** or lower trunk, is made up primarily of the pelvis, stomach, and lumbar vertebrae. The **neck** (cervical vertebrae) and **head** (cranium) are separate segments.

Body segments are rarely used to describe joint motion. For example, flexion occurs at the shoulder, not the arm. The motion occurs at the joint (shoulder), and the body segment (arm) just goes along for the ride! An exception to this concept is the forearm. It is a body segment but functions as a joint as well. Technically, joint motion occurs at the proximal and distal radioulnar joints; however, common practice refers to this as *forearm pronation* and *supination.*

Descriptive Terminology

The human body is active and constantly moving; therefore, it is subject to frequent changes in position. The relationship of the various body parts to each other also changes. To be able to describe the organization of the human body, it is necessary to use some arbitrary position as a starting point from which movement or location of structures can be described. This is known as the **anatomical position** (Fig. 1-2) and is described as the human body standing in an upright position, eyes facing forward, feet parallel and close together, and arms at the sides of the body with the palms facing forward. Although the position of the forearm and hands is not a natural one, it does allow for accurate description.

Specific terms are used to describe the location of a structure and its position relative to other structures (Fig. 1-3). **Medial** refers to a location or position toward the midline, and **lateral** refers to a location or position farther from the midline. For example, the ulna is on the medial side of the forearm, and the radius is lateral to the ulna.

Anterior refers to the front of the body or to a position closer to the front. **Posterior** refers to the back of the body or to a position more toward the back. For example, the sternum is located anteriorly on the chest wall, and the scapula is located posteriorly. **Ventral** is a synonym (a word with the same meaning) of *anterior,*

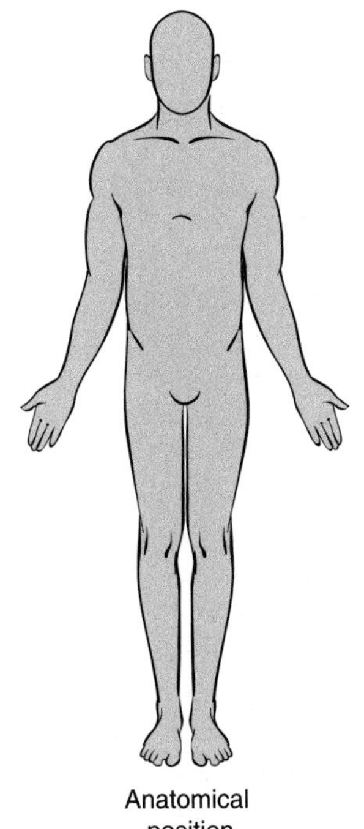

Figure 1-2. Descriptive position.

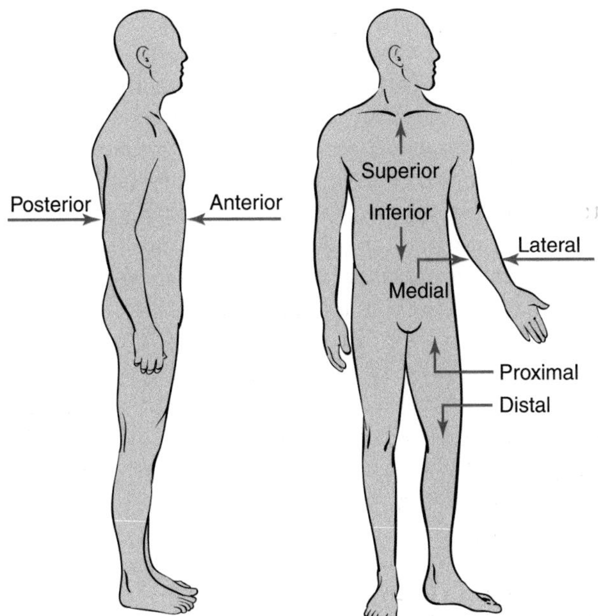

Figure 1-3. Descriptive terminology.

and **dorsal** is a synonym of *posterior; anterior* and *posterior* are more commonly used in kinesiology. *Front* and *back* also refer to the surfaces of the body, but these are considered lay terms and are not widely used by healthcare professionals.

Distal and *proximal* are used to describe locations on the extremities. **Distal** means away from the trunk, and **proximal** means toward the trunk. For example, the humeral head is located on the proximal end of the humerus. The elbow is proximal to the wrist but distal to the shoulder.

Superior is used to indicate the location of a body part that is above another or to refer to the upper surface of an organ or a structure. **Inferior** indicates that a body part is below another or refers to the lower surface of an organ or a structure. For example, the body of the sternum is superior to the xiphoid process but inferior to the manubrium. Sometimes people use **cranial** or *cephalad* (from the word root *cephal,* meaning "head") to refer to a position or structure close to the head. **Caudal** (from the word root *cauda,* meaning "tail") refers to a position or structure closer to the feet. For example, *cauda equina,* which means "horse's tail," is the bundle of spinal nerve roots descending from the inferior end of the spinal cord. Like *dorsal* and *ventral, cranial* and *caudal* are terms that are best used to describe positions on a quadruped (a four-legged animal). Humans are bipeds, or two-legged animals. You can see that if the dog in Figure 1-4 were to stand on its hind legs, dorsal would become posterior and cranial would become superior, and so on.

A structure may be described as **superficial** or **deep,** depending on its relative depth. For example, in describing the layers of the abdominal muscles, the external oblique is deep to the rectus abdominis but superficial to the internal oblique. Another example is the scalp being described as superficial to the skull.

Supine and *prone* are terms that describe body position while lying flat. When **supine,** a person is lying straight, with the face, or anterior surface, pointed upward. A person in the **prone** position is horizontal,

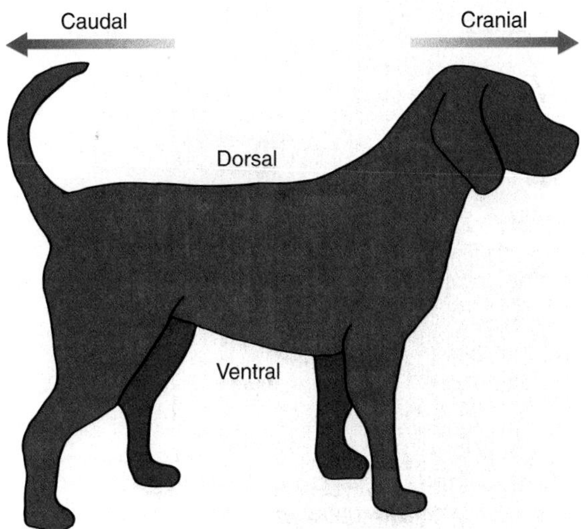

Figure 1-4. Descriptive terminology for a quadruped.

with the face, or anterior surface, pointed downward (the child in Fig. 1-5 is lying prone on the sled).

Bilateral refers to two, or both, sides. For example, bilateral above-knee amputations refer to both right and left legs being amputated above the knee. **Contralateral** refers to the opposite side. For example, a person who has had a stroke affecting the right side of the brain may have contralateral paralysis of the left arm and left leg. In contrast, **ipsilateral** refers to the same side of the body.

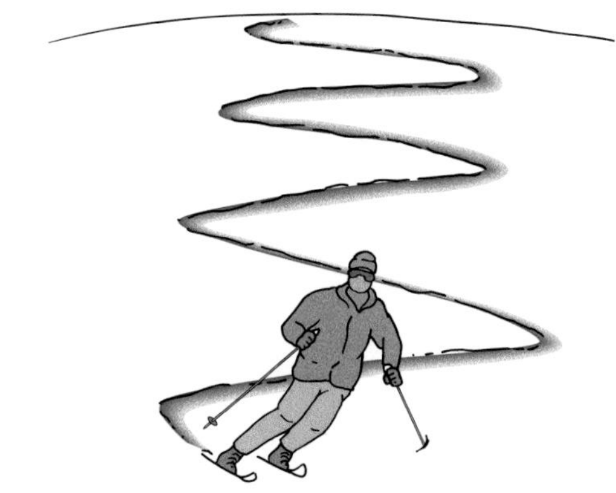

Figure 1-6. Curvilinear motion.

Types of Motion

Linear motion, also called *translatory motion,* occurs in a more or less straight line from one location to another. All parts of the object move the same distance, in the same direction, and at the same time. Movement that occurs in a straight line is called **rectilinear motion,** such as the motion of a child sledding down a hill (Fig. 1-5) or a sailboarder moving across the water. If movement occurs in a curved path that is not necessarily circular, it is called **curvilinear motion.** The path a diver takes after leaving the diving board until entering the water is curvilinear motion. Figure 1-6 demonstrates the curvilinear path a skier takes coming down a ski slope. Other examples of curvilinear motion are the path of a thrown ball, a javelin thrown across a field, or the earth's orbit around the sun.

Movement of an object around a fixed point (axis) is called **angular motion,** or *rotary motion* (Fig. 1-7). In the human body, our joints serve as the axis around which angular motion occurs. With angular motion, all parts of the object move through the same angle, in the same direction, and at the same time, but they do not move the same distance. When a person flexes his or her knee, the knee joint serves as the axis of rotation and the foot travels farther through space than does the ankle or leg.

Generally speaking, most movement within the body is angular; movement outside the body tends to be linear. It is not uncommon to see both types of movement occurring at the same time—the entire object moving in a linear fashion through space and the individual parts (within the body) moving in an angular fashion. In Figure 1-8, the skateboarder's whole body moves down the street (linear motion), whereas individual joints on the "pushing" leg (i.e., the hip, knee, and ankle) rotate around their axes (angular motion). Another example of combined motions is walking. The whole body

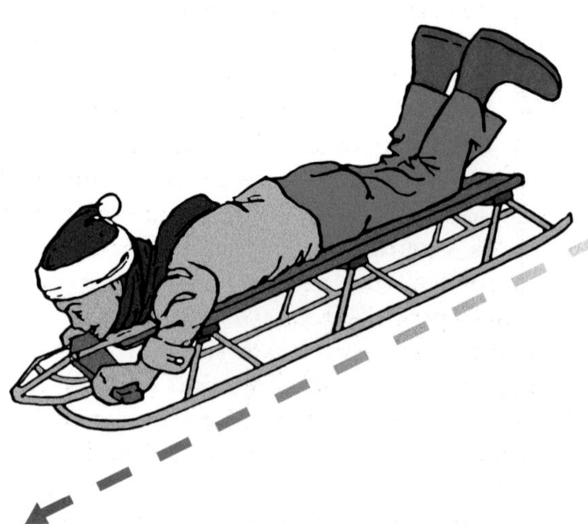

Figure 1-5. Rectilinear motion.

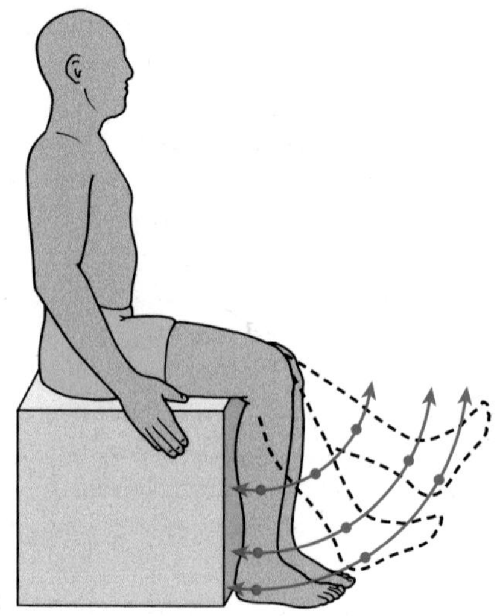

Figure 1-7. Angular motion.

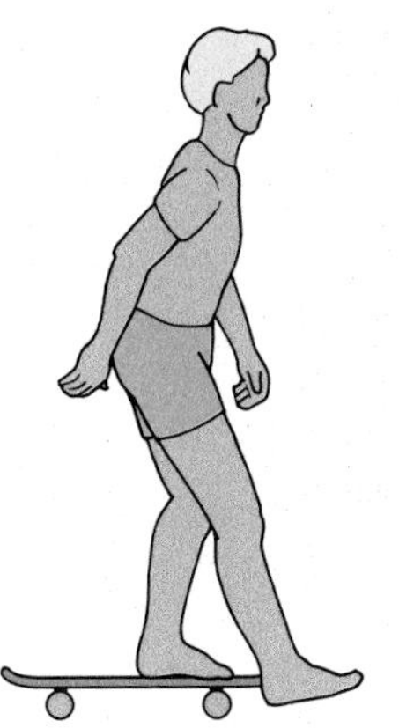
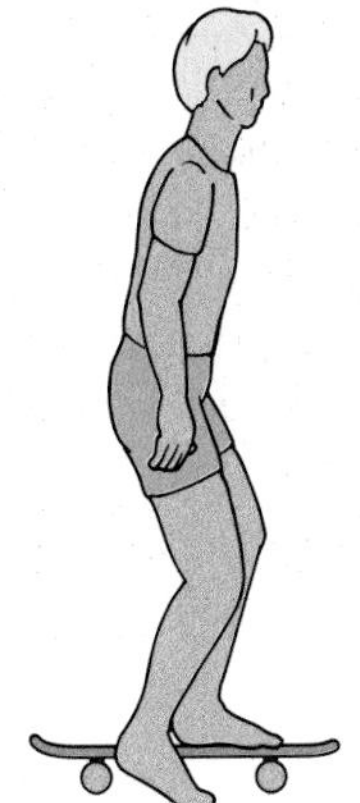
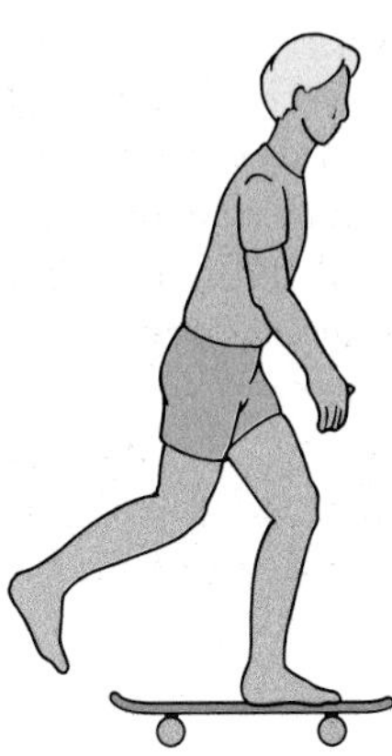

Figure 1-8. Combination of linear and angular motion.

exhibits linear motion when walking from point A to point B, whereas the hips, knees, and ankles exhibit angular motion. A person throwing a ball uses the upper extremity joints in an angular fashion, whereas the ball travels in a curvilinear path.

Exceptions to this statement can be found. For example, as will be described in Chapter 9, the movement of the scapula in elevation/depression and protraction/retraction is essentially linear. However, the movement of the clavicle, which is attached to the scapula, is angular and gets its angular motion from the sternoclavicular joint.

Joint Movements (Osteokinematics)

Joints move in many different directions. As will be discussed in Chapter 3, movement occurs around joint axes and through joint planes. *Flexion/extension, abduction/adduction,* and *rotation* are terms used to describe the various movements that occur at synovial joints. This type of joint motion is called **osteokinematics,** which deals with the relationship of the *movement of bones around a joint axis* (e.g., humerus moving on scapula). The relationship of *joint surface movement* (spin, glide, roll), called **arthrokinematic** motion, will be discussed in Chapter 4.

Flexion/extension, abduction/adduction, and *rotation* are general terms used to describe the osteokinematic movements that occur at synovial joints. *Inversion/eversion* and *protraction/retraction* are specific terms that apply only to specific synovial joints.

Flexion is the bending movement of one bone on another, bringing the two segments together and causing a decrease in the joint angle. Usually this occurs between anterior surfaces of adjacent bones, causing the anterior surfaces to move toward each other. In the case of the neck, flexion is a "bowing down" motion (Fig. 1-9A) in which the head moves toward the anterior chest. With elbow flexion, the anterior surfaces of the forearm and arm move toward each other. With hip flexion, the anterior thigh moves toward the anterior trunk. The knee is an exception in that flexion occurs when the posterior surfaces of the thigh and leg move toward each other. Flexion at the wrist may be called **palmar flexion** (Fig. 1-9F), and flexion at the ankle may be called **plantar flexion** (Fig. 1-9H).

Conversely, **extension** is the straightening movement of one bone away from another, causing an increase of the joint angle. This motion usually returns the body part to the anatomical position after it has been flexed (Fig. 1-9B, E). With extension, the anterior aspects of the joint surfaces tend to move away from each other. Extension occurs when the head moves up and away from the anterior chest, and the anterior thigh moves away from the trunk and returns to the anatomical position. **Hyperextension** is the continuation of extension beyond the anatomical position (Fig. 1-9C). The shoulder, hip, wrist, neck, and trunk can hyperextend. Extension at the wrist and ankle joints may be called **dorsiflexion** (Fig. 1-9G, I). Wrist or ankle **dorsiflexion** (Fig. 1-9G, I) refers to movement toward the dorsum (superior aspect) of the arm or foot.

Abduction is movement away from the midline of the body (Fig. 1-10A), and **adduction** (Fig. 1-10B) is movement toward the midline. The shoulder and hip can abduct *and* adduct. Exceptions to this midline definition are the fingers and toes. The reference point for the fingers is the middle finger. Movement away from the middle finger is abduction (see Fig. 13-5).

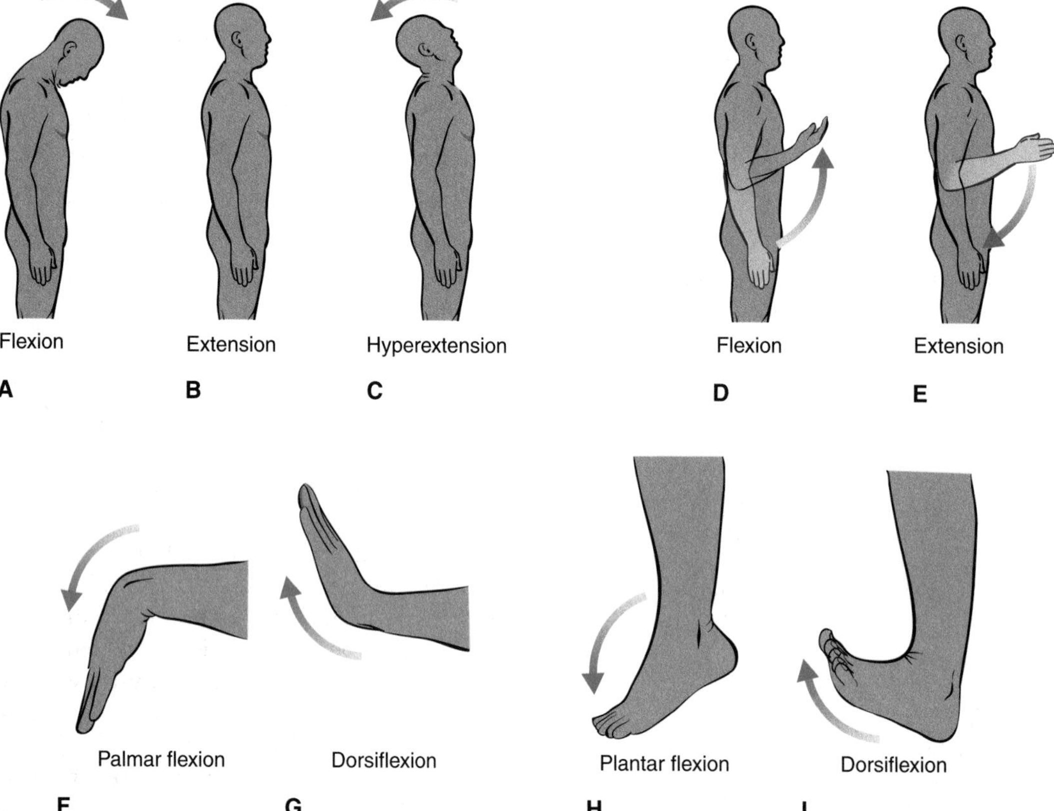
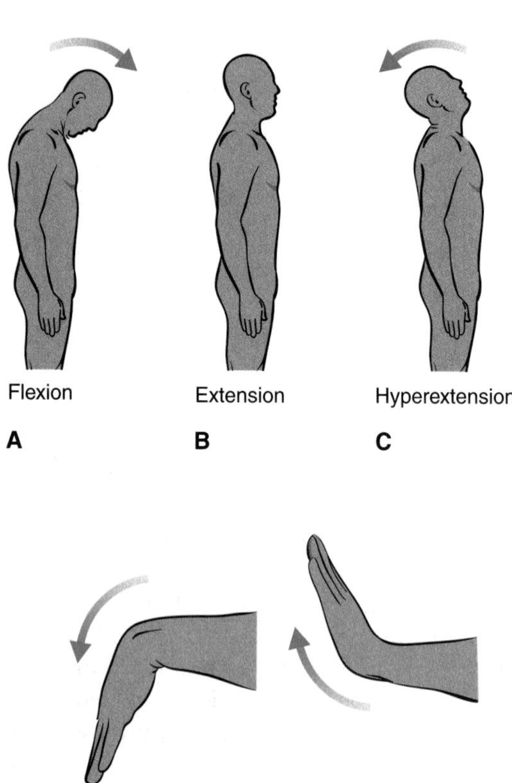
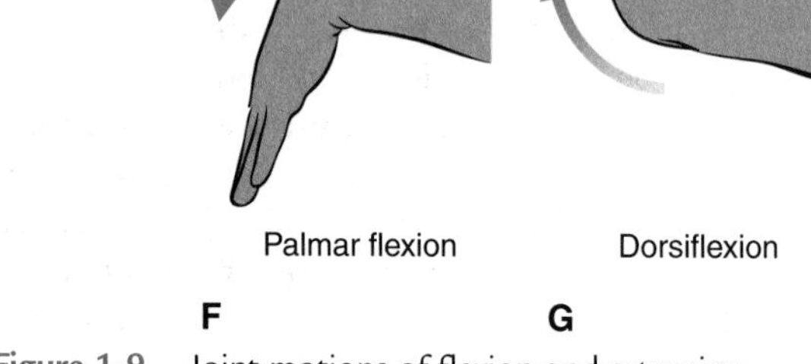

Figure 1-9. Joint motions of flexion and extension.

It should be noted that the middle finger abducts (to the right and to the left) but adducts only as a return movement from abduction to the midline. The point of reference for the toes is the second toe (see Fig. 20-14). Similar to the middle finger, the second toe abducts to the right and the left but does not adduct, except as a return movement from abduction. Horizontal abduction and adduction are motions that cannot occur from the anatomical position. They must be preceded by either flexion or abduction of the shoulder joint so that the arm is at shoulder level. From this position, shoulder movement backward is **horizontal abduction** (Fig. 1-10C) and movement forward is **horizontal adduction** (Fig. 1-10D). There are similar movements at the hip, but the ranges of motion are not usually as great.

Radial deviation and *ulnar deviation* are terms more commonly used to refer to wrist abduction and adduction. When the hand moves laterally, or toward the thumb side, it is **radial deviation** (Fig. 1-10E). When the hand moves medially from the anatomical position toward the little finger side at the wrist, it is **ulnar deviation** (Fig. 1-10F).

Lateral bending is the term used when the trunk moves sideways. The trunk can laterally bend to the right or the left (Fig. 1-10G, H). If the right side of the trunk bends, moving the shoulder toward the right hip, it is called *right lateral bending*. The neck also laterally bends in the same way. The term *lateral flexion* is sometimes used to describe this sideward motion. However, because this term is easily confused with *flexion,* it will not be used in this book.

Circumduction is motion that describes a circular, cone-shaped pattern. It involves a combination of four joint motions: (1) flexion, (2) abduction, (3) extension, and (4) adduction. For example, if the shoulder moves in a circle, the hand would move in a much larger circle. The entire arm would move in a cone-shaped sequential pattern of flexion to abduction to extension to adduction, bringing the arm back to its starting position (Fig. 1-11).

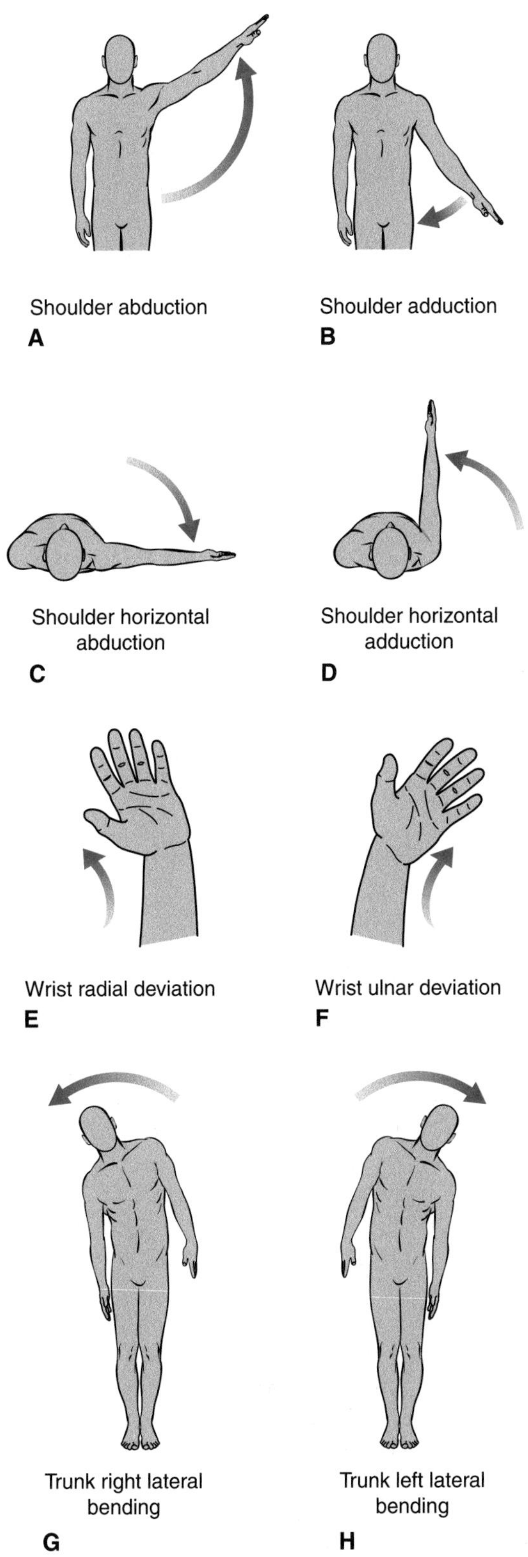

Figure 1-10. Joint motions of abduction and adduction.

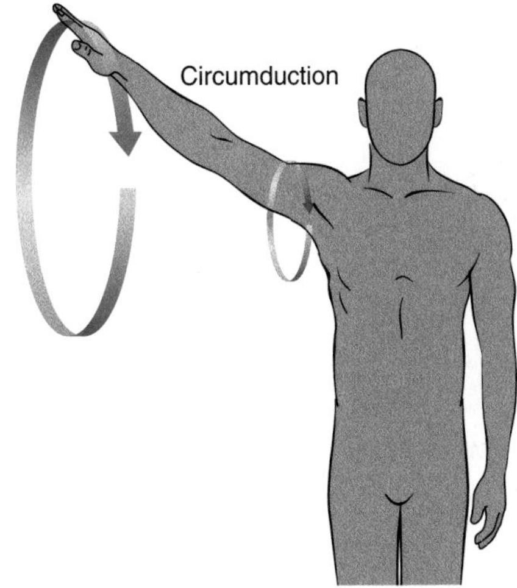

Figure 1-11. Circumduction motion.

Rotation is movement of a bone or part around its longitudinal axis. If the anterior surface rolls inward toward the midline, the motion is called **medial rotation** (Fig. 1-12A). This is sometimes referred to as *internal rotation.* Conversely, if the anterior surface rolls outward, away from the midline, the motion is called **lateral rotation** (Fig. 1-12B), or *external rotation.* Joints capable of performing medial and lateral rotation are the shoulder and the hip. The neck and trunk can also rotate to either the right or left side (Fig. 1-12C, D). Visualize the neck rotating as you look over your right shoulder. This would be "right neck rotation."

Rotation of the forearm is referred to as *supination* and *pronation.* In the anatomical position (see Fig. 1-2), the forearm is in **supination** (Fig. 1-12E). This faces the palm of the hand forward, or anteriorly. In **pronation** (Fig. 1-12F), the palm is facing backward, or posteriorly. When the elbow is flexed, the "palm up" position refers to supination and "palm down" refers to pronation.

The following are terms used to describe motions specific to certain joints. **Inversion** is moving the sole of the foot inward at the ankle (Fig. 1-13A), and **eversion** is the outward movement (Fig. 1-13B). **Protraction** is mostly a linear movement along a plane parallel to the ground and away from the posterior midline (Fig. 1-14A), and **retraction** is mostly a linear movement in the same plane but toward the posterior midline (Fig. 1-14B). Protraction of the shoulder girdle moves the scapula away from the posterior midline, as does protraction of the jaw, whereas retraction in both of these cases returns the body part toward the posterior midline, or back to the anatomical position.

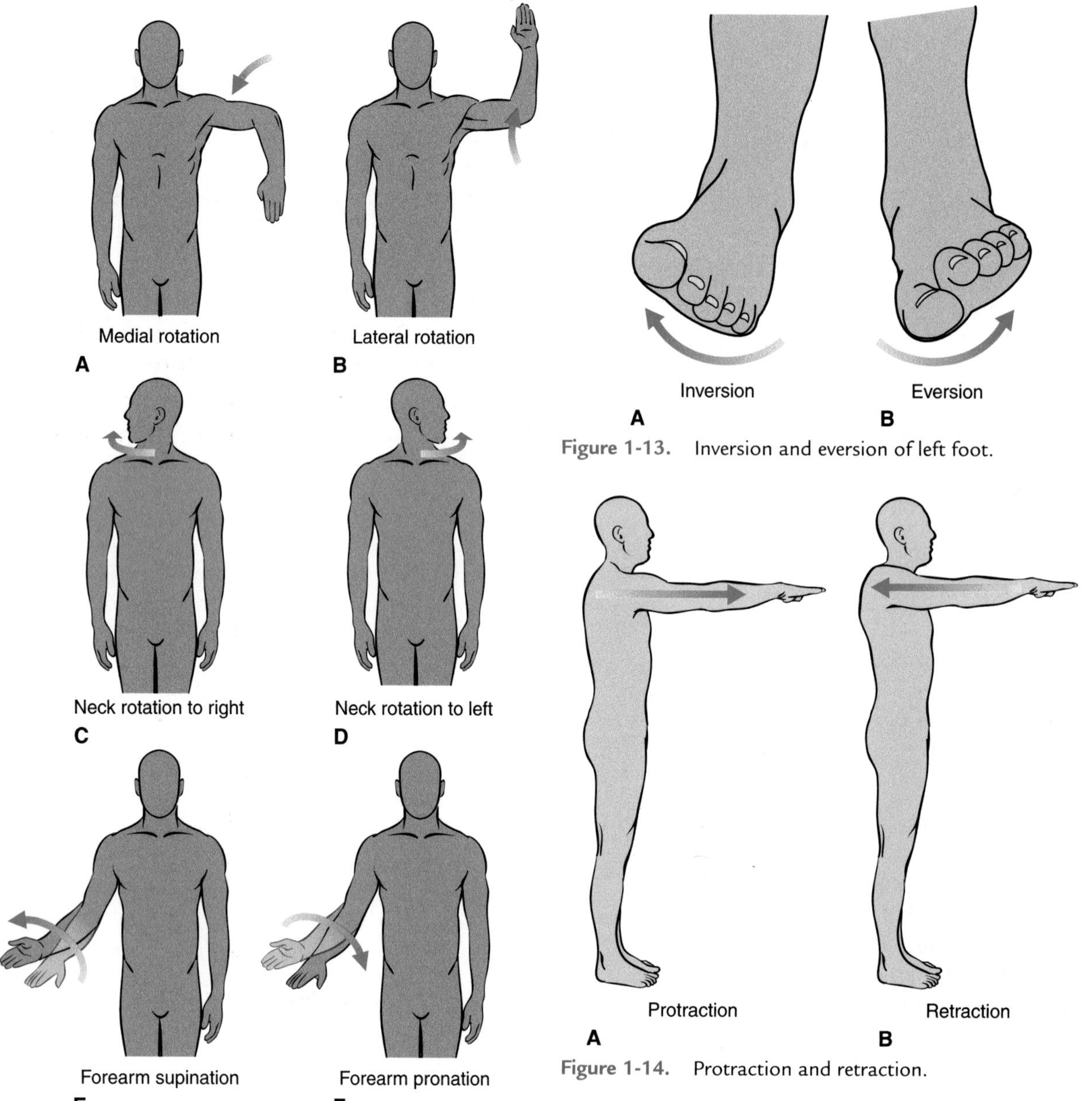

Figure 1-12. Joint rotation motions. In A & B, the shoulder is abducted to 90 degrees only to demonstrate the rotation more clearly.

Figure 1-13. Inversion and eversion of left foot.

Figure 1-14. Protraction and retraction.

Review Questions

1. Using descriptive terminology, complete the following:
   a. The sternum is ___Anterior___ to the vertebral column.
   b. The calcaneus is on the ___~~Plantar fascia~~ Posterior___ portion of the foot.
   c. The hip is ___inferior___ to the chest.
   d. The femur is ___Proximal___ to the tibia.
   e. The radius is on the ___lateral___ side of the forearm.
2. When a football is kicked through the goalposts, what type of motion is being demonstrated by the football? By the kicker? Angular motion
3. Looking at a spot on the ceiling directly over your head involves what joint motion? Hyperextension
4. Putting your hand in your back pocket involves what shoulder joint rotation? Shoulder extension
5. Picking up a pencil on the floor beside your chair involves what trunk joint motion? Flexion
6. Putting your right ankle on your left knee involves what type of hip rotation? lateral rotation
7. In the anatomical position, the forearms are in what position? Supination
8. If you place your hand on the back of a dog, that is referred to as placing it on what surface? If you place your hand on the back of a person, that is referred to as placing it on what surface? dorsal surface Posterior surface
9. A person wheeling across a room in a wheelchair uses both linear and angular motion. Describe when each type of motion is being used.
10. A person lying on a bed staring at the ceiling is in what position?
11. When touching the left shoulder with the left hand, is a person using the contralateral or ipsilateral hand?

Refer to Figure 1-15 below.

12. Identify the three main positions of the left hip.
13. What is the position of the left knee?
14. What is the position of the right forearm?
15. Identify the two main positions of the neck (not the head).

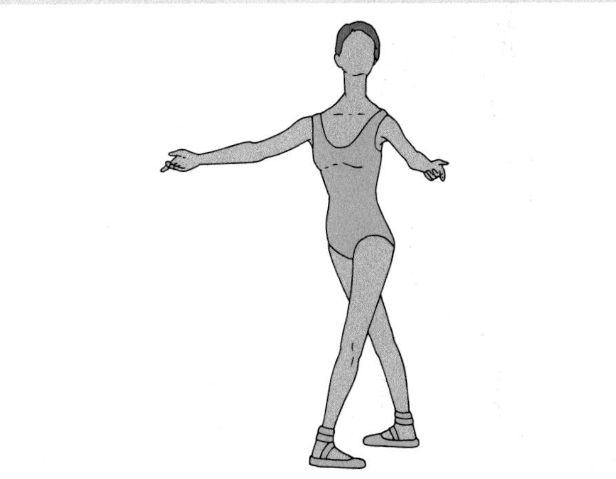

Figure 1-15. Ballet position.

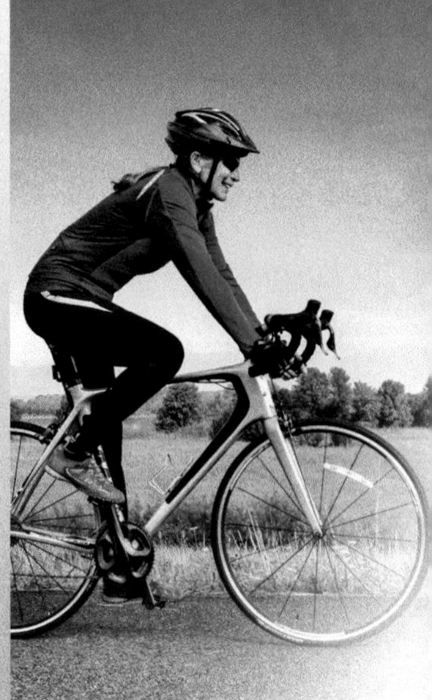

CHAPTER 2
Skeletal System

Functions of the Skeleton
Types of Skeletons
Composition of Bone
Structure of Bone
Types of Bones
Common Skeletal Pathologies
Review Questions

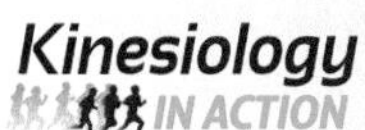

For additional practice activities and videos, please visit www.kinesiologyinaction.com

Functions of the Skeleton

The skeletal system, which is made up of numerous bones, is the rigid framework of the human body. It gives support and shape to the body; protects vital organs such as the brain, spinal cord, and heart; and assists in movement by providing a rigid structure for muscle attachment and leverage. The skeletal system also manufactures blood cells in various locations. The main sites of blood formation are the ilium, vertebrae, sternum, and ribs. This formation occurs mostly in flat bones. Calcium and other mineral salts are stored throughout all osseous tissue of the skeletal system.

Types of Skeletons

The bones of the body are grouped into two main categories: axial and appendicular (Fig. 2-1). The **axial skeleton** forms the upright part of the body. It consists of 80 bones of the head, thorax, and trunk. The **appendicular skeleton** attaches to the axial skeleton and contains the 126 bones of the extremities. There are 206 bones in the body. Individuals may have additional sesamoid bones, such as in the flexor tendons of the great toe and the thumb.

Table 2-1 lists the bones of the adult human body. The sacrum, coccyx, and innominate bones are each made up of several bones fused together. In the innominate bone, also called the os coxa or hip bone, these fused bones are known as the *ilium, ischium,* and *pubis.*

Composition of Bone

Bones can be considered organs because they are made up of several different types of tissue (fibrous,

Table 2-1 Bones of the Human Body

	Single	Paired	Multiple
Axial Skeleton			
Cranium (8)	Frontal Sphenoid Ethmoid Occipital	Parietal Temporal	None
Face (14)	Mandible Vomer	Maxilla Zygomatic Lacrimal Inferior concha Palatine Nasal	None
Other (7)	Hyoid	Ear ossicles (3)	None
Vertebral column (26)	Sacrum (5)* Coccyx (3)*	None	Cervical (7) Thoracic (12) Lumbar (5)
Thorax (25)	Sternum	Ribs (12 pairs = 24) True: 7 False: 3 Floating: 2	None
Appendicular Skeleton			
Upper extremity (64)	None	Scapula Clavicle Humerus Ulna Radius	Carpals (16) Metacarpals (10) Phalanges (28)
Lower extremity (62)	None	Innominate (3)* Femur Tibia Fibula Patella	Tarsals (14) Metatarsals (10) Phalanges (28)

*Denotes bones that are fused together.

cartilaginous, osseous, nervous, and vascular), and they function as integral parts of the skeletal system.

Bone is made up of one-third *organic* (living) material and two-thirds *inorganic* (nonliving) material. The organic material gives the bone elasticity, whereas the inorganic material provides hardness and strength, which makes bone opaque on an x-ray. Just how hard is bone? It has been estimated that if you took a human skull and slowly loaded weight onto it, the skull could support 3 tons before it broke!

Compact bone (Fig. 2-2A and Fig. 2-3) makes up the hard, dense outer layer of all bones. **Cancellous bone** (Fig. 2-2A and Fig. 2-3) is the porous and spongy inside portion made up of thin columns and plates called the *trabeculae,* which means "little beams" in Latin. The latticework network resists local stresses and strains (Fig. 2-2B). Trabeculae tend to be filled with marrow and make the bone lighter.

Structure of Bone

The **epiphysis** is the area at each end of a long bone. This area tends to be wider than the shaft (Fig. 2-3). In adult bone, the epiphysis is osseous; in growing bone, the epiphysis is cartilaginous material called the **epiphyseal plate.** Longitudinal growth occurs here through the manufacturing of new bone.

On an x-ray, a growing bone will show a distinct line between the epiphyseal plate and the rest of the bone (Fig. 2-4A). Because this line does not exist in the

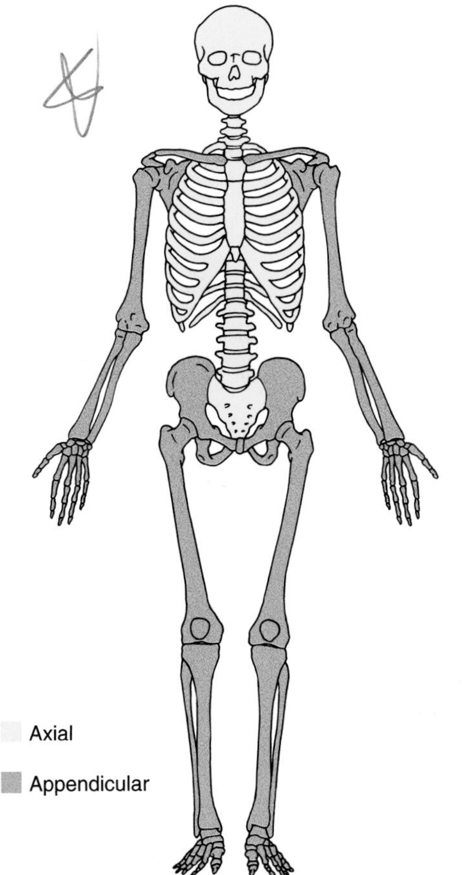

Figure 2-1. Axial and appendicular skeleton.

normal adult bone, its absence indicates that bone growth has stopped (Fig. 2-4B).

There are two types of epiphyses found in children whose bones are still growing (Fig. 2-5). A **pressure epiphysis** is located at the ends of long bones, where they receive pressure from the opposing bone making up that joint. This is where growth of long bones occurs. A **traction epiphysis** is located where tendons attach to bones and are subjected to a pulling, or traction, force.

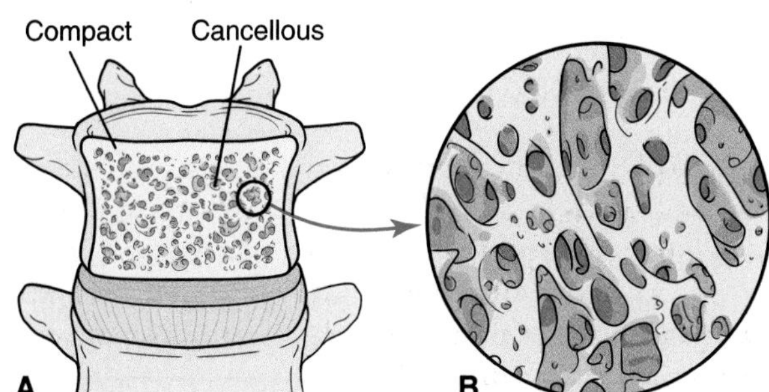

Figure 2-2. Normal bone structure: **(A)** compact and cancellous bone **(B)** trabeculae network within cancellous bone.

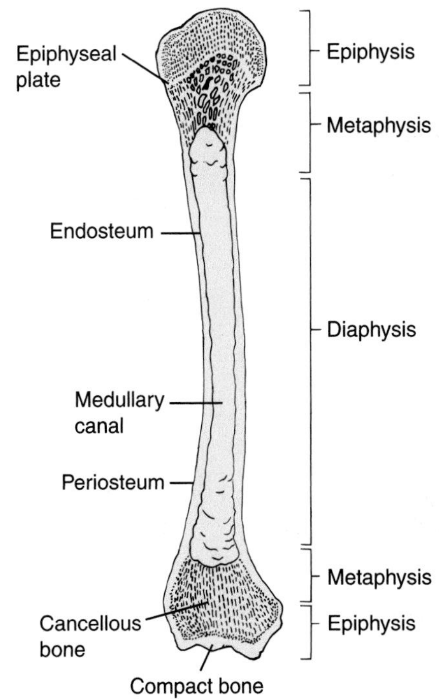

Figure 2-3. Longitudinal cross section of a long bone.

Examples would be the greater and lesser trochanters of the femur and tibial tuberosity.

The **diaphysis** (see Fig. 2-3) is the main shaft of bone. Its walls are made up mostly of compact bone, which gives it great strength. Its center, the **medullary canal,** is hollow, which, among other features, decreases the weight of the bone. This canal contains marrow and provides passage for nutrient arteries. The **endosteum** is a membrane that lines the medullary canal. It contains **osteoclasts,** which are mainly responsible for bone resorption—a process by which old bone is broken down so it can be replaced with new bone.

In long bones, the **metaphysis** is the flared part of the bone that serves as a transition from the end of each diaphysis to each epiphysis. It is made up mostly of cancellous bone and functions to support the epiphysis.

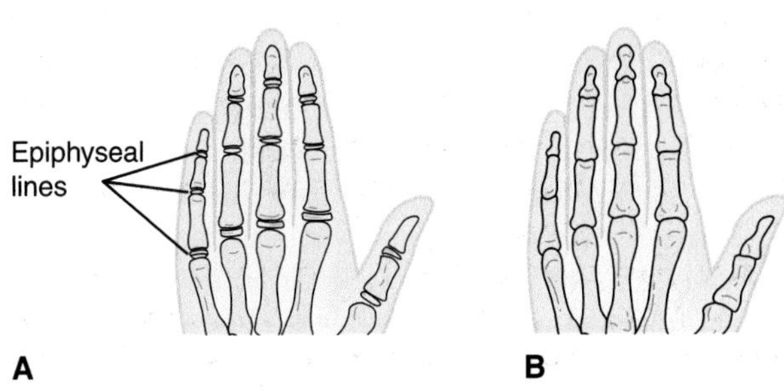

Figure 2-4. Epiphyseal lines in the hand bones of a child **(A)** and an adult **(B).**

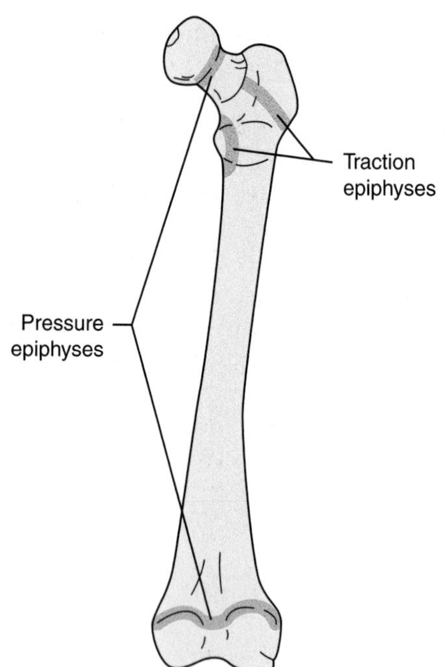

Figure 2-5. Types of epiphyses found in an immature bone.

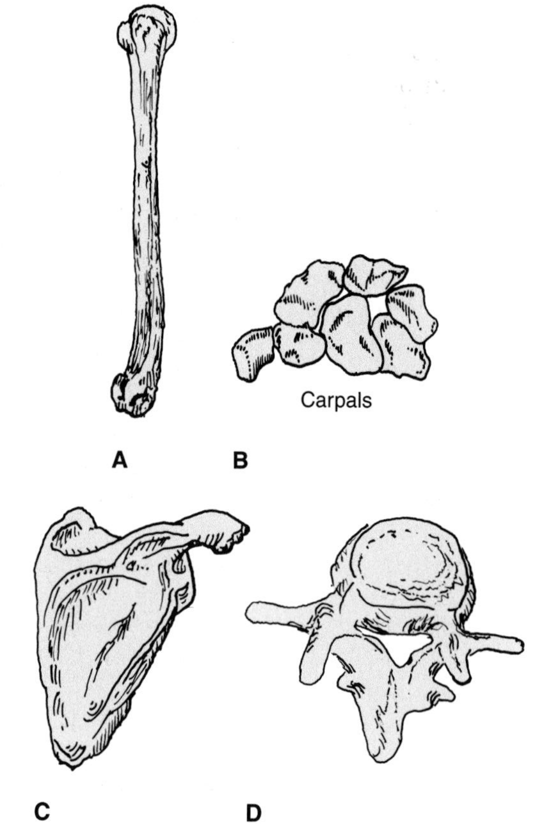

Figure 2-6. Types of bones.

Periosteum is the thin fibrous membrane covering all of the bone except the articular surfaces, which are covered with hyaline cartilage. The periosteum contains nerves as well as blood vessels that are important in providing nourishment, promoting growth in the diameter of immature bone, and repairing the bone. It also serves as an attachment point for tendons and ligaments. Compared with the surrounding bone tissue, the periosteum has a much greater number of pain receptors, which makes it exceedingly pain sensitive when it is overstressed, such as during a fracture or due to inflammation at the attachment site of a tendon.

Types of Bones

Long bones are so named because their length is greater than their width (Fig. 2-6A). They are the largest bones in the body and make up most of the appendicular skeleton. Long bones are basically tube-shaped, with a shaft (diaphysis) filled with bone marrow (medullary canal) and two bulbous ends (epiphysis). The wide part of the shaft nearest the epiphysis is called the *metaphysis* (see Fig. 2-3). As discussed previously, the diaphysis consists mainly of compact bone, whereas the metaphysis and epiphysis consist of cancellous bone covered by a thin layer of compact bone. While the body is still growing, bone growth occurs at the epiphyseal plate. Over the articular surfaces of the epiphysis is a thin layer of hyaline cartilage.

Short bones tend to have more equal dimensions of height, length, and width, giving them a cube shape (Fig. 2-6B). They have a great deal of articular surface and, unlike long bones, usually articulate with more than one bone. Their composition is similar to long bones: a thin layer of compact bone covering cancellous bone, which has a marrow cavity in the middle. Examples of short bones include the bones of the wrist (carpals) and ankle (tarsals).

Flat bones have a very broad surface but are not very thick. They tend to have a curved surface rather than a flat one (Fig. 2-6C). These bones are made up of two layers of compact bone with cancellous bone and marrow in between. The ilium, scapula, and many of the cranial bones are good examples of flat bones.

As their name implies, **irregular bones** have a variety of mixed shapes that do not fit into the other categories (Fig. 2-6D). Their unique shapes allow them to fulfill a particular function. For example, the opening in the center of the vertebrae houses and protects the spinal cord. Other irregular bones include the sacrum and bones of the skull that are not flat. They are also composed of cancellous bone and marrow encased in a thin layer of compact bone.

Sesamoid bones, which resemble the shape of sesame seeds, are small bones located where tendons cross the ends of long bones in the extremities. They develop within the tendon and protect it from excessive wear. For example, the tendon of the flexor hallucis longus spans the bottom (plantar surface) of the foot and attaches on the great toe. If this tendon were not protected in some way at the ball of the foot, it would constantly be stepped on. Mother Nature is too clever to allow this to happen. Sesamoid bones are located on either side of the tendon near the head of the first metatarsal, providing a protective "groove" for the tendon to pass through this weight-bearing area.

Sesamoid bones also change the angle of a tendon's attachment, which can increase its ability to generate force at the joints it crosses. (Chapter 8 will present the biomechanical rationale for this.) The sesamoid bones just discussed (in the flexor hallucis longus) greatly enhance this muscle's ability to produce force at the great toe when pushing off to take a step. The patella can also be considered a sesamoid bone because it is encased in the quadriceps tendon, and it improves the mechanical advantage of the quadriceps muscle, allowing it to generate more force at the knee. As previously mentioned, sesamoid bones are also found in the flexor tendons that pass posteriorly into the foot on either side of the ankle. Other sesamoid bones are found in the flexor tendons of the thumb, near the metacarpophalangeal and interphalangeal joints as well as at the wrist. Occasionally, a sesamoid bone is located near the metacarpophalangeal joint of the index and little fingers.

Table 2-2 summarizes the types of bones of the axial and appendicular skeletons. It should be noted that there are no long or short bones in the axial skeleton, and there are no irregular bones in the appendicular skeleton. Except for the patella, sesamoid bones are not included in Table 2-2 because they are considered accessory bones, and their shape and number vary greatly.

When looking at various bones, you will see holes, depressions, ridges, bumps, grooves, and various other kinds of markings. Each of these markings serves a different purpose. Table 2-3 describes the different kinds of bone markings and their purposes.

Common Skeletal Pathologies

Fracture, *broken bone,* and *cracked bone* are all synonymous. It is a break in the continuity of the bony cortex caused by direct force, indirect force, or pathology. Fractures in children tend to be incomplete ("greenstick") or at the epiphysis. Fractures in the elderly mostly happen in the hip joint (proximal femur), resulting from a fall, or in the upper extremity from falling on the outstretched hand. Fractures are often described by type (e.g., closed), direction of fracture line (e.g., transverse), or position of the bone fragments (e.g., overriding).

Table 2-2 Types of Bones

Type	Appendicular Skeleton		Axial Skeleton
	Upper Extremity	Lower Extremity	
Long bones	Clavicle Humerus Radius Ulna Metacarpals Phalanges	Femur Fibula Tibia Metatarsals Phalanges	None
Short bones	Carpals	Tarsals	None
Flat bones	Scapula	None	Cranial bones (frontal, parietal, occipital, temporal) Ribs Sternum
Irregular bones	None	Innominate	Vertebrae Sacrum Coccyx Mandible, facial bones
Sesamoid		Patella	

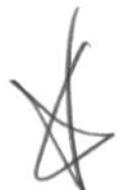

Table 2-3 Bone Markings

Depressions and Openings

Marking	Description	Examples
1. Foramen	Hole through which blood vessels, nerves, and ligaments pass	Vertebral foramen of cervical vertebra
2. Fossa	Hollow or depression	Glenoid fossa of scapula
3. Groove	Ditchlike groove containing a tendon or blood vessel	Bicipital (intercondylar) groove of humerus
4. Meatus	Canal or tubelike opening in a bone	External auditory meatus
5. Sinus	Air-filled cavity within a bone	Frontal sinus in frontal bone

Projections or Processes That Fit Into Joints

Marking	Description	Examples
1. Condyle	Rounded knucklelike projection	Medial condyle of femur
2. Eminence	Projecting, prominent part of bone	Intercondylar eminence of tibia
3. Facet	Flat or shallow articular surface	Articular facet of rib
4. Head	Rounded articular projection beyond a narrow, necklike portion of bone	Femoral head

Projections/Processes That Attach Tendons, Ligaments, and Other Connective Tissue

Marking	Description	Examples
1. Crest	Sharp ridge or border	Iliac crest
2. Epicondyle	Prominence above or on a condyle	Medial epicondyle of humerus
3. Line	Less prominent ridge	Linea aspera of femur
4. Spine	Long, thin projection (spinous process)	Scapular spine
5. Tubercle	Small, rounded projection	Greater tubercle of humerus
6. Tuberosity	Large, rounded projection	Ischial tuberosity
7. Trochanter	Very large prominence for muscle attachment	Greater trochanter of femur

Osteoporosis is a condition characterized by loss of normal bone density, or bone mass (Fig. 2-7). The bone density in this figure can be compared with that in Figure 2-2. This condition can weaken a bone to the point where it will fracture. The vertebrae of an elderly person are common sites for osteoporosis. Osteopenia is also a condition of reduced bone mass, though not as severe as osteoporosis. **Osteomyelitis** is an infection of the bone usually caused by bacteria. A fracture that breaks through the skin (open fracture) poses a greater risk of developing osteomyelitis than a fracture that does not break the skin (closed fracture).

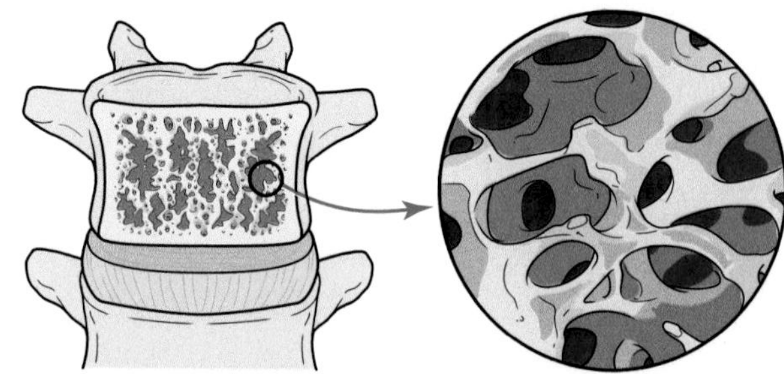

Figure 2-7. Osteoporotic bone.

Because the epiphysis of a growing bone is not firmly attached to the diaphysis, it can slip or become misshapen. The proximal head of the femur is a common site for problems such as **Legg-Calvé-Perthes disease,** which happens when blood supply is interrupted to the femoral head, causing necrosis of the bone, at the pressure epiphysis in growing children. A **slipped capital femoral epiphysis** occurs when the head of the femur becomes displaced due to a separation at the growth plate.

Overuse can cause irritation and inflammation of any traction epiphysis where tendons attach to bone. A common condition called Osgood-Schlatter disease occurs at the traction epiphysis of the tibial tuberosity in children whose bones are still growing. Problems at these pressure and traction epiphyses usually exist only during the bone-growing years and not after the epiphyses have fused and bone growth stops.

Review Questions

1. What are the differences between the axial and appendicular skeletons?
2. Give one example of compact bone and one of cancellous bone.
3. Which is heavier: compact bone or cancellous bone? Why?
4. What type of bone is mainly involved in an individual's growth in height? In what portion of the bone does this growth occur?
5. What is the purpose of sesamoid bones?
6. Name the bone markings that can be classified as
   a. depressions and openings
   b. projections or processes that fit into joints
   c. projections or processes that attach connective tissue such as tendons, ligaments, and fascia

In Questions 7 to 9, classify the bone markings.

7. Bicipital groove — ditch like grove
8. Humeral head – Round
9. Acetabulum – deep depression
10. What is the name of the membrane that lines the medullary canal?
11. The main shaft of bone is called what?
12. In children, does long bone growth occur at a traction epiphysis or at a pressure epiphysis?
13. Is the humerus part of the axial or appendicular skeleton?
14. Is the clavicle part of the axial or appendicular skeleton?
15. Is the sternum part of the axial or appendicular skeleton?

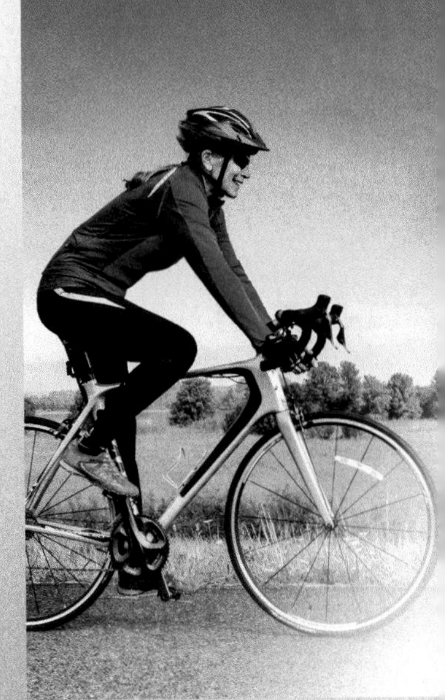

CHAPTER 3
Articular System

Types of Joints
Joint Structure
Planes and Axes
Degrees of Freedom
Common Pathological Terms
Review Questions

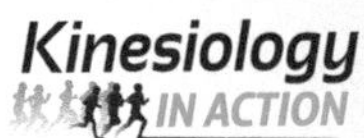

For additional practice activities and videos, please visit www.kinesiologyinaction.com

A joint is a connection between two bones. Although joints have several functions, perhaps the most important is to allow motion. Joints also help to bear the body's weight and to provide stability. This stability may be mostly due to the shape of the bones making up the joint, as with the hip joint, or may be due to soft tissue features, as seen in the shoulder and knee. Joints also contain synovial fluid, which lubricates the joint and nourishes the cartilage.

Types of Joints

A joint may allow a great deal of motion, as in the shoulder, or very little motion, as in the sternoclavicular joint. As with all differences, there are trade-offs. A joint that allows a great deal of motion will provide very little stability. Conversely, a joint that is quite stable tends to have little motion. There is often more than one term that can be used to describe the same joint. These terms tend to describe either the structure or the amount of motion allowed.

A **fibrous joint** has a thin layer of fibrous periosteum between the two bones, as in the sutures of the skull. There are three types of fibrous joints: synarthrosis, syndesmosis, and gomphosis. A **synarthrosis,** or suture joint, has a thin layer of fibrous periosteum between the two bones, as in the sutures of the skull. The ends of the bones are shaped to allow them to interlock (Fig. 3-1A). With this type of joint, there is essentially no motion between the bones; its purpose is to provide shape and strength. Another type of fibrous joint is a **syndesmosis,** or ligamentous joint. There is a great deal of fibrous tissue, such as ligaments and interosseous membranes, holding the joint together (Fig. 3-1B). A small amount of twisting or stretching movement can occur in this type of joint. The distal tibiofibular joint at the ankle and the distal radioulnar joint are examples. The third type of fibrous joint is called a **gomphosis,** which is Greek for "bolting together." This joint occurs between a tooth and the wall of its dental socket in the mandible and maxilla (Fig. 3-1C). Its structure is referred to as *peg-in-socket.*

A **cartilaginous joint** (Fig. 3-2) has either hyaline cartilage or fibrocartilage between the two bones. The vertebral joints are examples of joints in which fibrocartilage disks are directly connecting the bones. The first sternocostal joint is an example of the direct connection made by hyaline cartilage. Cartilaginous joints are also called **amphiarthrodial joints** because they allow a small amount of motion, such as bending or twisting, and some compression. At the same time, these joints provide a great deal of stability.

A **synovial joint** (Fig. 3-3) has no direct union between the bone ends. Instead, there is a cavity filled with synovial fluid contained within a sleevelike capsule. The outer layer of the capsule is made up of a strong fibrous tissue that holds the joint together. The inner layer is lined with a synovial membrane that secretes the synovial fluid. The articular surface is very smooth and covered with cartilage called *hyaline* or *articular cartilage.* The synovial joint is also called a **diarthrodial joint** because it allows free motion. It is not as stable as the other types of joints but does allow a great deal more motion. Table 3-1 provides a summary of the joint types. The number of axes, the shape of the joint, and the type of motion allowed by the joint could further classify synovial, or diarthrodial, joints (Table 3-2).

In a **nonaxial joint,** movement tends to be linear instead of angular (Fig. 3-4). The joint surfaces are relatively flat and glide over one another instead of one

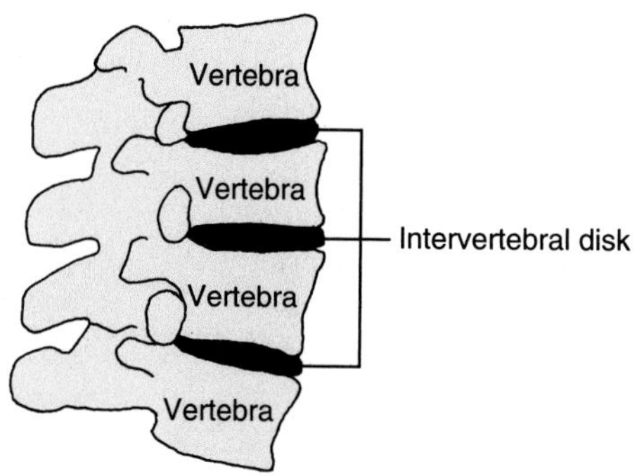

Figure 3-2. Cartilaginous joint.

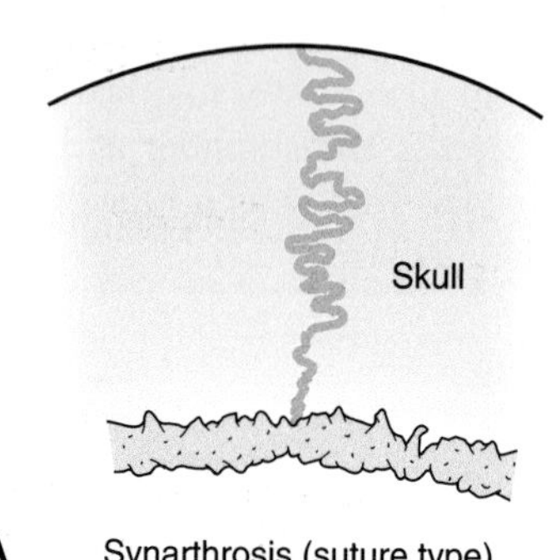

A Synarthrosis (suture type)

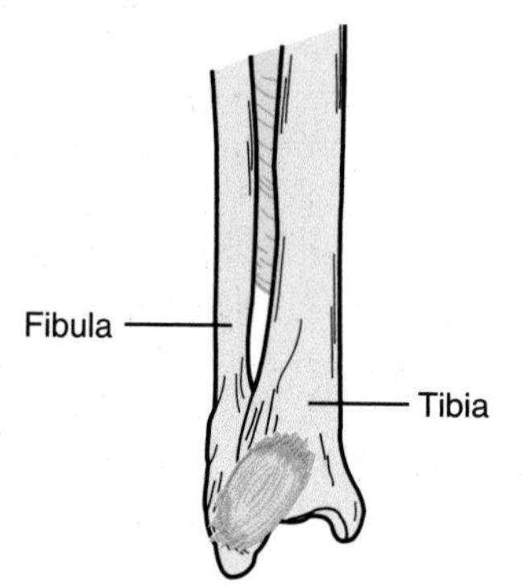

B Syndesmosis (ligamentous type)

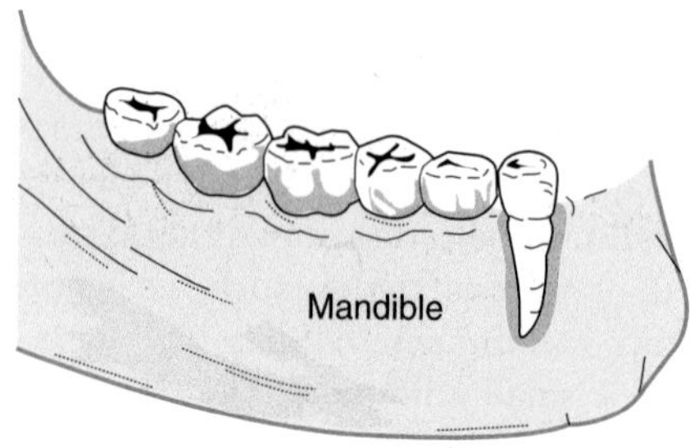

C Gomphosis (peg-in-socket)

Figure 3-1. Fibrous joints.

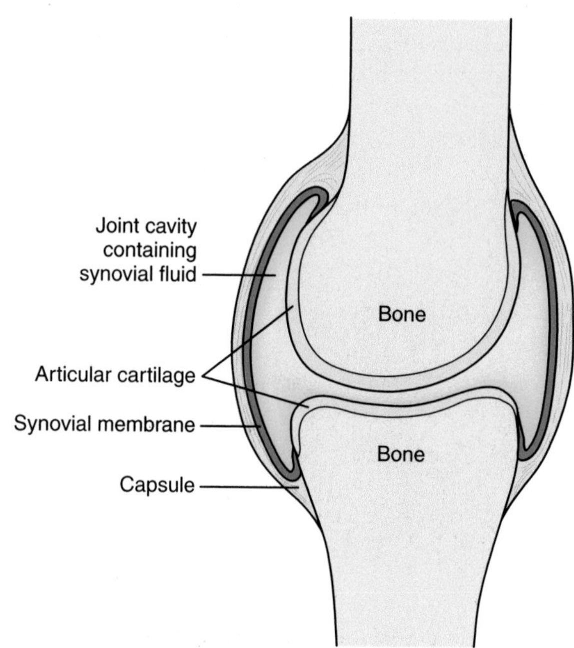

Figure 3-3. Synovial joint.

Table 3-1 Joint Classification

Type	Motion	Structure	Example
Synarthrosis	None	Fibrous—suture	Bones in the skull, except mandible
Syndesmosis	Slight	Fibrous—ligamentous	Distal tibiofibular
Gomphosis	None	Fibrous—peg-in-socket	Teeth in mandible and maxilla
Amphiarthrosis	Little	Cartilaginous	Symphysis pubis, vertebrae
Diarthrosis	Free	Synovial	Hip, elbow, knee

Table 3-2 Classification of Diarthrodial Joints

Number of Axes	Shape of Joint	Joint Motion	Example
Nonaxial	Plane (Irregular)	Gliding	Intercarpals
Uniaxial	Hinge	Flexion/extension	Elbow and knee
	Pivot	Rotation	Atlas/axis, radius/ulna
Biaxial	Condyloid (Ellipsoidal)	Flexion/extension, abduction/adduction	Wrist, MPs
	Saddle	Flexion/extension, abduction/adduction, rotation (accessory)	Thumb CMC
Triaxial (multiaxial)	Ball and socket	Flexion/extension, abduction/adduction, rotation	Shoulder, hip

moving around the other and can be described as a **plane joint.** The motion that occurs between the carpal bones is an example of this type of motion. Unlike most other types of diarthrodial joint motion, nonaxial motion occurs secondarily to other motion. For example, you can flex and extend your elbow without moving other joints; however, you cannot move your carpal bones by themselves. Motion of the carpals occurs when the wrist joint moves in either flexion and extension or abduction and adduction.

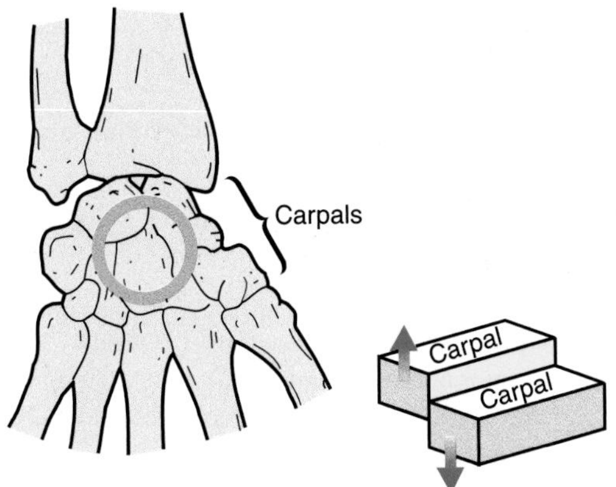

Figure 3-4. Plane joint demonstrates gliding motion between bones.

A **uniaxial joint** has angular motion occurring in one plane around one axis, much like a hinge. The elbow, or humeroulnar joint, is a good example of a **hinge joint** with the convex shape of the humerus fitting into the concave-shaped ulna (Fig. 3-5). The only motions possible are flexion and extension, which occur in the sagittal plane around the frontal axis. Planes and axes will be described later in this chapter. No other motions are possible at this joint. The interphalangeal joints of the hand and foot also have this hinge motion. The knee is a hinge joint, but this example must be clarified. During the last few degrees of extension, the femur rotates medially on the tibia. This rotation is not an active motion but rather

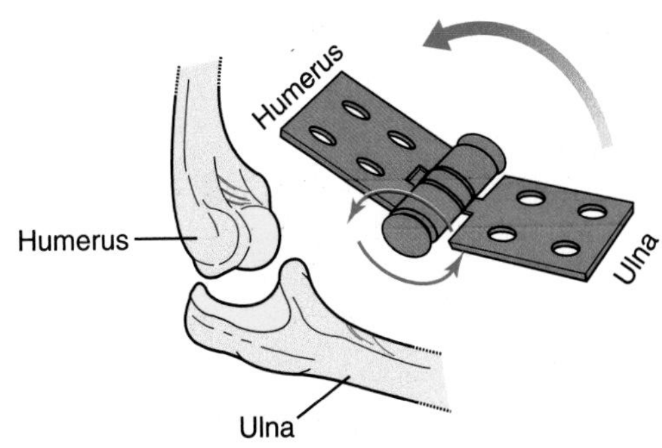

Figure 3-5. Hinge joint has anterior-posterior motion allowing flexion and extension.

the result of certain mechanical features present. Therefore, the knee is best classified as a uniaxial joint, because it has *active* motion around only one axis.

Also at the elbow is the radioulnar joint, which as a **pivot joint** demonstrates another type of uniaxial motion. The head of the radius pivots on the stationary ulna during pronation and supination of the forearm (Fig. 3-6). This pivot motion is in the transverse plane around the longitudinal axis. The motion of the atlantoaxial joint of C1 and C2 is also pivotal. The first cervical vertebra *(atlas),* on which the head rests, rotates around the odontoid process of the second cervical vertebra *(axis).* This allows the head to rotate.

Biaxial joint motion, such as that found at the wrist, occurs in two different directions (Fig. 3-7). Flexion and extension occur around the frontal axis, and radial and ulnar deviation occur around the sagittal axis. This bidirectional motion also occurs at the metacarpophalangeal (MCP) joints. The wrist and MCP joints are referred to as **condyloid joints,** or sometimes *ellipsoid joints* because of their shape.

The carpometacarpal (CMC) joint of the thumb is biaxial but differs somewhat from the condyloid joint. In this joint, the articular surface of each bone is concave in one direction and convex in the other. The bones fit together like a horseback rider in a saddle, which is why this joint is also descriptively called a **saddle joint** (Fig. 3-8).

Unlike the condyloid joint, the CMC joint allows a slight amount of rotation. Like the motion within the carpal bones, this rotation cannot occur by itself. If you try to rotate your thumb without also flexing and abducting, you find that you cannot do it. Yet, rotation does occur. Look at the direction to which the pad of your thumb is pointing when it is adducted. Abduct and flex your thumb and notice that the direction to which the pad is pointing has changed by approximately

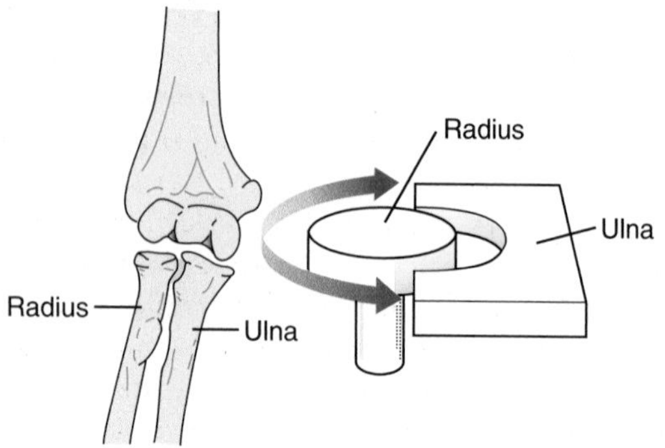

Figure 3-6. Pivot joint has rotation of one bone around another. At the elbow, this allows for pronation and supination of the forearm.

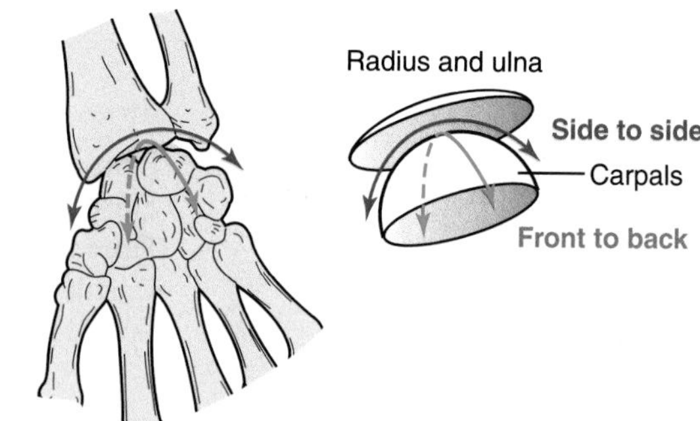

Figure 3-7. Condyloid joint has motion in two planes: posterior/anterior (allowing flexion/extension) and lateral/medial (allowing abduction/adduction).

90 degrees. This rotation has not occurred actively; rotation has occurred because of the joint's shape. Therefore, although the CMC joint of the thumb is not a true biaxial joint due to the rotation allowed, it fits best into this category because the *active* motion allowed is around two axes.

With a **triaxial joint,** sometimes referred to as a *multiaxial joint,* motion occurs actively around all three axes (Fig. 3-9). This joint allows more motion than any other type of joint. The hip and shoulder allow motion around the frontal axis (flexion and extension), around the sagittal axis (abduction and adduction), and around the vertical axis (rotation). The triaxial joint is also referred to as a **ball-and-socket joint** because in the hip, for example, the ball-shaped femoral head fits into the concave socket of the acetabulum.

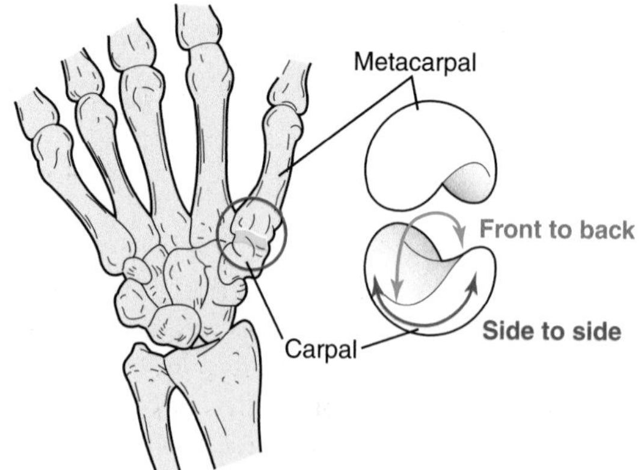

Figure 3-8. Saddle joint, while although to the condyloid joint, is uniquely different. Its two planes of motion: anterior-posterior allows carpometacarpal (CMC) joint abduction and adduction; medial-lateral motion allows CMC flexion/extension. The planes of this joint are the exception to the rule. Anterior-posterior motion usually occurs in the sagittal plane, whereas medial-lateral motion occurs in the frontal plane.

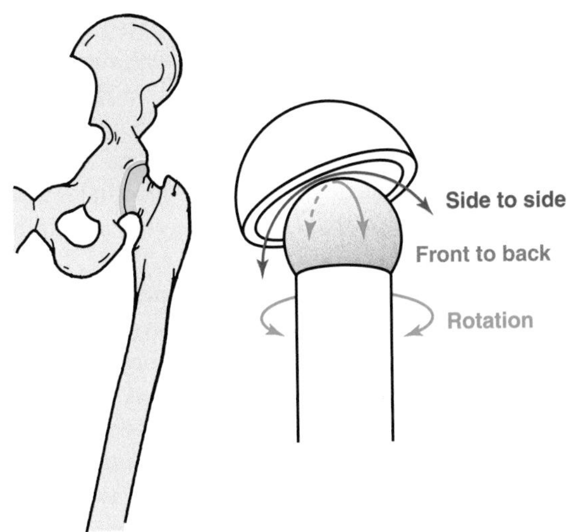

Figure 3-9. Ball-and-socket joint allows for motion in three directions: anterior-posterior (allowing flexion/extension), medial-lateral (allowing adduction/abduction), and rotation (allowing medial rotation/lateral rotation).

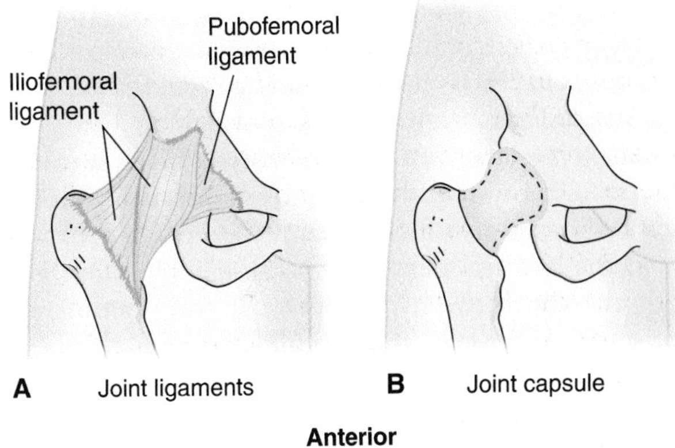

Figure 3-10. Support structures of a synovial joint: ligaments **(A)** and capsule **(B)**, which lies immediately deep to the surrounding ligaments.

Joint Structure

There are many components of a synovial joint (see Fig. 3-3). First, there are **bones,** usually two, that articulate with each other. The amount and direction of motion allowed at each joint are dictated by the shape of the bone ends and by the articular surface of each bone.

The two bones of a joint are held together and supported by **ligaments,** which are bands of fibrous connective tissue. Ligaments also provide attachment for cartilage, fascia, or, in some cases, muscle. Ligaments are flexible but not elastic. This flexibility is needed to allow joint motion, but the nonelasticity is needed to keep the bones in close approximation to each other and to provide some protection to the joint. In other words, ligaments prevent excessive joint movement. When ligaments surround a synovial joint, they are called *capsular ligaments* (Fig. 3-10A).

Every synovial joint has a **capsule** that surrounds and encases the joint and protects the articular surfaces of the bones. Figure 3-10B shows the capsule of the hip joint. It lies deep to, and is encased and supported by, the ligaments. In the shoulder joint, the capsule completely encases the joint, forming a partial vacuum that helps hold the head of the humerus against the glenoid fossa. In other joints, the capsule may not be as complete.

As was described earlier, there are several components within a synovial joint (see Fig. 3-3). The joint capsule has two layers: an outer layer and an inner layer. The outer layer consists of fibrous tissue and supports and protects the joint. This layer is usually reinforced by ligaments (see Fig. 3-10A). The inner layer is lined with a **synovial membrane,** a thick, vascular connective tissue that secretes synovial fluid. **Synovial fluid** is a thick, clear fluid (resembling an egg white) that lubricates the articular cartilage; this reduces friction and helps the joint move freely. This fluid provides some shock absorption and is the major source of nutrition for articular cartilage.

Cartilage is a dense, fibrous connective tissue that can withstand great amounts of pressure and tension. The body has three basic types of cartilage: hyaline, fibrocartilage, and elastic. **Hyaline cartilage,** also called **articular cartilage,** covers the ends of opposing bones within a synovial joint. With the help of synovial fluid, it provides a smooth articulating surface in all synovial joints. Because hyaline cartilage lacks its own blood or nerve supply and must get its nutrition from the synovial fluid, it cannot repair itself if it is damaged.

Fibrocartilage acts as a shock absorber and is present in both synovial and cartilaginous joints. Shock absorption is especially important in weight-bearing joints such as the knee and vertebrae. At the knee, the semilunar-shaped cartilage called the **meniscus** builds up the sides of the relatively flat articular surface of the tibia. Intervertebral **disks** (see Fig. 3-2) lie between the vertebral bones. Because of their very dense structure, these disks are capable of absorbing an amazing amount of shock that is transmitted upward from weight-bearing forces.

In the upper extremity, a fibrocartilaginous disk located between the clavicle and sternum is important for absorbing the shock transmitted along the clavicle to the sternum should you fall on your outstretched hand. This disk helps prevent dislocation of the sternoclavicular joint and is also important in allowing motion. The disk, which is attached to the sternum at one end and the clavicle at the other, is much like a swinging door hinge that allows motion in both directions. This double-hung hinge allows the clavicle to move on the sternum as the acromial end is elevated and depressed or protracted and retracted. In effect, the fibrocartilage divides the joint into two cavities, allowing two sets of motion.

There are other functions of fibrocartilage in joints. The shoulder fibrocartilage, called the **labrum,** deepens the shallow glenoid fossa, making it more of a socket to hold the humeral head (Fig. 3-11). Fibrocartilage also fills the gap between two bones. If you examine the wrist, you will notice that the ulna does not extend all the way to the carpal bones, as does the radius. A small triangular disk located in this gap acts as a space filler and allows force to be exerted on the ulna and carpals without causing damage.

The third type of cartilage, **elastic cartilage,** is designed to help maintain a structure's shape. Elastic cartilage is found in the external ear and eustachian (auditory) tube, and is also found in the larynx, where its motion is important to speech.

Muscles provide the contractile force that causes joints to move. Therefore, they must span the joint to have an effect on that joint. Muscles are soft and cannot attach directly to the bone. A **tendon** must connect them to bone. The tendon may be a cylindrical cord, like the long head of the biceps tendon, or a flattened band, like the rotator cuff. In certain locations, tendons are encased in **tendon sheaths.** These fibrous sleeves surround the tendon when it is subject to pressure or friction, such as when it passes between muscles and bones or through a tunnel between bones. The tendons passing over the wrist all have tendon sheaths. These sheaths are lubricated by fluid secreted from their lining.

An **aponeurosis** is a broad, flat tendinous sheet. Aponeuroses are found in several places where muscles attach to bones. The large, powerful latissimus dorsi muscle is attached at one end over a large area to several bones by means of an aponeurosis. In the anterior abdominal wall, aponeuroses provide a base of muscular attachment where no bone is present but where great strength is needed. As the abdominal muscles approach the midline from both sides, they attach to an aponeurosis called the **linea alba.**

Bursae are small, padlike sacs found around most joints. They are located in areas of excessive friction, such as between tendons and bony prominences (Fig. 3-12). Lined with synovial membrane and filled with a clear fluid, bursae reduce friction between moving parts. For example, in the shoulder, the deltoid muscle passes directly over the acromion process. Repeated motion would cause excessive wearing of the muscle tissue. However, the subdeltoid bursa that is located between the muscle and acromion process prevents excessive friction and reduces the likelihood of damage. The same arrangement occurs in the elbow, where the triceps tendon attaches to the olecranon process. Some joints, such as the knee, have many bursae. There are two types of bursae: natural bursae (which have just been described) and acquired bursae. In an area that normally does not have excessive friction, a bursa can appear in the event that abnormal friction does occur. These *acquired bursae* tend to occur in places other than joints. For example, a person may develop a bursa on the lateral side of the third finger of the writing hand. This is often called the "student's bursa," because students often do a lot of writing and note-taking. These bursae disappear when the activity or friction is stopped or greatly reduced.

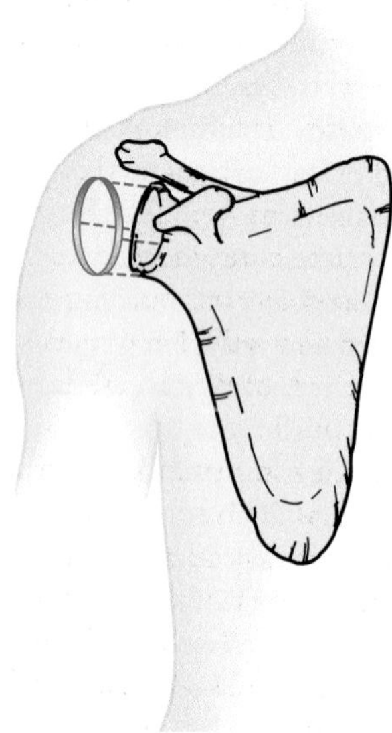

Figure 3-11. Labrum.

Planes and Axes

Planes of action are fixed lines of reference along which the body is divided. There are three planes, and each plane is at right angles, or perpendicular, to the other two planes (Fig. 3-13).

The **sagittal plane** passes through the body from front to back and divides the body into right and left parts. Think of it as a vertical wall that the extremity moves along. Motions occurring in this plane are flexion

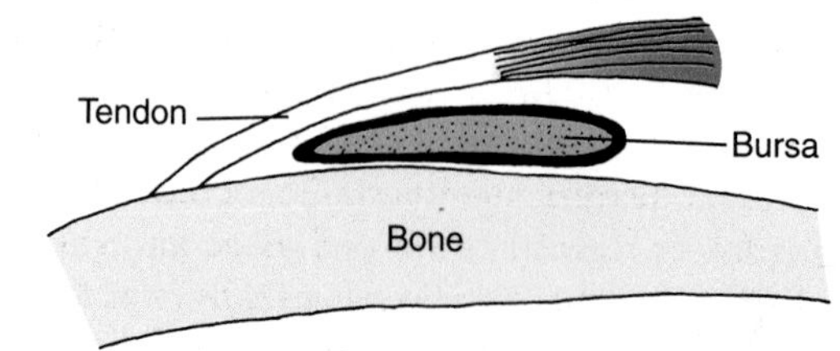

Figure 3-12. Bursa.

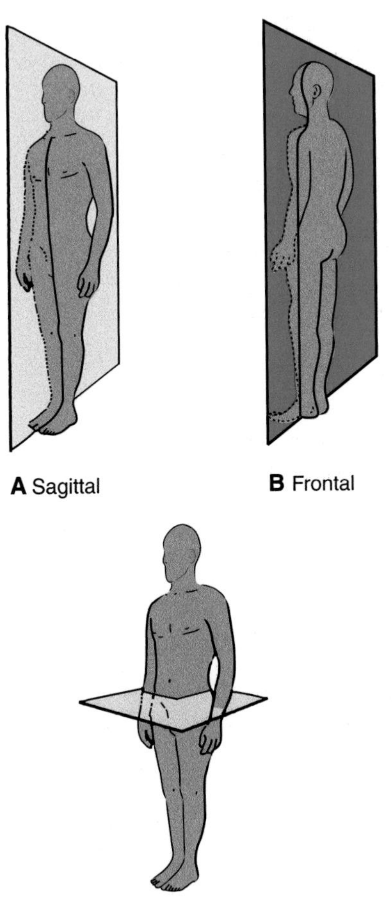

Figure 3-13. Planes of the body. **(A)** Sagittal plane. **(B)** Frontal plane. **(C)** Transverse plane.

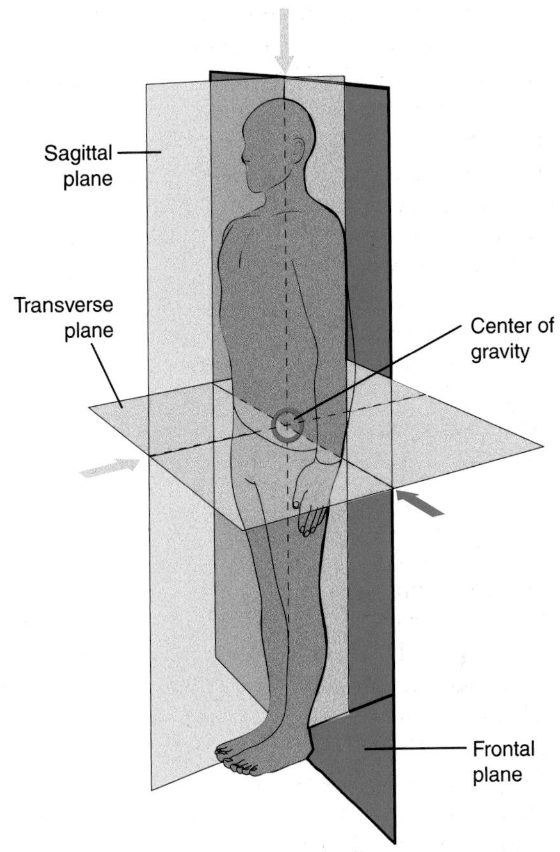

Figure 3-14. The center of gravity is the point at which the three cardinal planes intersect.

and extension. A mid-sagittal plane would divide the body in the middle into equal right and left parts. For example, a mid-sagittal section of the brain (see Fig. 6-5) would view the brain that has been cut in half from front to back (i.e., in the sagittal plane).

The **frontal plane** passes through the body from side to side and divides the body into front and back parts. It is also called the *coronal plane.* Motions occurring in this plane are abduction and adduction.

The **transverse plane** passes through the body horizontally and divides the body into top and bottom parts. It is also called the *horizontal plane.* Rotation occurs in this plane.

Whenever a plane passes through the midline of a part, whether it is the sagittal, frontal, or transverse plane, it is referred to as a *cardinal plane* because it divides the body into equal parts. The point where the three cardinal planes intersect each other is the **center of gravity.** In the human body, that point is in the midline at about the level of, though slightly anterior to, the second sacral vertebra (Fig. 3-14).

Axes are points that run through the center of a joint around which a part rotates (Fig. 3-15). The **sagittal axis** is a point that runs through a joint from front to back. The **frontal axis** runs through a joint from side to side. The **vertical axis,** also called the *longitudinal axis,* runs through a joint from top to bottom.

Joint movement occurs around an axis that is always perpendicular to its plane. Another way of stating this is that joint movement occurs *in a plane* and *around an axis.* A particular motion will always occur in the same plane and around the same axis. For example, flexion/extension will always occur in the sagittal plane around the frontal axis. Abduction/adduction will always occur in the frontal plane around the sagittal axis. Similar motions, such as radial and ulnar deviation of the wrist, will also occur in the frontal plane around the sagittal axis. The thumb is the exception, because flexion/extension and abduction/adduction do not occur in these traditional planes. (These thumb motions, and their planes and axes, will be described in Chapter 13.) Table 3-3 summarizes joint motion in relation to planes and axes.

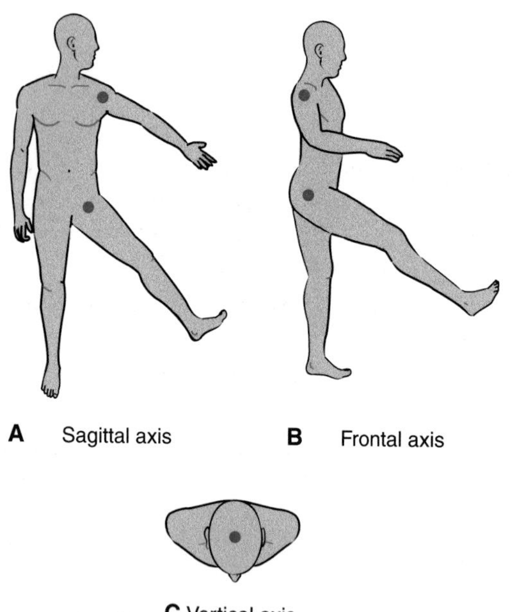

Figure 3-15. Axes of the body. **(A)** Sagittal axis. **(B)** Frontal axis. **(C)** Vertical axis.

Table 3-3 Joint Motions

Plane	Axis	Joint Motion
Sagittal	Frontal	Flexion/extension
Frontal	Sagittal	Abduction/adduction Radial/ulnar deviation Eversion/inversion
Transverse	Vertical	Medial-lateral rotation Supination/pronation Right/left rotation Horizontal abduction/adduction

Degrees of Freedom

Joints can also be described by the degrees of freedom, or number of planes, in which they can move. For example, a uniaxial joint has motion around one axis and in one plane. Therefore, it has one degree of freedom. A biaxial joint would have two degrees of freedom, and a triaxial joint would have three, the maximum number of degrees of freedom that an individual joint can have.

This concept becomes significant when dealing with one or more distal joints. For example, the shoulder has three degrees of freedom, the elbow and radioulnar joints each have one, and together they have five degrees of freedom. The entire limb from the finger to the shoulder would have 11 degrees of freedom.

Common Pathological Terms

Dislocation refers to the complete separation of the two articular surfaces of a joint. A portion of the joint capsule surrounding the joint will be torn. **Subluxation,** a partial dislocation of a joint, usually occurs over a period of time. A common example is a shoulder subluxation that develops after a person has had a stroke. Muscle paralysis and the weight of the arm slowly subluxes the shoulder joint.

Osteoarthritis is a type of arthritis that is caused by the breakdown and eventual loss of the cartilage of one or more joints. Also known as *degenerative arthritis,* it occurs more frequently as we age and commonly affects the hands, feet, spine, and large weight-bearing joints, such as the hips and knees.

Sprains are a partial or complete tearing of ligament fibers. A *mild* sprain involves the tearing of a few fibers with no loss of function. With a *moderate* sprain, there is partial tearing of the ligament with some loss of function. In a *severe* sprain, the ligament is completely torn (ruptured) and no longer functions. In contrast to a sprain, which affects a ligament, a **strain** refers to the overstretching of muscle fibers. As with sprains, strains are graded depending on severity.

Tendonitis is an inflammation of a tendon. **Synovitis** is an inflammation of the synovial membrane. **Tenosynovitis** is an inflammation of the tendon sheath and is often caused by repetitive use. The tendon of the long head of the biceps and the flexor tendons of the hand are common sites. **Bursitis** is an inflammation of the bursa. **Capsulitis** is an inflammation of the joint capsule. When a joint capsule is inflamed for an extended time, it begins to lose its extensibility, and loss of joint motion results. Each joint has a characteristic pattern of lost motion that presents when capsular tightness is present. This is referred to as the **capsular pattern** of motion restriction. There are many reasons why loss of motion may occur. When the capsular pattern is present, it aids the clinician in identifying the capsule as the *source* of the motion restriction and in directing appropriate treatment toward that structure. Some common capsular patterns are presented in Table 3-4.

Table 3-4 Common Capsular Patterns

Joint	Capsular Pattern
Shoulder	Severe loss of lateral rotation Moderate loss of abduction Slight loss of medial rotation
Wrist	Equal loss of flexion and extension
Knee	More loss of flexion than extension

Review Questions

1. What are the three types of joints that allow little or no motion?
2. What are the two terms for a joint that allows a great deal of motion?
3. What are the three features that describe diarthrodial joints?
4. What type of joint structure connects bone to muscle?
5. What type of joint structure pads and protects areas of great friction?
6. How does hyaline cartilage differ from fibrocartilage? Give an example of each type of cartilage.
7. When the anterior surface of the forearm moves toward the anterior surface of the humerus, what joint motion is involved? In what plane is the motion occurring? Around what axis?
8. What joint motions are involved in turning the palm of the hand down and up? In what plane and around what axis do these joint motions occur?
9. What joint motion is involved in returning the fingers to anatomical position from the fully spread position? In what plane and around what axis does the joint motion occur?
10. Identify the 11 degrees of freedom of the upper extremity.
11. Give an example of a synarthrodial joint in the axial skeleton.
12. *Diarthrodial, synovial, triaxial,* and *ball-and-socket* are all terms that could be used to describe which joint of the upper extremity? Could these same terms apply to a joint in the lower extremity? If so, what joint is it?
13. *Diarthrodial, synovial, biaxial,* and *saddle* are all terms that could be used to describe which joint?
14. What are two joint terms that could be used to describe the symphysis pubis?
15. What joint structure surrounds and encases the joint and protects the articular surfaces?

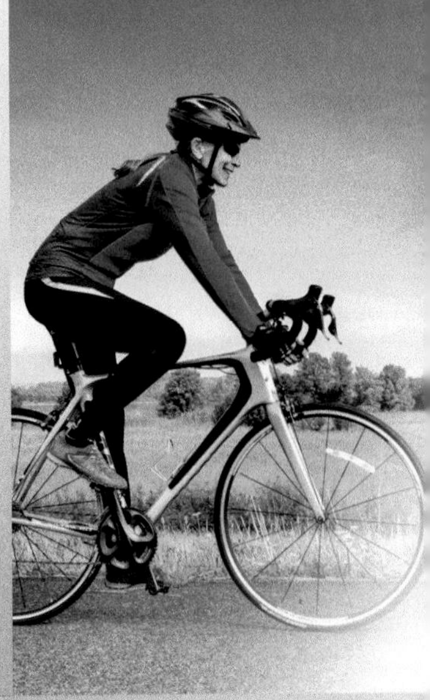

CHAPTER 4 Arthrokinematics

Osteokinematic Motion
End Feel
Arthrokinematic Motion
Accessory Motion Terminology
Joint Mobilization
Accessory Motion Forces
Joint Surface Shape
Types of Arthrokinematic Motion
Convex-Concave Rule
Joint Surface Positions (Joint Congruency)
Points to Remember
Review Questions

Kinesiology IN ACTION For additional practice activities and videos, please visit www.kinesiologyinaction.com

Osteokinematic Motion

Joint movement is commonly thought of as one bone moving on another, causing such motions as flexion, extension, abduction, adduction, or rotation. These movements, which are done under voluntary control, are often referred to as **classical, physiological,** or **osteokinematic motion** and were described in Chapter 1. Osteokinematic motion can occur actively or passively. Active range of motion (AROM) occurs when muscles contract to move joints through their ranges of motion (ROM). As we move our joints throughout the day, we are actively performing osteokinematic movements. Passive range of motion (PROM) occurs when a person's joint is moved passively through its range of motion. When a clinician moves a patient's joint passively through its range of motion, it is usually done to maintain or restore range of motion (e.g., stretching technique) or to determine the nature of the resistance the clinician feels at the end of the range. The latter is called the *end feel* of a joint.

End Feel

End feel is the type of the resistance that a clinician feels when bringing a patient's joint to the end of its passive range of motion, then applying a slight overpressure. It was first described by James Cyriax, who used this principle to identify what tissue was responsible for limiting further motion at the end range of a joint.

An end feel may be either normal or abnormal. A normal end feel exists when there is full PROM at a joint, and the motion is limited by the expected anatomical structure(s) for that particular joint (e.g., bone, capsule, muscle, and ligament). Abnormal end feel may be present when pain, muscle guarding, swelling, or abnormal anatomy stops the joint movement. When an abnormal end feel is noted, it can help to identify the "tissue at fault," or the tissue creating the dysfunction. This knowledge, in turn, helps clinicians to direct treatment toward the true anatomical source of the problem.

The three types of normal end feel are soft, firm, and hard. A **soft end feel** occurs when muscle bulk is compressed, and it is sometimes called *soft tissue approximation.* For example, elbow flexion is stopped by the approximation of the forearm and arm. This is particularly evident on a person with well-developed muscles or who is extremely obese. A **firm end feel** results from tension in the surrounding ligaments, capsule, and/or muscles and is perceived as a firm stop to the motion with only a "slight give" on overpressure. This is the most common end feel and is usually qualified by labeling the tissue type that limits the motion (e.g., firm muscular end feel, firm capsular end feel, firm ligamentous end feel). Examples would be shoulder medial and lateral rotation, hip and knee extension, and ankle dorsiflexion. A **hard end feel** is characterized by a hard and abrupt limit to passive joint motion with no give on overpressure. This occurs when bone contacts bone at the end of the ROM, and sometimes it is called a *bony end feel.* An example would be end range elbow extension as the bony olecranon process contacts the bony olecranon fossa.

Any of the normal end feels can be considered abnormal if they occur at the wrong joint or if they occur at the wrong point in the range. A firm capsular end feel is normal for shoulder lateral rotation. Soft tissue approximation is the normal end feel for elbow flexion. Therefore, a firm capsular end feel for elbow flexion is considered abnormal. A firm capsular end feel for elbow flexion may be due to capsular shortening after wearing a long arm cast. A hard end feel can result from abnormal bony structures (e.g., osteophyte) limiting joint motion.

Some end feels are always considered abnormal and may be present when pain, muscle guarding, swelling, or abnormal anatomy stops the joint movement. Abnormal end feels can be described as boggy, muscle spasm, empty, and springy block. These terms can be used to explain the source of the limitation of joint motion. **Boggy end feel** is often found in acute conditions in which soft tissue edema is present, such as immediately after a severely sprained ankle or with synovitis. It has a soft, "wet sponge" feel. **Muscle spasm** is a reflexive muscle guarding during motion. It is a protective response seen with acute injury. Palpation of the muscle will reveal the muscle in spasm. The clinician's ability to palpate normal end feel and to distinguish changes from normal end feel is important in protecting joints during ROM exercises. **Empty end feel** occurs when movement produces considerable pain and the patient stops the clinician from moving the joint beyond the painful point. Because the clinician does not bring the joint to the end of its physiologic range of motion, there is no way to tell if a limitation may exist past the point of pain, or to determine the tissue type that would have been the cause of any potential limitation. With **springy block,** a rebound movement is felt at the end of the ROM. It usually occurs with internal derangement of a joint, such as torn cartilage.

Arthrokinematic Motion

Another way of viewing joint movement is to look at what is taking place within the joint at the joint surfaces. Called **arthrokinematic motion,** it is defined as the manner in which adjoining joint surfaces move on each other during osteokinematic joint movement. Therefore, osteokinematic motion is referred to as *joint motion,* and arthrokinematic motion is referred to as *joint surface motion.*

Accessory Motion Terminology

Terminology can be somewhat confusing because various experts use words somewhat differently. That said, there are two types of accessory arthrokinematic motions that must be described: those that occur during active motion and those that occur during passive motion. Neither is under voluntary control, but both are necessary for normal functional motion to occur. **Component movements** are the small arthrokinematic joint motions that accompany active osteokinematic motion. For example, the head of the humerus must glide inferiorly in order for the shoulder to perform full flexion. The medial tibial condyle glides anteriorly on the medial femoral condyle during the last few degrees of knee extension. The joint surface of the first metacarpal glides posteriorly on the trapezium during thumb abduction. None of these component motions can be done independently; they must accompany osteokinematic motions for normal joint motion to occur. **Joint play** is the arthrokinematic movement that happens between joint surfaces when an external force creates passive motion at the joint. Regardless of whether the accessory motion occurs actively (component motion) or passively (joint play), the arthrokinematic motions that result can be described using the terms *roll, glide,* and *spin,* which will be defined later.

Joint Mobilization

If an accessory motion is limited, reduced joint motion usually results. **Joint mobilization** is a technique that applies an external force to a patient's joint to generate a passive oscillatory motion or sustained stretch between the joint surfaces. Joint mobilization can be used to restore joint mobility or decrease pain originating from joint structures. When used to restore ROM, the force is most commonly applied by generating passive arthrokinematic movement into the direction of restriction. A joint that presents with a capsular pattern of motion restriction (see Chapter 3) is one that will commonly present with reduced joint play and will be treated with joint mobilization to stretch the joint capsule. Another technique for restoring joint mobility is a high-velocity, low-amplitude (HVLA) thrust **manipulation.** This technique involves moving the joint with high speed through a very slight and calculated range that is just past where the joint play ends. Both techniques are beyond the scope of this book.

Accessory Motion Forces

When performing joint mobilization, three main types of force are used to create movement between the joint surfaces: traction, compression, and shearing. **Traction forces** cause *joint distraction* in which the joint surfaces pull apart from one another (Fig. 4-1). Carrying a heavy suitcase or hanging from an overhead bar causes distraction at the shoulder, elbow, and wrist joints. You can demonstrate this on another person by grasping their index finger at the proximal end of the middle phalanx with one thumb and index finger. Next, grasp the distal end of the proximal phalanx with your other thumb and index finger. Move the proximal interphalangeal (PIP) joint into a slightly flexed position (loose-packed position), and pull gently in opposite directions. This description, and others to follow, is meant to illustrate the various forces and is not a description of therapeutic technique. *Care must be exercised when performing these motions.*

Compression forces cause *joint approximation* in which the joint surfaces are pushed closer together (Fig. 4-2). Doing a chair or floor push-up causes the joint surfaces of the shoulder, elbow, and wrist joints to be approximated.

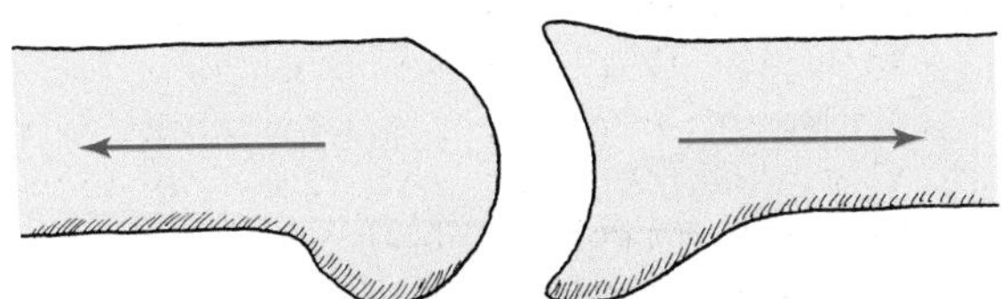

Figure 4-1. Traction force causes joint distraction in which joint surfaces move apart from each other.

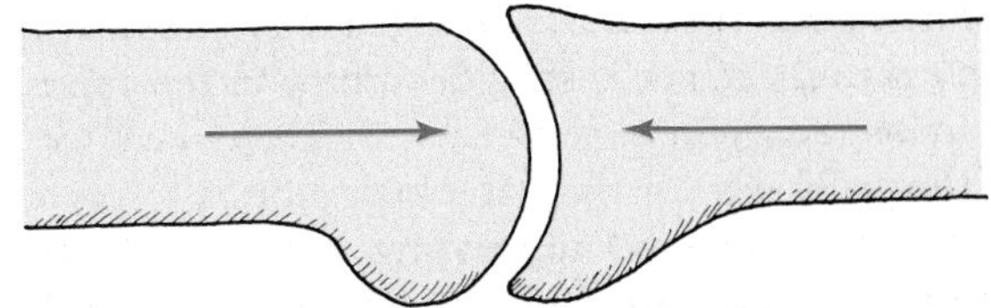

Figure 4-2. Compression force causes joint approximation in which joint surfaces move toward each other.

Shearing forces cause a *gliding motion* in which the joint surfaces move parallel to one another (Fig. 4-3). Using the positions described with distraction, grasp another person's index finger at the proximal end of the middle phalanx with one thumb and index finger. Next, grasp the distal end of the proximal phalanx with your other thumb and index finger. With the PIP joint slightly flexed, gently move your two hands in an opposite up-and-down motion. This motion describes anterior-posterior glide of the PIP joint (a shearing force).

Bending and torsional forces are actually a combination of forces. **Bending** occurs when an other-than-vertical force is applied, resulting in compression on the concave side and distraction on the convex side (Fig. 4-4). Rotary or torsional forces involve a twisting motion. One force is

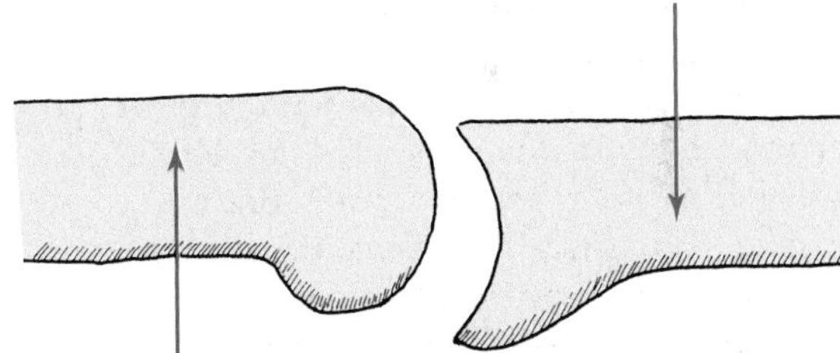

Figure 4-3. Shear force causes a glide between the joint surfaces in which bone ends move parallel to, and in opposite directions from, each other.

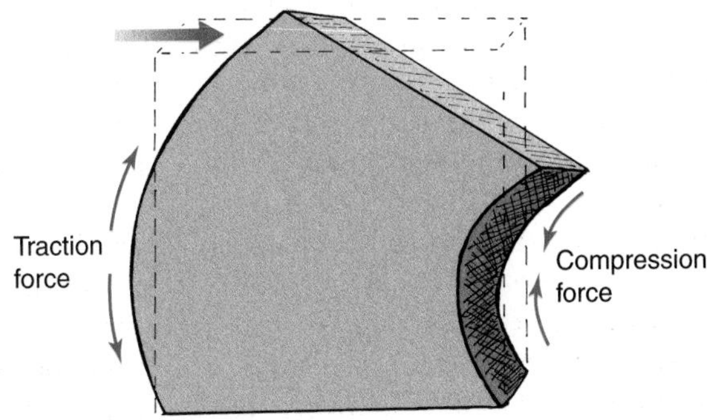

Figure 4-4. Bending force causes compression on one side and traction on the other side.

trying to turn one end or part about a longitudinal axis while the other force is fixed or turning in the opposite direction (Fig. 4-5).

Clinically, why are these accessory motion forces relevant? Distraction, gliding, bending, and torsional forces are often used to assist in restoring a joint's mobility, whereas approximation can assist in promoting joint stability.

Joint Surface Shape

To understand arthrokinematics, one must recognize that the type of motion occurring at a joint depends on the shape of the articulating surfaces of the bones. Most joints have one concave bone end and one convex bone end (Fig. 4-6). A convex surface is rounded outward, much like a mound. A concave surface is "caved" in, much like a cave.

All joint surfaces are either ovoid or sellar. An **ovoid joint** has two bones forming a convex-concave relationship. For example, in the metacarpophalangeal joint, one surface is concave (proximal phalanx) and the other is convex (see Fig. 4-6). Most synovial joints are ovoid. In an ovoid joint, one bone end is usually larger than its adjacent bone end. This permits a greater ROM on a lesser articular surface, which reduces the size of the joint.

In a **sellar,** or **saddle-shaped, joint,** each joint surface is concave in one direction and convex in another. The carpometacarpal (CMC) joint of the thumb is perhaps the best example of a sellar joint (Fig. 4-7). If you look at the carpal bone (trapezium), it is concave in an anterior-posterior direction and convex in a medial-lateral direction. The first metacarpal bone that articulates with this carpal bone has just the opposite shape. It is convex in an anterior-posterior direction and concave in a medial-lateral direction. Figure 13-2 compares the shape of this joint with the shape of two Pringles® potato chips stacked one atop the other.

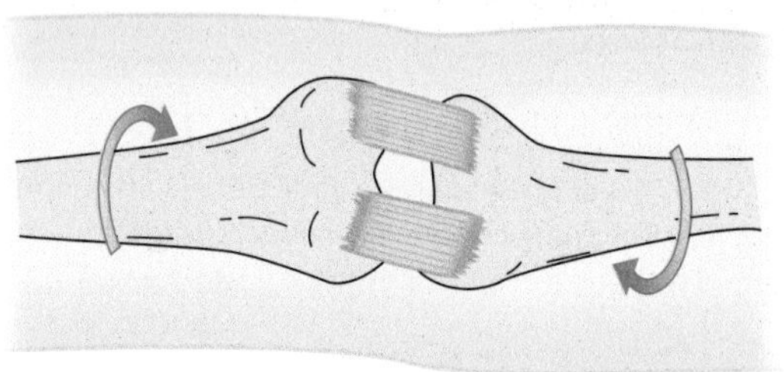

Figure 4-5. Rotary or torsional force is a twisting motion.

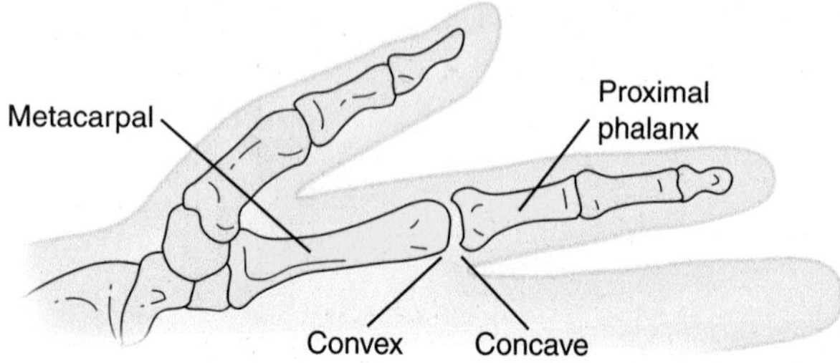

Figure 4-6. Shape of bone surfaces of an ovoid joint—MCP joint of finger.

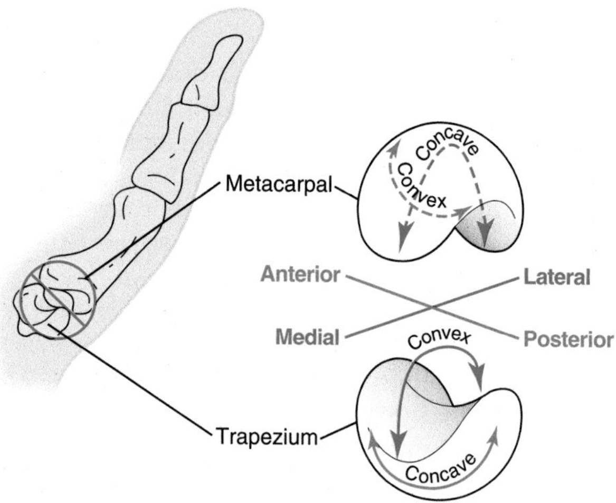

Figure 4-7. Shape of bone surfaces of a sellar joint—CMP joint of thumb.

Types of Arthrokinematic Motion

The types of arthrokinematic motion are roll, glide, and spin. Most joint movement involves a combination of all three of these motions. **Roll** is the rolling of one joint surface on another. New points on each surface come into contact throughout the motion (Fig. 4-8). Examples include the surface of your shoe on the floor during walking, or a ball rolling across the ground. **Glide,** or slide, is linear movement of a joint surface parallel to the plane of the adjoining joint surface (Fig. 4-9). In other words, one point on a joint surface contacts

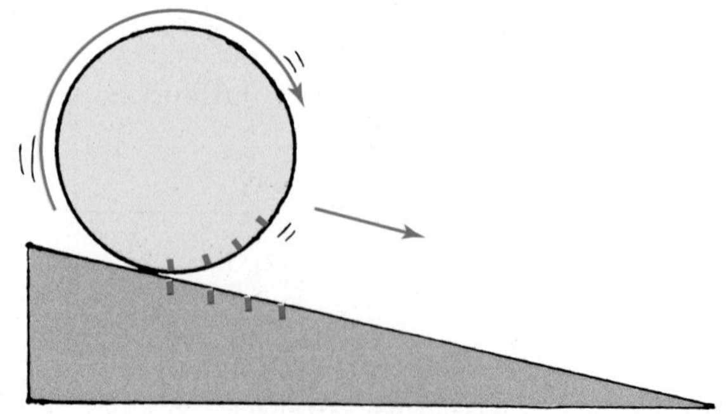

Figure 4-8. Roll—movement of one joint surface on another. New points on each surface make contact.

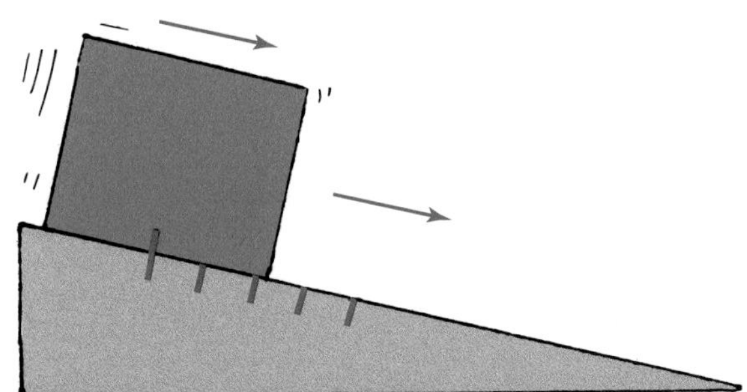

Figure 4-9. Glide—linear movement of one joint surface parallel to the other joint surface. One point on one surface contacts new points on other surface.

new points on the adjacent surface. An ice-skater's blade (one point) gliding across the ice surface (many points) demonstrates the glide motion. **Spin** is the rotation of the movable joint surface on the fixed adjacent surface (Fig. 4-10). Essentially the same point on each surface remains in contact with each other. An example of this type of movement would be a top spinning on a table. If the top remains perfectly upright, it spins in one place. Examples in the body would be any pure (relatively speaking) rotational movement, such as the humerus rotating in the glenoid fossa during shoulder medial and lateral rotation, or the head of the radius spinning on the capitulum of the humerus during forearm pronation and supination.

Analyzing the direction in which a joint surface glides during functional movement of the body is important because a glide is often the arthrokinematic motion that is passively introduced by the clinician during a joint mobilization technique. Be aware, however, that during normal joint motion, gliding is usually accompanied by rolling. Although rolling is needed to utilize all available articular surfaces, and thus to produce full range of motion at a given joint, it is the concurrent gliding that prevents one joint surface from rolling off the edge of the other before the joint motion was complete. The knee joint is a good example of how roll and glide work together to keep the joint surfaces aligned (Fig. 4-11). When an individual stands up from a chair, the convex femoral condyles begin to roll anteriorly on the concave tibial condyles. However, the tibial condyles possess far less articular surface than the femoral condyles, and because of the large range of flexion and extension permitted at the knee, the femur would roll off the tibia if the femoral condyles did not also glide posteriorly on the tibia. There is also an important spin component that is necessary during the last portion of knee extension. The nature and direction of this spin will be discussed further in Chapter 19.

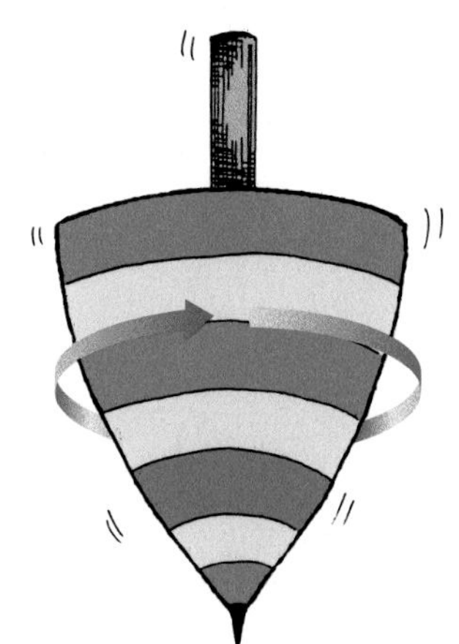

Figure 4-10. Spin—rotation of one joint surface on another. Same point on each surface remains in contact.

Convex-Concave Rule

Knowing whether the shape of a joint surface is concave or convex is important because shape determines motion. The **concave-convex rule** describes how the differences in shapes of bone ends require joint surfaces to move in a specific way during joint movement. The rule expresses the relationship between the osteokinematics and arthrokinematics for a given movement. To properly analyze the link between these two types of movement, one must observe the motion occurring at two locations: the joint surface of the moving bone (arthrokinematics) and the distal/opposite end of the moving bone (osteokinematics).

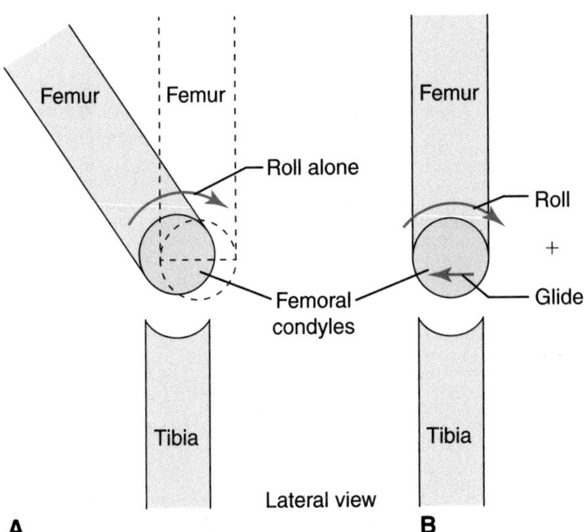

Figure 4-11. Roll and glide of femoral condyles on tibial condyles at knee joint.

The rule is described as follows: A concave joint surface will glide on a fixed convex surface in the same direction as the distal end of the moving bone. For example, the distal portion of the metacarpal is convex, and the proximal portion of the proximal phalanx is concave (Fig. 4-12). During finger extension (from finger flexion), the concave articular surface of the proximal phalanx moves in the same direction as the distal end of the proximal phalanx while moving on the fixed convex metacarpal. In this case, the joint surface of the proximal phalanx is gliding posteriorly (arthrokinematics) while the proximal phalanx is also extending posteriorly through the sagittal plane (osteokinematics). To summarize, the **concave joint surface** glides in the **same direction** as the distal end of the same bony segment.

Conversely, a convex joint surface will glide on a fixed concave surface in the opposite direction as the distal end of the moving bone. For example, the glenoid fossa of the scapula is concave, and the head of the humerus (with which it articulates) is convex (Fig. 4-13). During shoulder abduction, the convex surface of the humeral head moves inferiorly, or in the opposite direction from, the distal end of the humerus, which is moving superiorly. Thus, the **convex joint surface** glides in the **opposite direction** as compared with the distal end of the same bony segment.

There is an easy visual way to remember this rule. To represent a joint, make a fist with your left hand and place it inside your cupped right hand. Your left fist represents a convex joint surface of one bone. The left forearm represents the bone. Your cupped right hand represents a concave surface of the other bone. Keeping your hands at the same level, your wrist straight, and your left fist rotating inside the cupped hand, raise your left elbow. Note that as your forearm (body segment) moves up, your fist (joint surface) glides down. In other words, the convex surface glides in the opposite direction as the distal (opposite) end of the same bony segment. Repeat the action with the cupped hand moving on the fist. Raise your right elbow and note that your cupped right hand is gliding up and over the left fist. The concave surface (cupped hand) glides in the same direction as the distal (opposite) end of the same bony segment (right forearm).

A conceptual motion analysis uses the convex-concave rule to provide a comparison of whether joint surface motions are happening in the "same" or the "opposite" direction as compared with the distal end of the bony segment. Table 4-1 identifies the steps for such an analysis.

Although a conceptual motion analysis is theoretical in nature, it is a stepping stone to performing a real clinical motion analysis that pairs *actual* osteokinematic and arthrokinematic motions together. Note that arthrokinematic motions are expressed by naming the actual direction in which the joint surface is gliding. Table 4-2 gives a step-by-step guide to performing a clinical motion analysis.

Joint Surface Positions (Joint Congruency)

How well joint surfaces match or fit is called *joint congruency*. The surfaces of a joint are congruent in one position and incongruent in all other positions. When a joint is **congruent,** the joint surfaces have maximum contact with each other, are tightly compressed, and are difficult to distract (separate). The ligaments and capsule holding the joint together are taut. This is known as the **close-packed,**

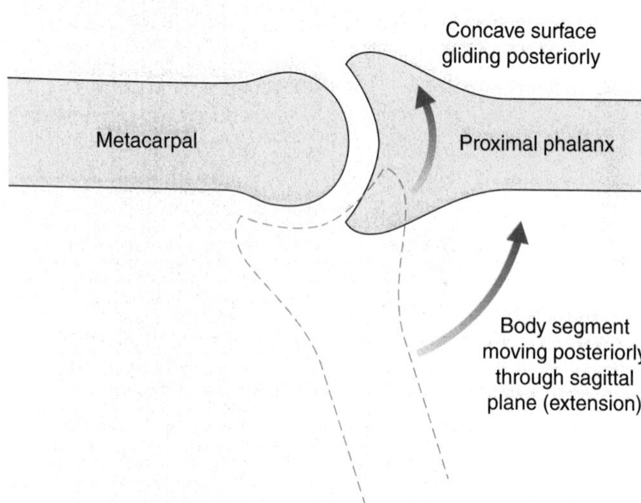

Figure 4-12. The concave surface glides in the same direction as the distal end of the moving bone. In this example, both types of motions are occurring posteriorly.

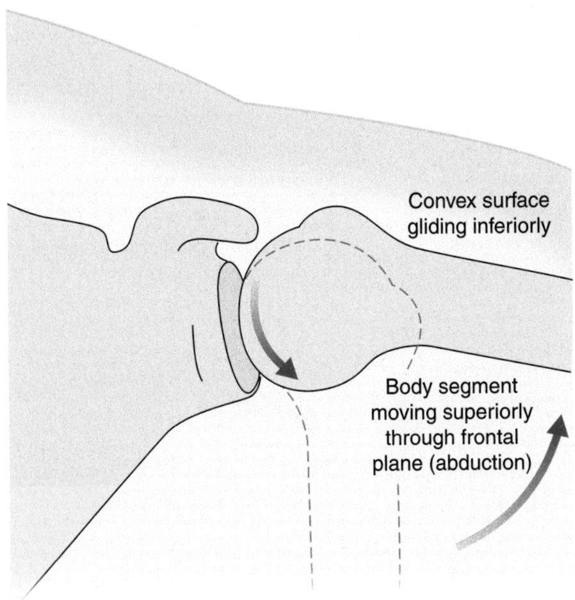

Figure 4-13. The convex surface glides in the opposite direction from the distal end of the moving bone.

or **closed-pack, position.** It usually occurs at one extreme of the ROM. For example, if you place your knee in the fully extended position, you can manually move the patella slightly from side to side and up and down. However, if you flex your knee, such patellar movement is *not* possible. Therefore, the close-packed position of the patellofemoral joint is knee flexion. Other close-packed positions are ankle dorsiflexion; metacarpophalangeal flexion; and extension of the elbow, wrist, hip, knee, and interphalangeal joints. Table 4-3 gives a more detailed listing of the close-packed positions of joints.

When ligaments and capsular structures are tested for stability and integrity, the joint is usually placed in the close-packed position. By the nature of the characteristics of a close-packed position, a joint is often in this position when injured. For example, a knee joint that sustains a lateral force when it is extended (close-packed position) is much more likely to be injured than when it is in a flexed or semiflexed position (loose-packed position). Also, when a joint is swollen, it cannot be moved into the close-packed position.

In all other positions, the joint surfaces are incongruent. The position of maximum incongruence is called the **open-packed** or **loose-packed position.** It is also referred to as the **resting position.** Parts of the capsule and supporting ligaments are lax. There is minimal congruency between the articular surfaces. Further passive separation of the joint surfaces can occur in this position. Because the ligaments and capsular structures tend to be more relaxed, joint mobilization techniques are best applied in the open-packed position. It is these open-packed positions that allow for the roll, spin, and glide

Table 4-1 Steps to Perform a Conceptual Motion Analysis

STEPS	1. Name the joint surfaces and identify which is convex and which is concave.	2. Identify the more movable bony segment (usually the more distal one).	3. Identify if the motion is convex-on-concave or concave-on-convex.	4. Determine if the more movable joint surface will glide in the same or opposite direction as the rest of that bone.
Example #1: Glenohumeral joint	• Glenoid fossa (concave) • Head of the humerus (convex)	Head of the humerus is more movable	Convex head of the humerus is *moving on* concave glenoid fossa (convex-on-concave)	Head of humerus glides in *opposite* direction from distal end of humerus
Example #2: MCP joint	• Metacarpal (convex) • Proximal phalanx (concave)	Proximal phalanx is more movable	Concave proximal phalanx is *moving on* convex metacarpal (concave-on-convex)	Proximal phalanx glides in *same* direction as distal end of proximal phalanx

Table 4-2 Steps to Perform a Clinical Motion Analysis

STEPS	1. Select an osteokinematic motion through which the joint is able to move. (These steps can all be repeated for any osteokinematic motions that the joint can perform.)	2. Identify the actual direction in which *the bone* moves when that osteokinematic motion occurs.	3. Identify the arthrokinematic motion that occurs by describing the actual direction in which the *joint surface* is gliding (e.g., anterior, posterior, lateral or medial glide).
Example #1: Glenohumeral joint	Shoulder abduction	Superior movement of humerus	Inferior glide of head of humerus
Example #2: MCP joint	MCP flexion	Anterior movement of proximal phalanx	Anterior glide of proximal end of proximal phalanx

Table 4-3 Comparison of Close-Packed and Loose-Packed Position of Joints

Joint(s)	Close-Packed Position	Loose-Packed Position
Facet (spine)	Extension	Midway between flexion and extension
Temporomandibular	Clenched teeth	Mouth slightly open (freeway space)
Glenohumeral	Abduction and lateral rotation	55 degrees abduction, 30 degrees horizontal adduction
Acromioclavicular	Arm abducted to 30 degrees	Arm resting by side in anatomical position
Ulnohumeral (elbow)	Extension	70 degrees flexion, 10 degrees supination
Radiohumeral	Elbow flexed 90 degrees, forearm supinated 5 degrees	Full extension and supination
Proximal radioulnar	5 degrees supination	70 degrees flexion, 35 degrees supination
Radiocarpal (wrist)	Extension with ulnar deviation	Neutral with slight ulnar deviation
Carpometacarpal	N/A	Midway between abduction/adduction and flexion/extension
Metacarpophalangeal (fingers)	Full flexion	Slight flexion
Metacarpophalangeal (thumb)	Full opposition	Slight flexion
Interphalangeal	Full extension	Slight flexion
Hip	Full extension and medial rotation*	30 degrees flexion, 30 degrees abduction, and slight lateral rotation
Knee	Full extension and lateral rotation of tibia	25 degrees flexion
Talocrural (ankle)	Maximum dorsiflexion	10 degrees plantar flexion, midway between maximum inversion and eversion
Metatarsophalangeal	Full extension	Neutral
Interphalangeal	Full extension	Slight flexion

*Some authors include abduction.

Adapted from Magee, DJ: *Orthopedic Physical Assessment,* ed 4. WB Saunders, Philadelphia, 2002, p 50, with permission.

that are necessary for normal joint motion. Table 4-3 gives a more detailed listing of the loose-packed positions of joints and compares these positions with those of the close-packed positions.

A certain amount of **joint play** can be demonstrated in these open-packed positions. Joint play is the passive movement of one articular surface over another. Because joint play is not a voluntary movement, it requires relaxed muscles and the external force of a trained practitioner to correctly demonstrate it.

Points to Remember

- Normal end feel can be described as soft, firm, or hard.
- Abnormal end feel can be described as bony, boggy, empty, springy block, or muscle spasm.
- Joint surface shape can be ovoid or sellar.
- Types of arthrokinematic motion are roll, glide, and spin.
- According to the concave-convex rule, concave joint surfaces glide in the same direction as the distal end of the same bony segment, whereas convex surfaces glide in the opposite direction from the distal end of the same bony segment.
- When a joint is congruent, it is in the close-packed position. When the joint is incongruent, it is in the open-packed position.
- When mobilizing a joint, distraction, gliding, bending, or torsional forces may be used.
- Joint approximation may be used to promote joint stability.

Review Questions

1. a. Is shoulder flexion and extension an arthrokinematic or osteokinematic type of motion?
   b. Is shoulder distraction an arthrokinematic or osteokinematic type of motion?
2. You would feel what type of end feel at the end of the knee flexion range?
3. Starting in anatomical position, move the shoulder into flexion.
   a. Is the humerus moving on the scapula, or is the scapula moving on the humerus?
   b. Is the proximal end of the humerus a concave or convex joint surface?
   c. Does the glenoid fossa of the scapula have a concave or convex joint surface?
   d. Is the concave surface gliding on a fixed convex surface, or is a convex surface gliding on a fixed concave surface?
   e. Is the joint surface gliding in the same or opposite direction as the distal end of the moving bone?
4. Identify the accessory motion force(s) occurring in the following activities:
   a. At the shoulder when leaning on a table with your elbows extended
   b. At the knee when a football player is hit on the front of the shin
   c. At the elbow when picking up one end of a table
   d. At the wrist when opening a jar
   e. To the shoulders of a child when they are being swung around by their arms
5. Is the temporomandibular joint (TMJ) (jaw) in the close-packed position when the teeth are clenched or when the mouth is slightly open?
6. In terms of joint congruency, describe how a stack of Pringles potato chips fits together (see Fig. 13-2). Place a stack of two chips in front of you with the long end pointing toward you in an anterior-posterior position. Consider the joint surfaces of each chip in contact with the other:
   a. Is the anterior-posterior shape of the bottom surface of the top chip concave or convex?
   b. Is the anterior-posterior shape of the top surface of the bottom chip concave or convex?
   c. Is the medial-lateral shape of the bottom surface of the top chip concave or convex?
   d. Is the medial-lateral shape of the top surface of the bottom chip concave or convex?
   e. If these chips represented a joint, would the shape of the joint be ovoid or sellar?

(continued on next page)

Review Questions—cont'd

7. You stand a quarter on its edge and give it a small push so that it travels slowly across to the other side of the table. What type of arthrokinematic motion does this represent?
8. Lay the quarter flat on the table and hit it with your finger, sending it across the table. This would be representative of what type of arthrokinematic motion?
9. In comparing the size of a quarter and a nickel, note that the quarter is larger. Place a pencil mark on the quarter at the 6 and 12 o'clock positions. Lay a nickel flat on the table. Roll the quarter across the flat surface of the nickel, starting with the quarter at the 6 o'clock position at the edge of the nickel.
   a. Will the quarter reach the edge of the nickel before reaching the 12 o'clock position?
   b. Which arthrokinematic motion will you have to use on the quarter, in addition to roll, so that the 12 o'clock mark can reach the opposite side of the nickel?
10. Hold a pencil vertically with the lead end on the table. Holding the eraser end between your thumb and index finger, roll the pencil between your fingers, keeping the lead end in contact with the table. This is representative of which type of arthrokinematic motion?
11. Assuming muscles are of normal length and bringing a person's ankle into dorsiflexion, you would expect what type of end feel?
12. A person bends down to touch the floor in the sagittal plane.
    a. What type of force is applied to the anterior part of the vertebra?
    b. What type of force is applied to the posterior part of the vertebra?
13. Sitting in a chair, a man turns around to look behind him. What type of force is being applied to the vertebral column?
14. The surfaces of the thumb metacarpophalangeal (MCP) joint are what shape?
15. When the joint surface of the first metacarpal glides posteriorly on the trapezium during thumb abduction, is this considered an osteokinematic movement or an arthrokinematic movement? Why?
16. Using the steps described in Table 4-1, analyze the motion at the elbow joint:
    a. Name the joint surfaces and identify whether each surface is concave or convex. (Do not worry about actual landmark names; use "proximal" and "distal" end.)
    b. Identify the more movable bony segment.
    c. Is the motion concave-on-convex or convex-on-concave?
    d. Will the more movable bony segment glide in the same or opposite direction as the rest of the bone?
17. For the following two steps, select elbow flexion as the motion to analyze:
    a. Identify the direction in which the bone moves during elbow flexion.
    b. Identify the arthrokinematic motion that occurs by describing the direction in which the joint surface is gliding.

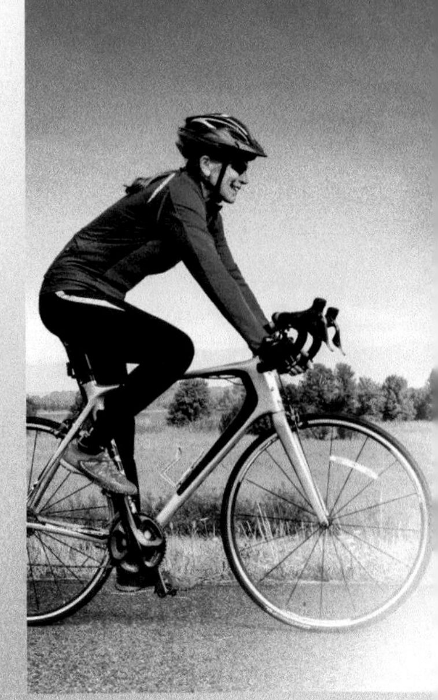

CHAPTER 5 Muscular System

Muscle Attachments

Muscle Names

Muscle Fiber Arrangement

Functional Characteristics of Muscle Tissue

Sliding Filament Theory

Length-Tension Relationship in Muscle Tissue

Optimal Length

Active and Passive Insufficiency

Adaptive Shortening & Lengthening of Muscle Tissue

Stretching

Tendon Action of a Muscle (Tenodesis)

Types of Muscle Contraction

Roles of Muscles

Line of Pull

Kinetic Chains

Common Muscle Pathologies

Points to Remember

Review Questions

Muscle Attachments

A muscle is a bundle of elastic tissue that has the ability to contract, producing movement or maintaining the position of a body part. As was described in Chapter 3, muscles are connected to bone via tendon. The **tendon** is fibrous connective tissue that connects muscle to bone, unlike a ligament (also fibrous connective tissue), which connects bone to bone. Often when discussing musculoskeletal pathology, the point where the muscle meets tendon is referred to as the **musculotendinous junction,** and the point where tendon meets bone is called the **tenoperiosteal junction** (Fig. 5-1).

When a muscle contracts, it knows no direction—it simply shortens. If a muscle is unattached at both ends and stimulated, the two ends would move toward the middle. However, muscles are attached to bones and cross at least one joint, so when a muscle contracts, one end of the joint moves toward the other. The more movable bone, often referred to as the **insertion,** moves toward the more stable bone, called the **origin.** For example, when the biceps brachii muscle contracts, the forearm moves toward the humerus, as when bringing a glass toward your mouth (Fig. 5-2A). The humerus is more stable because it is attached to the axial skeleton at the shoulder joint. The forearm is more movable because it is attached to the hand, which is free to move through space. Therefore, the insertion is moving toward the origin; explained another way, the more movable end is traveling toward the more stable end. Another point that can be made about muscle attachments on the appendicular skeleton is that origins tend to be closer to the trunk, and insertions tend to be closer to the distal end of the extremity.

The direction of movement can be reversed if the more movable end is stabilized by some external force or by another muscle contraction. For example, what happens when the hand is holding on to a pull-up bar when the biceps contracts? The biceps muscle still flexes the elbow,

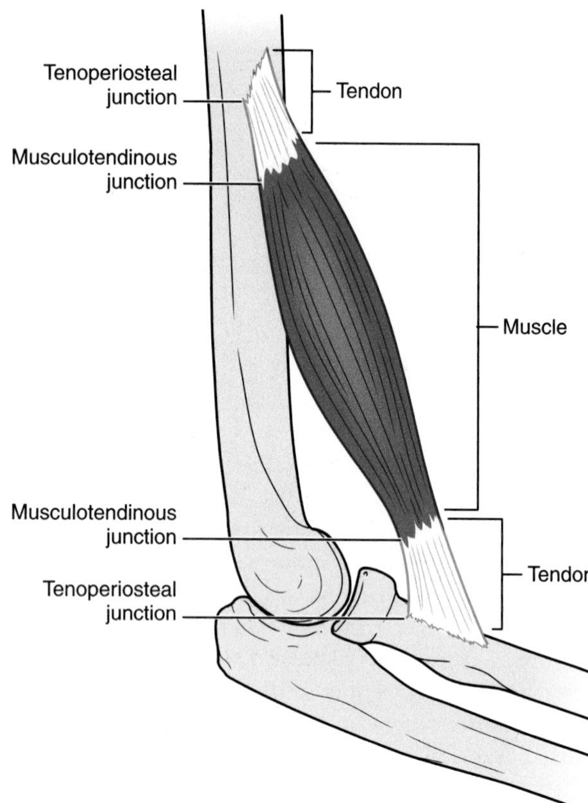

Figure 5-1. Muscle-tendon unit.

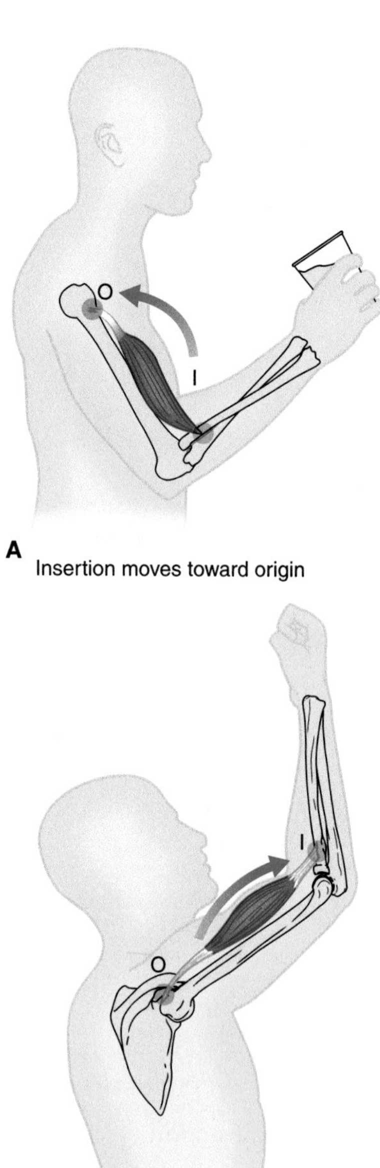

Figure 5-2. **(A)** Direction of movement of biceps muscle attachments when bringing a glass toward your mouth. **(B)** Direction of movement of biceps muscle attachments when the body moves up toward the pull-up bar in a reverse muscle action.

but now the humerus moves toward the forearm. In other words, the proximal bone (humerus), which is usually more stable, has become more movable compared with the distal bone (forearm), which is stabilized by the bar. So instead of the insertion moving toward the origin, the origin is now moving toward the insertion (Fig. 5-2B). This is referred to as **reverse muscle action.**

In the previous example, the direction of movement was reversed, but the joint motion (elbow flexion) remained the same. In some cases of reverse muscle action, a different joint motion can result. For example, the upper trapezius, which typically elevates the shoulder girdle, can, in a reverse muscle action, laterally bend the neck. The upper trapezius originates on the occiput and cervical vertebrae and inserts on the lateral clavicle and scapula. Typically the insertion (scapula and clavicle) moves toward the origin (occiput and cervical vertebrae) (Fig. 5-3A). However, if the scapula is stabilized by other muscles and can't move, the insertion is more stable, and the origin is more movable (Fig. 5-3B). Consequently, the upper trapezius laterally bends the neck in a reverse muscle action. The stabilization function mentioned above will be further described.

Muscle Names

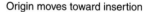

The name of a muscle can often tell you a great deal about that muscle such as location, shape, action, number of heads/divisions, attachment points, fiber orientation, and size.

The tibialis anterior, as its name indicates, is located on the anterior surface of the tibia. The rectus (meaning "straight" in Latin) abdominis muscle is a vertical muscle

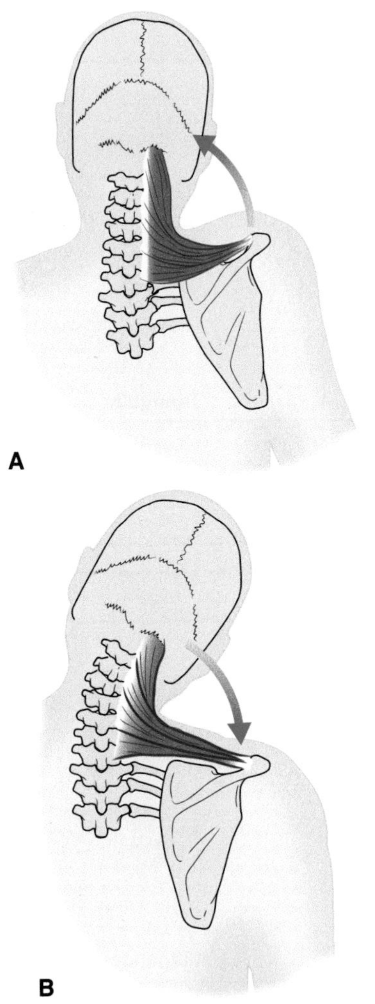

Figure 5-3. Upper trapezius; **(A)** muscle action (moving insertion toward origin, resulting in scapular elevation); **(B)** reverse muscle action (moving origin toward insertion, resulting in head and neck lateral bending).

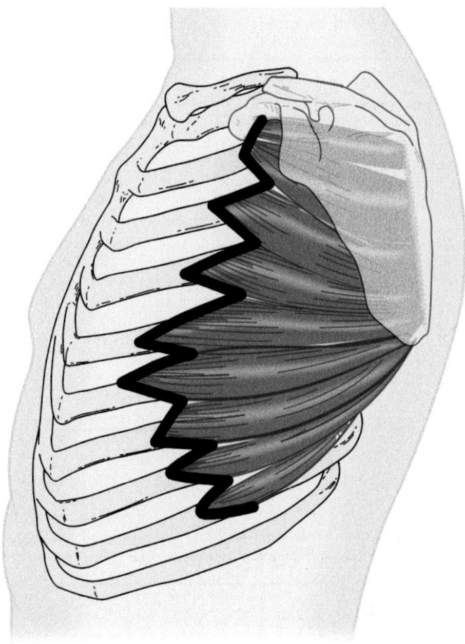

Figure 5-4. The serratus anterior muscle has a saw-toothed shape.

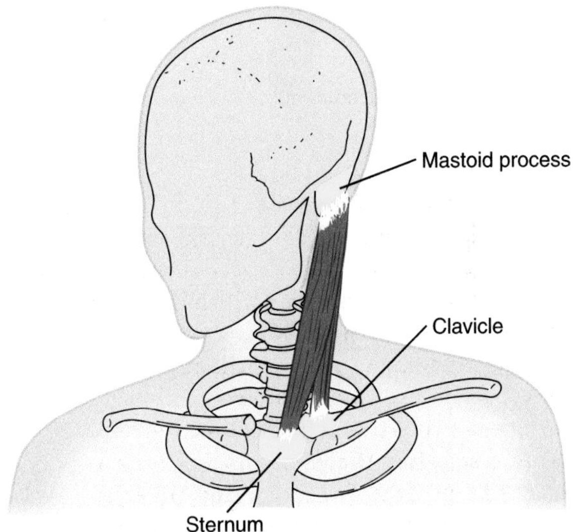

Figure 5-5. The sternocleidomastoid muscle is named for its attachments on the sternum, clavicle, and mastoid bone.

located on the abdomen. The trapezius muscle has a trapezoid shape, and the serratus anterior muscle (Fig. 5-4) has a serrated or jagged-shaped attachment anteriorly. The name of the extensor carpi ulnaris muscle tells you that its action is to extend the wrist (carpi) and that it attaches on the ulnar side. The triceps brachii muscle is a three-headed muscle on the arm (brachium), and the biceps femoris muscle is a two-headed muscle that attaches to the femur. The sternocleidomastoid muscle (Fig. 5-5) attaches on the sternum, clavicle, and mastoid bones. The names of the external and internal oblique muscles describe the diagonal direction of the fibers, and their relative depth to one another. In the same way, the names *pectoralis major* and *pectoralis minor* indicate that although both of these muscles are in the chest (pectoral) area, one is larger than the other.

Muscle Fiber Arrangement

Muscle fibers are arranged within the muscle in a direction that is either parallel or oblique to the muscle's long axis (Fig. 5-6). **Parallel muscle** fibers tend to be longer and thus have a greater potential for shortening and producing more range of motion. **Oblique muscle** fibers tend to be shorter but are more numerous per given area than parallel fibers, which means they tend

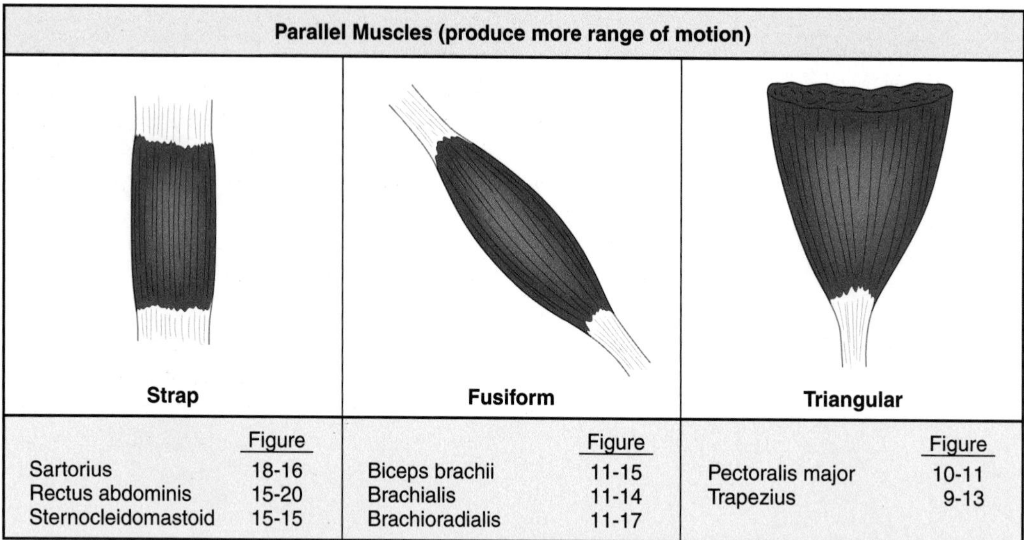

Parallel Muscles (produce more range of motion)
Strap
Fusiform
Triangular
Figure
Sartorius 18-16
Rectus abdominis 15-20
Sternocleidomastoid 15-15
Figure
Biceps brachii 11-15
Brachialis 11-14
Brachioradialis 11-17
Figure
Pectoralis major 10-11
Trapezius 9-13

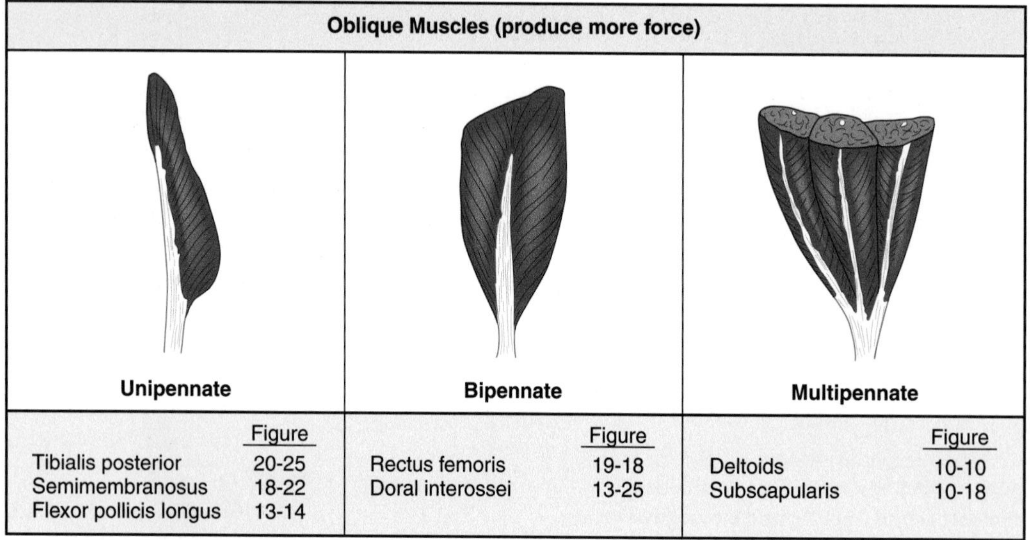

Oblique Muscles (produce more force)
Unipennate
Bipennate
Multipennate
Figure
Tibialis posterior 20-25
Semimembranosus 18-22
Flexor pollicis longus 13-14
Figure
Rectus femoris 19-18
Doral interossei 13-25
Figure
Deltoids 10-10
Subscapularis 10-18

Figure 5-6. Muscle fiber arrangements, parallel and oblique.

to have a greater strength potential but a smaller range-of-motion potential than parallel-fibered muscles. There are many types of each muscle fiber arrangement in the body.

Parallel-fibered muscles can be strap, fusiform, rhomboidal (rectangular), or triangular in shape. **Strap muscles** are those that are long and thin with fibers running the entire length of the muscle. A **fusiform muscle** has a shape similar to that of a spindle. It is wider in the middle and tapers at both ends where it attaches to tendons. Most, but not all, fibers run the length of the muscle. The muscle may be any length or size, from long to short or large to small. A **rhomboidal muscle** is four-sided, usually flat, with broad attachments at each end. **Triangular muscles** are flat and fan-shaped, with fibers radiating from a narrow attachment at one end to a broad attachment at the other (see Fig. 5-6).

Oblique-fibered muscles have a feather arrangement in which a muscle attaches at an oblique angle to its tendon, much like feather tendrils attach to the quill. The different types of oblique-fibered muscles are unipennate, bipennate, and multipennate. **Unipennate muscles** look like one side of a feather. There are a series of short fibers attaching diagonally along the length of a central tendon. The **bipennate muscle** pattern looks like that of a common feather. Its fibers are obliquely attached to both sides of a central tendon. **Multipennate muscles** have many tendons with oblique fibers in between (Fig. 5-6).

Functional Characteristics of Muscle Tissue

Muscle tissue has the properties of irritability, contractility, extensibility, and elasticity. No other tissue in the body has all of these characteristics. To better understand these properties, it helps to know that muscles have a **normal resting length.** This is defined as the length of a muscle when it is not shortened or lengthened—that is, when there are no forces or stresses placed upon it. **Irritability** is the ability to respond to a stimulus. A muscle contracts when stimulated. This can be a natural stimulus from a motor nerve or an artificial stimulus such as from an electrical current. **Contractility** is the muscle's ability to contract and generate force when it receives adequate stimulation. This may result in the muscle shortening, staying the same, or lengthening. **Extensibility** is the muscle's ability to stretch or lengthen when a force is applied. **Elasticity** is the muscle's ability to recoil or return to normal resting length when the stretching or shortening force is removed. Saltwater taffy has extensibility but not elasticity. You can stretch it, but once the force is removed, the taffy will remain stretched. A wire spring has both extensibility and elasticity. Stretch the spring, and it will lengthen. Remove the stretch, and the spring will return to its original length. The same can be said of a muscle. However, unlike the taffy or the wire spring, a muscle is able to shorten beyond its normal resting length.

The properties of a muscle are summarized as follows: Stretch a muscle, and it will lengthen (extensibility). Remove the stretch, and it will return to its normal resting position (elasticity). Stimulate a muscle, and it will respond (irritability) by generating force (contractility); then remove the stimulus and it will return to its normal resting position (elasticity).

Sliding Filament Theory

Muscles are comprised of groups of **muscle fibers** that are bound together into bundles called **fascicles.** Each individual muscle fiber is composed of smaller bundles called **myofibrils** (Fig. 5-7). The myofibril is partitioned longitudinally into functional divisions called **sarcomeres,** which are capable of shortening when stimulated. Sarcomeres are separated from one another by **z-lines.** At its smallest functional level, each sarcomere comprises a network of contractile proteins: the thinner **actin** filaments and the thicker **myosin** filaments. The myosin filaments have myosin heads, which are projections. When a muscle receives a stimulus to contract, myocin heads reach out and bind to the actin filaments (Fig. 5-8A). Once bound, these projections exert force on the actin filaments as they move like windshield wipers to pull the actin filaments closer together (Fig. 5-8B). This force causes the entire sarcomere to shorten. During a normal muscle contraction all sarcomeres in a given muscle fiber are shortening at the same time. Furthermore, this process of contraction is occurring in multiple muscle fibers within a given muscle belly, which in turn produces an overall shortening effect of the entire muscle. The **sliding filament theory** describes this interaction between the actin and myosin and explains how force is produced during a muscle contraction and how the sarcomere is shortened.

Length-Tension Relationship in Muscle Tissue

Tension refers to the force built up within a muscle. Stretching a muscle builds up *passive tension,* much like stretching a rubber band, and involves the noncontractile units of a muscle. *Active tension* comes from the contractile units and the force generated can be compared with releasing one end of a stretched rubber band. The total tension of a muscle is a combination of passive and active tension. **Tone** is the slight tension that is present in a muscle at all times, even when the muscle is resting. Tone is a state of readiness that allows the muscle to act more easily and quickly when needed.

Although there is variation between muscles, it can generally be said that a muscle is capable of being shortened to approximately half of its normal resting length. For example, a muscle that is approximately 6 inches long at rest can shorten to approximately 3 inches. Also, a muscle can be stretched to 1.5 times its normal resting length. Therefore, this same muscle can be stretched 3 inches beyond its resting length to an overall length of 9 inches. The **excursion** of a muscle is that distance from maximum lengthening to maximum shortening. In this example, the excursion would be 6 inches (Fig. 5-9).

Usually a muscle has sufficient excursion to allow the joint to move through its entire range. This is certainly true of muscles that span only one joint. However, a muscle spanning two or more joints may not have sufficient excursion to allow it to move through the combined range of all the joints it crosses.

Figure 5-7. Muscle fiber anatomy.

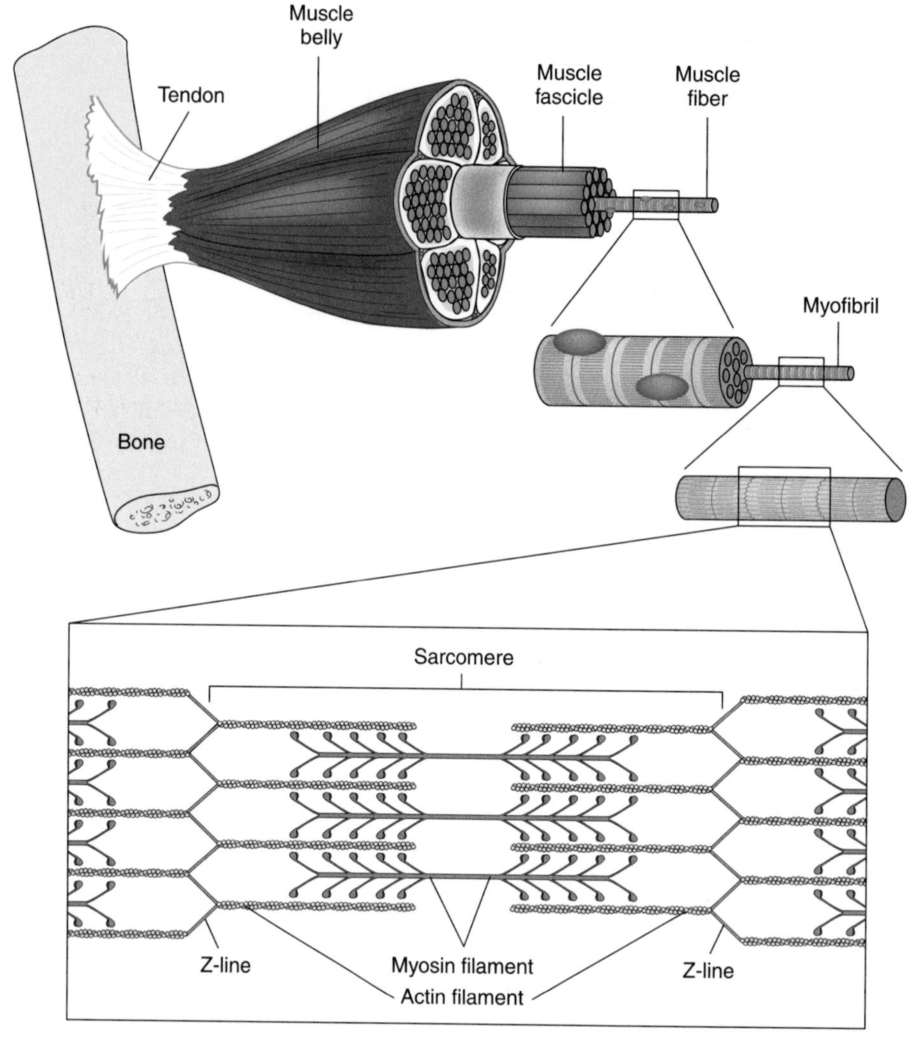

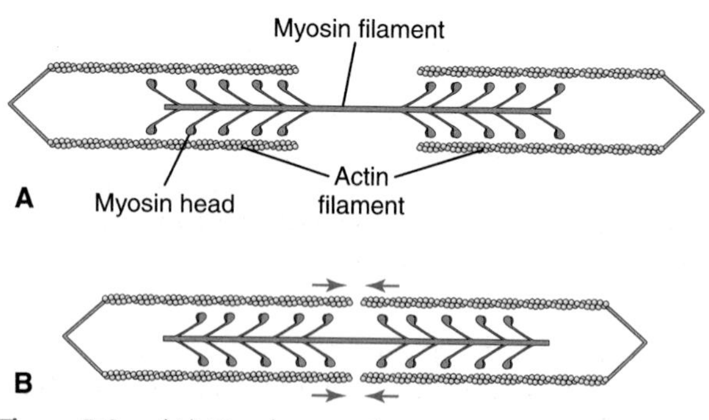

Figure 5-8. **(A)** Muscle preparing to contract: myosin heads bind to actin filaments. **(B)** Muscle contracts: myosin heads exert force and pull actin filaments closer together.

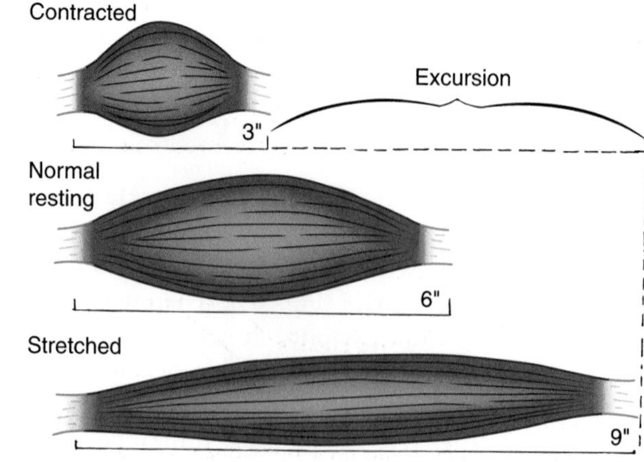

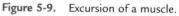

Figure 5-9. Excursion of a muscle.

There are several ways a muscle can be lengthened or shortened. A muscle can be shortened if it contracts concentrically (where the origin and insertion move closer together). A muscle is lengthened when it contracts eccentrically (where the origin and insertion move farther apart) or when a stretching force is applied to the muscle.

Optimal Length

One of the factors determining the amount of force a muscle can generate is its length. When a muscle is on a slight stretch (but not overstretched), it is said to be at **optimal length.** Being at optimal length increases the muscle's force-generating capacity in two ways. First, at optimal length there is maximum interface between actin and myosin filaments. Every myosin head is bound to an actin filament. Maximizing the number of myosin heads bound to and pulling on the actin filaments results in more force generated during the contraction (Fig. 5-10). Second, at optimal length there is some passive tension in the muscle. As with the stored energy in a stretched rubber band, a muscle is capable of generating its strongest contraction when stretched but then loses power quickly as it shortens. There are many examples of this concept. For instance, think of what you do when kicking a ball. First you hyperextend your hip and then forcefully flex it. In other words, you put the hip flexors on a slight stretch over the anterior aspect of the hip (lengthening) (Fig. 5-11A). The slight stretch creates passive muscle tension, which is similar to pulling back on a rubber band before snapping it. As the contraction (shortening) progresses (Fig. 5-11B), the muscle's ability to generate force decreases because the muscle loses its stretch (passive tension decreases).

The contraction force of a muscle is reduced when a muscle is either shortened or lengthened beyond optimal length. Picture the hip extended back even farther behind the body than what is illustrated in Figure 5-11A. If you hyperextend the hip flexors beyond the optimal length, the muscle's ability to generate force is decreased.

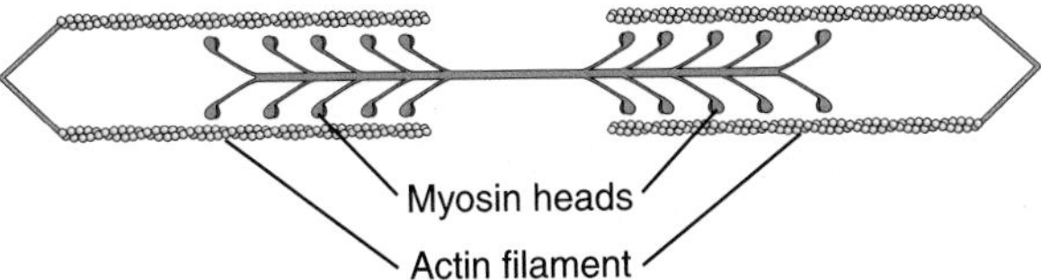

Figure 5-10. Actin and myosin at optimal length. At optimal length, every myosin head has an actin filament with which to bind.

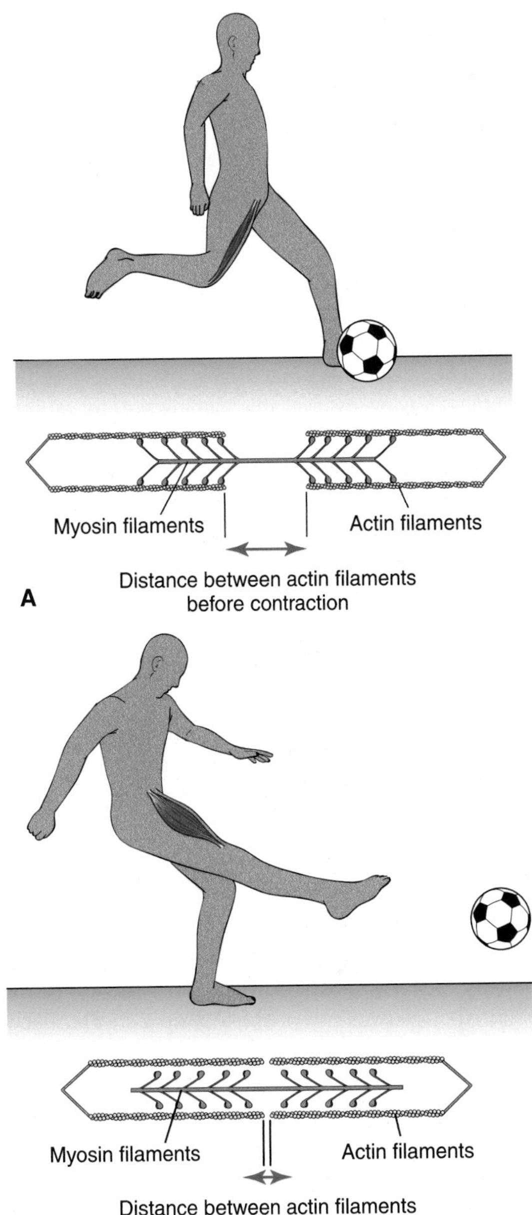

Figure 5-11. Using optimal length to enhance muscle contraction. **(A)** Muscle loaded with passive tension and actin and myosin positioned for maximum binding. **(B)** Passive tension decreases as muscle shortens, and actin filament are closely approximated.

When a muscle is stretched too far, there are myosin heads that cannot reach a binding site on the actin filament and therefore cannot contribute to the production of force (Fig. 5-12A). On the contrary, when a muscle is shortened too far, some of the actin filaments are overlapping, thus reducing the available binding sites

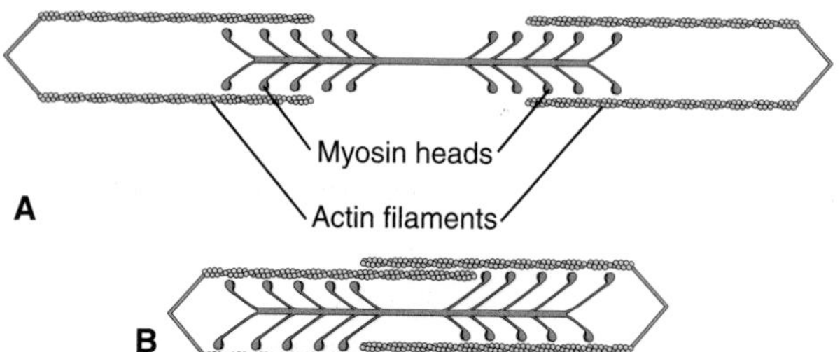

Figure 5-12. Influence of actin and myosin on length-tension relationship. **(A)** Lengthened beyond optimal length, some myosin heads not able to bind to actin filaments. **(B)** Shortened beyond optimal length, actin filaments are overlapping, leaving less available binding sites for myosin heads.

for the myosin heads (Fig. 5-12B). For example, if the hip were flexed even farther than what is illustrated in Figure 5-11B, there would be less binding between actin and myosin and less force generated as the muscle continues to shorten.

Multijoint muscles have an advantage over one-joint muscles in that they maintain greater contractile force through a wider range of motion. They can do so because they maintain "optimal length" by contracting (shortening) over one joint while being lengthened over another. Consider your hamstring muscles when climbing stairs. The hamstring muscles are two-joint muscles located on the posterior thigh. The actions produced by the hamstrings are hip extension and knee flexion. When you go up stairs, you start by flexing the hip and knee (Fig. 5-13A). This position stretches (lengthens) the hamstrings over the posterior hip and places them on slack (shortens them) over the posterior knee. As you move your body up, your hip goes into extension (concentric contraction = shortening the hamstrings at hip joint) while your knee also goes into extension (stretching = lengthening the hamstrings at the knee joint; Fig. 5-13B). In other words, the hamstring muscles are being shortened over the hip while they are being lengthening over the knee. This allows the muscle to maintain its optimal length as well as maximum force-generating capacity throughout the functional activity by: 1) keeping the muscle under the tension of a slight stretch and 2) allowing for maximal overlap of actin and myosin. See Table 5-1 for an analysis of how optimal length is maintained in the hamstrings while ascending a step.

The activity of ascending a step can also be used to analyze how the rectus femoris maintains optimal length during movement. The rectus femoris crosses the anterior aspect of the hip and the anterior aspect of the knee. When it contracts concentrically, it flexes the hip and extends the knee. In the starting position for this activity, the rectus femoris is shortened (on slack) over the hip and lengthened (stretched) over the knee. When ascending the step, the hip extends, which lengthens the rectus femoris. Concurrently the knee is extending due to a concentric contraction of the rectus femoris, which creates shortening of the muscle. This combination of a shortening and lengthening allows the muscle to maintain optimal length (and optimal strength) during this functional activity (see Fig. 5-14 and Table 5-1).

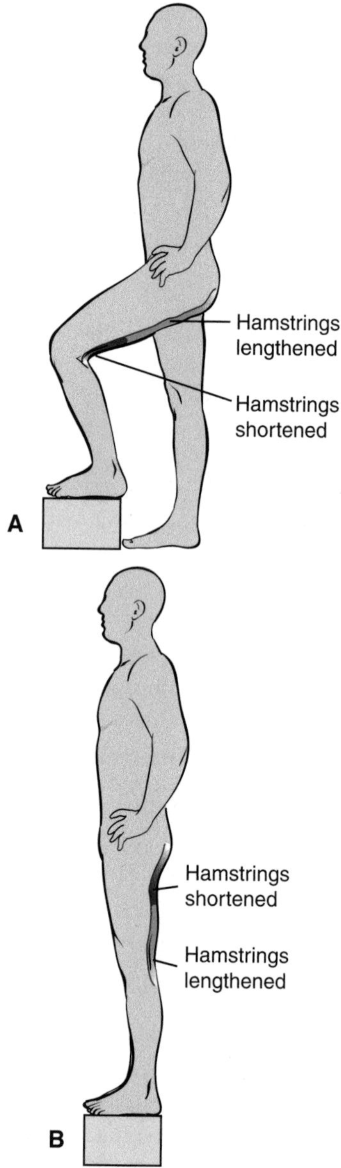

Figure 5-13. Hamstrings maintain optimal length while ascending step. **(A)** Hamstrings lengthened over hip and shortened over knee. Relationship reverses: **(B)** Hamstrings lengthened over knee and shortened over hip.

Table 5-1 Change of Muscle Length While Ascending a Step

Joint Motion Analysis	Hip	Knee
While ascending step	Hip joint is extending	Knee joint is extending
Hamstring Muscle Analysis	**Hip**	**Knee**
Normal action of hamstrings	Extension	Flexion
Change of hamstring muscle length	Shortening Hamstring contracts concentrically to produce hip extension.	Lengthening Hamstring is lengthened over knee, offsetting the shortening at the hip and allowing optimal length to be maintained.
Rectus Femoris Muscle Analysis	**Hip**	**Knee**
Normal action of rectus femoris	Flexion	Extension
Change of rectus femoris muscle length	Lengthening Rectus femoris is lengthened over hip, offsetting the shortening at the knee and allowing optimal length to be maintained.	Shortening Rectus femoris contracts concentrically to produce knee extension.

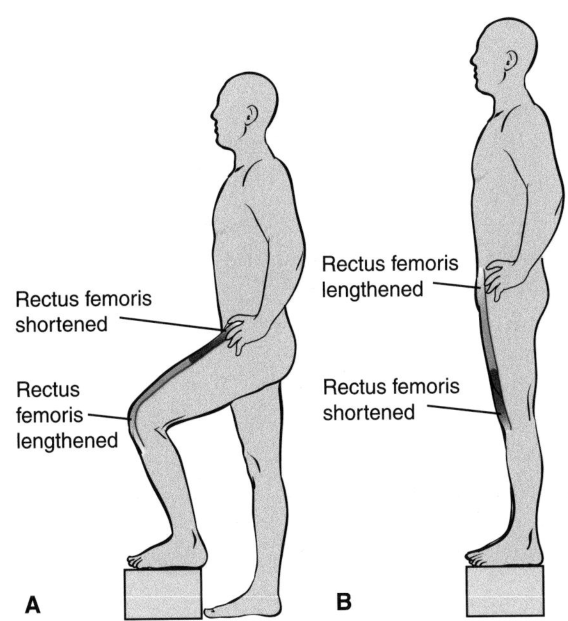

Figure 5-14. Rectus femoris maintains optimal length while ascending a step. **(A)** Rectus femoris shortened over hip and lengthened over knee. Relationship reverses: **(B)** Rectus femoris is shortened over knee and lengthened over hip.

Active and Passive Insufficiency

In a one-joint muscle, the excursion of the muscle will be greater than the range of motion allowed by the joint. For example, the brachialis, which crosses the anterior aspect of the elbow, has plenty of excursion to bring the elbow through its full range of motion—starting in a fully extended position and moving into full flexion (see Fig. 11-14). However, with a multijoint muscle, the muscle's excursion is less than the combined range allowed by the joints. Brunnstrom uses the terms *active* and *passive insufficiency* to describe conditions in which a multijoint muscle cannot be shortened or lengthened far enough to allow all of the joints the muscle crosses to move through their full range of motion.

The point at which a muscle cannot shorten any farther is called **active insufficiency.** Active insufficiency occurs to the agonist (the muscle that is contracting/shortening). Consider again the hamstrings as an example. The hamstrings can perform either hip extension or knee flexion but cannot shorten enough to perform both simultaneously. Notice that if you flex your knee while your hip is extended, you cannot complete the full knee flexion range (Fig. 5-15A, B). The inability to complete full knee flexion happens because the hamstrings are being asked to shorten over the hip *and* over the knee at the same time, and the muscle does not have the capability to shorten that much. The hamstrings have become actively insufficient. The myosin filaments are contacting the z-lines, and the sarcomere cannot get any shorter (see Fig. 5-15B). While the muscle has run out of ability to shorten, the joint has not run out of range of motion. To see that an increased range of motion can be obtained passively, grab your ankle and pull the knee into increased flexion (Fig. 5-15C). Be careful when

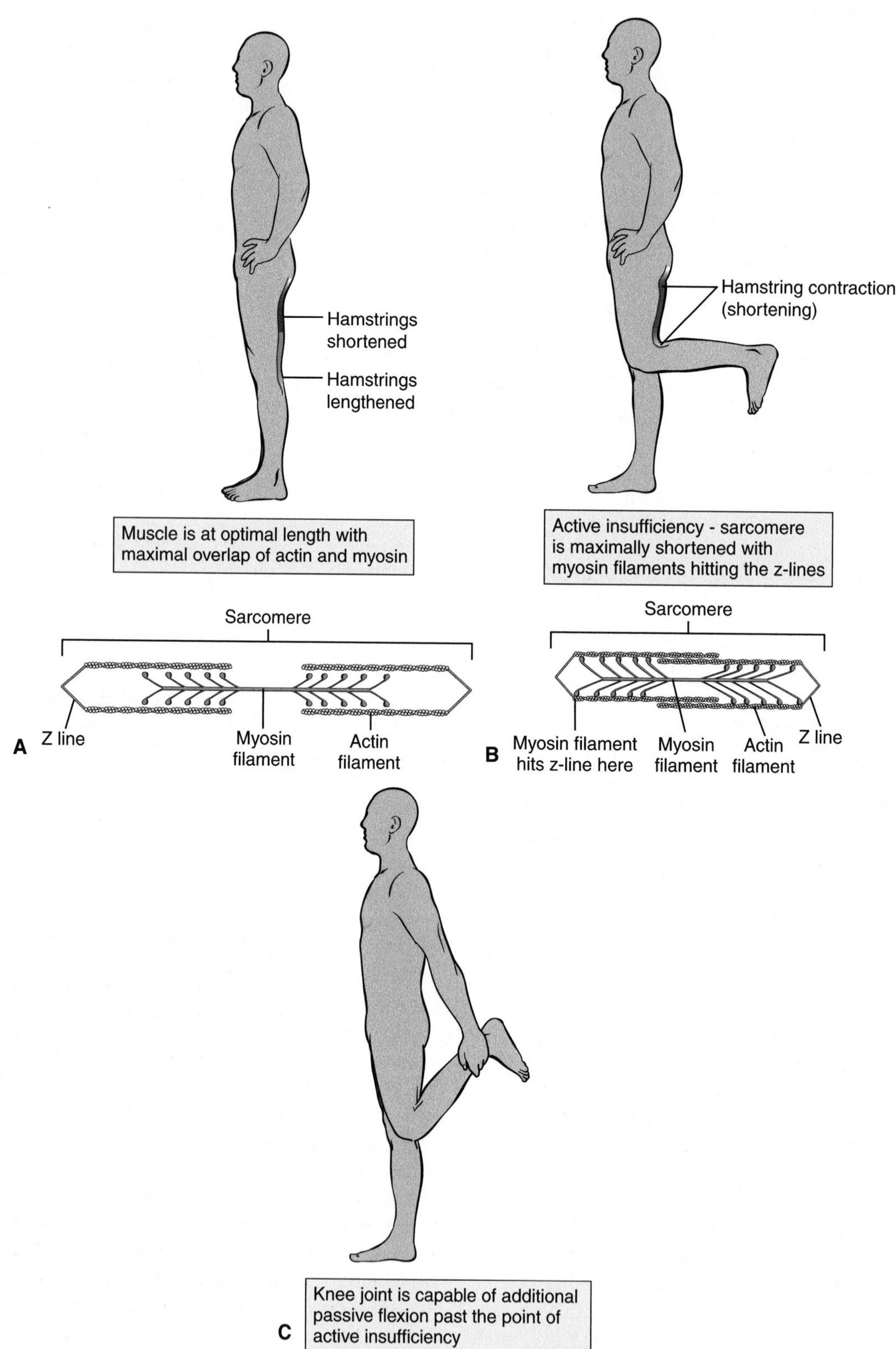

Figure 5-15. Active insufficiency of the hamstring muscle. **(A)** Muscle is at optimal length with maximal overlap of actin and myosin. **(B)** Active insufficiency; sarcomere is maximally shortened with myosin filaments hitting the z-lines. **(C)** Knee joint is capable of additional passive flexion past the point of active insufficiency.

trying this exercise that you do not get a muscle cramp. In other words, in this two-joint muscle that is contracting over both joints at the same time, the muscle (hamstrings) will run out of contractility before the joints (hip and knee) run out of range of motion.

Passive insufficiency occurs when a multijoint muscle cannot be lengthened any farther without damage to its fibers. Passive insufficiency occurs to the antagonist (the relaxed muscle that is on the opposite side of the joint from the agonist—the contracting muscle).

Consider an example where the hamstring muscles are of passive insufficiency. The hamstring is long enough to be stretched over each joint individually (hip flexion or knee extension), but not both simultaneously. If you flex your hip with your knee flexed, you can complete the range. As you can see in Figure 5-16A, the individual can touch the toes by flexing both the hip and the knee. The hamstrings are being stretched over only one joint (the hip). You can also extend your knee fully when the hip is extended (Fig. 5-15B) because the hamstrings are being lengthened over only the knee. However, if you try to flex your hips to touch your toes with your knee extended (Fig. 5-16C), you will probably experience a stretch in the posterior thigh well before you reach full hip flexion. Your hamstring muscles are telling you to stop. They are being stretched over both joints at the same time and have become passively insufficient. They cannot be stretched any farther.

The benefits and drawbacks of single versus multijoint muscles are summarized in Table 5-2. Note that the benefit of a single joint muscle is a drawback of a multijoint muscle and vice-versa.

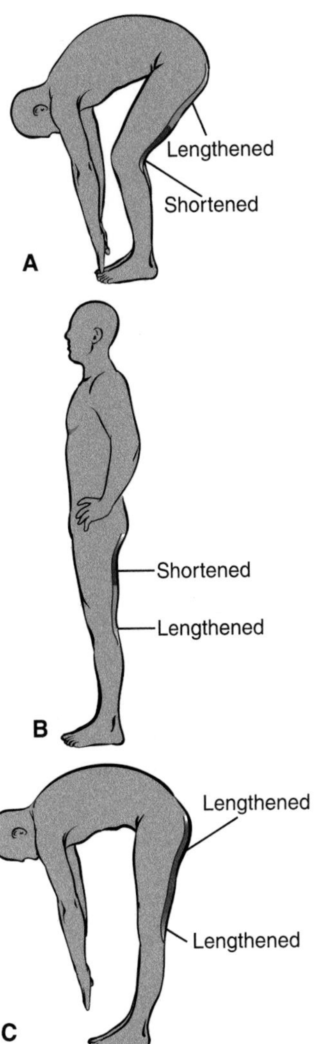

Figure 5-16. Passive insufficiency of the hamstring muscle. **(A & B)** There are no range of-motion restrictions, because the hamstring is being stretched (lengthened) over only one joint at a time). **(C)** Stretching the muscle over both joints (the hip and knee) allows less individual joint range of motion (person cannot touch toes).

Adaptive Shortening & Lengthening of Muscle Tissue

Poor posture can often result in a muscle being in a chronically overstretched (lengthened) state where it adopts an abnormally long resting length. Figure 5-17 illustrates how the scapular retractors become overstretched with forward-head, rounded-shoulder posture. Just as we saw when a *normal* muscle is placed on stretch, a muscle that is *chronically* overstretched also experiences a decrease in the overlap of actin and myosin (see Fig. 5-12A). The muscle is not able to generate as much force during contraction. Therefore an overstretched muscle is also considered a weak muscle. Strengthening exercises are often performed for muscles that have undergone this **adaptive lengthening**. Posture causing chronic overstretched muscles needs correcting to regain appropriate overlap of actin and myosin filaments.

On the contrary, in situations when a muscle is left in a shortened position for a prolonged period of time without moving through its full excursion, it undergoes **adaptive shortening** in which the resting length and amount of extensibility decrease. This would commonly be called a "tight muscle," and if taken to the extreme point of permanent shortening, would be called a "contracture." Development of muscle tightness can happen due to immobilization following an injury or due to poor posture. Figure 5-17 illustrates how forward-head, rounded-shoulder posture causes the pectoral muscles to become short and tight due to their chronically

Table 5-2 Benefits and Drawbacks of Single vs. Multijoint Muscles

	Single Joint Muscles	Multijoint Muscles
Benefits	Capable of moving a joint through its full ROM (not subject to active and passive insufficiency)	Can maintain optimal length during contraction by shortening over one joint while lengthening over another
Drawbacks	Less powerful at ends of joint ROM (when moving away from optimal length)	Subject to active and passive insufficiency, which can limit ROM and movements in the joints the muscle crosses

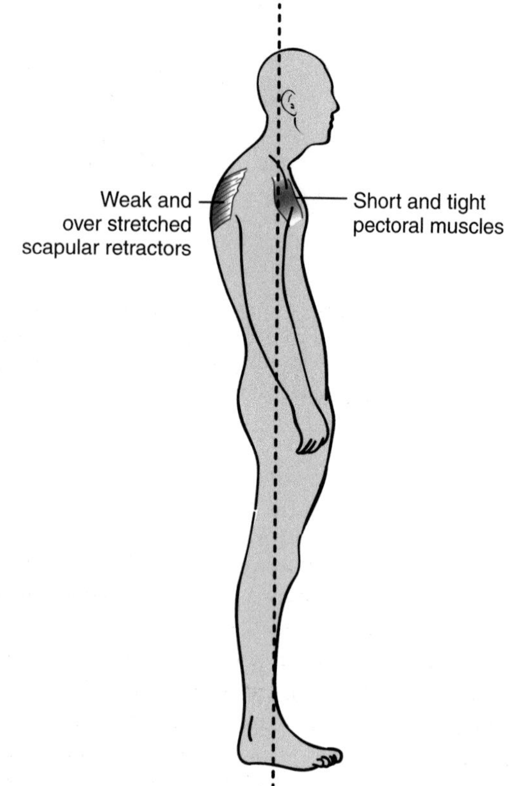

Figure 5-17. Effect of forward-head, rounded-shoulder posture on muscle resting length.

shortened state. Stretching techniques are often used for muscles that have undergone adaptive shortening.

Stretching

Generally speaking, an agonist usually becomes actively insufficient (cannot contract any farther) before the antagonist becomes passively insufficient (cannot be stretched farther). This concept can be used to our advantage when we purposely want to stretch a muscle to either maintain or regain its normal resting length. Some activities require a great deal of flexibility, so stretching is done to increase the resting length of a muscle. In all of these situations, stretching should be performed on relaxed muscles. The joint(s) the muscle crosses should be placed in a position that is opposite from the action of that muscle. In the case of a multi-joint muscle, the muscle must be lengthened over all joints simultaneously in order to achieve a stretch. For example, you will recall the action of the hamstrings is hip extension and knee flexion (contraction = shortening), therefore to *stretch* the hamstring muscles, put the knee in extension (lengthening over posterior knee) and slowly flex the hip (additional lengthening—over posterior hip) to the point where you feel a stretching discomfort but not to the point of pain (Fig. 5-18 and Table 5-3).

To stretch a one-joint muscle, it is necessary to put any two-joint muscles on a slack over the joint(s) not crossed by the one joint-muscle. For example, to stretch the soleus muscle (which crosses the ankle only), the gastrocnemius muscle (which crosses the ankle and knee) must be put on a slack over the knee. This can be

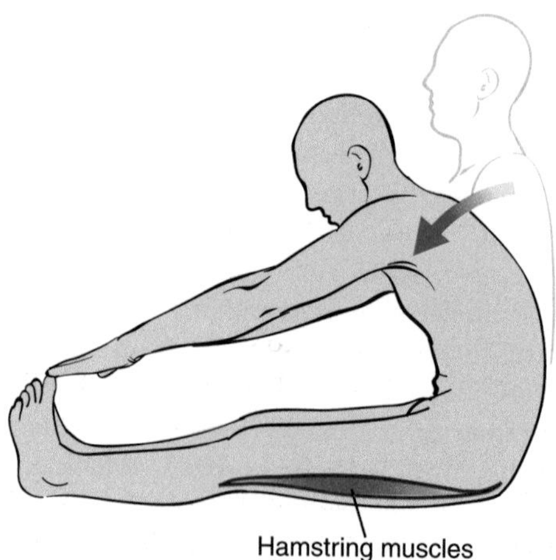

Figure 5-18. Stretching of the hamstring muscle. To place the hamstring muscle on stretch over the posterior side of the hip and knee, start with the knee in extension, and then slowly flex the hip by leaning forward.

Table 5-3 Comparison of Muscle Action vs. Muscle Stretching Position

	Hip	Knee
Normal action of hamstrings *(Action = Concentric Contraction = Shortening)*	Extension	Flexion
Joint position for hamstring stretch *(Stretching = Lengthening)*	Flexion	Extension

accomplished by flexing the knee while dorsiflexing the ankle (Fig. 5-19A). Otherwise, if you attempt to dorsiflex the ankle when the knee is extended, you may be stretching the gastrocnemius (two-joint muscle) more than the soleus (Fig. 5-19B). If the intent is to stretch the gastrocnemius, it must be stretched over both joints at the same time, as Figure 5-19B illustrates.

There are various methods of stretching used for different situations and sometimes for different results. These different methods are important but are beyond the scope of this discussion.

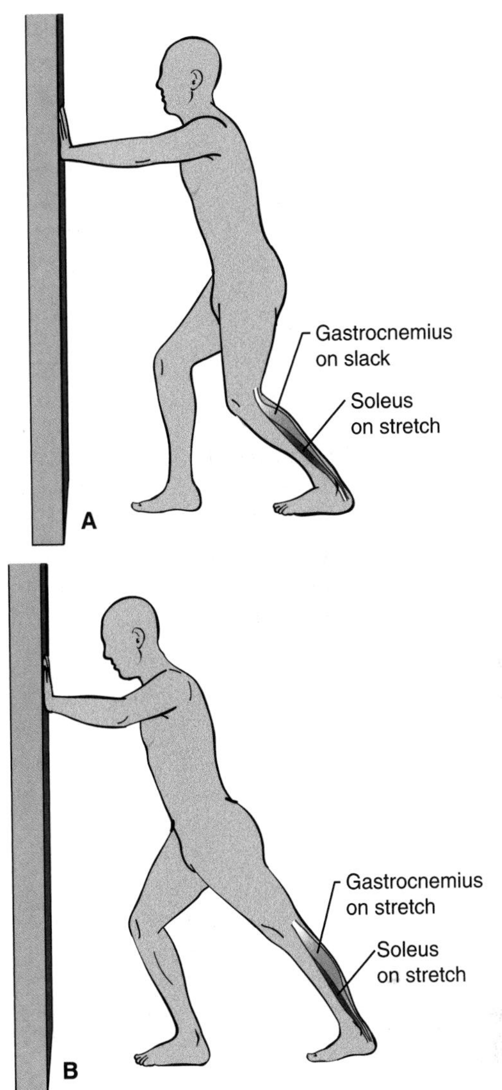

Figure 5-19. Stretching soleus versus gastrocnemius muscle. **(A)** Flex the knee to put the gastrocnemius on slack allows the soleus to be stretched. **(B)** Simultaneous stretch of gastrocnemius and soleus.

Tendon Action of a Muscle (Tenodesis)

Some degree of opening and closing the hand can be accomplished by using the principle of passive insufficiency. The finger flexors and extensors are multijoint muscles. They cross the wrist, the metacarpophalangeal (MCP) joints, the proximal interphalangeal (PIP) joints, and sometimes the distal interphalangeal (DIP) joints. We have already noticed that a two-joint or multijoint muscle does not have sufficient length to be stretched over all joints simultaneously. Something has to give. If you rest your flexed elbow on the table in a pronated position, relax, and let your wrist drop into flexion, you will notice that your fingers have a tendency to extend passively (Fig. 5-20A). Conversely, if you supinate your forearm and relax your wrist into extension, your fingers will have a tendency to close (Fig. 5-20B). If these tendons were a little tight, this opening and closing would be more pronounced. This is called **tenodesis** or **tendon action of a muscle.** A person who is quadriplegic and has no voluntary ability to open and close the fingers can use this principle to grasp and release light objects. By supinating the forearm, the weight of the hand and gravity causes the wrist to fall into hyperextension. This closes the fingers, creating a slight grasp. Pronating the forearm causes the wrist to fall into flexion, thus opening the fingers and releasing an object.

Types of Muscle Contraction

There are three basic types of muscle contraction: isometric, isotonic, and isokinetic. An **isometric contraction** occurs when a muscle contracts, producing force without changing the length of a muscle (Fig. 5-21A). The term *isometric* originates from the Greek word meaning "same length." To demonstrate this action, get in a sitting position and place your right hand under your thigh and place your left hand on your right biceps muscle. Now, pull up with your right hand—in other words, attempt to flex your right elbow. Note that there was no real motion at the elbow joint, but you did feel

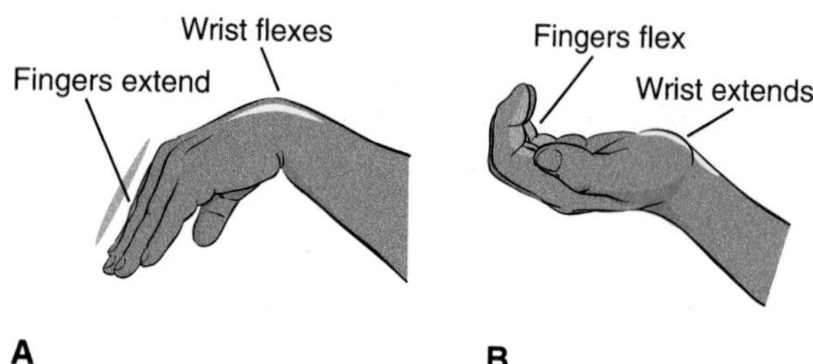
Wrist flexes
Fingers extend
Fingers flex
Wrist extends
A
B

Figure 5-20. Tenodesis, the functional use of passive insufficiency, is demonstrated on the finger flexor and extensor muscles. None of the muscle groups can be stretched over all of the wrist and finger joints at the same time. **(A)** Passive insufficiency of the finger extensors occurs when the wrist is flexed, causing the fingers to extend. **(B)** Passive insufficiency of the finger flexors occurs when the wrist is extended, causing the fingers to flex.

the muscle contract. This is an isometric contraction of your right biceps muscle. The muscle contracted, but no joint motion occurred.

Next, hold a weight in your hand while flexing your elbow to bring the weight up toward your shoulder (Fig. 5-21B). You will feel the biceps muscle contract, but this time there is joint motion. A **concentric contraction** occurs when there is joint movement, the muscles shorten, and the muscle attachments (origin [*O*] and insertion [*I*]) move toward each other (Fig. 5-21B). It is sometimes referred to as a *shortening contraction.* The biceps shortens as it brings the hand toward the shoulder.

If you continue to palpate the biceps muscle while setting the weight back down on the table, you will feel that the biceps muscle (not the triceps muscle) continues to contract, even though the joint motion is elbow extension. What is occurring is an eccentric contraction of the biceps muscle. An **eccentric contraction** occurs when there is joint motion but the muscle appears to lengthen; that is, the muscle attachments separate (Fig. 5-21C). After fully flexing the elbow, realize that if you relaxed your biceps muscle, the pull of gravity on your hand, forearm, and the weight would cause them to drop to the table. If you used your triceps muscle to extend the elbow (concentrically), your hand and weight would crash onto the tabletop with great force and speed. However, what you did by slowly returning the weight to the tabletop was to slow down (decelerate) the pull of gravity. You did this by eccentrically contracting the biceps (elbow flexor). Your biceps "lengthened" while contracting as your elbow moved into extension.

Although eccentric contractions are sometimes referred to as *lengthening contractions,* the muscle is actually returning to its normal resting position from a shortened position. An eccentric contraction can produce much greater force than can a concentric contraction.

Frequently, different types of muscle contractions are used in various exercises. Quadriceps "setting" exercises are isometric contractions of the quadriceps muscle. Flexing and extending the knee use concentric and eccentric contractions. Sitting on a chair and extending the knee is a concentric contraction of the quadriceps muscle (Fig. 5-22), whereas flexing the knee and returning it to

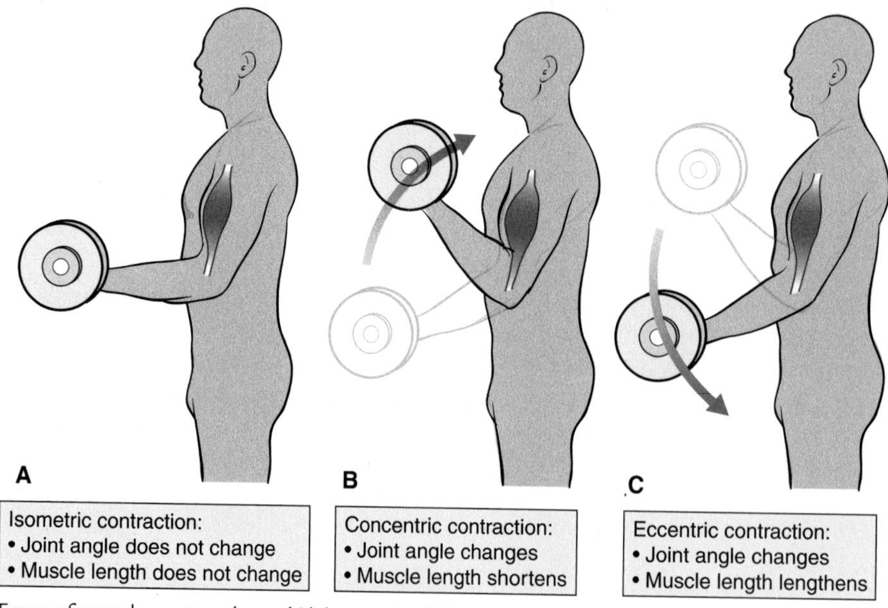
A
Isometric contraction:
• Joint angle does not change
• Muscle length does not change
B
Concentric contraction:
• Joint angle changes
• Muscle length shortens
C
Eccentric contraction:
• Joint angle changes
• Muscle length lengthens

Figure 5-21. Types of muscle contractions: **(A)** isometric, **(B)** concentric, and **(C)** eccentric.

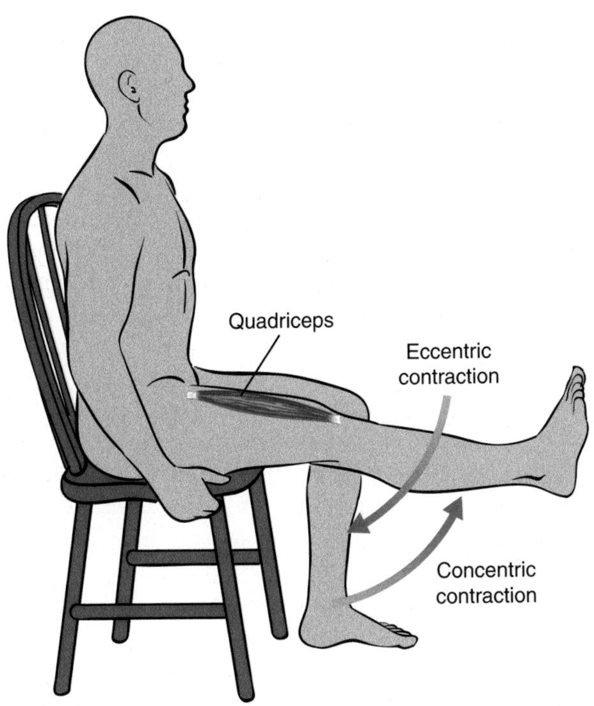

Figure 5-22. Concentric (shortening) contraction of quadriceps muscles causes knee extension (up arrow). Gravity causes knee flexion, but it is controlled (slowed) by an eccentric (lengthening) contraction of the quadriceps muscles (down arrow).

the starting position is an eccentric contraction of the quadriceps muscle. Similarly, if you lie on the floor in a prone position and flex your knee to 90 degrees, you are performing a concentric contraction of the hamstring muscles. Straightening your knee while in that same position is an eccentric contraction of the same muscles. What is happening? Both examples involve moving the lower leg *against gravity* and *with gravity*. Muscles need to accelerate to move against gravity. This is a concentric contraction, whereas muscles need to decelerate when moving with gravity to slow down the effects (pull) of gravity. In general, concentric contractions are used in acceleration activities, whereas eccentric contractions are used in deceleration activities.

The differences between the three types of muscle contractions have been summarized in Table 5-4.

Table 5-5 shows many examples to emphasize the difference between concentric and eccentric contractions and how they change depending on the action performed. You could say the same thing about any two opposing muscle actions (e.g., supinators and pronators).

However, not all concentric and eccentric contractions work against or with gravity. There are exceptions. Here is an example: In the sitting position with the knee extended, have someone give resistance while you flex your knee. You would be performing a concentric contraction of the hamstring muscles (knee flexors). In this case, your lower leg is moving down (the same direction as the pull of gravity). However, the external force (the other person's resistance) is greater than the pull of gravity and must be overcome with a muscle contraction. So, the knee flexors are contracting concentrically against an external resistance, even though the lower leg moves in the same direction as gravity.

Consider another example: Normally, you use your shoulder flexors to lower your arm into extension in an eccentric contraction because you are slowing down gravity. However, if you hold on to the handle of an overhead pulley and pull down into shoulder extension, you are performing a concentric contraction of the shoulder extensors. While your arm is moving in the same direction as gravity, you are overcoming a force greater than gravity (i.e., the overhead pulley weight). To prove this, keep holding the pulley handle, but relax your shoulder muscles. Notice that your arm does not fall toward the ground. Why? The pulley weight is greater than the gravity weight (force of gravity).

Next, if you slowly, and under control, return the pulley handle to the starting position (shoulder flexion), you are performing an eccentric contraction of the shoulder extensors. Why? You are moving against

Table 5-4 Characteristics of Isometric, Concentric and Eccentric Contractions

Isometric Contractions	Concentric Contractions	Eccentric Contractions
Muscle attachments do not move.	Muscle attachments move closer together.	Muscle attachments move farther apart.
Gravity is not a factor.	Movement is usually occurring against gravity (a "raising" motion).	Movement usually occurs with gravity (a "lowering" motion).
It is neither an acceleration or deceleration movement.	It is an acceleration activity.	The contraction is used to decelerate movement caused by gravity.

Table 5-5 Concentric and Eccentric Contractions and Resulting Joint Motion

Muscle Group (Contracting)	Joint Motion Occurring with Concentric Contraction	Joint Motion Occurring with Eccentric Contraction
Flexors	Flexion	Extension
Extensors	Extension	Flexion
Abductors	Abduction	Adduction
Adductors	Adduction	Abduction
Medial rotators	Medial rotation	Lateral rotation
Lateral rotators	Lateral rotation	Medial rotation

the force of gravity, acting on the pulley weight. In this case, you are decelerating the external force (the pulley weights) moving with gravity. To prove this, picture holding on to a pulley handle with the arm pulled down into shoulder extension. If you were to relax your shoulder muscles, the pulley weight would crash down, causing your shoulder to quickly flex. To prevent this, you would need your shoulder extensors to contract eccentrically and control the flexion motion being imposed by the force of the weights.

Elastic tubing is a common method of providing resistance while exercising. Although it can be used effectively with concentric contractions, it has greater limitations with eccentric contractions. If you attached elastic tubing over the top of a door and pulled down, you would be duplicating the action of the overhead pulley. Pulling down would be a concentric contraction of the shoulder extensors. However, returning to the starting position using elastic tubing is not as effective as an eccentric contraction with the pulleys. The initial motion is a strong eccentric contraction, but the elasticity quickly loses its tension. Therefore, using tubing for eccentric contractions must be done only in the early part of the motion and must not be considered effective throughout the entire range. It is possible to have effective eccentric contraction through smaller ranges using elastic tubing, such as forearm pronation and supination, but not with wider ranges, such as elbow flexion and extension.

If a muscle is too weak to move against gravity, the clinician might put the person in a **gravity-eliminated** position to exercise. For flexion and extension, the gravity-eliminated position is side-lying with the arm supported. The muscle may have enough strength to move but not to overcome or slow down gravity. Sit or kneel next to a table and rest your arm at shoulder level on the table. Another example of a gravity-eliminated motion is moving your arm forward and backward in horizontal adduction and abduction with the weight of your arm being supported by the table.

Another, though less common, type of muscle contraction is an **isokinetic contraction.** In this case "kinetic" refers to speed, so an isokinetic contraction is one in which the speed of the motion stays the same for the duration of the contraction. This can be done only with special equipment that regulates the speed of motion. In an isokinetic contraction, the body part to be exercised is usually connected to a machine that does not produce any movement itself, but limits the speed it will allow the body part to move when a contraction is performed. If the person tries to move faster than the speed limit, they will end up generating more resistance against the machine, whereas if a person does not push as fast/hard, there will be less resistance.

With an isokinetic contraction, resistance to the part varies, but the speed stays the same. This differs from a concentric or eccentric contraction, in which the resistance remains constant but the speed varies. Consider the example of a person sitting in a chair with a 5-pound weight attached to the leg. While the person extends (concentric contraction of quadriceps) and flexes (eccentric contraction of same muscle) the knee, the amount of resistance stays the same. That 5-pound weight remains 5 pounds throughout the range. Because of other factors, such as the angle of pull, it is easier to move the leg in the middle and at the end of the range than at the beginning, which causes the speed at which the person is able to move the leg to vary throughout the range.

Why are isokinetic muscle contractions significant? A complete discussion of the merits of isokinetic exercise in comparison with other forms of exercise is best covered in a more detailed discussion of therapeutic exercise, which is beyond the scope of this book. However, there are two significant advantages. Isokinetic exercises can alter or adjust the amount of resistance given through the range of motion, whereas a concentric/eccentric exercise cannot. This is important because a muscle is not as strong at the beginning or end of its range as it is in the middle. Because the muscle is strongest in the midrange, more resistance should be given there, and less resistance should be given at the beginning and end. An isotonic exercise cannot do this; therefore, there may be too much resistance in the weaker parts of the range and not enough resistance in the stronger parts.

Accommodating resistance is also important because of the pain factor. If pain suddenly develops during the exercise, the person's response is to stop exercising or not work as hard. With an isotonic contraction, this response cannot happen quickly or even safely. With an isokinetic exercise, if the person stops working, the machine also stops. If the person does not contract as hard, the machine does not give as much resistance.

Hopefully this will give you some idea of the value of isokinetic exercise. However, there are some drawbacks. For example, isokinetic exercise requires special equipment, and that equipment is large and expensive. There is a time and place for all of these types of muscle contractions. It is important that you recognize the differences among them. Table 5-6 summarizes the major differences among these three types of muscle contractions.

Roles of Muscles

Muscles assume different roles during joint motion, depending on such variables as the motion being performed, the direction of the motion, and the amount of resistance the muscle must overcome. If any of these variables change, the muscle's role may also change. The roles a muscle can assume are those of an agonist, antagonist, stabilizer, or neutralizer. An **agonist** is a muscle or muscle group that causes the motion. It is sometimes referred to as the **prime mover.** A muscle that is not as effective but does assist in providing that motion is called an **assisting mover.** Factors that determine whether a muscle is a prime mover or an assisting mover include size, angle of pull, leverage, and contractile potential and will be discussed in more detail later in this chapter. During elbow flexion, the biceps muscle is an agonist, and because of its size and angle of pull, the pronator teres muscle is an assisting mover.

An **antagonist** is a muscle that performs the opposite motion of the agonist. In the case of elbow flexion, the antagonist is the triceps muscle. Keep in mind that the role of a muscle is specific to a particular joint action. In the case of elbow extension, the triceps muscle is the agonist, and the biceps muscle is the antagonist.

Table 5-6 Types of Muscle Contraction

Type	Speed	Resistance	Joint Motion
Isometric	Fixed	Fixed (0 degrees/sec)	No
Isotonic	Variable	Fixed	Yes
Isokinetic	Fixed	Variable (accommodating)	Yes

The antagonist has the potential to oppose the agonist, but it is usually relaxed while the agonist is working. When the antagonist contracts at the same time as the agonist, a **cocontraction** results. A cocontraction occurs when there is a need for accuracy. Some experts feel that cocontractions are common when a person learns a task, especially a difficult one; thus, as the task is learned, cocontraction activity tends to disappear.

A **stabilizer** is a muscle or muscle group that supports, or makes firm, a part allowing the agonist to work more efficiently. For example, when you do a push-up, the agonists are the elbow extensor muscles. The abdominal muscles (trunk flexor muscles) act as stabilizers to keep the trunk straight, whereas the arms move the trunk up and down. A stabilizer is sometimes referred to as a *fixator.*

Remember, a muscle knows no direction when it contracts. If a muscle can do two (or more) actions but only one is wanted, a **neutralizer** contracts to prevent the unwanted motion. For example, the biceps muscle can flex the elbow and supinate the forearm. If only elbow flexion is wanted, the supination component must be canceled out. Therefore, the pronator teres muscle, which pronates the forearm, contracts to counteract the supination component of the biceps muscle, allowing only elbow flexion to occur. A neutralizer may also allow a muscle to perform more than one role. Wrist ulnar deviation is such an example. The flexor carpi ulnaris muscle causes flexion and ulnar deviation of the wrist. The extensor carpi ulnaris muscle causes extension and ulnar deviation. In ulnar deviation, these muscles contract and accomplish two things: The extensor carpi ulnaris and flexor carpi ulnaris neutralize each other's flexion/extension component while acting as agonists in wrist ulnar deviation.

A **synergist** is a nonspecific term describing a muscle that works with one or more other muscles to enhance a particular motion. Some authors use this term to encompass the role of agonists, assisting movers, stabilizers, and neutralizers. The disadvantage of this term is that, although it indicates that the muscle is working, it does not indicate how.

Line of Pull

The line of pull between the origin and insertion of a muscle will dictate its action. To analyze the line of pull of a muscle, one must know the muscle's attachment points, the relative position of these attachments to one another, which point is more moveable, the side of the joint(s) that the muscle crosses, the available motions at the joint(s) it crosses, the angle at which it pulls, including whether it wraps around any bony prominences between its origin and insertion. In most cases, with this information, one can essentially *figure out* what a muscle's action might be. In addition, by looking at the muscle's distance from the axis of rotation of the joint, and the size of the muscle belly, and comparing those factors with other muscles that perform the same action, one can estimate whether a muscle is a prime mover or assisting mover for a given motion.

For example, compare the size of the triceps with that of the anconeus (see Figs. 11-17 and 11-18). It is easy to see that the anconeus will have little effect on joint motion compared with the triceps. Next, you know the motions that a particular joint allows. In the case of the elbow, the motions possible are flexion and extension. The triceps and anconeus cross the joint posterior to the joint axis, which, during contraction would produce elbow extension. Because the triceps is much larger than the anconeus and because it crosses the elbow posteriorly, it is logical that the triceps is a prime mover in elbow extension.

Line of pull can also be a major factor. As will be discussed in Chapter 8, regarding torque, most muscles have a diagonal line of pull. That diagonal line of pull is the resultant force of a vertical force and a horizontal force. In the case of the shoulder girdle, muscles with a greater vertical angle of pull will be effective in pulling the scapula up or down (elevating or depressing the scapula). Muscles with a greater horizontal pull will be more effective in pulling the scapula in or out (protracting or retracting). Muscles with a more equal horizontal and vertical pull will have a role in both motions. Figure 5-23 gives an example of each. The levator scapula has a stronger vertical component, the middle trapezius has a stronger horizontal component, and the rhomboids have a more equal pull in both directions. As you will see when these muscles are described later in Chapter 9, the levator scapula is a prime mover in scapular elevation, and the middle trapezius is a prime mover in retraction, whereas the rhomboids are prime movers in both elevation and retraction.

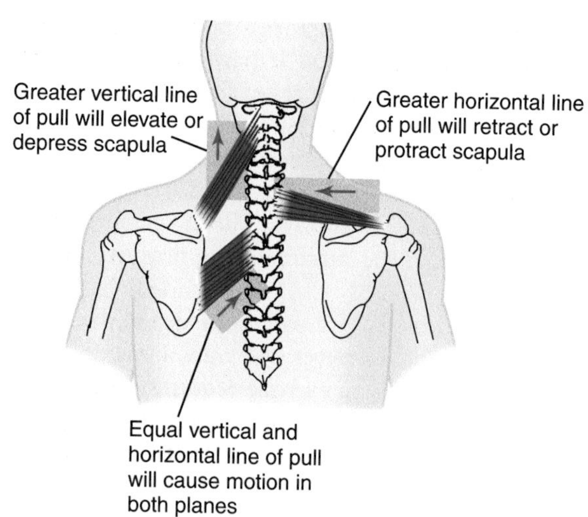
Greater vertical line of pull will elevate or depress scapula
Greater horizontal line of pull will retract or protract scapula
Equal vertical and horizontal line of pull will cause motion in both planes

Figure 5-23. Line of pull as a determinant of muscle action. The line of pull of the levator scapula is more vertical, middle trapezius is horizontal, whereas the rhomboids pull equally horizontally and vertically.

Kinetic Chains

The concept of open versus closed kinetic chain exercises has evolved into movement and exercise. In engineering terms, a kinetic chain consists of a series of rigid links connected in such a way as to allow motion. Because these links are connected, movement of one link causes motion at other links in a predictable way. Applying this to the human body, a **closed kinetic chain** requires that the distal segment is fixed (closed) and the proximal segment(s) moves (Fig. 5-24). For example, when you rise from a sitting position, your

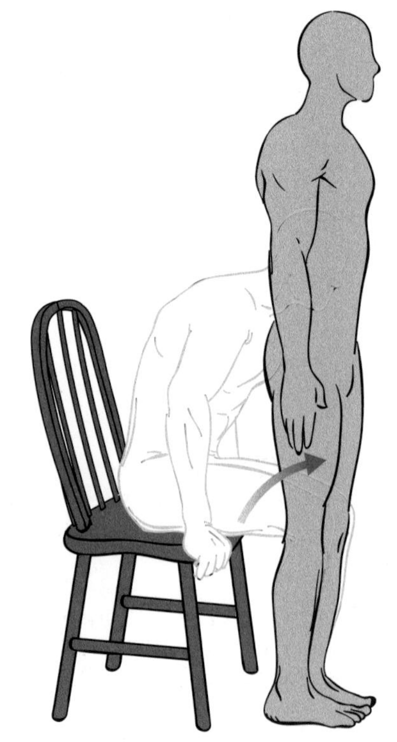
Proximal segment moves
Distal segment fixed

Figure 5-24. Closed kinetic chain.

knees extend, causing your hips and ankles to move as well. With your foot fixed on the ground, there is no way you can move your knee without causing movement at the hip and ankle.

If you were to remain seated and extend your knee, your hip and ankle joint would not move. This is an **open kinetic chain** activity. The distal segment(s) is free to move while the proximal segment(s) can remain stationary (see Fig. 5-24). With open-chain activities, the limb segments are free to move in many directions (Fig. 5-25). For example, if you are lying on a bed with your arm in the air, you can move your shoulder, elbow, wrist, and hand in many directions, either together or individually. This is open-chain activity. The distal segment is not fixed but is free to move.

If you grab an overhead trapeze, your hand, the distal segment, is fixed, or closed. As you flex your elbow, your shoulder has to go into some extension. As your elbow extends, your shoulder must go into some flexion. With closed-chain activities, the limb segments move in limited and predictable directions. Other examples of upper extremity closed-chain activities occur during crutch walking and pushing a wheelchair. The crutch tip (distal segment) is fixed on the ground, and the body (proximal segment) moves. The hands on the wheelchair rims are the distal segments, and joints proximal to the hands move in a connected fashion (i.e., the elbows extend and the shoulders flex).

Closed-chain exercise equipment includes such things as the bench press, rowing machine, stationary bicycle, and stair stepper. Examples of open-chain exercise equipment include free weights and any resistance training machines found in a gym that allow the hands or feet to move through space. Manual muscle testing is almost always open-chain movement. An exception would be testing the gastrocnemius/soleus group by doing a standing heel raise. The treadmill is a combination of both open- and closed-chain exercise. The weight-bearing portion is the closed-chain movement, and the non-weight-bearing portion is the open-chain movement.

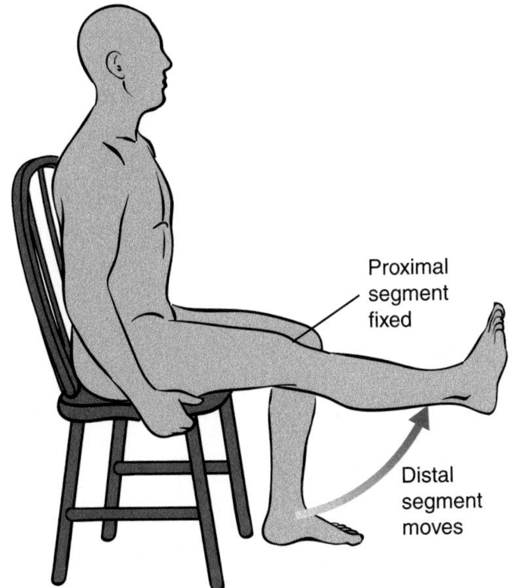

Figure 5-25. Open kinetic chain.

Common Muscle Pathologies

Dysfunction in the muscular system is very common. A muscle **strain** is an overstretching of muscle fibers and can happen with different degrees of severity. Strains to the hamstring muscle group are common. **Trigger points** are hyperirritable points within a tight band of muscle that refer pain to other areas of the body when they are active or when they are palpated. Trigger points can be found in overworked muscle, such as the upper trapezius in an individual who does a lot of computer work without proper ergonomics. **Tendonitis** is inflammation of a tendon and can present at either the musculotendinous junction, the tenoperiosteal junction, or within the body of the tendon (See Fig. 5-1). Common sites for tendonitis at the tenoperiosteal junction are at the origin of the extensor carpi radialis brevis (this is the site for "tennis elbow"), and the insertion of the supraspinatus. In contrast, when the Achilles tendon is affected with tendonitis, the inflammation is typically located within the body of the tendon.

Table 5-7 illustrates the interrelationships of the concepts discussed in this chapter. Keep in mind that these are general statements and are not absolute.

Table 5-7 Exercise Terminology

Concentric	Eccentric
Usually open chain	Can be open or closed chain
Usually non-weight-bearing	Can be weight-bearing or non-weight-bearing
Open Chain	**Closed Chain**
Can be concentric or eccentric	Can be concentric or eccentric
Usually non-weight-bearing	Usually weight-bearing
Non-Weight-Bearing	**Weight-Bearing**
Can be concentric or eccentric	Usually eccentric
Usually open chain	Usually closed chain

Points to Remember

- The two ends of a muscle are referred to as the origin or insertion.
- Usually the insertion moves toward the origin.
- When the origin moves toward the insertion, it is referred to as reverse muscle action.
- Active insufficiency is when a muscle cannot contract any farther.
- Passive insufficiency is when a muscle cannot be lengthened any farther.
- Muscle tissue has the properties of irritability, contractility, extensibility, and elasticity.
- Muscle fibers are arranged in either a parallel or an oblique pattern, which favor range or power, respectively.
- Muscle contractions are of three basic types: isometric, concentric, or eccentric.
- A muscle can assume the role of agonist, antagonist, stabilizer, or neutralizer, depending on a particular situation.
- Concentric contraction results in active muscle shortening.
- Eccentric contraction results in active muscle lengthening, whereas stretching results in passive muscle lengthening.
- An overstretched muscle is a weak muscle, whereas a muscle that has undergone adaptive shortening is a tight muscle.

Kinetic chain movement depends on whether the distal segment is fixed (closed-chain) or free to move (open-chain).

Review Questions

1. Usually when a muscle contracts, the distal attachment moves toward the proximal attachment.
   a. What is another name to describe the distal attachment?
   b. What is another name for the proximal attachment?
2. What is the term that describes a muscle contraction in which the proximal end moves toward the distal end?
3. The flexor carpi radialis performs wrist flexion and radial deviation. The flexor carpi ulnaris performs wrist flexion and ulnar deviation.
   a. In what wrist action do the two muscles act as agonists?
   b. In what wrist action do they act as antagonists?
4. The following chart identifies the hip motions of three muscles. Hip extension is the desired motion.

Muscle	Extension	Lateral Rotation	Medial Rotation
Gluteus maximus	X	X	
Hamstrings	X		
Gluteus minimus			X

   a. Which of these muscles are acting as agonists in hip extension?
   b. What motion must be neutralized so the agonists can do only hip extension?
   c. What muscle must act as a neutralizer to rule out the undesired motion?
5. What is the term for the situation in which a muscle contracts until it can contract no farther, even though more joint range of motion is possible?
6. Is walking downhill a concentric or an eccentric contraction of your quadriceps muscle?
7. Sitting with a weight in your hand, forearm pronated, elbow extended, and shoulder medially rotated, slowly move your hand out to the side and raise it.
   a. What is the joint motion at the shoulder?
   b. Is an isometric, concentric, or eccentric muscle contraction occurring at the shoulder?
   c. What muscle group is contracting at the shoulder?
   d. What type of muscle contraction is occurring at the elbow?
   e. What muscle group is contracting at the elbow?
8. While lying supine with your arm at your side and with a weight in your hand, raise the weight up and over your shoulder. (*Hint:* Think about gravity's effect throughout the range.)
   a. What is the joint motion at the shoulder?
   b. Is the muscle action during the first 90 degrees of the motion concentric or eccentric?

Review Questions—cont'd

c. Are the shoulder flexors or extensors responsible for this action?
d. Is the muscle action during the second 90 degrees of the motion concentric or eccentric?
e. Are the shoulder flexors or extensors responsible for this action?

9. Identify the following in terms of open- or closed-kinetic chain activities:
   a. Wheelchair push-ups
   b. Exercises with weight cuffs
   c. Overhead wall pulleys
10. What position would a person have to be in to perform shoulder abduction and adduction in a gravity-eliminated position?
11. For a muscle to have an effective angle of pull to be a shoulder flexor and not a shoulder abductor, it would have to span the shoulder on what surface?
12. The rectus femoris flexes the hip and extends the knee. The vastus medialis extends only the knee. In what position must the hip and knee be placed to be able to stretch only the vastus medialis?
13. If you wanted a muscle to lift a very strong load, what muscle fiber arrangement would you want?
14. If you wanted a muscle to contract through a very great range, what muscle fiber arrangement would you want?
15. In terms of muscle tissue characteristics:
    a. What can a muscle do that a rubber band cannot?
    b. What characteristic does a rubber band have that chewing gum does not?
16. Please perform an analysis of what is happening to the length of the rectus femoris muscle at both the hip and the knee when an individual moves from a seated position to a standing position.

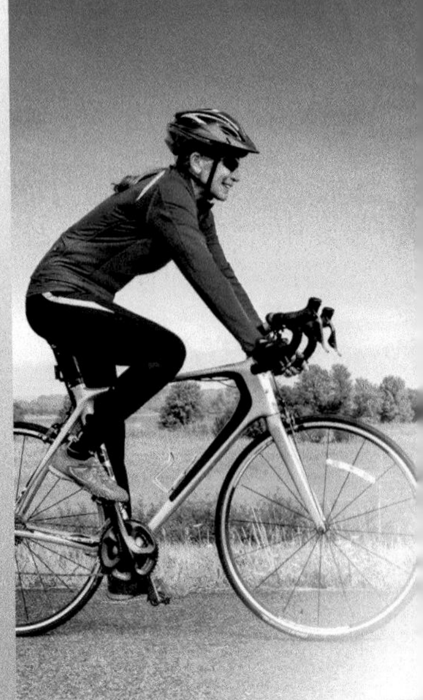

CHAPTER 6
Nervous System

Introduction

Nervous Tissue (Neurons)

The Central Nervous System

Brain

Spinal Cord

The Peripheral Nervous System

Cranial Nerves

Spinal Nerves

Functional Significance of Spinal Cord Level

Plexus Formation

Common Pathologies of the Central and Peripheral Nervous Systems

Common Pathologies of the Central Nervous System

Common Pathologies of the Peripheral Nerves

Review Questions

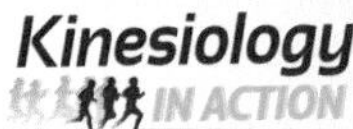

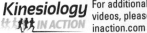

For additional practice activities and videos, please visit www.kinesiologyinaction.com

Introduction

The nervous system is the highly complex mechanism in our bodies that controls, stimulates, and coordinates all other body systems. As outlined in Figure 6-1, it can be divided anatomically into the central nervous system (CNS), which includes the brain and spinal cord; the peripheral nervous system (PNS), which includes nerves outside the spinal cord; and the autonomic nervous system (ANS), which controls mostly visceral structures. The subdivisions of the ANS are the sympathetic and the parasympathetic nervous systems. These operate as a check-and-balance system for each other. The sympathetic system deals with stress and stimulation, and the parasympathetic system deals with conserving energy.

A specific description of the various parts of each system and their functions is beyond the scope of this text. However, we will provide a fairly brief anatomical and functional description of the CNS and PNS as they affect muscle movement. This description will be focused at the gross, not the cellular, level.

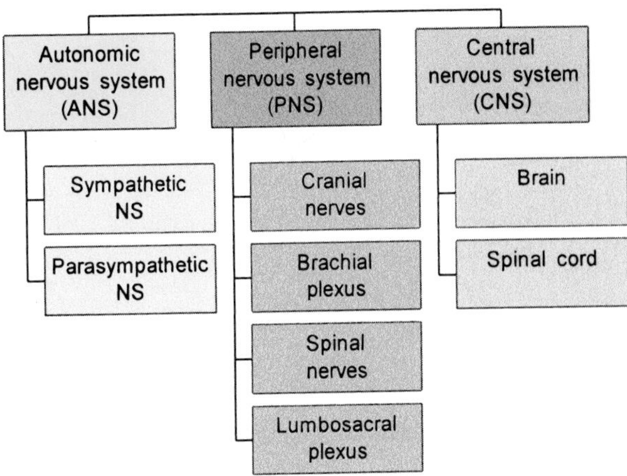

Figure 6-1. Nervous system.

Nervous Tissue (Neurons)

The fundamental unit of nervous tissue is the neuron (Fig. 6-2). Each neuron contains a **cell body** from which extends a single process, called an *axon,* and a variable number of branching processes, called *dendrites.* The term *nerve cell* is synonymous with *neuron* and includes all of its processes (dendrites and axons).

Dendrites are fiber branches that receive impulses from other parts of the nervous system and bring those impulses toward the cell body. **Axons** transmit impulses away from the cell body. They are located on the side opposite the dendrites and usually consist of a single branch. The axon is often surrounded by a fatty sheath called **myelin.** The myelin is interrupted approximately every half millimeter. The breaks in the myelin are referred to as the **node of Ranvier.**

Myelin is a white, fatty substance found in the CNS and PNS. One function is to increase the speed of impulse conduction in the myelinated fiber. Myelin does not cover cell bodies or certain nerve fibers. Areas that contain mostly unmyelinated fibers are referred to as **gray matter,** and areas that contain mostly myelinated fibers are called **white matter** (Fig. 6-3).

Areas of gray matter include the cerebral cortex and the central portion of the spinal cord. White matter includes the major tracts within the spinal cord and fiber systems, such as the internal capsule within the brain.

A **nerve fiber** is the conductor of impulses from the neuron. Transmission of impulses from one neuron to another occurs at a **synapse,** which is a small gap between neurons involving very complex physiological actions.

A **tract** is a group of myelinated nerve fibers within the CNS that carries a specific type of information from one area to another. Depending on the tract's location within the CNS, the group of fibers may be referred to as a *fasciculus, peduncle, brachium, column,* or *lemniscus.* A group of fibers within the PNS may be called a *spinal nerve, nerve root, plexus,* or *peripheral nerve,* depending on its location. (An example of the pathway of a tract can be seen in Fig. 6-15.)

Motor and sensory neurons are the two major types of nerve fibers in peripheral nerves. A **motor (efferent) neuron** has a large cell body with multibranched dendrites and a long axon (see Fig. 6-2A). This cell body and its dendrites are located within the anterior horn of the spinal cord (see Fig. 6-3). Depending on an author's use of terms, *anterior* and *ventral* are synonymous, as are *posterior* and *dorsal.* The axon leaves the anterior horn and is organized with other similar axons in the **anterior root,** which is located just outside the spinal cord in the area of the intervertebral foramen. The axon continues down the peripheral nerve to its termination in a **motor endplate (axon terminal)** of a muscle fiber. A motor neuron conducts **efferent** impulses from the spinal cord to the periphery (see Figs. 6-3 and 6-4).

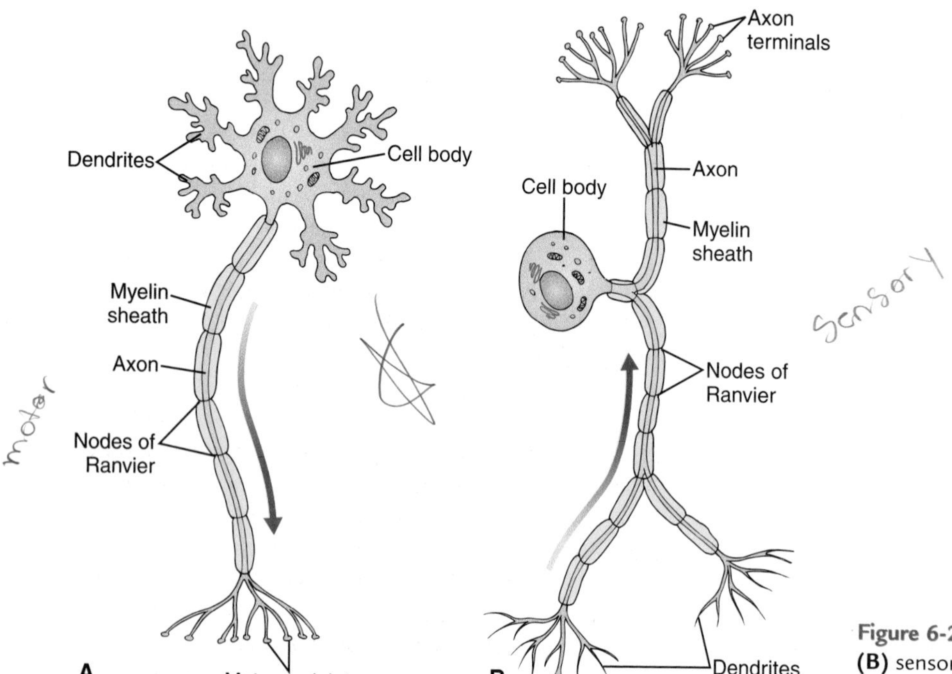

Figure 6-2. Typical **(A)** motor and **(B)** sensory neurons. Arrows indicate the direction that impulses travel.

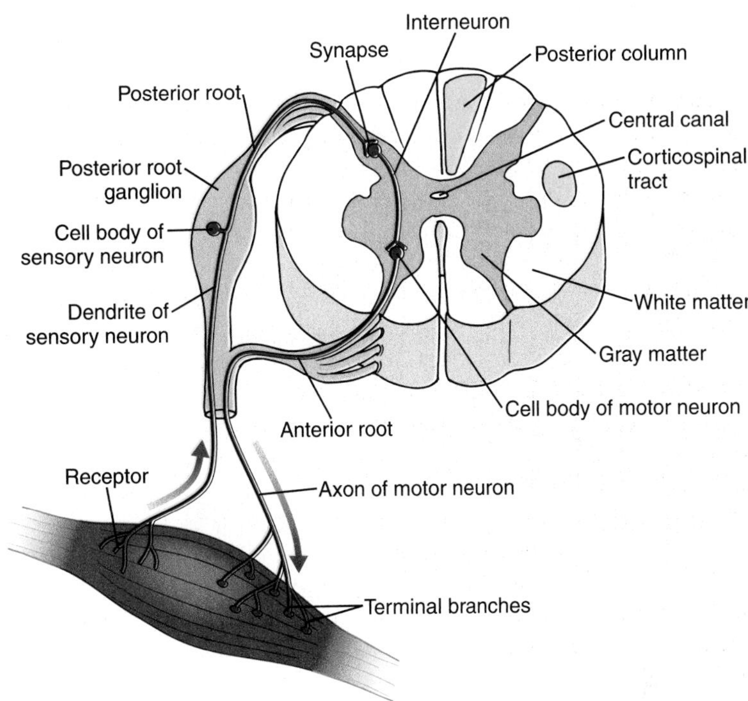

Figure 6-3. Cross section of spinal cord. Note the sensory neuron going into the cord, the motor neuron coming out, and the interneuron connecting the two neurons.

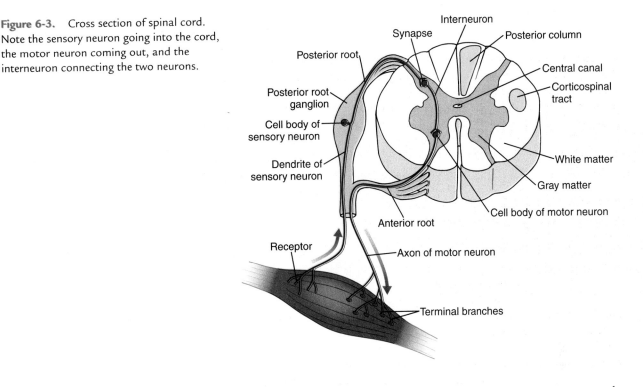

The **sensory (afferent) neuron** has a dendrite, which arises from sensory receptors located in skin, muscles, and joints and runs all the way to its cell body in the posterior root ganglion (Figs. 6-2B and 6-3), located in the intervertebral foramen. The axon travels through the posterior (dorsal) root of the spinal nerve and into the spinal cord through the posterior horn. The axon may end at this point, or it may enter the white matter and ascend to a different level of the spinal cord or to the brainstem. A sensory neuron sends **afferent** impulses from the periphery to the spinal cord (see Figs. 6-3 and 6-4).

Both sensory and motor impulses travel along nerve fibers located outside the spinal cord but within peripheral nerves. As described earlier, motor impulses travel from the CNS to the periphery. Sensory impulses travel from the periphery to the CNS (see Fig. 6-4).

A third type of neuron is an **interneuron** (see Fig. 6-3). It is found within the CNS. Its function is to transmit or integrate signals from one or more sensory neurons and relay impulses to motor neurons.

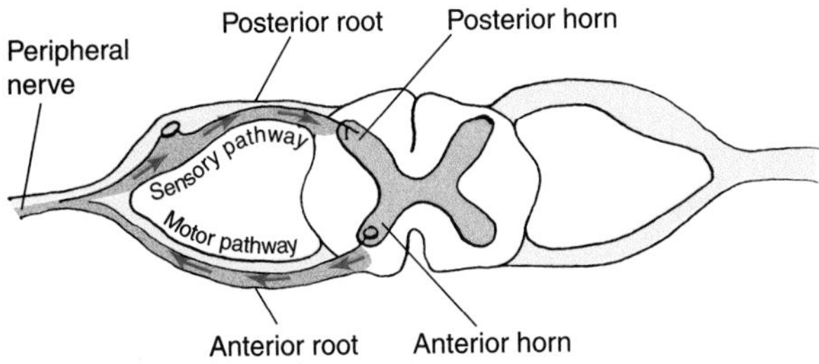

Figure 6-4. Sensory and motor pathways within the spinal cord.

The Central Nervous System

The main components of the CNS are the brain and the spinal cord. The brain is made up of the cerebrum, brainstem, and cerebellum. (Trivia fans will note that the adult brain weighs about 3 pounds.)

Brain

Cerebrum

The **cerebrum** is the largest and main portion of the brain (Fig. 6-5), and it is responsible for the highest mental functions. It occupies the anterior and superior areas of the cranium above the brainstem and cerebellum. The cerebrum is made up of right and left **cerebral hemispheres** joined across the midline by the **corpus callosum.**

Each cerebral hemisphere has a **cortex,** or outer coating, that is many cell layers deep, and each hemisphere is divided into four **lobes** (Fig. 6-6). Each lobe has specific functions. Specific locations of some functions remain undetermined. The **frontal lobe** occupies the anterior portion of the skull. The area of brain activity that controls personality is located here. The frontal lobe also controls motor movement and expressive speech. The **occipital lobe** takes up the posterior portion of the skull. It is responsible for vision and recognition of size, shape,

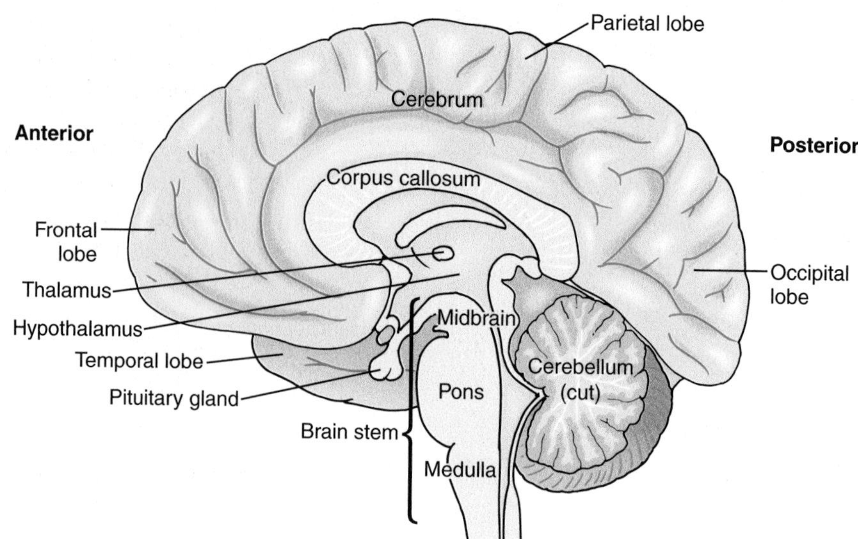

Figure 6-5. Midsagittal section of the brain.

and color. The **parietal lobe** lies between the frontal and occipital lobes. These nerve cells control gross sensation, such as touch and pressure. It also controls fine sensation, such as the determination of texture, weight, size, and shape. Brain activity associated with reading skills is also located in the parietal lobe. The **temporal lobe** lies under the frontal and parietal lobes, just above the ear. This is the center for behavior, hearing, language reception, and understanding.

Deep within the cerebral hemispheres, beneath the cortex, is the **thalamus** (see Fig. 6-5). This mass of nerve cells serves as a relay station for body sensations; it is here where pain is perceived. Deep inside the brain is the **hypothalamus,** which is important for hormone function and behavior. Also in this area is the **basal ganglia** (not shown in figure), which is important in coordination of motor movement.

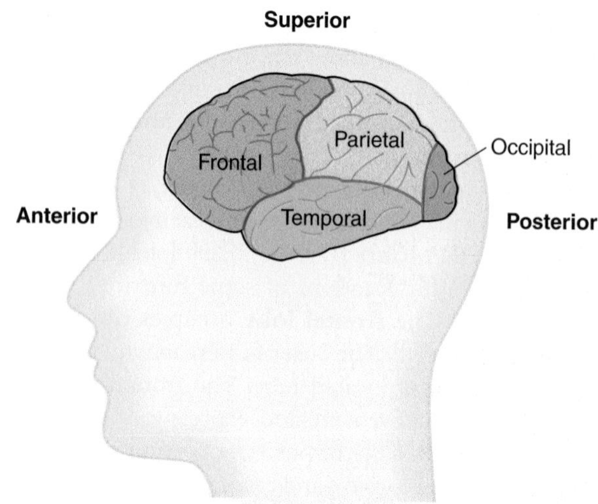

Figure 6-6. Four lobes of the cerebral hemisphere.

Brainstem

Lying below the cerebrum is the brainstem, which can be divided into three parts: the midbrain, the pons, and the medulla (see Fig. 6-5). The upper portion of the brainstem is the midbrain, located somewhat below the cerebrum. The **midbrain** is the center for visual reflexes. Pons is Latin for "bridge" and is located between the midbrain and the medulla. The **medulla oblongata** is the most caudal, or inferior, portion of the brainstem. It is usually referred to simply as the *medulla.* The medulla is continuous with the spinal cord. The transition from the medulla to the spinal cord occurs at the foramen magnum. The medulla is the center for automatic control of respiration and heart rate.

Most of the cranial nerves come from the brainstem, and all fiber tracts from the spinal cord and peripheral nerves to and from higher centers of the brain go through the brainstem.

Cerebellum

In Latin, **cerebellum** means "little brain." It is located in the posterior portion of the cranium behind the pons and medulla (see Fig. 6-5). It is covered superiorly by the posterior portion of the cerebrum. The main functions of the cerebellum are control of muscle coordination, tone, and posture.

Brain Protection

The brain has three basic levels of protection: bony, membranous, and fluid. Surrounding the brain is the **skull,** which is made up of several bones with joints fused together for greater strength (Fig. 6-7).

Within the skull are three layers of membrane called *meninges* (Fig. 6-8). The meninges cover the

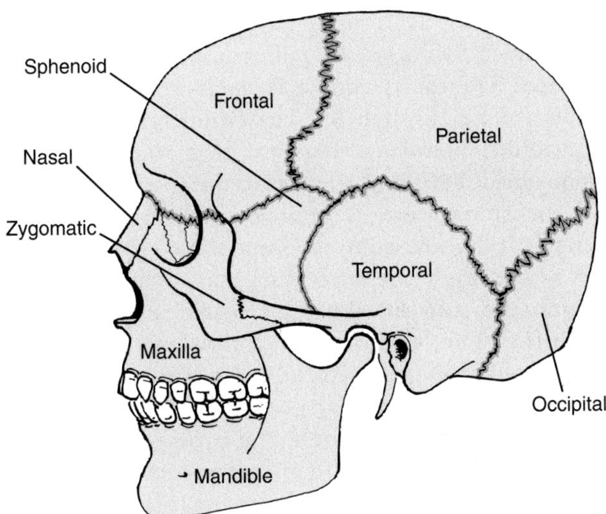

Figure 6-7. Bones of the skull. The fibrous, immovable joints between these bones offer maximum protection.

brain and provide support and protection. The thickest, most fibrous, tough outer layer is called the **dura mater,** which means "hard mother" in Latin. The middle, thinner layer is called **arachnoid** or, less commonly, *arachnoid mater.* (*Arachnoid,* from Greek for *spider,* means "spiderlike.") The inner, delicate layer is called the **pia mater** (Latin for "tender mother"), which carries blood vessels to the brain. These cranial meninges are continuous with the spinal meninges that surround the spinal cord, which will be described later in the chapter.

Between the layers of the arachnoid and pia mater is the **subarachnoid space** through which circulates **cerebrospinal fluid** (see Fig. 6-8). This fluid surrounds the brain and fills the four **ventricles** within the brain. The ventricles are four small cavities containing a capillary network that produces cerebrospinal fluid. There are two lateral ventricles, a third ventricle, and a fourth

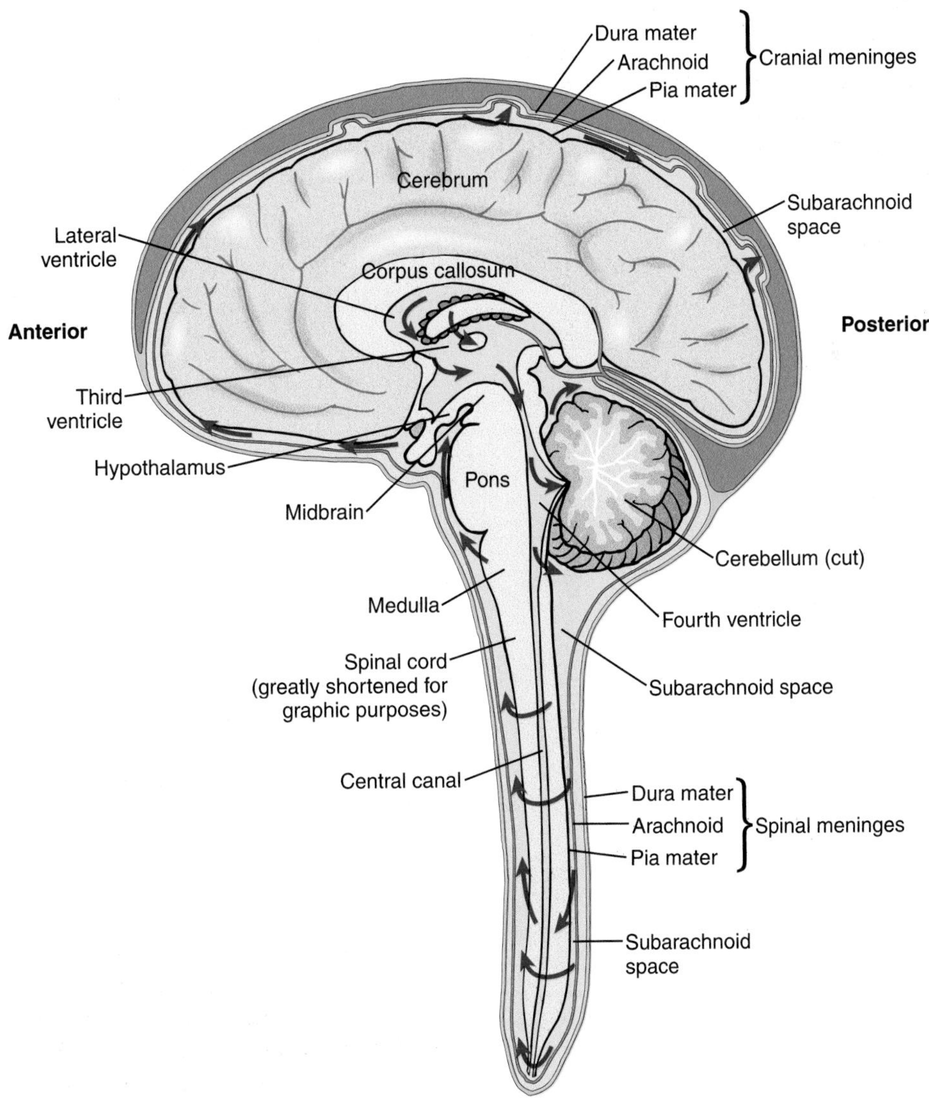

Figure 6-8. Circulation of cerebrospinal fluid. The arrows indicate direction of flow.

ventricle. The main function of the cerebrospinal fluid is shock absorption.

Spinal Cord

A continuation of the medulla, the spinal cord runs within the vertebral canal from the foramen magnum to the cone-shaped **conus medullaris** at approximately the level of the second lumbar vertebra in an adult (Fig. 6-9). Below this level is a collection of nerve roots running down from the spinal cord; these nerve roots look much like a horse's tail, hence the name **cauda equina.** The cauda equina is made up of the nerve roots for L2 through S5. The **filum terminale** is a threadlike, nonneural filament that runs from the conus medullaris and attaches to the coccyx.

The spinal cord is approximately 17 inches in length. It is enclosed in the same three protective layers as the brain: the outer dura mater, the arachnoid membrane, and the inner pia mater (Fig. 6-10). As with the brain, cerebrospinal fluid flows in the subarachnoid space between the arachnoid layer and the pia mater (see Fig. 6-8).

The **vertebral foramen,** the passageway for the spinal cord, is surrounded and protected by the bony structures of each individual vertebra (Fig. 6-11). Each vertebra is made up of the **body,** which is the anterior weight-bearing portion, and the posterior **neural arch** (Fig. 6-12). The opening formed between these two parts is the vertebral foramen. The vertebral foramen is not to be confused with the **intervertebral foramen,** located on the sides of the vertebral column. The intervertebral foramen is the opening formed by the superior vertebral notch of the vertebra below and the inferior vertebral notch of the vertebra above (Fig. 6-13). Through the intervertebral foramen, the spinal nerve exits the vertebral canal.

A cross-sectional view of the spinal cord reveals peripheral white matter and central gray matter

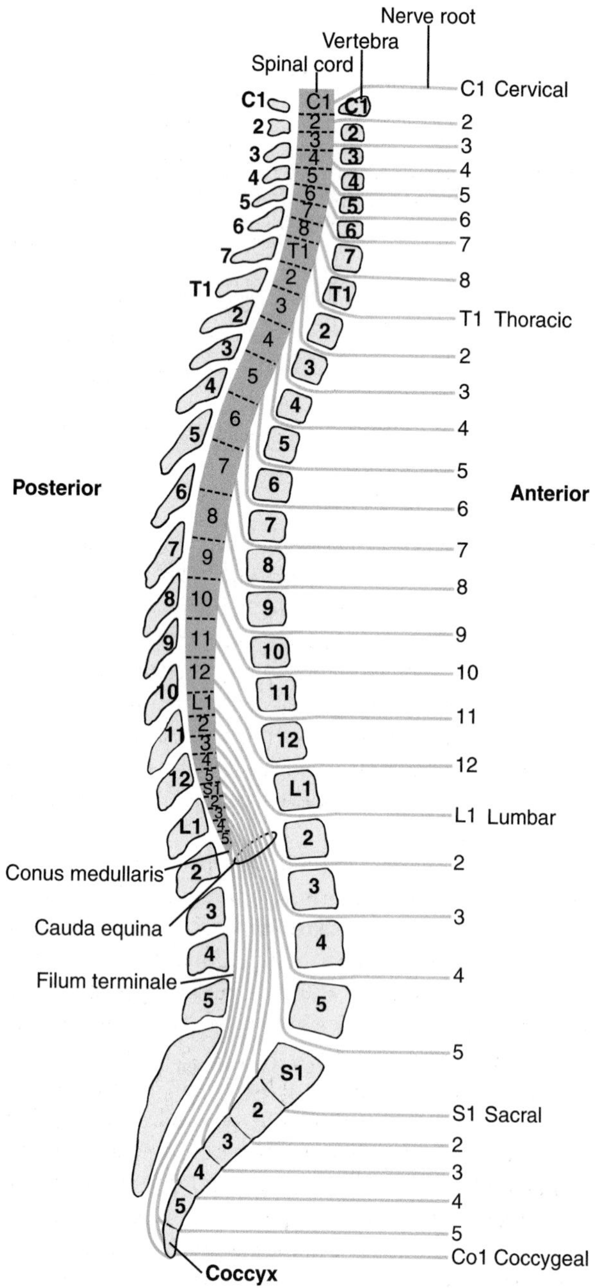

Figure 6-9. Spinal cord.

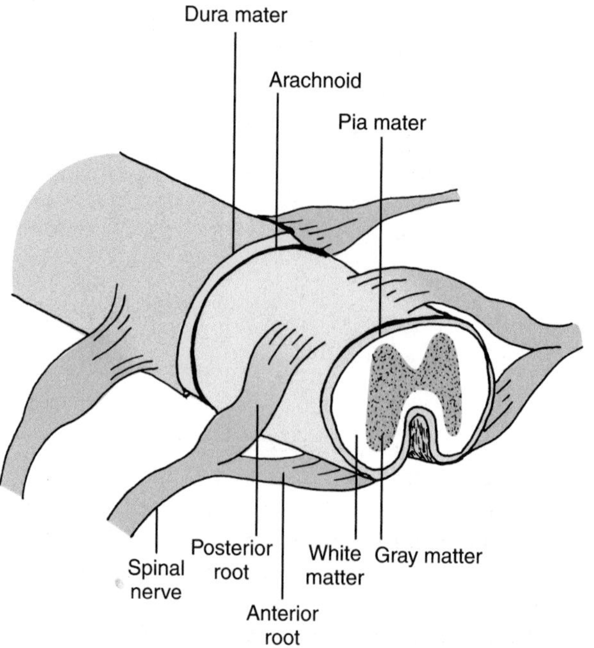

Figure 6-10. The three layers of the meninges are shown as they surround the spinal cord.

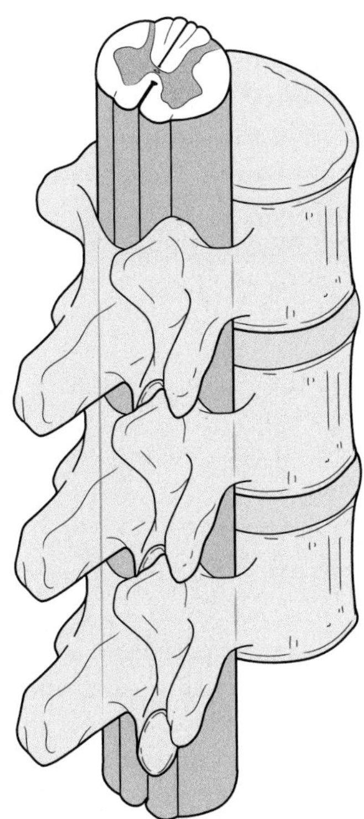

Figure 6-11. The spinal cord runs through the bony vertebral foramen.

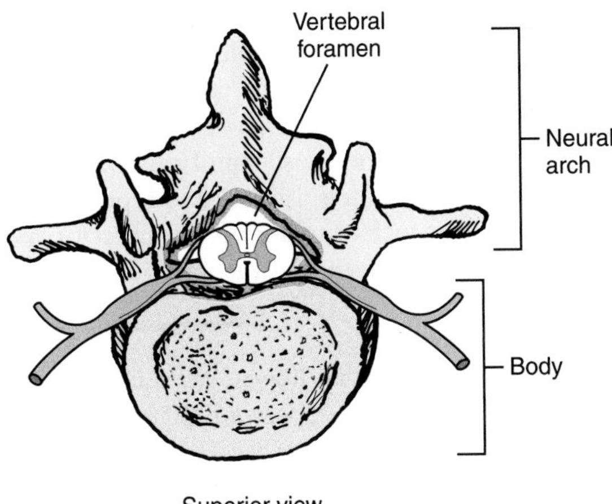

Figure 6-12. The vertebra provides bony protection for the spinal cord.

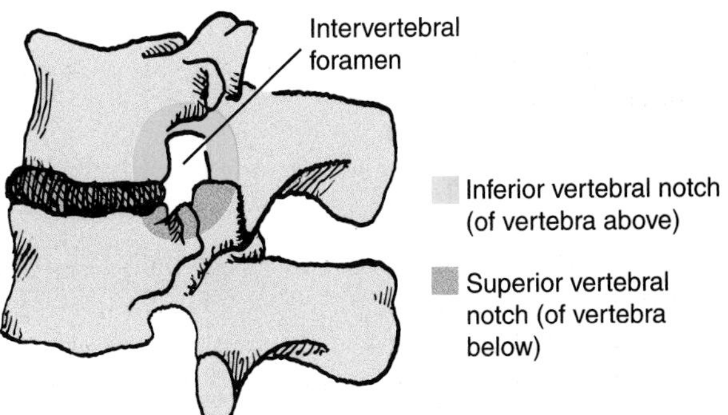

Figure 6-13. Two vertebrae combine to form an opening (intervertebral foramen) on each side through which passes a spinal nerve root.

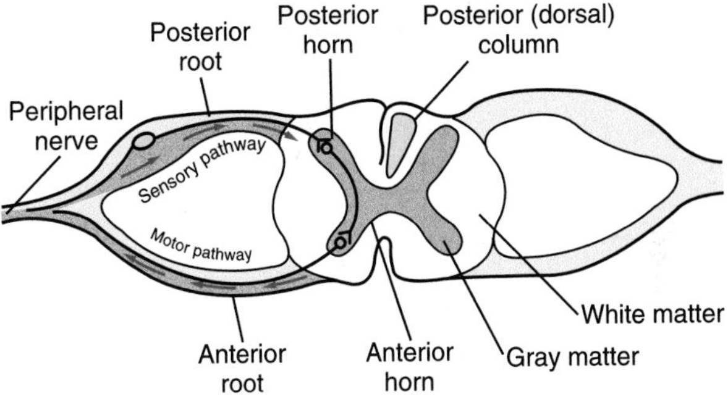

Figure 6-14. Cross section of spinal cord showing gray and white matter.

(Fig. 6-14). The **gray matter** is in the middle of the cord in an **H** or "butterfly" shape. It contains neuronal cell bodies and synapses. The top portion of the **H** is the **posterior horn,** which receives and transmits sensory impulses. The lower portion, the **anterior horn,** transmits motor impulses.

White matter contains ascending (sensory) and descending (motor) fiber pathways. Each pathway carries a particular type of impulse, such as touch, from and to a specific area. These various pathways cross over from one side of the body to the other at different levels. It is this crossover phenomenon that results in a stroke on the left side of the brain affecting the right side of the body.

The **posterior columns,** also called the *dorsal columns,* are located in the posterior medial portions of the spinal cord and are white matter. These columns transmit the sensations of proprioception, pressure, and vibration (see Fig. 6-14).

The pathway of particular significance to muscle control is the **lateral corticospinal tract** (Fig. 6-15). It is located in the lateral column. As its name implies, it runs from the motor area of the cerebral cortex to the spinal cord, crossing over at about the level of the lower part of the brainstem. Corticospinal pathways synapse in the anterior horn just before leaving the spinal cord.

Motor neurons whose cell bodies are located in the cerebral cortex, brainstem, and cerebellum are called **upper motor neurons.** Motor neurons whose cell bodies are located in the anterior horn are called **lower motor neurons.** Injury to these two types of neurons results in quite different clinical signs. In other words, if a lesion occurs proximal to the anterior horn, it is

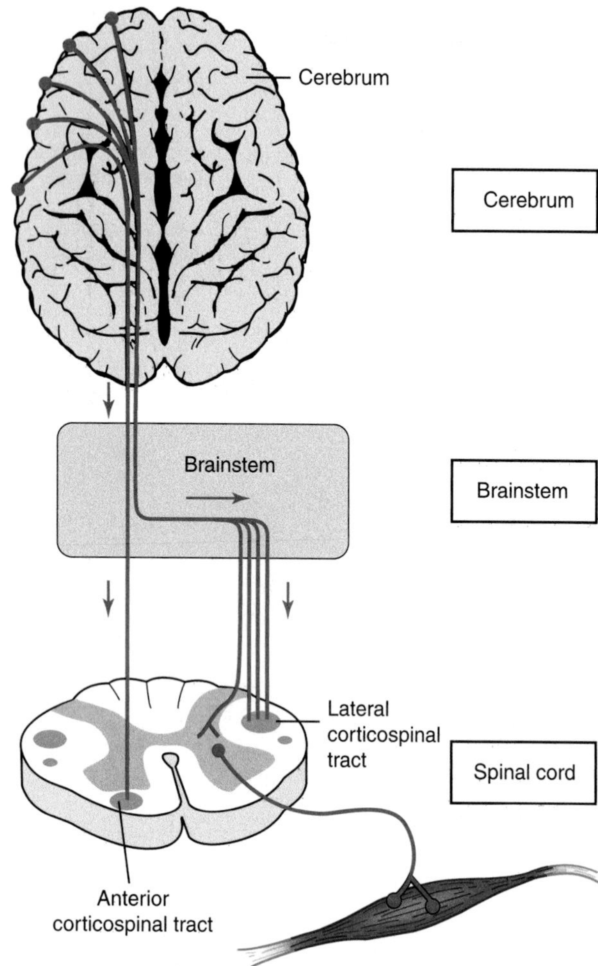

Figure 6-15. Pathway of corticospinal tract from the brain's motor cortex to the spinal cord.

considered an upper motor neuron lesion. If the lesion occurs to the cell bodies or axons of lower motor neurons, it is considered a lower motor neuron lesion. Paralysis will usually result in either case; however, clinical signs differ greatly (these are contrasted in Table 6-1).

Examples of diagnoses involving upper motor neuron lesions include spinal cord injuries, multiple sclerosis, parkinsonism, cerebrovascular accident, and various types of head injuries. Examples of diagnoses involving lower motor neuron lesions are muscular dystrophy, poliomyelitis, myasthenia gravis, and peripheral nerve injuries.

To summarize, motor impulses travel from the brain, down the spinal cord, through the anterior horn, and out to the muscles via peripheral nerves. Sensory impulses from the periphery travel via the peripheral nerves into the spinal cord to the posterior (or dorsal) horn, then up the spinal cord to the brain.

Table 6-1 Clinical Differences Between Upper and Lower Motor Neuron Lesions

Sign	Upper Motor Neuron Lesion	Lower Motor Neuron Lesion
Paralysis	Spasticity present	Flaccid
Muscle atrophy	Not significant	Marked
Fasciculations and fibrillations	Not present	Present
Reflexes	Hyperreflexia	Hyporeflexia
Babinski reflex	Present	Not present
Clonus	Present	Not present

The Peripheral Nervous System

The PNS is, for the most part, made up of all the nervous tissue outside the vertebral canal and brainstem. It actually begins at the anterior horn of the spinal cord, sending motor impulses out to the muscles and receiving sensory impulses from the skin.

Cranial Nerves

There are 12 pair of cranial nerves, which are numbered and named (Fig. 6-16). They are sensory nerves, motor nerves, or mixed nerves (a combination of both). Their functions are summarized in Table 6-2.

Of the 12 cranial nerves, the trigeminal (V), facial (VII), and spinal accessory (XI)—often shortened to *accessory*—nerves are the most significant in terms of their control over certain muscles. The chapters in Parts 2, 3, and 4 will identify innervation of muscles, along with a summary description of each muscle.

Spinal Nerves

There are 31 pair of spinal nerves, including 8 cervical nerves, 12 thoracic nerves, 5 lumbar nerves, 5 sacral nerves, and 1 coccygeal nerve (see Fig. 6-9). The first seven cervical nerves (C1 to C7) exit the vertebral column *above* the corresponding vertebra. For example, the C3 nerve exits above the C3 vertebra. Because there is one more cervical nerve than cervical vertebra, this arrangement changes with the eighth cervical nerve. The C8 nerve exits *under* the C7 vertebra and *over* the T1 vertebra. The T1 nerve exits *under* the T1 vertebra, and so on down the vertebral column (Fig. 6-17).

Branches of Spinal Nerves

Once outside the spinal cord, the anterior (motor) and posterior (sensory) roots join together to form the spinal nerve (Fig. 6-18), which passes through the bony intervertebral foramen. Almost immediately, the nerve

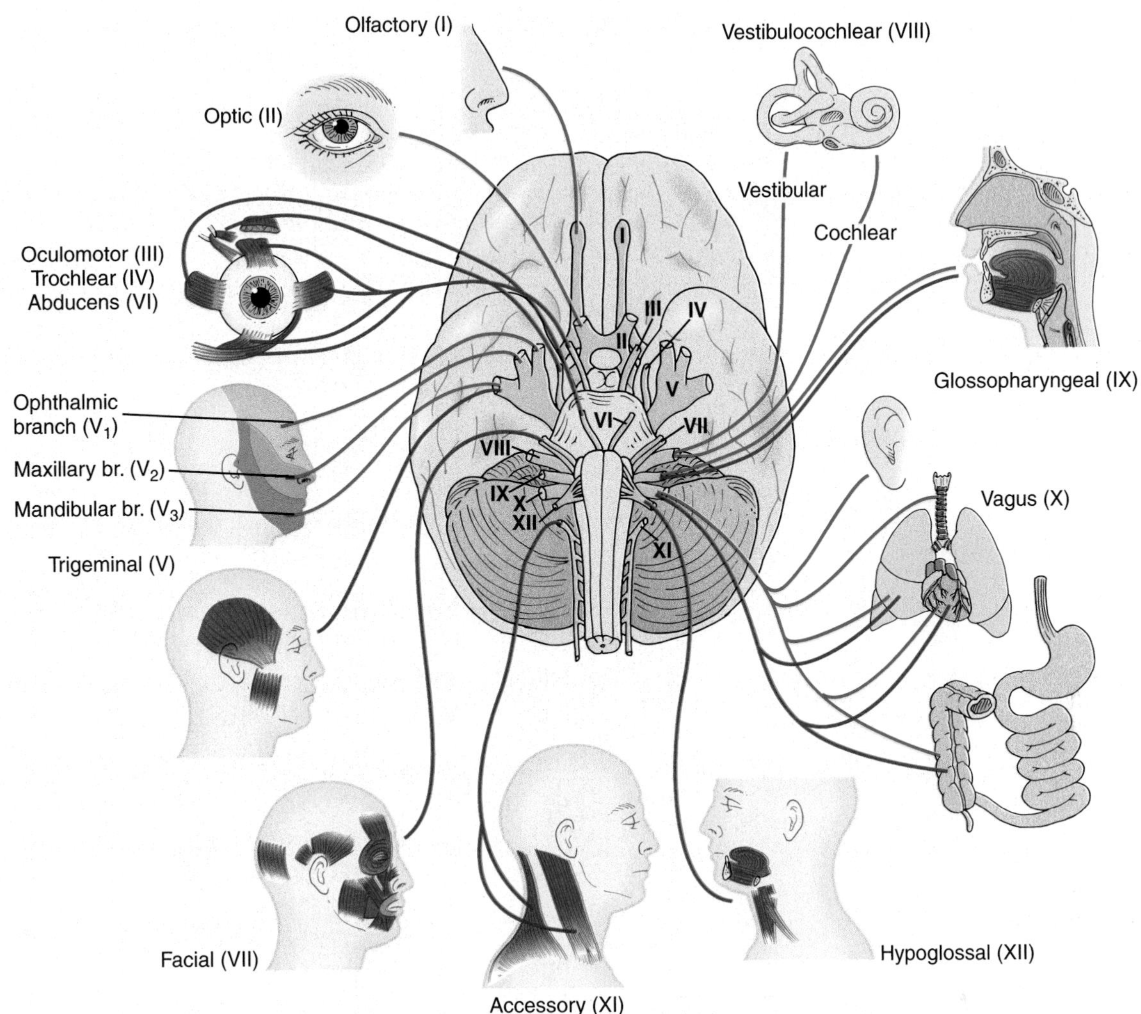

Figure 6-16. Cranial nerves and their distributions.

Table 6-2 Cranial Nerves

Number	Name	Type	Function	Mnemonic*
I	Olfactory	Sensory	Smell	**O**n
II	Optic	Sensory	Vision	**O**ld
III	Oculomotor	Motor	Muscles of eye	**O**lympus
IV	Trochlear	Motor	Muscles of eye	**T**owering
V	Trigeminal	Mixed	Sensory: Face area Motor: Chewing muscles	**T**ops
VI	Abducens	Motor	Muscles of eye	**A**
VII	Facial	Mixed	Sensory: Tongue area Motor: Muscles of facial expression	**F**inn
VIII	Vestibulocochlear (auditory)	Sensory	Hearing Equilibrium sensation	**A**nd
IX	Glossopharyngeal	Mixed	Sensory: Taste, pharynx, middle ear Motor: Muscles of pharynx	**G**erman

Continued

Table 6-2 Cranial Nerves—cont'd

Number	Name	Type	Function	Mnemonic*
X	Vagus	Mixed	Sensory: heart, lungs, GI tract Motor: heart, lungs, GI tract	**V**iewed
XI	Spinal accessory	Motor	Sternocleidomastoid and trapezius muscles	**S**ome
XII	Hypoglossal	Motor	Muscles of tongue	**H**ops

*A mnemonic (pronounced "neh-mon-ik") is a learning aid. In this case, the first letter of each word of the saying is also the first letter of the cranial nerve.

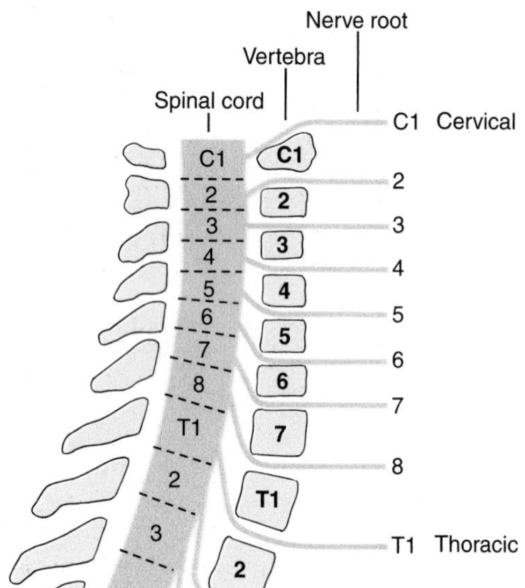

Figure 6-17. Cervical nerve–vertebra relationship.

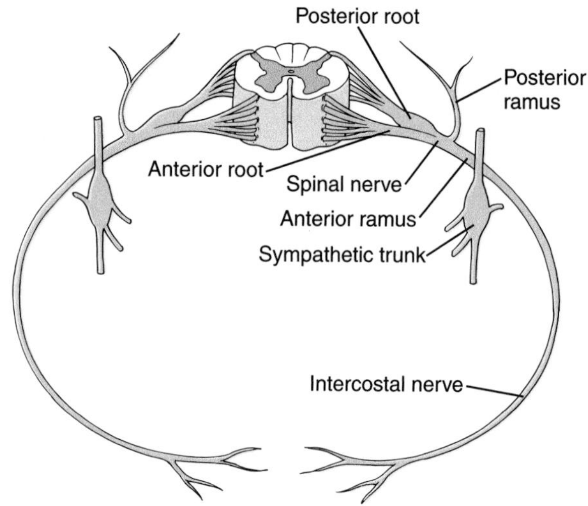

Figure 6-18. Formation of a spinal nerve. In the thoracic region, the spinal nerves form the intercostal nerves.

sends a branch called the **posterior (dorsal) ramus.** As a rule, this branch tends to be smaller than the anterior ramus. It innervates the muscles and skin of the posterior trunk. The spinal nerve continues as the **anterior (ventral) ramus.** These rami (plural of *ramus*) innervate all muscles and skin areas not innervated by the posterior ramus, which includes the anterior and lateral trunk and all the extremities. Located just peripheral to the posterior ramus is a branch to the autonomic nervous system (sympathetic trunk). It is involved with such functions as blood pressure regulation. Although these functions are vital, they will not be discussed here. Instead, we emphasize the motor functions that occur mostly via the anterior ramus. In the thoracic region, the spinal nerves form the intercostal nerves.

Dermatomes

The area of skin supplied with the **sensory fibers** of a spinal nerve is called the **dermatome** (Fig. 6-19). Contiguous dermatomes often overlap. Complete anesthesia of the area will not occur unless more than two spinal nerves have lost function. If an injury involves only one spinal nerve, sensation will be decreased or altered, but it will not be lost.

Thoracic Nerves

There are 12 pairs of thoracic nerves. With the exception of T1, which is part of the brachial plexus, thoracic nerves maintain their segmental relationship and do not join with the other nerves to form a plexus. As described, each nerve branches into a posterior and anterior ramus (see Fig. 6-18). The posterior rami innervate the muscles of the back (motor) and the overlying skin (sensory). The anterior rami become **intercostal nerves,** innervating the anterior trunk and intercostal muscles (motor) as well as the skin of the anterior and lateral trunk (sensory).

Functional Significance of Spinal Cord Level

Remember that the spinal nerves in the cervical region exit the spinal cord *above* the vertebra (see Fig. 6-17). The C8 spinal nerve comes out *below* the C7 vertebra

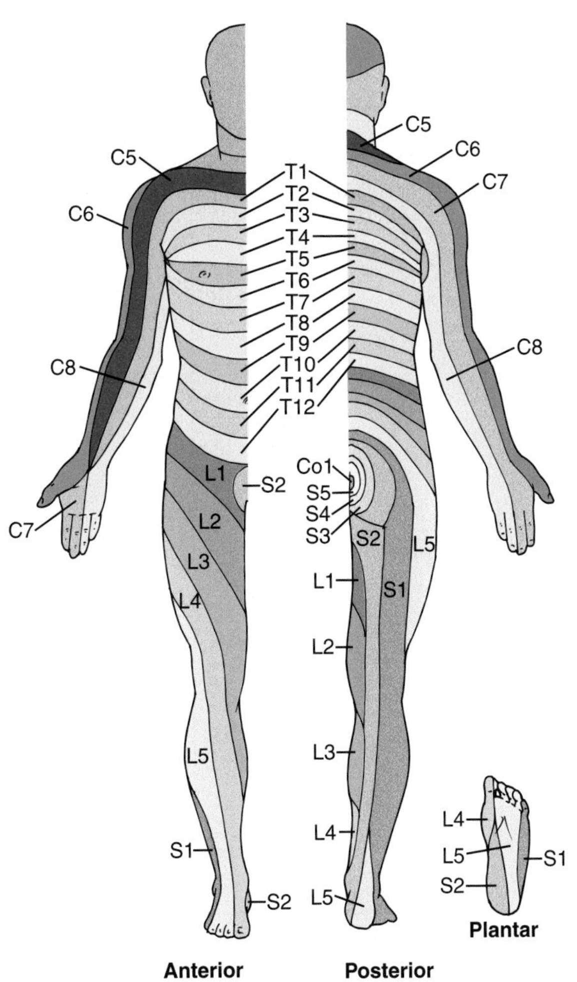

Figure 6-19. Dermatomes: segmental areas of innervation of the skin.

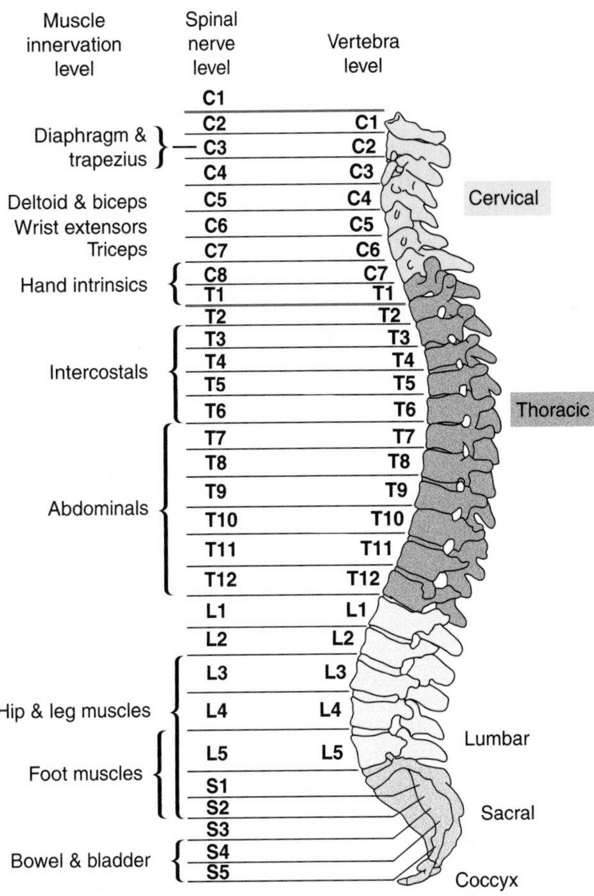

Figure 6-20. General innervation levels of major muscles. Lateral view of vertebral column.

because there is one more cervical nerve than there are vertebrae. Starting with the T1 spinal nerve, all spinal nerves below T1 come out below the same-numbered vertebra.

In Figure 6-20, one can gain an appreciation for the general innervation level of major muscles. It should be noted that most muscles take innervation from more than one spinal level. Therefore, an injury at one spinal level may weaken a muscle, but some function will remain. For example, the elbow flexors receive innervation from the C5 and C6 spinal levels. An injury at the C5 vertebral level will weaken elbow flexion, but function will not be completely lost. This is because the C5 spinal nerve exits the spinal cord above the C5 vertebra, whereas the C6 spinal nerve exits below the C5 vertebra. Therefore, the C5 spinal nerve may not be injured, allowing the elbow flexors to continue to receive partial innervation.

Although there is slight variation among individuals, some general statements can be made about the level of function at various levels of the spinal cord. A person with a spinal cord injury at C3 or above would not have the function of the diaphragm and would be unable to breathe without assistance. Below that level, although breathing would be compromised, a person would probably be able to breathe without assistance. With C5 spinal cord involvement, some innervation of the shoulder abductors and elbow flexors may be present, allowing some function of the upper extremities. The wrist extensors receive innervation from C6 to C8, whereas the triceps are innervated at C7 to C8. The intrinsic muscles of the hand are the lowest to be innervated in the upper extremity at C8 to T1.

In the thoracic level, muscles receive innervation at each spinal level. Because the intercostal and erector spinae muscles receive innervation throughout the thoracic region, the lower the level of injury, the more muscles remain intact. The abdominal muscles receive innervation from the lower thoracic levels.

The muscles of the lumbar and sacral regions are controlled by plexus innervation, so once again the level of injury will be important in knowing which muscles are functioning. The hip flexors and knee extensors are innervated between L2 and L4. Next are the hip adductors at L2 to L4 and the hip abductors at L4 to L5. The hip extensors and knee flexors are innervated at L5 through S2. The ankle muscles are innervated between L4 and S2. Last to receive innervation is bowel and bladder control at S4 to S5.

Sensation changes as one proceeds down the spinal cord. Figure 6-19 shows the sensory innervation (dermatomes) at various levels. A person with a C3 spinal cord injury will have sensation only from the top of the head to the neck. At T3, both entire upper extremities and the chest, level with the axilla, are innervated. An injury at L3 would show loss of sensation in an irregular pattern to approximately the midthigh level.

Plexus Formation

Except for the thoracic nerves, the anterior rami of the spinal nerves will join together and/or branch out, forming a network known as a **plexus.** There are three major plexuses (Fig. 6-21):

1. The cervical plexus, made up of C1 through C4 spinal nerves, innervates the muscles of the neck.
2. The brachial plexus, made up of C5 through T1, innervates muscles of the upper limb.
3. The lumbosacral plexus, made up of L1 through S5, innervates muscles of the lower limb.
   a. The lumbar portion, L1 through L4, supplies mostly muscles of the thigh.
   b. The lumbosacral trunk, made up of L4 and L5.
   c. The sacral portion, S1 through S3, supplies mostly muscles of the leg and foot.

Cervical Plexus

The anterior rami of the first four cervical nerves (C1 to C4) split and join together in a specific pattern to form the **cervical plexus** (see Fig. 6-21). This plexus will not be described in detail because only a few muscles covered in this text receive their innervation from the cervical plexus.

A branch from C2 goes to the sternocleidomastoid, and branches from C3 and C4 supply the trapezius. The levator scapula receives innervation from C3 through C5. The anterior scalene gets some innervation from C4, and the middle scalene gets innervation from C3 and C4. Perhaps one of the most significant nerves of the cervical plexus is the *phrenic nerve,* which is formed by branches of C3 through C5 and innervates the diaphragm.

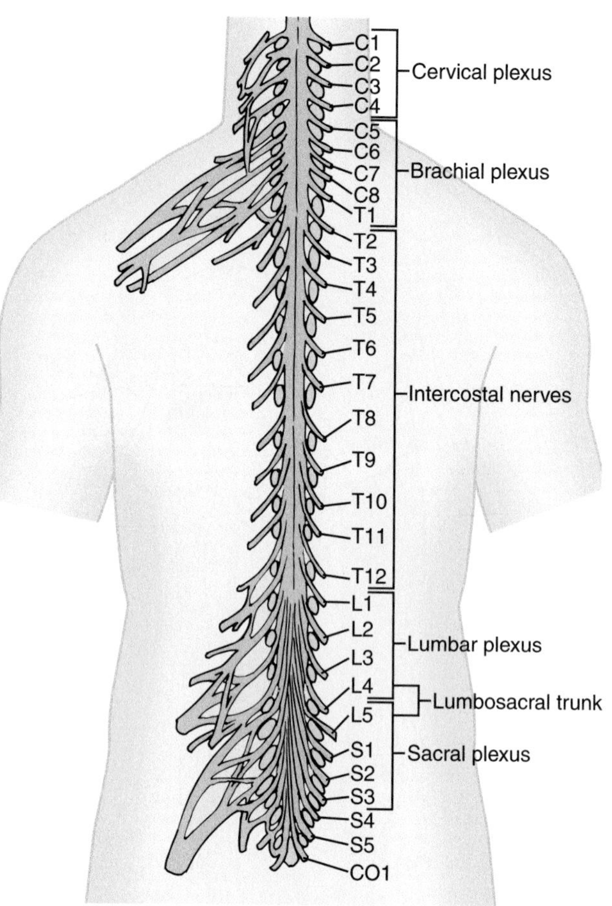

Figure 6-21. Spinal nerves and plexuses.

Brachial Plexus

The **brachial plexus** is formed by the anterior rami of C5 through T1 spinal nerves (see Fig. 6-21). It splits and joins several times before ending in five main peripheral nerves. Its network arrangement consists of roots, trunks, divisions, cords, and peripheral (terminal) nerves, as shown in Figure 6-22.

There are five **roots** made up of the anterior rami of C5, C6, C7, C8, and T1. These roots join together, forming three **trunks.** The three trunks, named for their position relative to each other, are the following:

1. The superior trunk coming from C5 and C6
2. The middle trunk coming from C7
3. The inferior trunk coming from C8 and T1

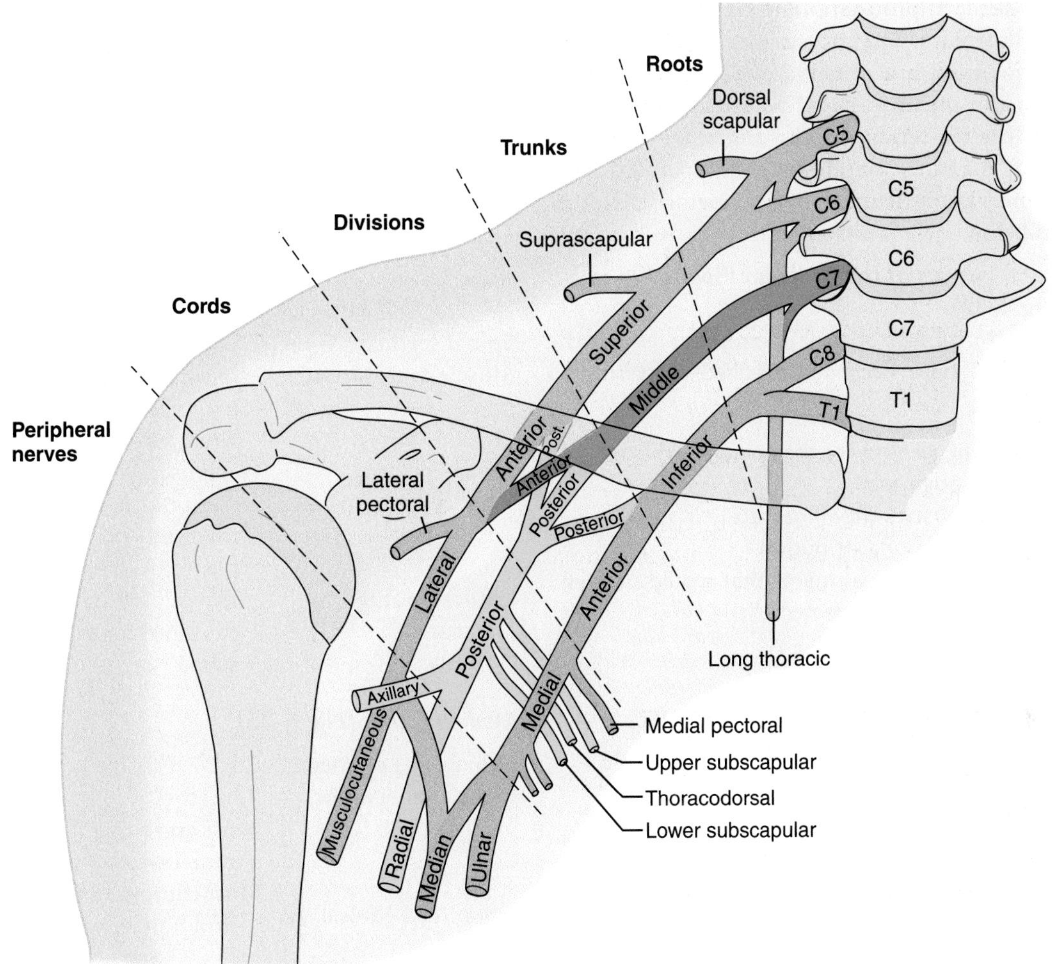

Figure 6-22. Organization of the brachial plexus from the nerve roots to the peripheral nerves. Some lesser motor and sensory nerves have been omitted.

Each trunk splits into an anterior and posterior **division,** named for their positions relative to each other.

Next are the three **cords,** named according to their relationship to the axillary artery. They are formed by the joining of trunk divisions. The lateral cord is formed by the anterior division of the superior and middle trunks. The posterior cord originates from the posterior divisions of all three trunks, and the medial cord comes from the anterior division of the inferior trunk. The five **peripheral nerves,** which are branches of the cords, form the terminal nerves of the plexus as follows:

1. Musculocutaneous nerve: from the lateral cord
2. Axillary nerve: a branch of the posterior cord
3. Radial nerve: a branch of the posterior cord
4. Median nerve: from the lateral and medial cords
5. Ulnar nerve: from the medial cord

This network arrangement provides muscles with innervation from more than one level. In the event of trauma or disease, perhaps not all levels of innervation will be involved. This would result in a muscle being weakened but not completely paralyzed.

For the most part, these five peripheral nerves innervate the muscles of the upper limb; however, some muscles receive innervation from nerves that have branched off the plexus superior to the formation of the peripheral nerves (not shown). The dorsal scapular nerve comes off the anterior ramus of C5 and innervates the rhomboids and levator scapulae muscles. The suprascapular nerve comes off the superior trunk and innervates the supraspinatus and infraspinatus muscles. The medial pectoral nerve comes off the medial cord and innervates the pectoralis major and minor muscles, whereas the lateral pectoral nerve comes off the lateral cord to provide additional innervation to the pectoralis major. The subscapular nerve comes off the posterior cord and innervates the subscapularis and teres major muscles. The thoracodorsal nerve also comes off the posterior cord to innervate the latissimus dorsi. All other muscles of the upper extremity receive innervation from the five terminal nerves described below.

Terminal Nerves of the Brachial Plexus (see Fig. 6-22)

The five terminal, or peripheral, nerves of the brachial plexus have been summarized according to the following:

1. The segment, or root, of the spinal cord from which they originate
2. The major muscles they innervate
3. The major sensory distribution
4. The main motor impairments that would be seen following damage to the nerve

Axillary Nerve (Fig. 6-23)

Spinal cord segment	C5, C6
Muscle innervation	Deltoid, teres minor
Sensory distribution	Lateral arm over lower portion of deltoid
Clinical motor features of paralysis	Loss of shoulder abduction Weakened shoulder lateral rotation

Musculocutaneous Nerve (Fig. 6-24)

Spinal cord segment	C5, C6, C7
Muscle innervation	Coracobrachialis, biceps, brachialis
Sensory distribution	Anterior lateral surface of forearm
Clinical motor features of paralysis	Loss of elbow flexion, weakened supination

Radial Nerve (Fig. 6-25)

Spinal segment	C5, C6, C7, C8, T1
Muscle innervation	Triceps; anconeus; brachioradialis; supinator; wrist, finger, and thumb extensors and abductors
Sensory distribution	Posterior arm, posterior forearm, and radial side of posterior hand
Clinical motor features of paralysis	Loss of elbow, wrist, finger, and thumb extension (commonly called "wrist drop")

Median Nerve (Fig. 6-26)

Spinal cord segment	C6, C7, C8, T1
Muscle innervation	Pronators Wrist and finger flexors on radial side Most thumb muscles, 1st and 2nd lumbricals

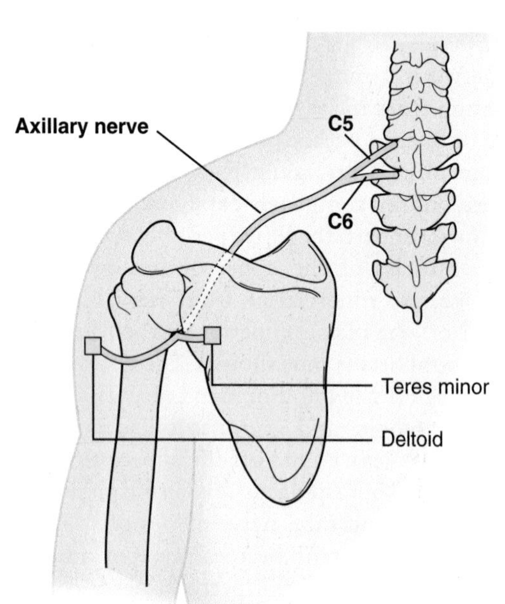

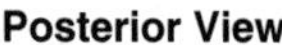

Figure 6-23. Axillary nerve.

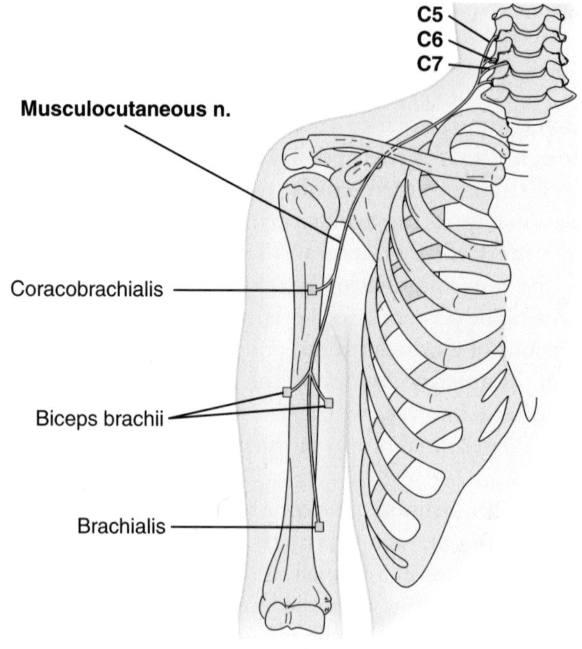

Figure 6-24. Musculocutaneous nerve.

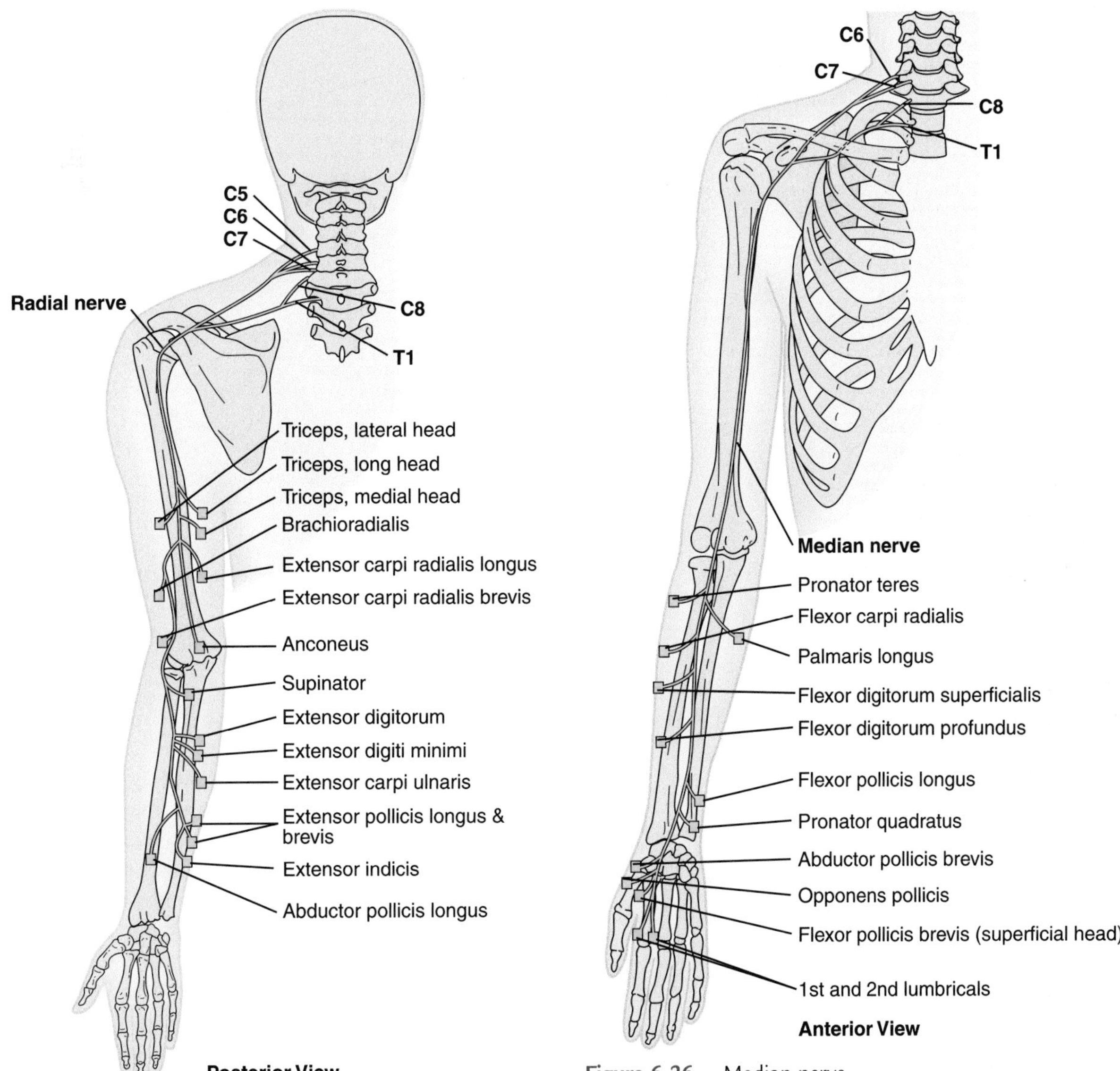

Figure 6-25. Radial nerve.

Figure 6-26. Median nerve.

Sensory distribution	Palmar aspect of thumb, second, third, fourth (radial half) fingers
Clinical motor features	Loss of forearm pronation
	Loss of thumb opposition, flexion, and abduction (“ape hand”), weakened wrist flexors (radial side), weakened wrist radial deviation
	Weakened second and third finger flexion (“pope’s blessing” or “hand of benediction”)

Ulnar Nerve (Fig. 6-27)

Spinal cord segment	C8, T1
Muscle innervation	Flexor carpi ulnaris
	Flexor digitorum profundus (medial half)
	Interossei
	3rd and 4th lumbricals, muscles of 5th finger
Sensory distribution	Fourth finger (medial portion), fifth finger
Clinical motor features of paralysis	Loss of wrist ulnar deviation
	Weakened wrist, finger flexion
	Loss of thumb adduction
	Loss of most intrinsics (“claw hand”)

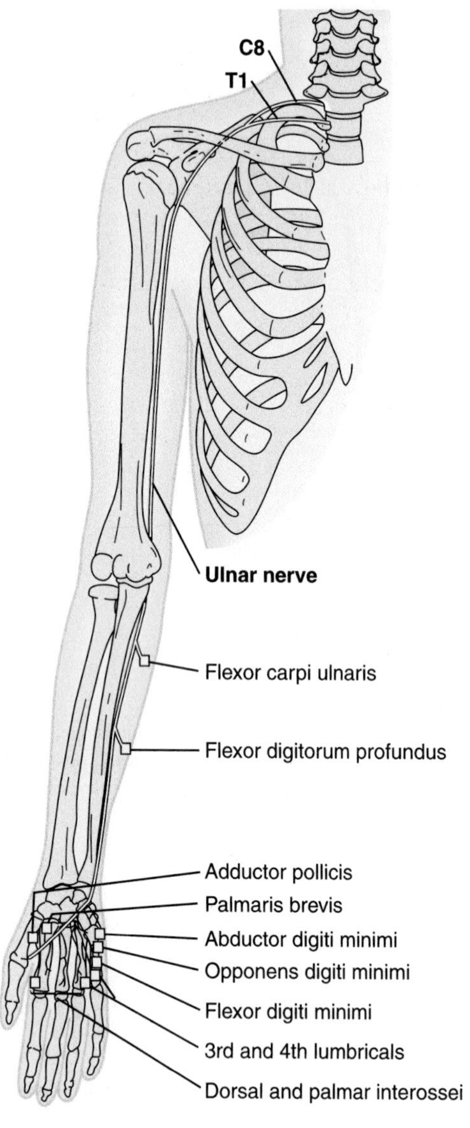

Figure 6-27. Ulnar nerve.

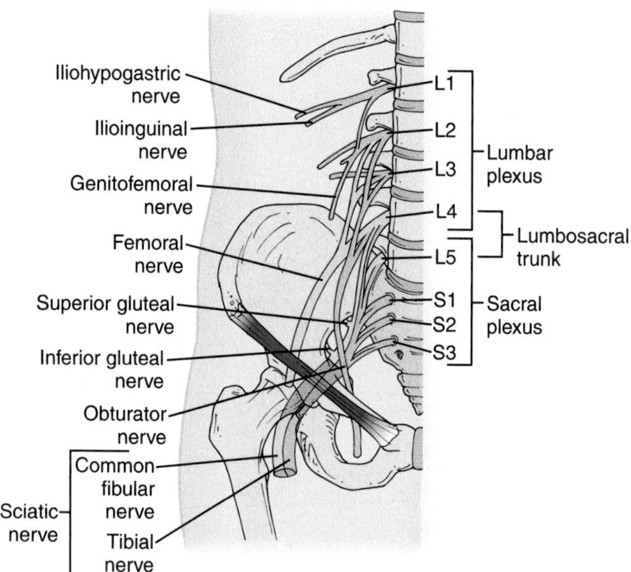

Figure 6-28. Lumbosacral plexus (anterior view). Note that anterior divisions are in yellow and posterior divisions are in green. Some lesser motor and sensory nerves have been omitted.

Lumbosacral Plexus

The lumbosacral plexus is formed by the anterior rami of L1 through S3 (Fig. 6-28). Some sources separate the lumbosacral plexus into a **lumbar plexus** (L1 through L4), which innervates most muscles of the thigh and the **sacral plexus** formed by the lumbosacral trunk (L4 and L5) and the anterior rami of S1 through S3, which innervates mostly muscles of the leg and foot. Because there are several muscles of the lower limb that receive innervation from both the lumbar and sacral plexuses, they will be discussed here as one, the lumbosacral plexus. S3 through S5 innervate the perineum and pelvic floor.

The lumbosacral plexus does not have as much dividing and joining of nerve fibers as does the brachial plexus, although there are some. This plexus has eight roots, each dividing into upper and lower rami. Most of these rami divide into an anterior and posterior division. These divisions join in a specific pattern to form the seven main peripheral nerves.

The upper branch of L1 divides into the iliohypogastric and ilioinguinal nerve fibers. The lower branch of L1 and the upper branch of L2 form the genitofemoral nerve. These three nerves are primarily sensory in nature and will not be discussed in detail.

The anterior divisions of L2, L3, and L4 form the **obturator nerve.** Posterior divisions of the same roots form the **femoral nerve.** The posterior divisions of L4 through S1 form the **superior gluteal nerve,** and the posterior divisions of L5 through S2 make up the **inferior gluteal nerve.** The **sciatic nerve** is made up of branches from L4 through S3. It is actually the tibial and common fibular (peroneal) nerves joined by a common sheath, and it separates into the two nerves just above the knee. The **common fibular nerve** comes from posterior divisions of L4 through S2, whereas the **tibial nerve** is made up of anterior divisions of L4 through S3. If all of this is confusing, perhaps the illustrations in Figures 6-29 through 6-33, plus the summary that follows, will provide some clarity.

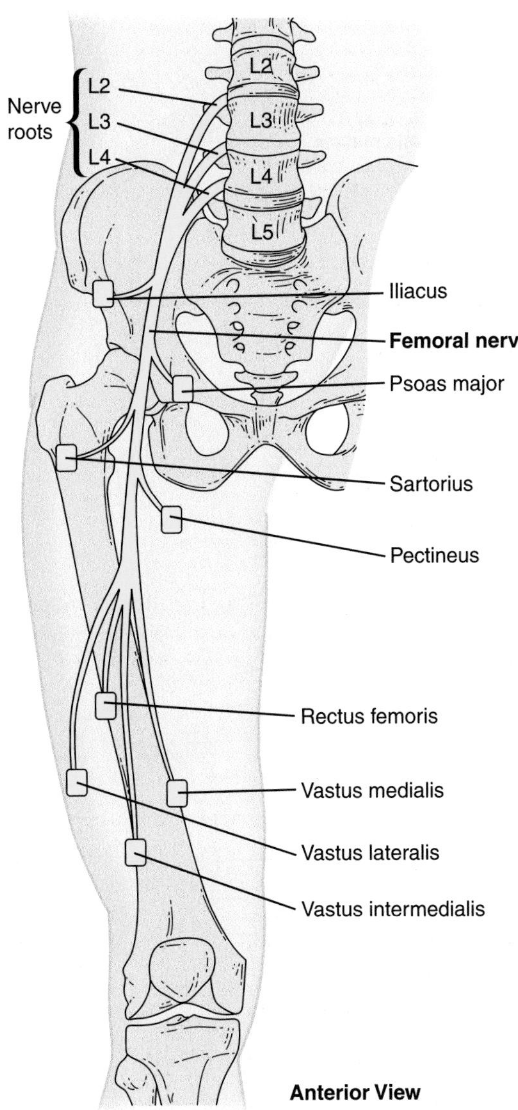

Figure 6-29. Femoral nerve.

This summary is similar to the one provided for the brachial plexus.

Terminal Nerves of the Lumbosacral Plexus

Like the nerves of the upper extremity, the nerves of the lower extremity have been summarized according to the following:

1. The segment, or root, of the spinal cord from which they come
2. The major muscles they innervate
3. The major sensory distribution
4. The main motor impairments that would be seen following damage to the nerve

Femoral Nerve (Fig. 6-29)

Spinal cord segment	L2, L3, L4
Muscle innervation	Iliopsoas (iliacus and psoas major), sartorius, pectineus, quadriceps femoris
Sensory distribution	Anterior and medial thigh, medial leg, and foot
Clinical motor features of paralysis	Weakened hip flexion, loss of knee extension

Obturator Nerve (Fig. 6-30)

Spinal cord segment	L2, L3, L4
Muscle innervation	Hip adductors Obturator externus

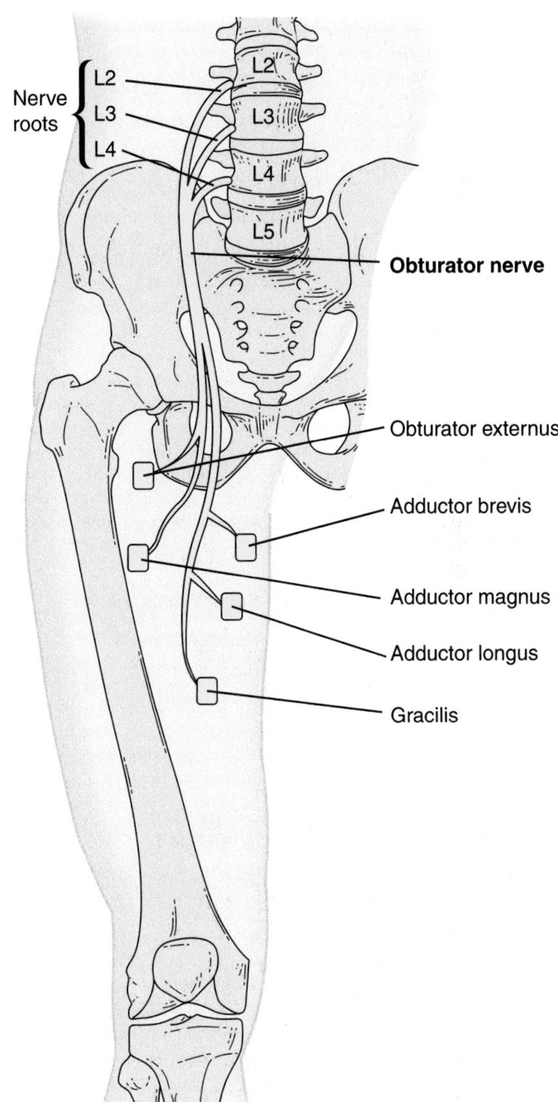

Figure 6-30. Obturator nerve.

Sensory distribution	Middle part of medial thigh
Clinical motor features of paralysis	Loss of hip adduction, weakened hip lateral rotation

Sciatic Nerve (Made up of Tibial and Common Fibular (Peroneal) Nerves; Fig. 6-31)

Spinal segment	L4, L5, S1, S2, S3
Muscle innervation	Hamstring muscles, adductor magnus
Sensory distribution	None
Clinical motor features of paralysis	Weakened hip extension, loss of knee flexion

Tibial Nerve (Divides into the Medial and Lateral Plantar Nerves; Fig. 6-32)

Spinal cord segment	L4, L5, S1, S2, S3
Muscle innervation	Popliteus Ankle plantar flexors (gastrocnemius & soleus) Tibialis posterior, flexor digitorum longus, flexor hallucis longus foot intrinsics (medial and lateral plantar)

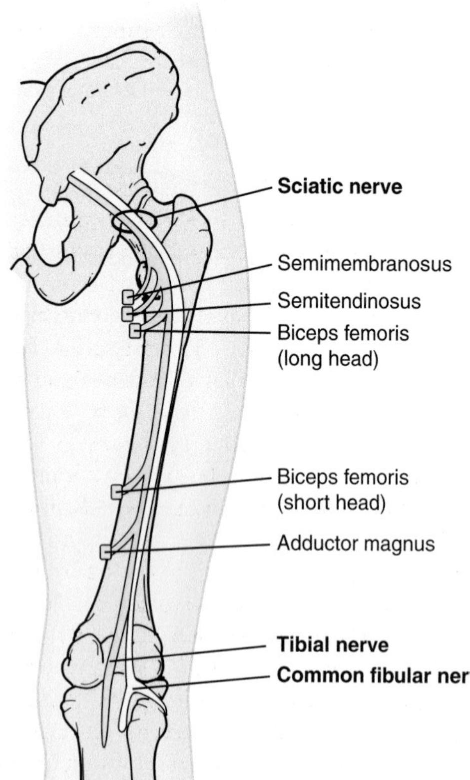

Figure 6-31. Sciatic nerve.

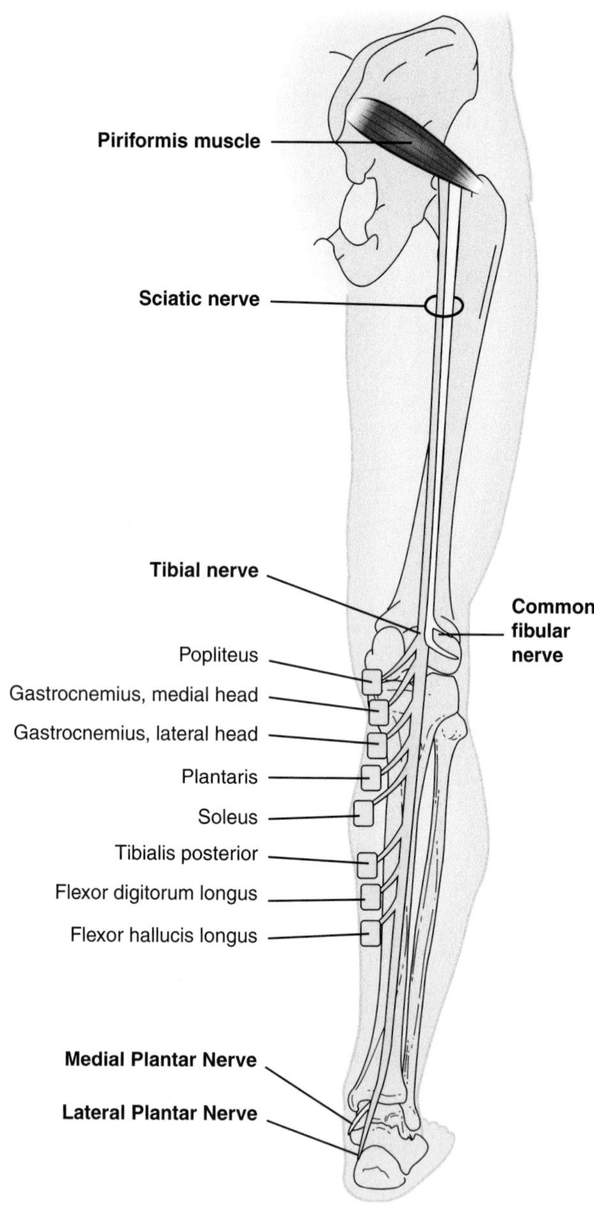

Figure 6-32. Tibial nerve. It divides into the medial and lateral plantar nerves.

Sensory distribution	Posterior lateral leg, lateral foot
Clinical motor features of paralysis	Loss of ankle plantar flexion, weakened ankle inversion, loss of toe flexion

Common Fibular (Peroneal) Nerve (Divides into Superficial and Deep Fibular [Peroneal] Nerves; Fig. 6-33)

Spinal segment	L4, L5, S1, S2
Muscle innervation	Fibularis longus and brevis (superficial fibular) Tibialis anterior (deep fibular) Toe extensors (deep fibular)

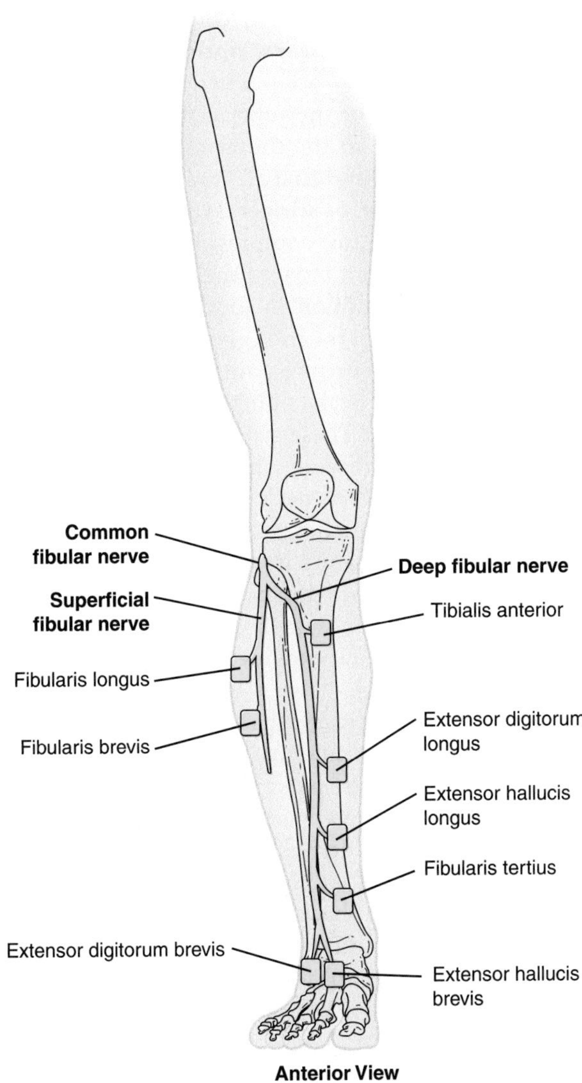

Figure 6-33. Fibular (peroneal) nerves. The common fibular nerve divides into the superficial and deep fibular nerves.

Sensory distribution	Anterior lateral aspect of leg and foot
Clinical motor features of paralysis	Loss of ankle dorsiflexion ("foot drop"), loss of toe extension, loss of ankle eversion

Common Pathologies of the Central and Peripheral Nervous Systems

The following is a very incomplete list of common central and peripheral nerve system pathologies. The very brief description focuses on the anatomical location or the functional implications of the defect or disease.

Common Pathologies of the Central Nervous System

Congenital Defects

Spina bifida is a congenital defect in which the posterior segments of some of the vertebrae fail to close during embryo development. There are three types, ranging from few or no signs and symptoms to quite severe symptoms. With **spina bifida occulta,** a small bony defect is present, but the spinal cord and nerves are usually normal. With **meningocele,** there is a bony defect through which the meninges protrude. There is usually little or no nerve damage. With **myelomeningocele,** the most severe form of spina bifida, the meninges and spinal nerves come through the bony defect. This causes nerve damage and severe disability.

Hydrocephalus, once called "water on the brain," is a congenital or acquired defect involving cerebrospinal fluid (CSF) production, absorption, and flow through the ventricles and subarachnoid space. An excessive accumulation of CSF results in an abnormal widening of the ventricles, which creates potentially harmful pressure on the brain tissues.

Cerebral palsy is a term used to describe a group of nonprogressive disorders of the brain that result from damage in utero, at birth, or soon after birth. It is not always congenital. The signs and symptoms of cerebral palsy are variable and depend on the area of the brain that is damaged.

Spinal Cord Trauma

Spinal cord injury (SCI) can take many forms, depending on (1) the spinal level and (2) the area of the damage. These injuries usually result in loss of sensation and muscle function. SCIs are divided into two categories, based on level. *Quadriplegia,* which refers to all four extremities, involves T1 and above. *Paraplegia* refers to lower extremity involvement of T2 and below.

An incomplete SCI can result when only part of the cord is damaged. **Central cord syndrome** is associated with greater loss of upper limb function compared with the lower limbs. **Brown-Séquard syndrome** results from injury to one side of the spinal cord, causing weakness and loss of proprioception on the side of the injury and loss of pain and thermal sensation on the opposite side. **Anterior cord syndrome** occurs when the injury affects the anterior spinal tracts. Because the posterior part of the cord is spared, proprioception that is carried in that part of the cord is preserved, but muscle function, pain sensation, and thermal sensation are lost.

Autonomic dysreflexia, also known as **hyperreflexia,** is a serious and potentially life-threatening complication associated with spinal cord injuries at or above T10. It is usually triggered by a noxious stimulus below the level of injury, such as a distended bladder. Symptoms include severe headache, sudden hypertension, facial flush, sweating, and gooseflesh. Blood pressure may rise to dangerous levels. Untreated, it can lead to stroke or death.

Disorders of Muscle and the Neuromuscular Junction

Myasthenia gravis is a disease that involves a defect at the neuromuscular junction, where the terminal axon synapses with the receptor site of muscles. This results in weakness and fatigue of skeletal muscles.

Muscular dystrophy is a hereditary and progressive disease of the muscle tissue. It is characterized by weakness of proximal muscles, followed by progressive involvement of distal muscles.

Degenerative Diseases

Amyotrophic lateral sclerosis (ALS) is a degenerative motor disease involving both upper and lower motor neurons. It is also known as Lou Gehrig's disease.

Alzheimer's disease is an irreversible, progressive brain disorder causing dementia and loss of cognitive functioning. It eventually destroys a person's ability to function.

Demyelinating Diseases

Multiple sclerosis is characterized by a breaking down of the myelin sheath around axons. This will interfere with normal nerve transmission. *Sclerosis* refers to scars or lesions in the white matter of the brain and spinal cord.

Common Pathologies of Peripheral Nerves

Neuropathy of a peripheral nerve is usually accompanied by neurological deficits along the nerve pathway. They are usually classified according to cause or anatomical location. Sensory distribution and clinical motor features of paralysis have been described earlier, with the individual nerves. The following is a very brief description of some of the more common peripheral nerve conditions.

Typical muscle paralysis patterns can be seen depending on the peripheral nerve involved and the level at which it is injured. **Bell's palsy** involves the facial nerve (cranial nerve VII), which controls movement of facial muscles. The condition is usually temporary and typically affects only one side of the face.

The following conditions commonly affect the upper extremities. **Scapular winging** occurs when an injury to the long thoracic nerve weakens or paralyzes the serratus anterior muscle, causing the medial border of the scapula to rise away from the rib cage.

There are three well-known conditions involving the brachial plexus. **Thoracic outlet syndrome** is a group of disorders that occur when the nerves of the brachial plexus and/or the subclavian artery and vein become compressed in the thoracic outlet—the space between the clavicle and first rib and possibly the scalene muscles. **Burner,** or **stinger, syndrome** can occur following a stretch or compression injury to the brachial plexus from a blow to the head or shoulder. This is relatively common in football players and is also seen in wrestlers and gymnasts. Symptoms include immediate burning pain, prickly paresthesia radiating from the neck, numbness, and even brief paralysis of the arm. These symptoms should resolve within minutes, although shoulder weakness and muscle tenderness of the neck may continue for a few days. **Erb's palsy** (sometimes known as *tip position*) is a traction injury to a baby's upper brachial plexus and occurs most commonly during a difficult childbirth. The affected arm hangs in shoulder extension and medial rotation, elbow extended, forearm pronated, and wrist flexed.

There are two conditions that affect the radial nerve in approximately the same location but have different causes. **Saturday night palsy** occurs when the radial nerve becomes compressed as it spirals around the midhumerus. The name derives from the nature of the injury—the person, often intoxicated, falls asleep with his or her arm over the back of a chair. **Wrist drop** (loss of wrist extension) and a weakened ability to release objects (finger extension) will result from a high radial nerve injury, which is often a complication of a midhumeral fracture.

Carpal tunnel syndrome is the result of compression of the median nerve as it passes within the carpal tunnel. The tunnel is formed by the transverse carpal ligament superficially and the bony floor of the carpal bones deeply. A similar condition called **cubital tunnel syndrome** occurs when the ulnar nerve crosses the medial border of the elbow as the nerve runs through a bony passageway called the *cubital tunnel*. When you "hit your funny bone" and have tingling in the small and ring fingers, you are hitting the ulnar nerve at the cubital tunnel. The ulnar nerve can also be compressed distally by sustained pressure on the hypothenar eminence such as leaning on handle bars during long bicycle rides.

The following conditions describe hand positions that result from specific nerve damage. Loss of thumb opposition *(median nerve injury)* is referred to as **ape hand** because, like apes, the person is unable to oppose the thumb. Inability to flex the thumb and index and middle fingers (also median nerve injury) gives the appearance of the **pope's blessing,** or **hand of benediction.** Loss of the intrinsic muscles due to ulnar nerve damage results in a **claw hand.** The proximal phalanges are hyperextended, and the middle and distal phalanges are in extreme flexion.

The following conditions commonly affect the lower extremity. **Sciatica** is caused by irritation of the sciatic nerve roots, with pain radiating down the back of the leg. It is often caused by compression from a herniated lumbar disc.

Damage to the common fibular (peroneal) nerve can result in **foot drop.** Compression of the common fibular nerve is often caused by cast pressure at the head of the fibula, where the nerve is quite superficial as it lies over the bony fibular head.

Morton's neuroma is an enlarged nerve and usually occurs between the third and fourth toes (branches of the tibial nerve). The enlargement usually involves nerve compression in a confined space. Compression could be from a flattening of the metatarsal arch; wearing high heels, which transfers weight forward, putting more pressure on the metatarsal arch area; or wearing a shoe with a tight toe box, creating compression on the nerves as they pass between the metatarsals.

Review Questions

1. The spinal cord extends to about what vertebral level?
2. What makes up gray matter? White matter?
3. Name the bony, membranous, and fluid features that protect the brain from trauma.
4. What are the differences between upper and lower motor neurons?
5. How do thoracic nerves differ from cervical or lumbar nerves?
6. What is the difference between an afferent and an efferent nerve fiber?
7. In an individual who has lost the ability to oppose the thumb, what nerve is involved? What is a common term for this condition?
8. In an individual who has lost the ability to pick up the toes (ankle dorsiflexion), what nerve is involved? What is a common term for this condition?
9. Claw hand involves the loss of what muscle group? What nerve is primarily involved?
10. If a person had a subdural hematoma from a blow to the head, where would that hematoma be located?
11. If a person had pressure on a nerve root, what bony area is likely to be involved?
12. If a person has a spinal cord injury at L4, would it be considered an upper or lower motor neuron lesion?
13. Would the spinal cord injury at L4 show clinical signs more like a spinal cord lesion or a peripheral nerve lesion? Why?
14. Does a motor nerve send impulses from the periphery to the spinal cord or from the spinal cord to the periphery?

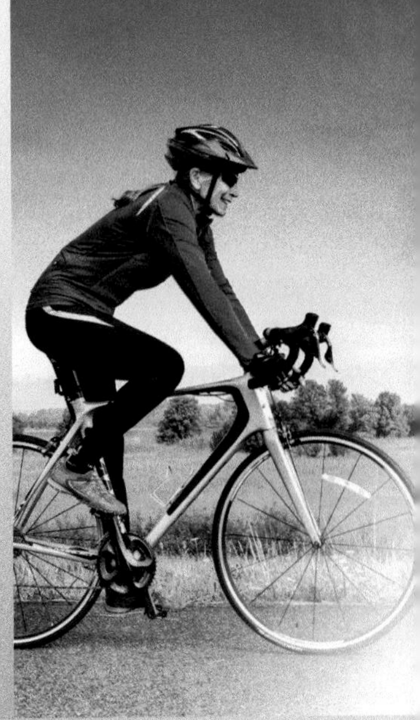

CHAPTER 7 Circulatory System

Cardiovascular System

Heart

Blood Vessels

Lymphatic System

Functions

Drainage Patterns

Common Pathologies

Review Questions

Cardiovascular System

Lymphatic System

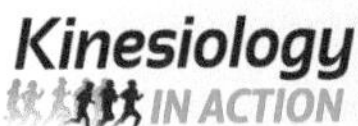

For additional practice activities and videos, please visit www.kinesiologyinaction.com

The circulatory system includes two types of transport systems: (1) the cardiovascular system and (2) the lymphatic system.

The **cardiovascular system,** which includes the blood vessels (arteries and veins) and the heart, transports blood throughout the body. Arteries and veins transport blood from the capillaries in the lungs—where carbon dioxide is exchanged for oxygen—to capillaries throughout the body, where oxygen is exchanged for carbon dioxide. The heart is the pump that pushes blood through the arteries and veins. Blood and lymph are the liquid mediums in which the materials are transported.

Linked directly to the circulatory system and the immune system, the **lymphatic system** is made up of lymph vessels and nodes. It collects excess extracellular fluid as lymph and transports it from the periphery to the venous system, thereby helping the cardiovascular system maintain adequate blood volume and pressure. In addition, the lymphatic system helps the immune system by filtering bacteria, viruses, waste products, and other foreign matter and by producing specific antibodies that help the immune system fight infection and defend against invasion by foreign material.

Cardiovascular System

Because blood never leaves the body's network of arteries, veins, and capillaries, the cardiovascular system is considered a closed system. It operates two different and distinct circuits, or loops—the pulmonary circuit and the systemic circuit (Fig. 7-1). The **pulmonary circuit** transports oxygen-depleted blood (shown in blue) from the body through the right side of the heart (right atrium and right ventricle) to the lungs via the pulmonary arteries. When blood reaches the lungs, carbon dioxide is exchanged for oxygen before returning to the left side of the heart via the pulmonary

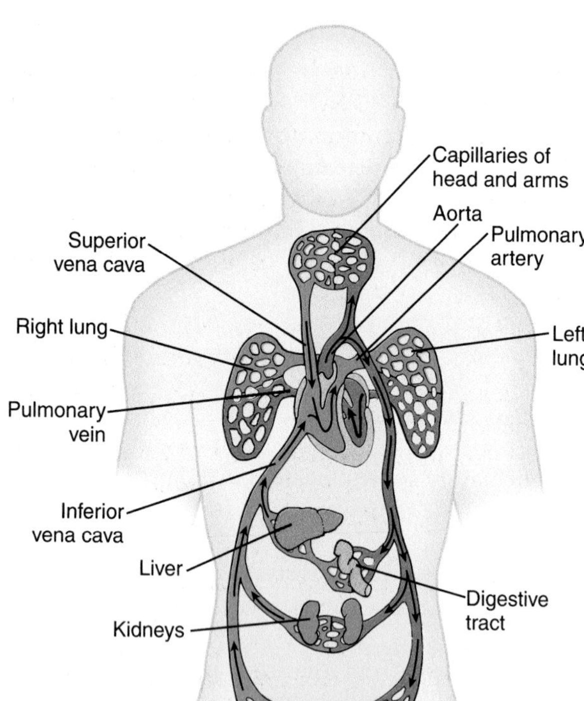

Figure 7-1. Pulmonary and systemic circulation (anterior view).

veins. The **systemic circuit** loops through the left side of the heart (left atrium and left ventricle), out to the rest of the body via the aorta and branching arteries, and then to capillary beds. It is here in the capillary beds that oxygenated blood (shown in red) is exchanged for deoxygenated blood, which then returns to the heart through a series of veins.

Heart

Unlike most other muscles discussed in this book, the heart is largely an involuntary muscle. For example, you cannot consciously decide whether to contract your heart muscle like you do, say, the biceps brachii muscle. This is a good thing. Imagine if you got busy doing a task and forgot to contract your heart, or if you went to sleep and didn't tell your heart to contract. In other words, the heart must be under involuntary control, because it needs to work constantly all day and all night. You can learn to control heart rate to some extent, but you cannot stop or start your heart.

How much does the heart work? Assume that your heart contracts 72 times per minute. At 60 minutes per hour, 24 hours per day, and 365 days per year, your heart contracts around 38 million times per year. If you live to the age of 80, your heart will contract over 3 trillion times without stopping.

The heart provides the pumping force to move blood though blood vessels (arteries, capillaries, and veins). It is not directly responsible for the exchange of oxygen and carbon dioxide. That function is carried out in the lungs.

Location

The heart is approximately the size of a closed fist. It is contained in the middle portion of the thoracic cavity known as the **mediastinum** (Fig. 7-2), with about two-thirds of its mass to the left of midline. The thoracic cavity also contains the left and right lungs, which lie on either side of the heart. All of the chest organs except the lungs are contained within the mediastinum, including the heart, aorta, thymus gland, chest portion of the trachea, esophagus, lymph nodes, and vagus nerves.

The heart lies between the sternum and the vertebral column (Fig. 7-3). Manual, rhythmic pressing and releasing on the sternum creates pressure differences within the thoracic cavity and allows blood to be pumped through the heart. These pressure differences are the basis for cardiac compression applied during cardiopulmonary resuscitation (CPR).

Chambers

The heart is made up of four separate chambers and is divided into right and left halves. Each half is again divided into an upper and lower part. The two top chambers are called **atria** (singular is *atrium*), and the two bottom chambers are called **ventricles** (Fig. 7-4).

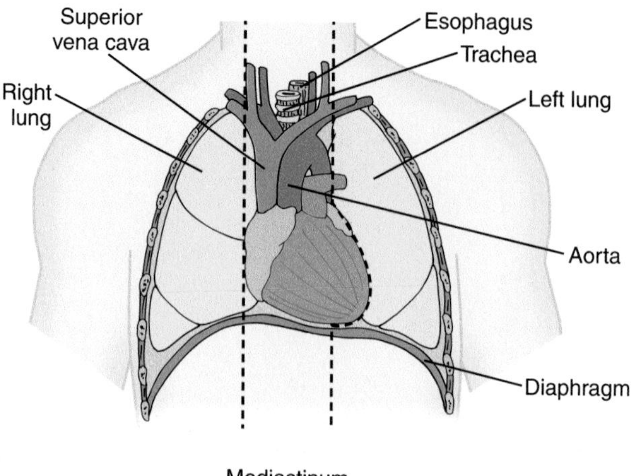

Figure 7-2. Location of the heart within the mediastinum—that area in the chest cavity between the two lungs.

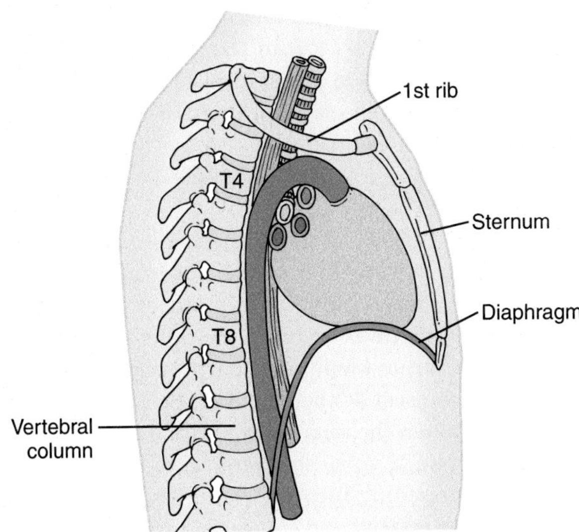

Figure 7-3. The position of the heart between two hard surfaces (sternum and vertebral column) within the thoracic cavity allows one to apply cardiac compression (CPR) that creates pressure differences in the heart to continue pumping blood to the brain.

The atria, which receive blood from veins, have relatively thin muscular walls, because they are required to propel blood only into the ventricles. Larger than the atria, the ventricles have thicker walls that provide a greater pumping force. The left ventricle is approximately three times thicker than the right ventricle. This thickness is necessary to withstand the greater pumping force needed to push blood out to all areas of the body, as opposed to just pumping blood from the heart to the lungs.

Valves

Heart valves function by allowing blood to flow through the heart in only one direction. Just as there are four heart chambers, there are four heart valves. These valves lead into and out of the ventricles. Two **atrioventricular** (AV) valves lie between the atria and the ventricles, and two **semilunar** (SL) valves lie between the ventricles and the arteries leading out of the heart (see Fig. 7-4).

When shut, AV valves prevent the backflow of blood from the ventricles into the atria. Because the AV valve between the right atrium and ventricle has three flaps, it is called the **tricuspid valve.** The AV valve between the left atrium and ventricle is called the **bicuspid valve** and has only two flaps. This bicuspid valve is also referred to as the **mitral valve** because it resembles the ceremonial headdress, consisting of two like parts (miter), worn by bishops and certain other clergy.

The SL valve, located between the right ventricle and the pulmonary arteries leading to the lungs, is also called the **pulmonic,** or **pulmonary, valve.** The valve between the left ventricle and the aorta is the **aortic valve.** These valves prevent blood from flowing backward into the heart.

Blood Flow Through the Heart

Deoxygenated blood (high in carbon dioxide and low in oxygen) from the peripheral tissues of the body returns to the heart via the superior and inferior vena cavae and enters the right atrium. This deoxygenated blood then passes through the right AV (tricuspid) valve into the right ventricle. Blood is pumped out of the right ventricle and through the pulmonic valve into the pulmonary

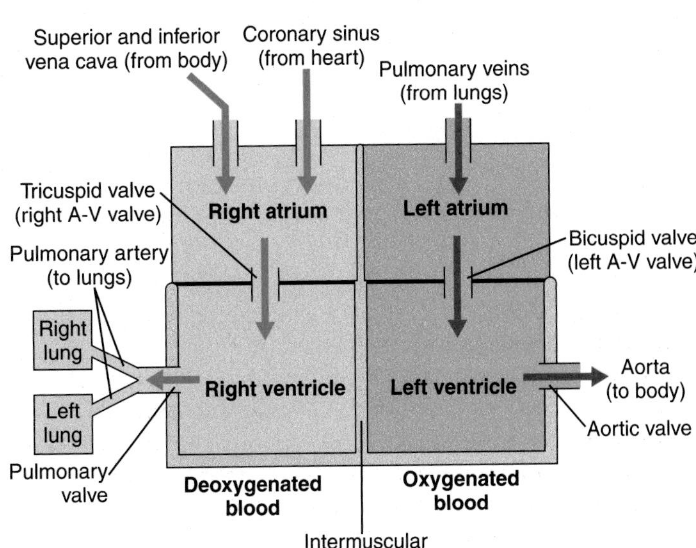

Figure 7-4. Schematic illustration of heart chambers, valves, and blood flow through the heart. Note that blood vessels have been shown in different positions within the chambers compared with a real heart.

trunk, which branches into the right and left pulmonary arteries and then on to the lungs. It is in the lungs that carbon dioxide is exchanged for oxygen. Oxygenated blood leaves the lungs via the pulmonary veins and enters the heart's left atrium. From the left artium, blood passes through the left AV (bicuspid) valve and into the left ventricle. The left ventricle pumps blood out of the heart through the aortic valve, into the aorta, and then out to the entire body, including the heart muscle itself (Fig. 7-5). Blood leaving the left ventricle is under the greatest pressure due to the powerful contraction needed to push blood throughout the body. In summary, the right side of the heart pumps deoxygenated blood to the lungs, and the left side pumps oxygenated blood throughout the body.

Heart Sounds

Heart sounds, which occur when the heart valves close, can be heard with a stethoscope. These sounds are often described as *lub-dub*. The right and left atria contract together, followed by contraction of the right and left ventricles. As stated above, blood returns to the atria, the AV valves (tricuspid and bicuspid) open, the atria contract, and blood flows into the ventricles. When the ventricles are full, the AV valves close, making the first heart sound (*lub*). Next, the SL valves open, the ventricles contract, and blood is pumped to the aortic and pulmonary arteries. The SL valves then close to prevent blood from flowing back into the ventricles when the ventricles relax making the second heart sound (*dub*). The cycle starts again and repeats itself approximately 72 times per minute.

Cardiac Cycle

The **cardiac cycle** is a series of mechanical events that we will begin tracing in the right atrium. When the right atrium relaxes, blood rushes out of the superior and inferior vena cavae and into the right atrium. Once filled, the atrium suddenly and sharply contracts, greatly reducing the size of the chamber. Because there are no valves between the vena cavae and the atrium, blood can go backward into the vena cavae or forward, through the opening into the right ventricle. Because the ventricle is relaxed and empty, and the superior and inferior vena cavae are still full of blood wanting to enter the right atrium, the path of least resistance is through the opening between the atrium and the ventricle. Therefore, contraction of the atrium drives the blood into the right ventricle.

As the ventricle fills, the AV valve closes, and the blood cannot flow backward into the atrium. Once full, the ventricle contracts and forces the blood out of the heart, through the pulmonic valve, and into the pulmonary arteries. The pulmonary arteries are already full

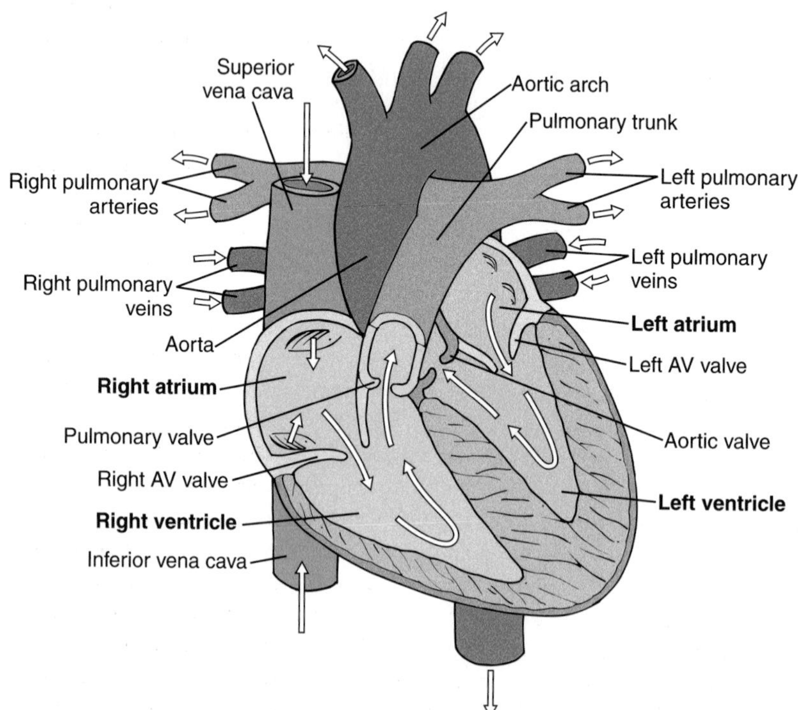

Figure 7-5. Blood flow through heart.

of blood, but the force of the contraction pushes the blood in the pulmonary arteries along to all other vessels "downstream" and eventually into the lung capillaries. The blood already in the capillaries is pushed onward into the pulmonary veins, and blood flow continues toward the left side of the heart.

What occurs on the right side of the heart also occurs *at the same time* on the left side. Blood enters the left atrium through the pulmonary veins. Once filled, the left atrium contracts, greatly reducing the size of its chamber. The blood takes the path of least resistance and enters the empty and relaxed left ventricle. When the left ventricle is full, the AV valve closes. The ventricle contracts and pushes the blood through the aortic valve into the aorta. The aorta is already full of blood, but the force of the contraction pushes blood into the aorta, along to all the other vessels "downstream," and eventually into the capillaries throughout the body. Blood already in the body's capillary beds is pushed into the veins and continues through the venous system toward the right side of the heart.

Blood Vessels

Types of Blood Vessels

There are three basic types of blood vessels: arteries, veins, and capillaries. The walls of arteries and veins are three layers thick. Capillaries are essentially one-layer endothelial tubes.

By definition, **arteries** carry blood away from the heart and to the rest of the body's tissues. The largest artery is the **aorta,** and the smallest ones are called **arterioles.** Because arteries carry blood *away* from the heart, that blood tends to be rich in oxygen. The exceptions are the pulmonary arteries, which carry deoxygenated blood away from the heart and to the lungs, where it is exchanged for oxygen-rich blood. Arterial walls must be very strong, muscular, and elastic to withstand the great pressure to which arteries are subjected.

Veins carry blood *toward* the heart. The largest are the superior and inferior **vena cavae,** and the smallest are **venules.** With the exception of the pulmonary veins, all veins carry deoxygenated blood (rich in carbon dioxide and poor in oxygen) toward the heart. The pulmonary veins carry blood to the heart, but this blood is high in oxygen. Veins tend to be larger in diameter, have thinner walls, and are less elastic than arteries. Veins that carry blood against the force of gravity usually contain valves to prevent backflow. For this reason, valves are more common in the lower extremities than in the upper extremities. They are also more common in the deeper veins than in the superficial ones. The valves are actually folds in the inner layer of the veins, usually arranged in two cusps. The valves allow blood to flow toward the heart, but they fill and come together to occlude the vessel when blood tries to reverse its direction of flow.

Generally speaking, veins are paired with arteries and share the same name. For example, there are the axillary artery and vein and the femoral artery and vein. Of course, there are exceptions. For example, the carotid artery and the jugular vein run together in the neck. (Some of these exceptions will be noted later in the chapter when describing the blood supply to various areas.) It is important to remember that although arteries and veins may parallel each other, blood is flowing in *opposite* directions.

Capillaries (capillary beds) form the link between arterioles and venules. They are microscopic, with walls only one endothelial cell layer thick. All exchange of oxygen and carbon dioxide occurs in the capillaries.

The cardiovascular system has many general similarities to a highway system. Both systems are involved in orderly two-way transport. Just like freeways, arteries and veins tend to run together throughout the body but in opposite directions—arteries move blood *away* from the heart, and veins move blood *toward* the heart. Visualize driving around the city on a freeway that leads to various destinations. There are many exits (branches and divisions) from the freeway that lead to smaller roads and streets (arteries) until you turn into the driveway (arteriole) of your destination (capillary bed). Once there, you unload the groceries (oxygen) and pick up the recycling (carbon dioxide). You then retrace your route, driving up increasingly larger streets (venules to veins to vena cava) until you return to where you began (the heart).

Arteries and veins generally run parallel throughout the body, connected with a weblike network of capillaries. This two-way transport system goes to every part of the body. To appreciate how vast, dense, and delicate this network of blood vessels is, consider the human body dissected of everything except blood vessels. What remains is a dense, mesh-like form of the body (Fig. 7-6).

Regardless of where in the body blood travels after leaving the heart, it gets there through a series of ever smaller arteries and returns via a series of ever larger veins. This anatomical concept is the key to understanding many clinical conditions. For example, a clot that formed in the heart due to turbulent blood flow from a faulty heart valve would travel through the heart and out into the arterial system until it reached an artery that was too small to allow the clot to travel any farther. There the

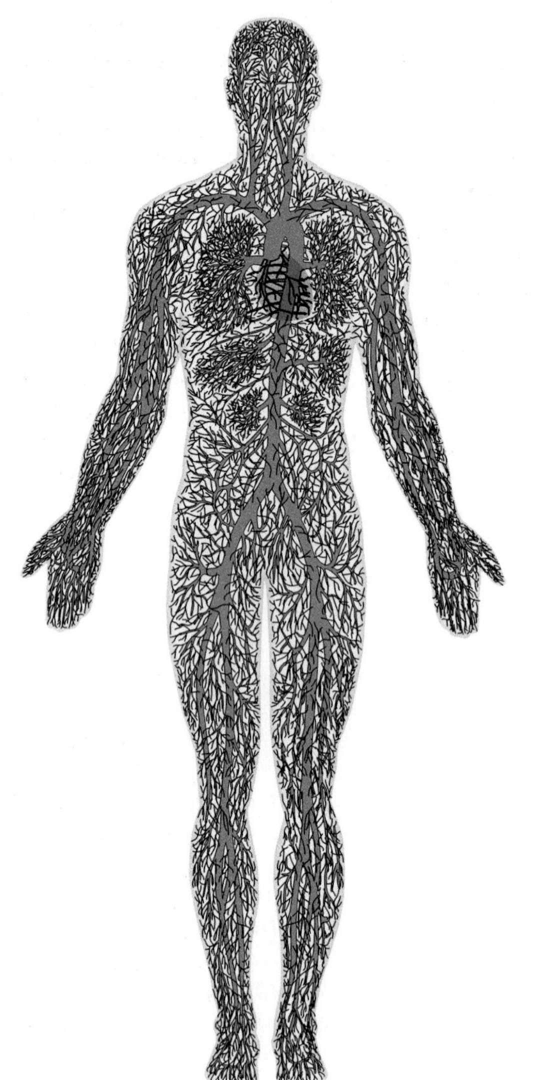

Figure 7-6. The body's vast system of blood vessels creates a dense and delicate web that mirrors the shape of the body.

clot would either decrease the flow of blood beyond that point or block it completely. A clot that originates on the heart's right side will end up in the pulmonary artery system. A clot that originates on the heart's left side will travel through the aorta and end up in a smaller artery somewhere in the body, depending on which branch of the aorta it travels. The clot could end up in the brain, in an extremity, or in another organ, or could enter one of the coronary arteries, the first branch off of the aorta. How far along the pathway the clot travels depends on the clot's size. The smaller the clot, the farther along the arterial system it will travel before becoming wedged.

If a clot dislodges from a vein, it will travel along the venous system, passing through ever larger vessels, through the right side of the heart, and will end up in the pulmonary artery system. Why? The clot travels until it reaches a vessel small enough to block further passage. In the venous system, vessel diameter increases along the passageway to the heart. The heart is basically a hollow organ through which blood is pumped. Vessel diameter decreases in size along the arterial system, in this case the pulmonary arteries to the lungs.

Pulse and Blood Pressure

A pulse is an important clinical feature of arteries. It is the "throbbing" that can be felt at various locations in the body, caused by the contraction and expansion of an artery as a wave of blood passes by a particular spot. A pulse can be palpated anywhere that an artery can be compressed against a bone and that is near enough to the surface to be felt. Common sites for feeling a pulse are at the wrist (radial artery), at the neck (carotid artery), and atop the ankle (dorsalis pedis artery, a branch of the posterior tibial artery). Figure 7-7 shows these and other sites where a pulse can be detected. The pulse is usually an accurate measure of heart rate. An average pulse is about 72 beats per minute.

Another important clinical feature of arteries is the measurement of **blood pressure.** You can "hear" your heart in action with a stethoscope. Heart ventricles work together and have two phases. When they contract, they send blood either to the lungs (from the right ventricle) or to the rest of the body (from the left ventricle). Blood pressure is highest during the contraction phase (systole) and lowest when the ventricles relax and fill with blood (diastole). Both phases of blood pressure can be measured using a sphygmomanometer (blood pressure cuff). Systolic pressure is the highest pressure

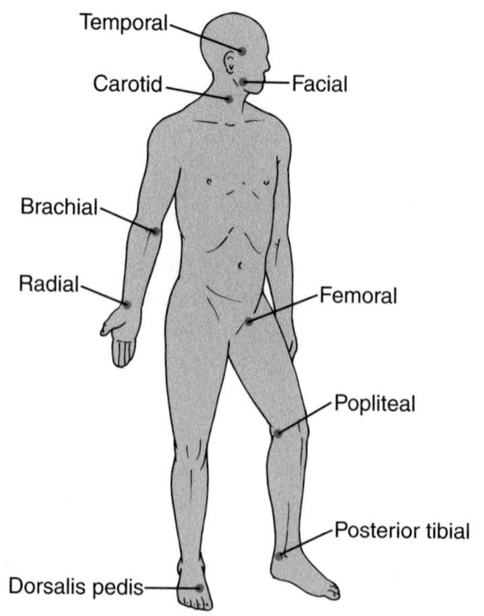

Figure 7-7. Major sites where pulse can be detected.

in an artery at the moment when the heart beats and pumps blood through the body. Systole is the first sound heard through the stethoscope as the pressure cuff deflates. Diastolic pressure is the lowest pressure in an artery between successive heartbeats, when heart sounds cannot be heard.

The average systolic pressure is about 120 mm of mercury (mm Hg), and an average diastolic pressure is about 80 mm Hg. Because systolic pressure is always recorded first, this would be recorded as 120/80.

Pathways

In the following section, the main arteries are described as they branch and divide, followed by a similar description of the main veins. Keep in mind that arteries and veins often run parallel to each other and often have the same name. However, it is important to remember that blood in these vessels is traveling in opposite directions. In arteries, blood travels *away* from the heart; in veins, blood travels *toward* the heart. Table 7-1 summarizes the major arteries, the main branches described in this chapter, and the areas they supply. Table 7-2 summarizes the major veins, the veins they empty into, and the regions drained.

The **ascending aorta** leaves the left ventricle of the heart, passes upward, and arches above the heart (Fig. 7-8). Immediately branching off the ascending aorta are the right and left **coronary arteries,** which supply blood to the heart muscle (myocardium) itself. The cardiac veins, which essentially parallel the coronary

Table 7-1 Summary of Major Arteries

Name	Main Branches	Area Supplied
Ascending aorta	Coronary	Heart
Aortic arch	Brachiocephalic	
	Left subclavian	Upper extremity—left
	Left common carotid	Neck—left side
Brachiocephalic	Right subclavian	Upper extremity—right
	Right common carotid	Neck—right side
Common carotid	Internal carotid	Brain
	External carotid	External head
Subclavian	Vertebral	Brain
	Axillary	Upper extremity
Axillary	Brachial	Arm
Brachial	Radial and ulnar	Forearm and hand
Descending aorta	Renal	Kidneys
	Common iliac	Lower abdomen
Common iliac	Internal iliac	Pelvic region
	External iliac	Lower extremity
External iliac	Femoral	Thigh
Femoral	Popliteal	Knee
Popliteal	Anterior and posterior tibial	Leg and foot

Table 7-2 Summary of Major Veins

Vein	Vein Joined	Region Drained
Trunk		
Brachiocephalic	Superior vena cava	Upper body
Renal	Inferior vena cava	Kidneys
Hepatic	Inferior vena cava	Liver
Internal iliac	Common iliac	Pelvic region
External iliac	Common iliac	Lower extremity
Common iliac	Inferior vena cava	Lower extremity and abdomen

Continued

Table 7-2 Summary of Major Veins—cont'd

Vein	Vein Joined	Region Drained
Lower Extremity		
Anterior and posterior tibial	Popliteal	Leg and foot
Popliteal	Femoral	Knee
Small saphenous	Popliteal	Superficial leg and foot
Great saphenous	Femoral	Superficial lower extremity
Femoral	External iliac	Thigh
Head and Neck		
Cranial venous sinuses	Internal jugular	Brain (including reabsorbed cerebral spinal fluid)
Internal jugular	Brachiocephalic	Cranium, face, and neck
External jugular	Subclavian	Face, neck, and scalp
Vertebral	Brachiocephalic	Posterior skull, cervical spinal cord, and cervical vertebrae
Subclavian	Brachiocephalic	Shoulder
Brachiocephalic	Superior vena cava	Upper body
Superior vena cava	Right atrium	Upper body
Upper Extremity		
Radial and ulnar	Brachial	Forearm and hand
Cephalic	Axillary	Superficial arm and forearm
Basilic	Axillary	Superficial arm
Median cubital	Basilic and cephalic	Cubital fossa
Brachial	Axillary	Arm
Axillary	Subclavian	Axilla
Subclavian	Brachiocephalic	Shoulder

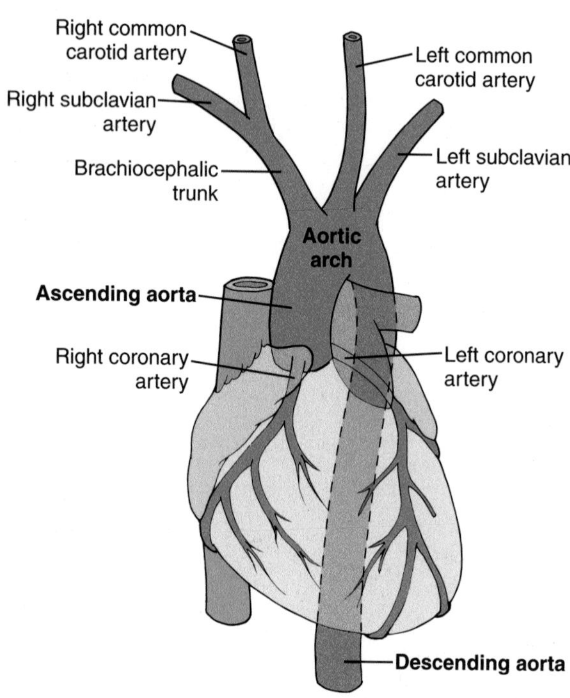

Figure 7-8. Main parts of aorta: ascending aorta, aortic arch, and descending aorta.

arteries, are the tributaries that drain most of the myocardium, emptying into the coronary sinus. The coronary sinus is the largest venous vessel of the heart and empties directly into the right atrium.

The **arch** of the aorta contains three branches: first, the brachiocephalic trunk, then the left common carotid artery, and lastly, the left subclavian artery. The **brachiocephalic trunk** (from the Latin *brachium,* meaning "arm," and *cephalicus,* meaning "head") is the major blood source for the right arm and right side of the head. This artery is very short, but its pathway allows the right-sided arteries to cross over the heart to the body's right side, where it divides into the right common carotid and right subclavian arteries. The second and third branches off the aortic arch are the left common carotid and left subclavian arteries, respectively, the major blood supply to the left side of the head and left arm. The carotid arteries travels up the neck, whereas the subclavian arteries go to the upper extremities. After these branches, the aorta turns downward and becomes the **descending aorta.** The aorta's huge diameter largely protects itself from blockage by clots, although high pressure within the aorta can make it susceptible to an aneurysm. The descending aorta runs down through the trunk to supply the lower extremities with multiple branches along the way to supply the trunk area as well. At approximately the fourth lumbar vertebra, the descending aorta divides into the right and left **common iliac** arteries (Fig. 7-9), which in turn divide into the **external and internal iliac** arteries. The external iliac arteries supply the lower limbs, whereas the internal iliac arteries supply the viscera and pelvis.

On the venous side, the **inferior vena cava** travels with the descending aorta through the trunk. Remember that blood flows away from the heart in the aorta and toward the heart in the vena cava. The inferior vena cava is formed at approximately the fifth lumbar vertebra by the confluence of the **right and left common iliac veins** (see Fig. 7-9). These common iliac veins are formed by the merging of the external and internal iliac veins. The **external iliac vein** receives blood flow from the abdominal wall and from the lower extremity via the **femoral vein.** The internal iliac vein receives blood from the viscera and the pelvic region.

Circulation of the lower extremity begins as the external iliac artery and vein pass under the inguinal ligament and become the **femoral artery and vein** (Fig. 7-10A, B). Because the artery is fairly superficial in the groin, the femoral pulse can be felt (see Fig. 7-7). The femoral triangle is bordered by the inguinal ligament superiorly, the sartorius laterally, and the adductor longus medially (Fig. 7-11). In addition to the femoral artery and vein, the femoral nerve, numerous lymph nodes, and the terminal portion of the great saphenous vein lie in this triangle. The pectineus and iliopsoas muscles form the floor of this triangle.

The femoral artery runs deep along the length of the thigh, passes posteriorly through the adductor hiatus, an opening in the insertion of the adductor magnus muscle (see Figs. 18-18 and 18-28), and enters the popliteal fossa on the posterior side of the knee. Here, its name changes to the **popliteal artery.** The popliteal pulse can be felt in the middle of the popliteal space (see Fig. 7-7).

Just distal to the knee, the popliteal artery divides into the **anterior and posterior tibial arteries** (see Fig. 7-10A). As their names imply, these arteries run down the anterior and posterior aspects of the tibia, branching off in numerous places. At the ankle on the dorsum of the foot, a branch called the **dorsalis pedis artery** can be palpated and a pulse felt (see Fig. 7-7).

Traveling in the opposite direction in the lower extremity are two main venous systems: the deep and superficial systems (see Fig. 7-10B). Deep veins tend to parallel arteries of the same name. The **anterior and posterior tibial and fibular veins** drain the foot and lower leg before emptying into the popliteal vein. The

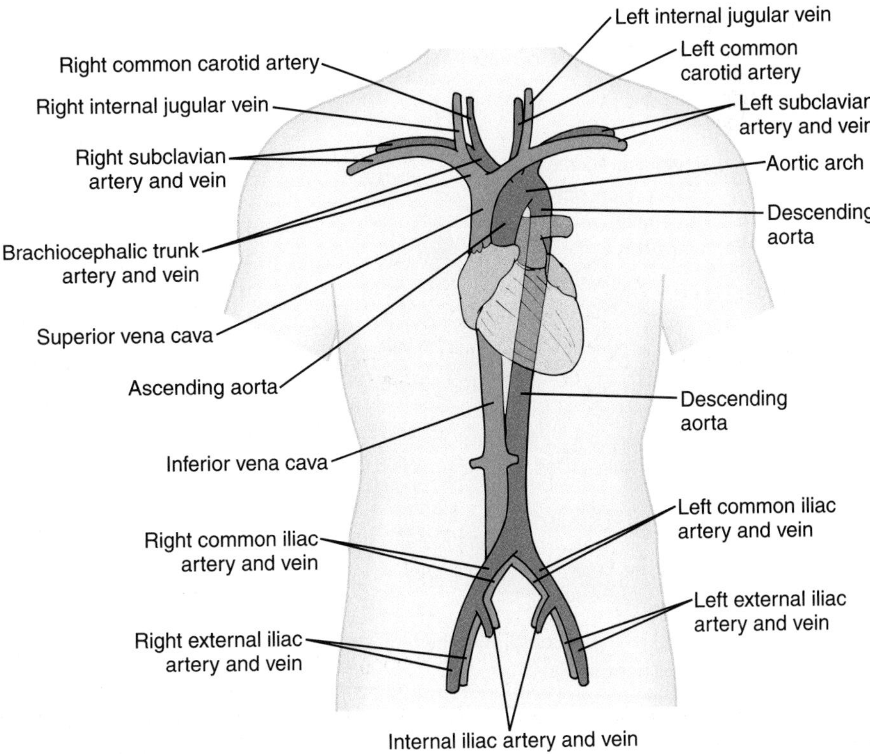

Figure 7-9. Major branches of aorta and vena cavae.

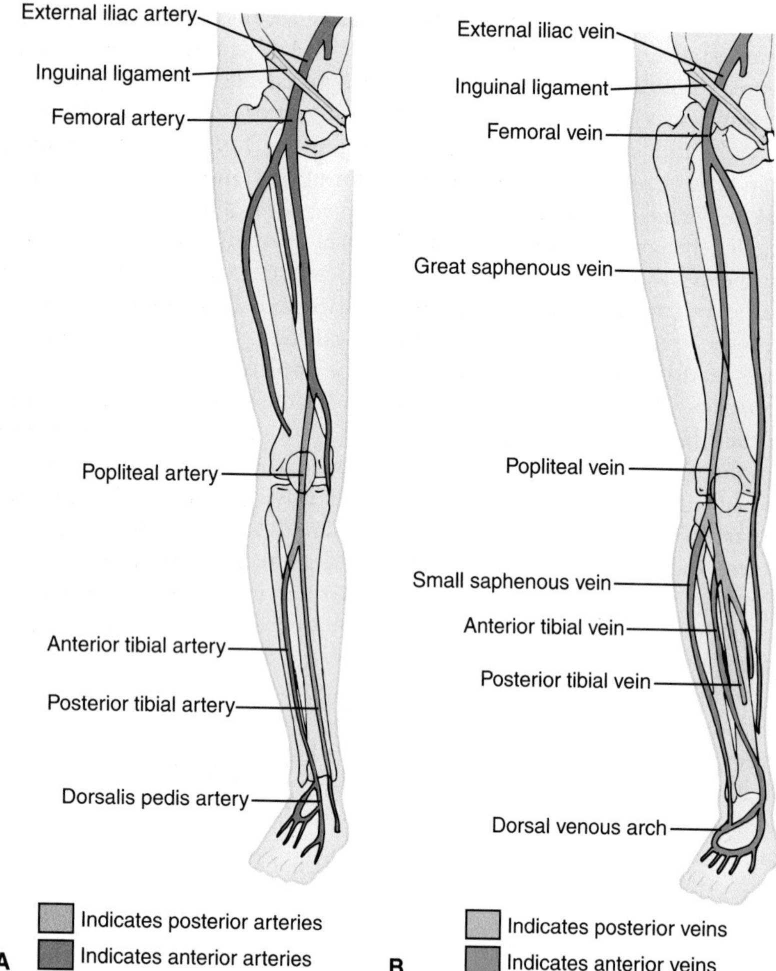

Figure 7-10. Major arteries **(A)** and veins **(B)** of the lower extremity (right side).

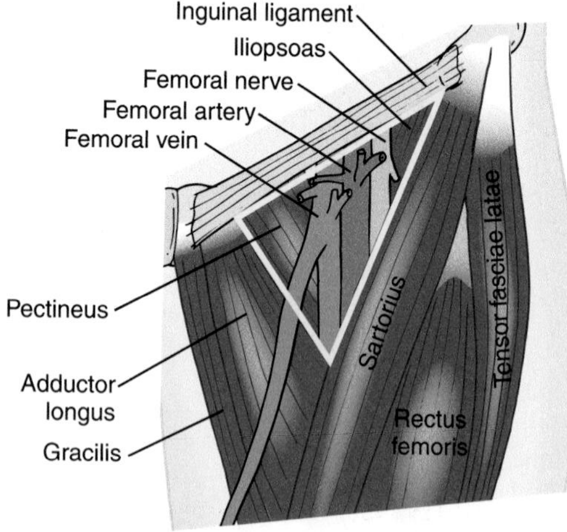

Figure 7-11. Femoral triangle, containing the femoral artery, vein, and nerve (right side).

popliteal vein drains the knee region before becoming the femoral vein after it passes through the adductor hiatus. The **femoral vein** drains the thigh area and joins the external iliac vein as it passes under the inguinal ligament. The two main superficial veins of the lower extremities are the saphenous veins. The **great saphenous vein,** the longest vein in the body, runs superficially along most of the length of the lower extremity on the medial side before emptying into the femoral vein. The **small saphenous vein** runs superficially from the lateral side of the foot and up the posterior lower leg to empty into the popliteal vein.

Circulation of the upper extremities begin as the subclavian artery and vein. The **subclavian artery** delivers arterial blood to the upper extremity, chest wall, and neck. The right subclavian artery comes off the aortic arch via the short brachiocephalic trunk, whereas the left subclavian artery comes directly off the aortic arch. The subclavian artery is clinically important when it becomes compressed between the clavicle and first rib in a crowded space called the *thoracic outlet,* producing symptoms.

At the lateral border of the first rib, the subclavian artery becomes the **axillary artery** (Fig. 7-12A). It runs through the axilla to the proximal end of the arm, where it becomes the **brachial artery** and runs the length of the arm. At the anterior elbow, the brachial artery is often used to measure blood pressure and is where it divides into the **radial and ulnar arteries.** These arteries run down the forearm on the radial and ulnar sides, respectively. Each artery has many branches in the forearm, and they all terminate by forming two arches in the palmar side of the hand.

Similar to the lower extremity, the upper extremity has both deep and superficial veins (Fig. 7-12B). The deep veins of the upper extremity eventually drain into the **subclavian vein,** which parallels the artery of the same name. The **radial and ulnar veins** drain the lateral and medial forearm and hand, respectively, and then join the **brachial vein,** which drains the upper arm. In addition to these deep veins, three superficial veins are worth noting. Draining the forearm is the **cephalic vein,** which runs laterally to empty into the axillary vein. The **basilic vein** runs medially up the forearm to empty into the brachial vein. Anteriorly in the cubital fossa is the **median cubital vein,** which unites the basilic and cephalic veins. It is here in the cubital fossa that one of these three veins is commonly used for drawing blood.

The description of the circulatory pathway to the head and neck will begin with the **common carotid artery.** It runs up each side of the neck beside the trachea, where its pulse can be palpated. The left common carotid artery arises directly from the aortic arch, whereas the right common carotid artery comes off the brachiocephalic trunk of the aortic arch (Fig. 7-13). At about the level of the jaw, each common carotid artery

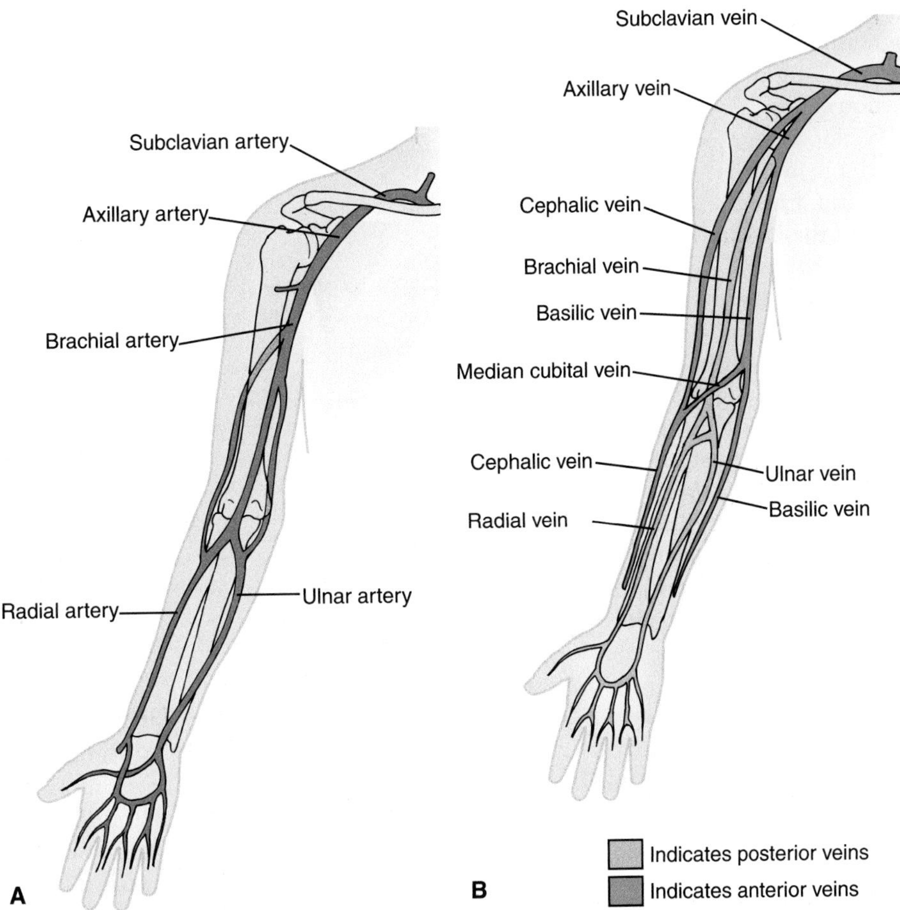

Figure 7-12. Major arteries **(A)** and veins **(B)** of the upper extremity (right side).

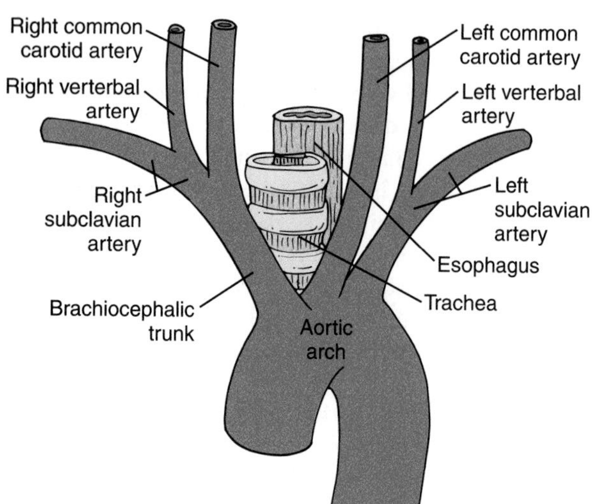

Figure 7-13. Branches of the aortic arch.

divides into the external and internal carotid arteries (Fig. 7-14A). The **external carotid artery** supplies the external head—the face, jaw, scalp, and skull. The **internal carotid artery** continues upward and enters the cranium through the carotid canal in the temporal bone, primarily supplying the anterior portion of the brain. Several venous sinuses within the layers of the dura mater receive blood from the brain. Eventually all of these sinuses drain into the internal jugular vein. Paralleling the carotid arteries and draining the head and neck regions are the **internal and external jugular veins** (Fig. 7-14B).

The **vertebral artery** is the first and largest branch of the subclavian artery (see Fig. 7-13). It runs upward in the cervical region, through the transverse foramen of the cervical vertebrae (see Fig. 7-14A and Fig. 15-7). It then enters the base of the brain through the foramen magnum, supplying the posterior portion of the brain. The right and left vertebral arteries supply blood to the medulla and cerebellum before joining together to form the **basilar artery** on the underside of the brainstem, which supplies parts of the cerebellum, pons, and midbrain. The **vertebral vein** parallels the vertebral artery in the neck within the transverse foramen of the cervical vertebrae (see Fig. 7-14B). However, the vertebral vein does not emerge through the foramen magnum with the vertebral artery. It drains blood from the cervical spinal cord, vertebrae, and posterior surface of the skull.

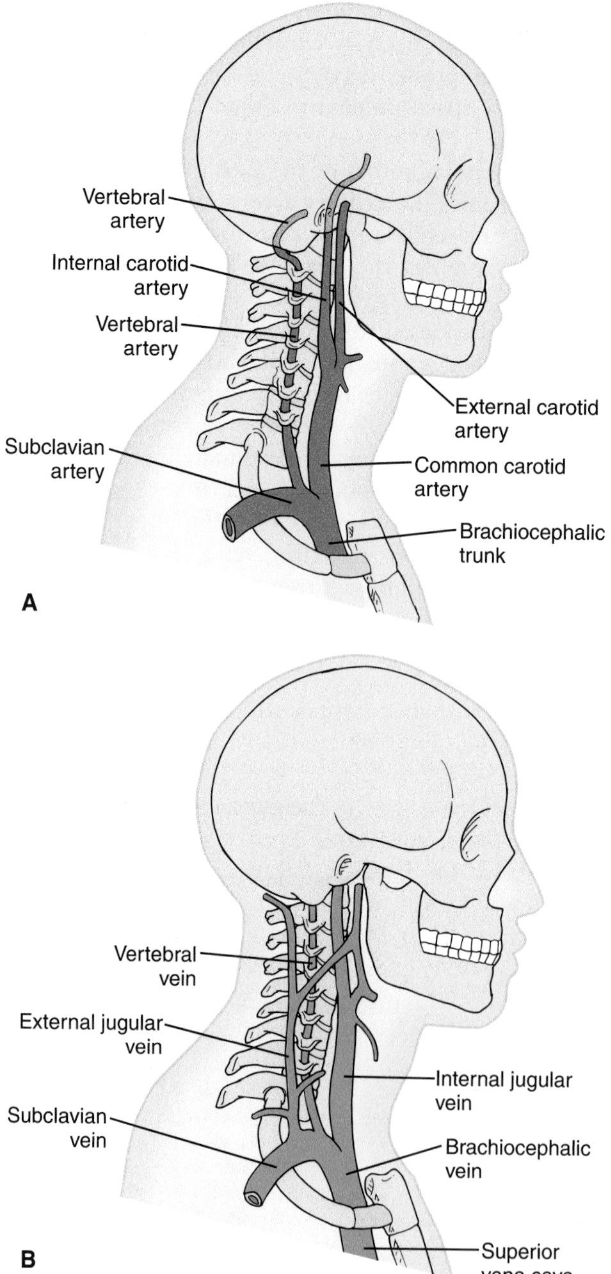

Figure 7-14. Main arteries **(A)** and veins **(B)** of the neck (right side).

Blood Supply to the Brain

At the base of the brain, the internal carotid arteries (anteriorly) and the basilar artery (posteriorly) are joined by communicating arteries, forming a circle that is often referred to as the **circle of Willis** (Fig. 7-15), after the English physician Thomas Willis, who first described this interconnection. Immediately upon entering the cranium, the internal carotid artery branches into the middle and anterior cerebral arteries. The **middle cerebral arteries** supply the lateral cerebral hemispheres. The **anterior cerebral arteries** supply the medial surface of the brain. The vertebral arteries join to form the basilar artery at the juncture of the pons and medulla on their anterior surfaces.

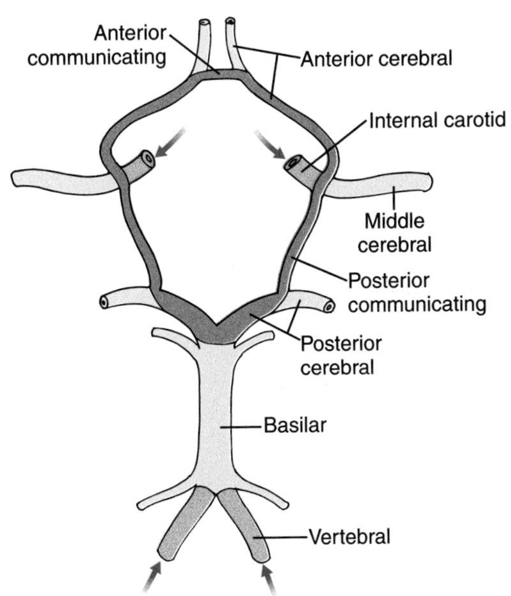

Figure 7-15. Circle of Willis.

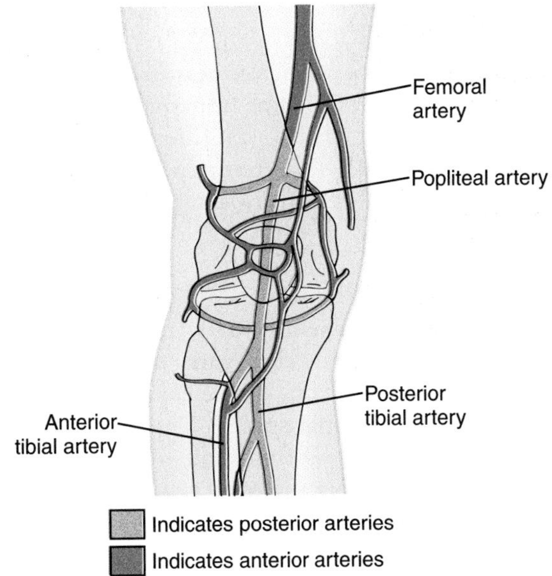

Figure 7-16. Arterial anastomosis around the knee.

The basilar artery divides to form the **posterior cerebral arteries,** which supply the occipital lobes and part of the temporal lobes.

The anterior cerebral artery (from the internal carotid) and the posterior cerebral artery (from the basilar) are joined at the base of the brain by the **posterior communicating artery.** The right and left anterior cerebral arteries are joined by the **anterior communicating artery.** The design of this circle is to ensure continued blood flow to the brain area should one of these major arteries fail. However, the circle of Willis is not always completely developed, so it does not ensure continued blood flow to the brain in every individual.

Clinical Significance of Anastomosis

An **anastomosis** is a joining of (or communication between) like vessels at their terminal ends, such as artery to artery or vein to vein. The purpose for this structural connection is to provide alternative circulation if one of the vessels becomes blocked. This helps ensure that blood will get to its intended destination (i.e., arterial blood will get to capillaries for exchange of oxygen and carbon dioxide, and venous blood will get back to the heart).

Within each extremity, smaller anastomosing branches are commonly found around each joint. These smaller alternative arterial pathways allow the distal part of the limb to receive vital oxygenated blood should a main artery in an area become blocked. With time, these communicating branches may become large enough to meet the needs of the area involved. In Figure 7-16, note that there are several smaller branches off the femoral artery around the knee. Many of these branches join with either the anterior or posterior tibial artery distal to the knee. There are also anastomoses between the major cerebral arteries.

Lymphatic System

The lymphatic system is linked to the cardiovascular system and the immune system. Lymphatic vessels collect fluid and proteins that have leaked out of the blood capillaries and return them back to the venous system as lymph. Knowing the lymphatic structures and how they drain into the cardiovascular system helps one understand the treatment of certain pathological conditions.

The lymphatic organs serve as staging areas for defense against infection from microbes and other foreign particles. En route to the venous system, lymph fluid filters through lymph nodes and other lymphatic tissue, where microbes are detected and an immune system attack can be launched.

Whereas the circulatory system is a closed system of veins and arteries, the lymphatic system is a partially open system that moves fluids only from the periphery to the subclavian veins. The blood vascular system is an ongoing circular loop (i.e., arteries to capillaries to veins, etc.). However, the lymphatic system begins as capillaries in the tissues and ends as major ducts emptying into the subclavian vein. Unlike the two-way cardiovascular system, the lymphatic system is a one-way route from the periphery to the venous system.

Functions

The vast network of lymphatic vessels has four main functions: (1) collecting lymph from the body's interstitial (intercellular) spaces, (2) filtering the lymph through lymph nodes, (3) detecting and fighting infection in the lymph nodes, and (4) returning the lymph to the bloodstream.

Lymph Collection

Blood capillaries generally deliver more fluid to peripheral tissues than they carry away. A certain amount of fluid leaks out of the capillaries into the tissue spaces (interstitial spaces). The lymphatic system collects this excess fluid and returns it to the venous system. In doing that, it plays a vital role in maintaining normal blood volume and blood pressure within the circulatory system.

Similar to blood capillaries in structure, lymph capillaries begin in the intercellular spaces of most tissues. These intercellular spaces are also referred to as **interstitial spaces,** or tissue spaces—the spaces between cells (Fig. 7-17). To better visualize this arrangement, think of your body as a vase full of marbles. The marbles are tissue cells, and the spaces between the marbles are interstitial spaces. If you pour water (interstitial fluid) into the container, you fill all the spaces. Removing this fluid requires a vast network of minute lymph capillaries woven throughout most of the body. Lymph capillaries act as if their walls have one-way valves. When pressure outside the lymph capillary is greater, the cells allow the interstitial fluid to seep in. When the pressure within the lymph capillary becomes greater, the cell walls stop allowing fluid into the lymph capillaries. Once inside the lymph capillary, the interstitial fluid is called **lymph.**

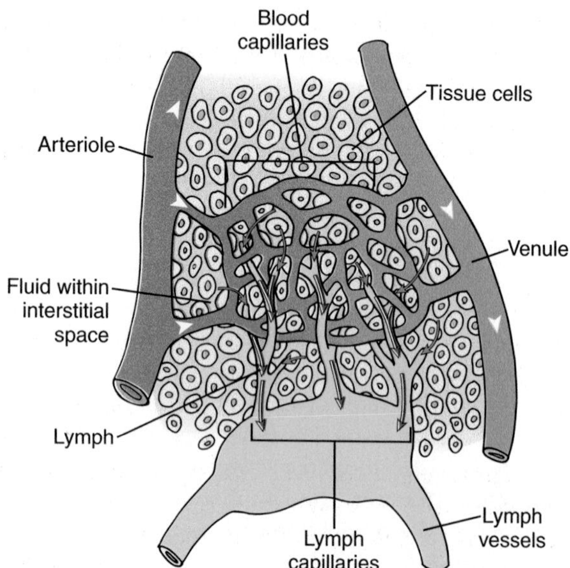

Figure 7-17. Lymph vessels from capillaries (beginning) to subclavian vein (end).

Lymph originates as plasma—the fluid portion of blood. As arterial blood enters the capillary bed, it slows down. This allows the plasma to move into the tissues, where it is called **intercellular** (or **interstitial**) **fluid.** Oxygen and nutrients are delivered to the cells. When the fluid leaves the cells, it collects waste products. Most of this fluid (approximately 90%) returns to blood circulation through the venules as plasma. The remaining 10% is now known as lymph, which is rich in protein. Approximately 2 liters of lymph flow into blood circulation daily.

Transport

The lymphatic system begins as minute capillaries in the tissues. These initial lymph vessels, or **lymph capillaries,** form a vast network throughout most of the body. Lymph capillaries are not found in the central nervous system, bones, teeth, epidermis, certain types of cartilage, or any avascular tissue.

Lymphatic capillaries join together into larger lymph vessels. Think of the leaves of a tree as the interstitial spaces. The leaves connect to the small branches that begin the drainage system. The branches join together on larger branches. Large branches join onto larger limbs, which then join the main trunk of the tree. This same idea of smaller vessels joining together on larger vessels is true of the lymphatic system. As lymph capillaries become larger and collect more lymphatic fluid, they are referred to as **lymph vessels.**

Lymph vessels are wider than veins, have thinner walls and more valves, and contain kidney bean–shaped sacs called **lymph nodes** that are located in various places along the route. The function of these nodes will be discussed later in this chapter.

While the cardiovascular system has the heart to pump blood along in the blood vessels, the lymphatic system has no such pump. Lymph is propelled through lymph vessels in several ways by actions both within and outside the lymphatic system. Like veins, lymphatic vessels have valves that prevent any backward flow of fluid. Between valves is a segment of lymph vessel called an **angion.** Smooth muscles in the walls of the lymphatic vessels cause a stretch reflex of the lymph angions (Fig. 7-18), resulting in sequential contractions that are activated by the nerves that encircle the angions. The continuing chain reaction of

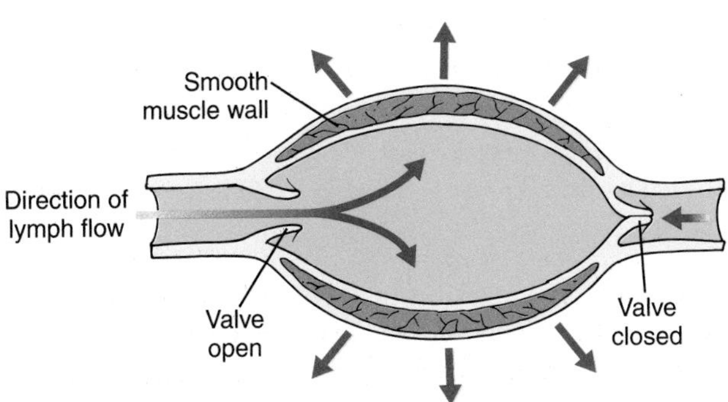

Figure 7-18. Stretch mechanism of a lymph angion.

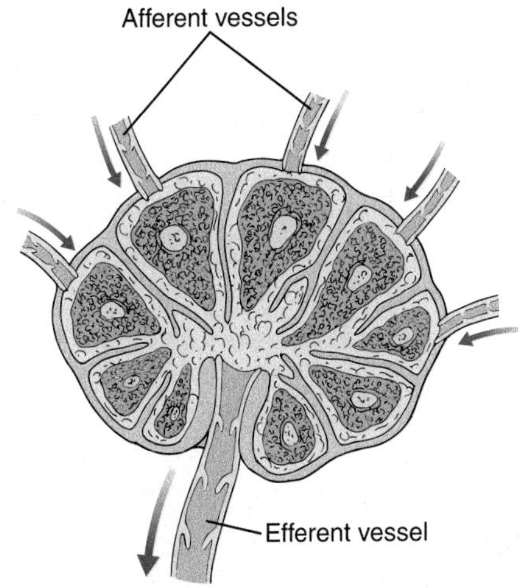

Figure 7-19. Lymph node and vessels.

contracting and stretching assists the onward flow of lymph from one angion to the next in a peristalsis-like movement controlled mainly by the filling state of each lymph angion. The pulsation helps move lymph onward from one lymph angion to the next. The motion is similar to the "wave" often done by the stadium crowd at sporting events.

There are also more subtle actions external to the lymphatic system that influence the movement of lymph within lymph vessels. The squeezing of the surrounding skeletal muscles assists in moving lymph along, much like the way blood is moved along in veins. This is especially true in the extremities during the pumplike movement of contracting and relaxing muscles. The movement of the diaphragm and the changes in thoracic cavity pressure during the phases of breathing—especially abdominal breathing (see Chapter 16)—can provide a subtle "pumping" effect on the lymphatic vessels within the trunk. Maintenance of good posture (see Chapter 21) allows more efficient abdominal breathing, hence greater pumping effect on the lymphatic vessels.

Filtration and Protection

As mentioned earlier, lymph passes through lymph nodes en route to its end point, the subclavian vein. Lymph nodes are frequently arranged in groups along the pathways of lymph vessels. The first node of a group is called the **sentinel node,** which can be considered the first line of defense. Lymph nodes filter out bacteria, cell debris, and other foreign particles from the lymph.

The lymph enters a node through several **afferent lymph vessels** and exits through one or two **efferent lymph vessels** (Fig. 7-19). Therefore, an efferent lymph vessel of one lymph node becomes an afferent lymph vessel of the next lymph node in a chain. As a general rule, lymph travels through one or more lymph nodes before entering the bloodstream.

As lymph passes through a lymph node, bacteria and other foreign particles are intercepted, engulfed, and digested by white blood cells (macrophages and lymphocytes). When infection is present, nodes enlarge and become tender to the touch as the accumulating bacteria and an increasing number of lymphocytes cause them to swell.

Lymph nodes are often erroneously called *lymph glands*. A distinguishing feature of a gland is secretion. For example, the pituitary gland secretes growth hormone, the pancreas secretes insulin, sweat glands secrete sweat, and salivary glands secrete saliva. Lymph nodes filter lymph as it passes through, but they don't secrete anything. Therefore, they are not considered glands.

There are a multitude of lymph nodes throughout the body; one estimate states there are 500 to 1000. Most nodes are concentrated in the cervical, axillary, and inguinal areas. Lymph nodes are able to increase or decrease in size, but a damaged or destroyed node cannot regenerate.

Drainage Patterns

Because lymph is really transported only from the periphery to the subclavian veins and not back to the periphery, one should think of lymph **drainage** rather than lymph circulation. There is a fairly predictable pattern of lymph drainage from tissues and organs, although some variation can be expected. Understanding these patterns is key to knowing the location of an infection or tumor and determining treatment.

Superficial lymph vessels drain the skin and subcutaneous tissue, forming a vast network that eventually drains into the deep lymph vessels. Deep lymph vessels drain the deeper structures. Deep lymph vessels tend to accompany the major blood vessels in the various regions.

Although there are lymph nodes throughout the body, there are three main groups of regional nodes: cervical (neck), axillary (upper extremity), and inguinal (lower extremity). These regional nodes are located at the junctions of the head and extremities with the trunk (Fig. 7-20). The cervical, axillary, and inguinal nodes drain into the jugular, subclavian, and lumbar **lymphatic trunks,** respectively.

These lymphatic trunks, plus those in the abdominal and chest area, drain in turn into one of two ducts that empty into the venous system (Fig. 7-21). The **right lymphatic duct** is by far the smaller of the two ducts. It is only about 1 to 2 inches long and is located at the base of the neck on the right side. Only the right head and neck, the right upper extremity, and the right upper trunk empty into the right lymphatic duct, which then empties into the right subclavian vein.

The rest of the body's lymph empties into the **thoracic duct.** For the most part, this includes the entire left side of the body as well as the right side below the diaphragm. All deep lymphatics in the thorax, abdomen, pelvis, perineum, and lower extremities enter the thoracic duct. To complete this lymph drainage, the thoracic duct enters the venous circulation at the left subclavian vein.

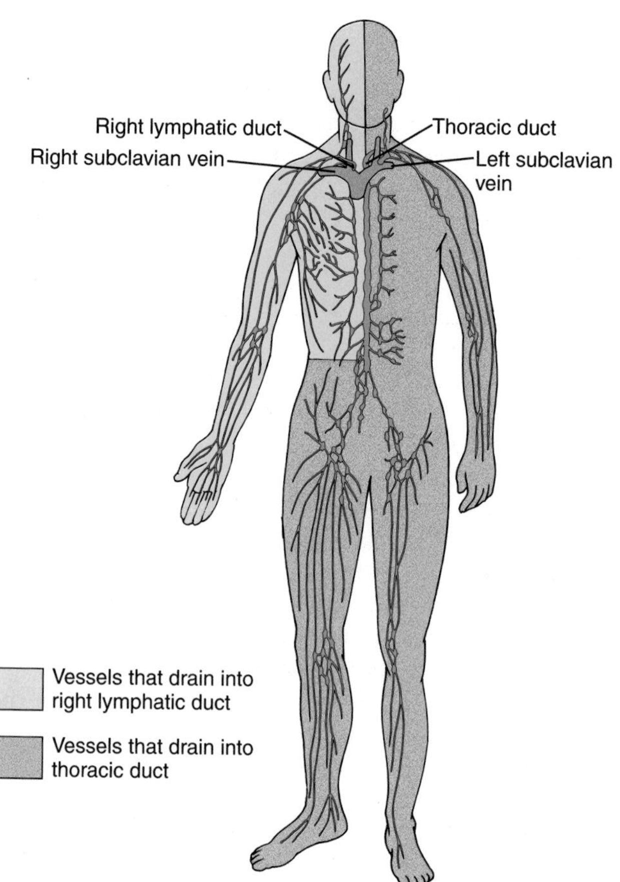

Figure 7-21. Lymphatic drainage into the two lymph ducts: the right lymphatic duct and the thoracic duct. Note that the superficial vessels are shown on the right side and the deep vessels on the left side.

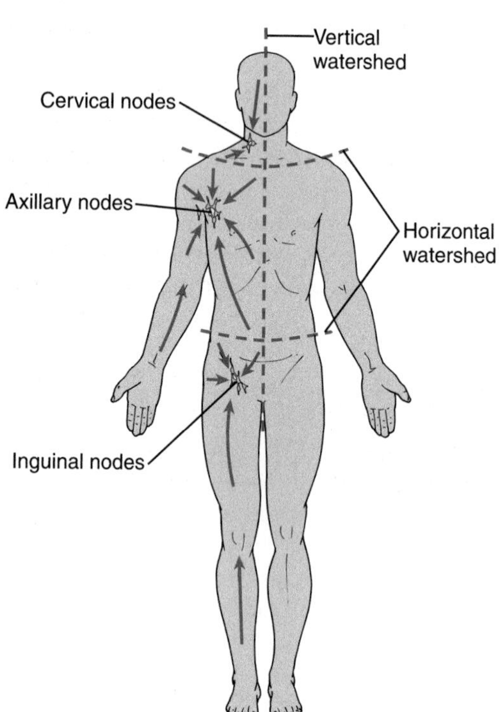

Figure 7-20. Regional lymph nodes and drainage watersheds.

In addition, the body has three main **watersheds** that separate the areas of lymph drainage (see Fig. 7-20). Visualize a mountain ridge; water will flow in opposite directions down each side of the ridge. The body has one vertical line at the midline that drains the right and left sides, and it has two horizontal lines, one at the level of the clavicle and the other at the level of the umbilicus. Lymph vessels draining above the clavicle enter the cervical lymph nodes. Those draining between the clavicle and the umbilicus enter the axillary nodes, whereas those draining below the umbilicus enter the inguinal nodes. The lymph collectors start at the watersheds and travel toward the regional lymph node bed. Because there are lymphatic capillary anastomoses between all the watersheds, this allows some crossover, if needed, to support drainage. The fact that this crossover is even possible is an important concept in the treatment of lymphedema.

Common Pathologies

Hemorrhage (bleeding) occurs when a break in a blood vessel allows blood to leak out of the closed system. A **cerebral hemorrhage** is particularly serious because it occurs within the confines of the bony skull. With nowhere for the blood to go, it can quickly put pressure on vital structures within the brain, causing a **stroke** or even death. A hemorrhage that occurs in an unconfined area like the abdomen, where blood loss volume can be great may also be serious. Hemorrhage that occurs from head trauma tends to be either epidural (between the skull and the dura mater) or subdural (under the dura mater). **Epidural bleeds** occur in arteries; therefore, symptoms develop more quickly due to higher pressure within the vessel. **Subdural bleeds** occur in veins, which are under less pressure, so symptoms tend to develop more slowly.

Congestive heart failure is a condition in which the heart can't pump strongly enough to push an adequate supply of blood out to the various parts of the body. As blood flowing from the heart slows, blood returning to the heart through the veins backs up, causing congestion in the body's tissues. This often results in edema, especially in the feet, ankles, and lungs.

A **heart murmur** is an extra or unusual heart sound in addition to the normal *lub-dub* sounds heard during a heart contraction. The *whooshing* that can be heard through a stethoscope is usually turbulent blood backflow. This whooshing sound may be normal for that individual or a sign of valve pathology that allows blood to flow in the wrong direction.

If an artery becomes narrow, blood flow will slow or stop. Narrowing can be from a blood clot traveling through an artery or from deposits within an artery. Another condition that will slow blood flow is **arteriosclerosis,** or "hardening" of the arteries. It is especially a problem in the legs and feet. The vessel wall becomes less elastic and cannot dilate to allow greater blood flow when needed. **Atherosclerosis,** a type of arteriosclerosis, is when fatty deposits in the artery wall cause narrowing or blockage of the vessel. The site of the blockage will determine the problem. For example, a partial blockage that occurs and slows blood flow in a **coronary artery,** which supplies blood to the heart muscle, can cause **ischemia,** resulting in chest pain **(angina).** If the blockage is complete, it can cause a heart attack **(myocardial infarction).** If the blockage occurs in an artery to or in the brain, it can cause a stroke **(cerebrovascular accident).** If the blockage occurs in a leg artery, it can cause ischemia, **pain,** and possible **occlusion**. These same conditions caused by fatty deposits in the artery wall can occur with a blood clot.

If a vein loses elasticity, it will stretch. As the vein enlarges, the valve flaps will no longer meet properly and blood that should be flowing toward the heart will flow backward. **Varicose veins** occur as the blood pools in the vein, enlarging it even more. This condition is more common in superficial veins of the leg, because standing subjects them to higher pressure. Deep veins tend to be surrounded by muscles that, as they contract, assist the veins in pumping the blood onward.

Phlebitis is an inflammation of a vein. **Thrombosis** is the formation of a blood clot that may partially or totally block a blood vessel (artery or vein). **Thrombophlebitis** (often shortened to *phlebitis*) occurs when a clot causes inflammation in a vein. **Embolism** is a blood clot (or other foreign matter, such as air, fat, or tumor) that becomes dislodged and travels to another part of the body through ever smaller vessels until becoming wedged, causing an obstruction.

An **aneurysm** is an abnormal outward bulging or ballooning that is often caused by a weakened area in the wall. An aneurysm may go undetected until it ruptures.

Thoracic outlet syndrome is a group of disorders involving compression of the brachial plexus and/or the subclavian artery and vein within in the spaced called the *thoracic outlet.* Various vascular, neurological, and muscular symptoms may result.

Why are drainage patterns important? When lymphatic tissue or nodes have been damaged, destroyed, or removed, lymph cannot drain normally from the involved area. Abnormal drainage will result in an accumulation of excess lymph and swelling, a condition known as **lymphedema,** and most commonly involves the arms or legs. Treatment of lymphedema is often based on the patterns of lymph drainage.

Review Questions

Cardiovascular System

1. The right atrioventricular (AV) valve is also referred to as the ________________ valve.
2. The left AV valve has two other names.
   a. Referring to the number of flaps, it is called the ________________ valve.
   b. Referring to its shape, it is called the ________________ valve.
3. The semilunar valve located at the exit of the right ventricle is also called the ________________ valve. The valve located at the exit of the left ventricle is called the ________________ valve.
4. The blood vessels that transport blood from the heart to the lungs are the ________________. Those that transport blood from the lungs to the heart are the ________________.
5. a. Veins carry which type of blood? (oxygenated/deoxygenated)
   b. What is the exception?
   c. Arteries carry which type of blood? (oxygenated/deoxygenated)
   d. What is the exception?
6. a. The first heart sound (*lub*) is heard when which valves close?
   b. The second heart sound (*dub*) is heard when which valves close?
7. If a clot breaks loose in a leg artery, where will it end up?
8. If a clot breaks loose in a leg vein, where will it end up?
9. At the inguinal ligament, the main artery and vein change name from ________________ (proximally) to ________________ (distally).
10. The head and neck regions are drained mostly by what two veins?
11. The pulse of which artery can be felt in the neck?
12. Name the 10 structures that a clot would travel through on its way from the left femoral vein (1) to the lung (10).
13. a. Which pressure is lowest in an artery? When does it occur?
    b. Which pressure is highest in an artery? When does it occur?

Lymphatic System

1. Does the lymph in an afferent or efferent lymph vessel contain more impurities?
2. At what point does lymph drain into the vascular system?
3. Lymph capillaries are found in
   a. brain.
   b. bone.
   c. muscle.
   d. all of the above.
4. Name five mechanisms that help move lymph from the periphery to the venous system.
5. Superficial lymph drainage goes into what three regional lymph node groups?
6. Which lymph duct drains a larger area of the body?
7. What are the three main functions of lymph vessels?

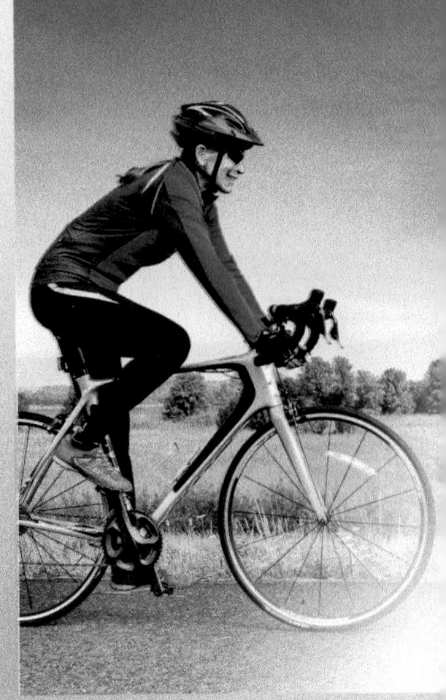

CHAPTER 8
Basic Biomechanics

Laws of Motion
Force
Torque
Stability
Simple Machines
Levers
Pulleys
Wheel and Axle
Inclined Plane
Points to Remember
Review Questions

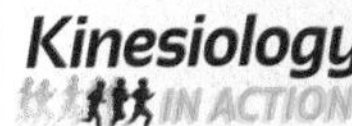

For additional practice activities and videos, please visit www.kinesiologyinaction.com

The human body, in many respects, can be referred to as a living machine. It is important when learning about *how* the body moves (kinesiology) to also learn about the forces placed on the body that *cause* the movement. As illustrated in Figure 8-1, **mechanics** is the branch of physics dealing with the study of forces and the motion produced by their actions. **Biomechanics** involves taking the principles and methods of mechanics and applying them to the structure and function of the human body. As mentioned in Chapter 1, mechanics can be divided into two main areas: statics and dynamics. **Statics** deals with factors associated with nonmoving or nearly nonmoving systems. **Dynamics** involves factors associated with moving systems and can be divided into kinetics and kinematics. **Kinetics** deals with *forces* causing movement in a system, whereas **kinematics** describes the *movement* created by the force which involves the time, space, and mass aspects of a moving system. Kinematics can be divided into osteokinematics and arthrokinematics. **Osteokinematics** focuses on the manner in which bones move in space without regard to the movement of joint surfaces, such as shoulder flexion/extension. **Arthrokinematics** deals with the manner in which adjoining joint surfaces move in relation to each other—that is, in the same or opposite direction.

Various mechanical terms must be defined before beginning to discuss these topics. **Force** is a push or pull action that can be represented as a vector. A **vector** is a quantity having both magnitude and direction. For example, if you were to push a wheelchair, you would push it with a certain speed and in a certain direction. **Velocity** is a vector that describes speed and is measured in units such as feet per second or miles per hour.

A **scalar** quantity describes only magnitude. Common scalar terms are *length, area, volume,* and *mass.* Everyday examples would be units such as 5 feet, 2 acres, 12 fluid ounces, and 150 pounds. **Mass** refers to the amount of matter that a body contains. In this example, the amount

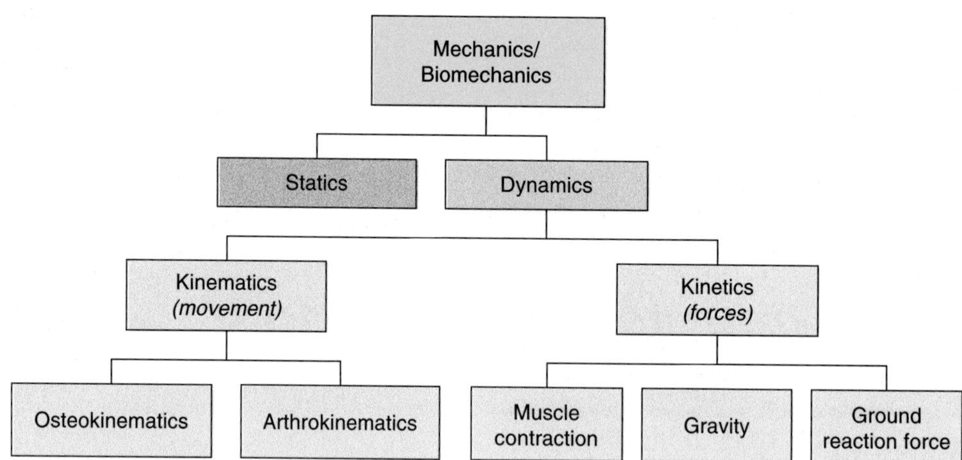

Figure 8-1. Mechanics/biomechanics relationship flowchart.

of matter within and making up the body is the mass. **Inertia** is the property of matter that causes it to resist any change of its motion in either speed or direction. Mass is a measure of inertia—its resistance to a change in motion.

With regard to kinetics, **torque** is the tendency of force to produce rotation around an axis. Muscles within the body produce motion around joint axes. Other forces that can cause movement within the body are gravity and ground reaction force. **Friction** is a force developed by two surfaces, which tends to prevent motion of one surface across another. For example, if you slide across a carpeted floor in your stocking feet, there will be so much friction between the two surfaces that you will not slide very far. However, if you slide across a highly polished hardwood floor in your stocking feet, there will be very little friction between these two surfaces and you will have a good slide.

Laws of Motion

Motion is happening all around you—people walking, cars traveling on highways, airplanes flying in the air, water flowing in rivers, balls being thrown, and so on. Isaac Newton's three laws explain all types of motion. Newton's first law of motion states that an object at rest tends to stay at rest, and an object in motion tends to stay in motion. This is sometimes referred to as the **law of inertia** because inertia is the tendency of an object to stay at rest or in motion. To demonstrate this law, consider riding in a car. If the car moves forward quickly from a starting position, your body pushes against the back of the seat and your neck probably hyperextends. Your body was at rest before the car moved, and it tended to stay at rest as the car started to move. If the car is moving and then stops suddenly, your body is thrown forward and your neck goes into extreme flexion, because your body was in motion and tended to stay in motion when the car stopped. Unfortunately, many of the people with neck injuries from automobile accidents have demonstrated this law.

A force is needed to overcome the inertia of an object and cause the object to move, stop, or change direction. The object's acceleration depends on the strength of the force applied and the object's mass. For example, kick a soccer ball and it will roll along the grass. If no forces act on it, the ball will roll forever. However, the force of friction acting on the ball causes the ball to eventually stop. There is friction between any two surfaces. In this case, it is the friction of the grass on the surface of the ball that causes the ball to stop rolling.

A soccer ball can also be used to demonstrate Newton's second law. First, mildly kick the ball and notice how far it travels. Next, kick the ball about twice as hard as the first kick. Notice that the ball will travel approximately twice as far. **Acceleration** is any change in the velocity of an object. The soccer ball is accelerating when it starts moving. If you were to kick the ball again even harder, it would travel proportionately farther. This is Newton's second law of motion, the **law of acceleration:** The amount of acceleration depends on the strength of the force applied to an object. Acceleration can also deal with a change in direction. Force is needed to change direction; according to the law, the change in an object's direction depends on the force applied to it.

Another part of Newton's second law deals with the mass of an object. *Mass* is the amount of matter in an object. Acceleration is inversely proportional to the mass of an object. If you apply the same amount of force to two objects of differing mass, the object with greater mass will accelerate less than the object with less mass. You can demonstrate this by first rolling a soccer ball, then rolling a bowling ball with the same amount of force. The heavier bowling ball will not travel nearly as far.

Newton's third law of motion, the **law of action-reaction,** states that for every action there is an equal and opposite reaction. The strength of the reaction is always equal to the strength of the action, and it occurs in the opposite direction. This can be demonstrated by jumping on a trampoline. The action is you jumping down on the trampoline. The reaction is the trampoline pushing back with the same amount of force, causing you to rebound up in the opposite direction that you jumped. The harder you jump, the higher you rebound. While not as visible as on the trampoline, the floor also pushed back on your leg while walking, with an equal amount of force, and in an opposite direction. If you jump down onto the floor off a small step, you can feel this force traveling up through your legs. This is called the **ground reaction force.**

As stated, no motion can occur without a force. There are basically two types of force that will cause the body to move. Forces can be internal, such as muscular contraction, ligamentous restraint, or bony support. Forces can also be external, such as gravity or any externally applied resistance such as weight, friction, and so on.

Force

Force is one of those concepts that everyone understands but is difficult to define. To create a force, one object must act on another. Force can be either a push, which creates compression, or a pull, which creates tension. Movement occurs if one opposing force pushes (or pulls) harder than the other or when two or more forces are working together.

Forces are vector quantities. A vector quantity describes both magnitude and direction. A person pulling a heavy load with a rope is an example of a vector. The tension in the rope represents the vector's magnitude, and the direction of the pull on the rope represents the vector's direction.

A vector force can be shown graphically by an arrow of appropriate length and direction. The longer the line of the arrow, the larger the force it represents. Figure 8-2 shows two people (representing forces) pushing on the chest of drawers, but at right angles to each other. The characteristics of force include the following:

1. Magnitude (each person is pushing equally in this case)
2. Direction (shown by the arrow)
3. Point of application (the same for both people)

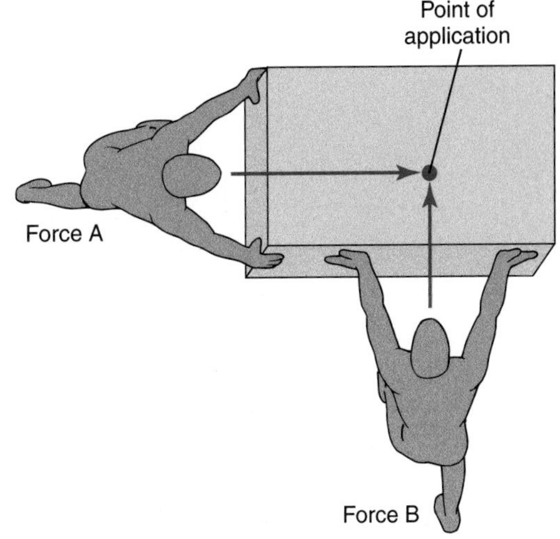

Figure 8-2. Concurrent force system. Two people pushing at different angles to each other through a common point of application.

Forces can be described by the effect they produce. A **linear force** results when two or more forces are acting along the same line. Figure 8-3A shows two people pulling a boat with the same rope in the same direction. Figure 8-3B shows two people pulling on the same rope but in opposite directions. **Parallel forces** occur in the same plane and in the same or opposite direction. An example of parallel forces would be the three-point pressures of bracing (Fig. 8-4). Two forces—in this case, *X* and *Y*—are parallel to each other and pushing in the same direction while a third parallel force *(Z),* the back brace, is pushing against them. This middle force must always be located between the two parallel forces. To be effective, the middle force must be of sufficient strength to resist the other two forces. You could also say that the two forces must be of sufficient strength to resist the middle force.

To produce **concurrent forces,** two or more forces must act on a common point but must pull or push in different directions, such as the two people pushing on the cabinet in Figure 8-5. The overall effect of these two different forces is called the **resultant force** and lies somewhere in between.

Because forces can be represented as vectors, they can be shown graphically using what is called the **parallelogram method.** Using Figure 8-5 as an example, first draw in vectors for the two forces (solid lines). Second, complete the parallelogram using dotted lines. Next, draw in the diagonal of the parallelogram (middle line and arrow). This diagonal line represents the resultant force, or in this case, the actual direction in which the cabinet will move.

An example of resultant force in the body is the anterior and posterior parts of the deltoid muscle

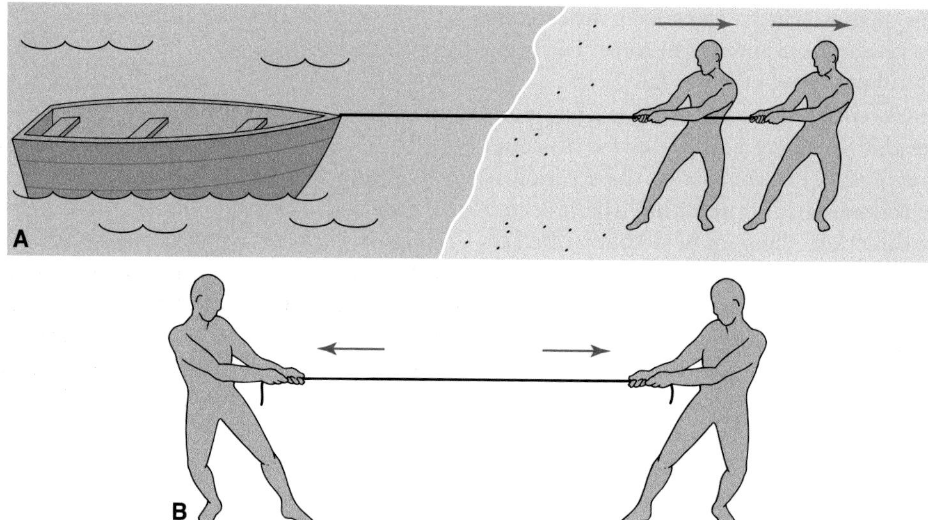

Figure 8-3. Linear forces. **(A)** Two people pulling in same direction. **(B)** Two people pulling in opposite directions.

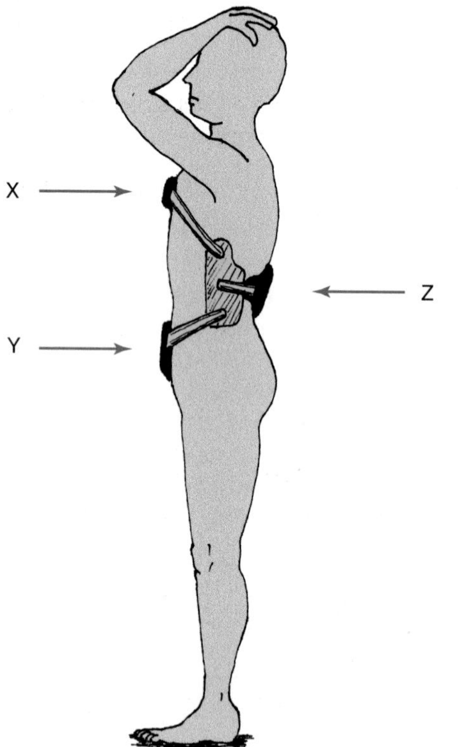

Figure 8-4. Parallel forces of body brace. Forces *X* and *Y* are parallel in the same direction while force *Z* is parallel but in the opposite direction. Force *Z* must be between forces *X* and *Y* to provide stability. If force *Z* was at either end, instead of in the middle, motion would occur.

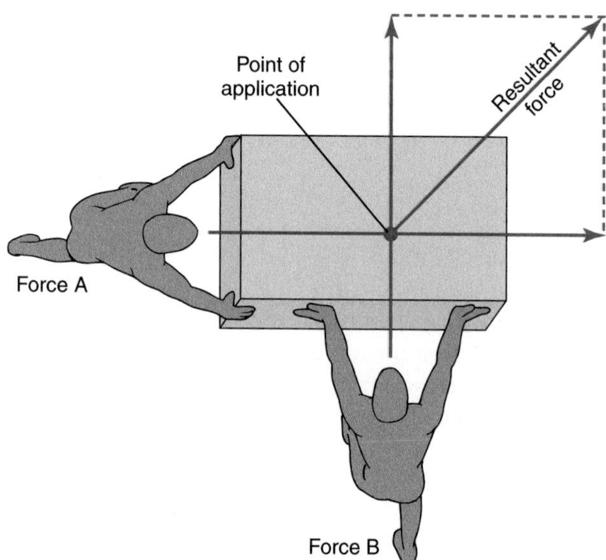

Figure 8-5. A parallelogram shows graphically the resultant force of two concurrent forces pushing on a chest of drawers.

(Fig. 8-6). Although both parts have a common attachment (the insertion), they pull in different directions. When both concurrent forces are equal, the resultant force will fall right in the center and cause the shoulder to abduct. If the pull of the two forces is not equal (i.e., if the pull of the anterior deltoid is stronger than that of the posterior), the resultant force will produce motion

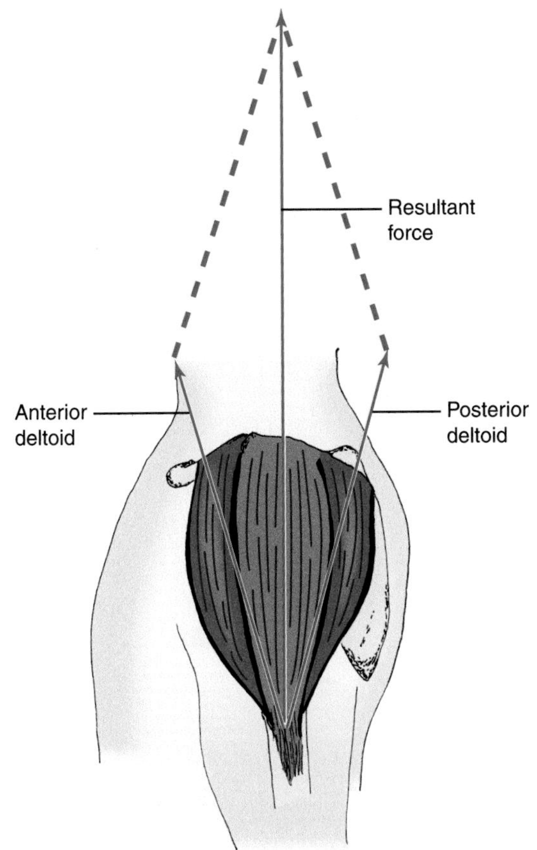

Figure 8-6. Resultant force of equal forces of anterior and posterior deltoid muscles.

more in the direction of the anterior deltoid (Fig. 8-7). Notice in Figure 8-7 that the anterior deltoid arrow is longer and therefore a stronger force than the posterior deltoid. This will cause the shoulder to flex and abduct diagonally in a forward and outward direction.

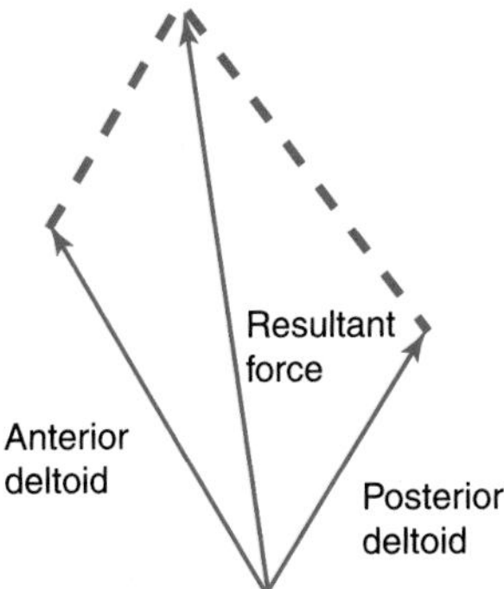

Figure 8-7. Resultant force of unequal forces moves toward the stronger force.

A **force couple** occurs when two or more forces act in different directions, resulting in a turning effect. This can be seen with two or more children pushing on opposite sides of a playground merry-go round (Fig. 8-8). A third child could be added between them on the right side of the wheel. This child would be pushing in a different direction, as would a fourth child positioned opposite the third child. They would all be pushing in different directions, but the merry-go-round would continue to rotate counter clockwise in this example. In Figure 8-9, notice that the upper trapezius pulls up and in, the lower trapezius pulls down, and the serratus anterior pulls out. The combined effect is that the scapula rotates.

Torque

Torque, also known as **moment of force,** is the ability of force to produce rotation around an axis. It can be thought of as rotary force. The amount of torque a lever has depends on the amount of force exerted and the distance the force is from the axis. Use of a wrench demonstrates torque. The twisting force (torque) exerted by the wrench can be increased either by

1. Increasing the force applied to the handle, or
2. Increasing the length of the handle.

Torque is also the amount of force needed by a muscle contraction to cause rotary joint motion.

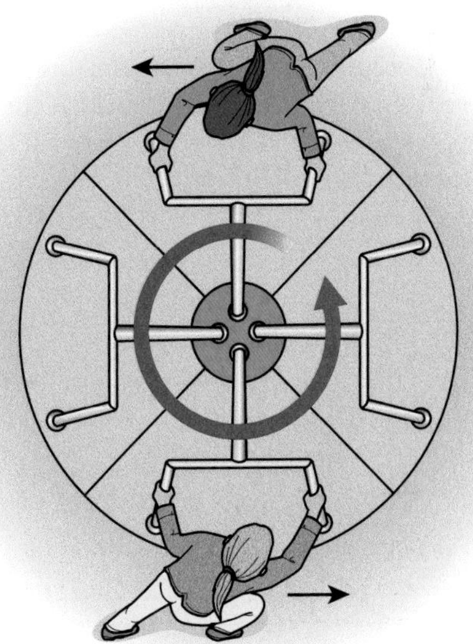

Figure 8-8. Force couple of a playground merry-go-round.

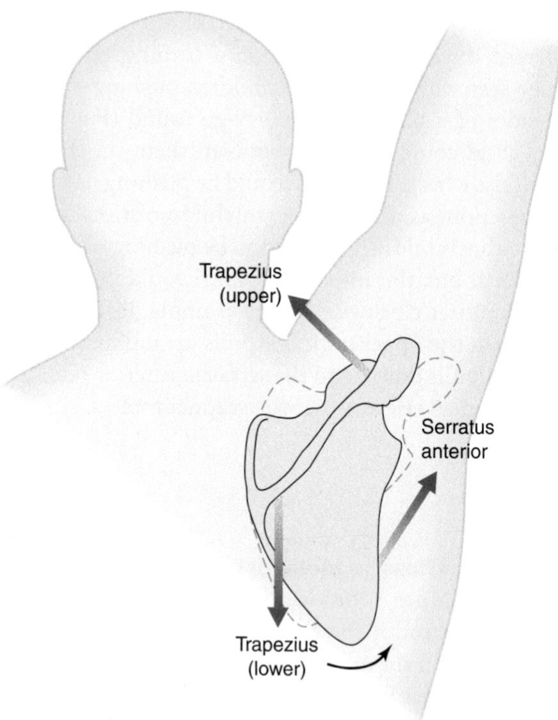

Figure 8-9. Force couple of muscles rotating the scapula.

How much torque can be produced depends on the strength of the force (magnitude) and its perpendicular distance from the force's line of pull to the axis of rotation. That perpendicular distance is called the **moment arm,** or *torque arm* (Fig. 8-10). Therefore, the moment arm of a muscle is the perpendicular distance between the muscle's line of pull and the center of the joint (axis of rotation). Torque is greatest when the angle of pull is at 90 degrees (Fig. 8-11A), and it decreases as the angle of pull either decreases (Fig. 8-11B) or increases (Fig. 8-11C) from that perpendicular position.

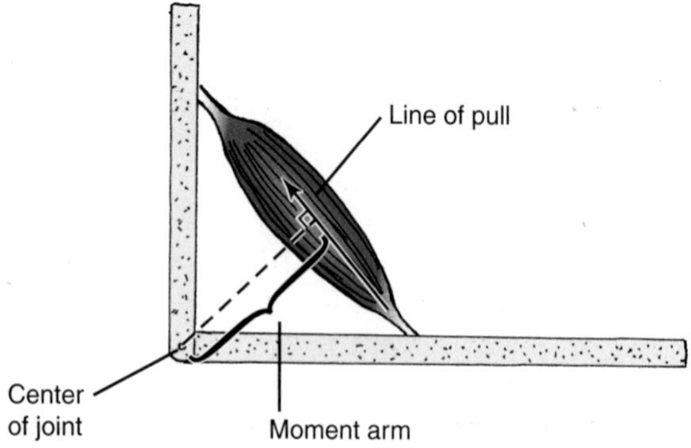

Figure 8-10. Moment arm of biceps is the perpendicular distance between the muscle's line of pull and the center of the joint.

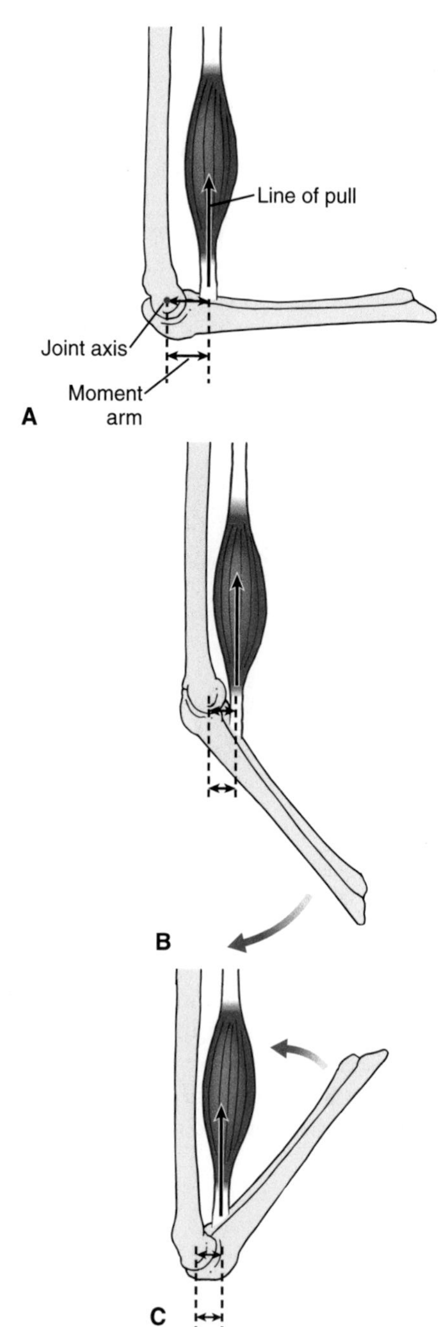

Figure 8-11. Effect of moment arm on torque. **(A)** Moment arm and angular force are greatest at 90 degrees. **(B)** As joint moves toward 0 degrees, moment arm decreases and stabilizing force increases. **(C)** As joint moves beyond 90 degrees and toward 180 degrees, moment arm decreases and dislocating force increases.

No torque is produced if the force is directed exactly through the axis of rotation. Although this is not quite possible for a muscle, it comes very close. For example, if the biceps contracts when the elbow is nearly or completely extended, there is very little torque produced (see

Fig. 8-11B). The perpendicular distance between the joint axis and the line of pull is very small. Therefore, the force generated by the muscle is primarily a **stabilizing force,** in that nearly all of the force generated by the muscle is directed back into the joint, pulling the two bones together.

When the angle of pull is at 90 degrees (see Fig. 8-11A), the perpendicular distance between the joint axis and the line of pull is much larger. Therefore, the force generated by the muscle is primarily an **angular force,** or movement force, in that most of the force generated by the muscle is directed at rotating, not stabilizing, the joint.

As a muscle contracts through its range of motion (ROM), the amount of angular or stabilizing force changes. As the muscle increases its angular force, it decreases its stabilizing force and vice versa. At 90 degrees, or halfway through its range, the muscle has its greatest angular force. Past 90 degrees, the stabilizing force becomes a **dislocating force** because the force is directed away from the joint (see Fig. 8-11C). In Figures 8-11B and C, when the stabilizing and dislocating forces are increasing, the angular (rotating) force is decreasing. Stated another way, a muscle is most efficient at moving, or rotating, a joint when the joint is at or near 90 degrees. A muscle becomes less efficient at moving or rotating when the joint angle is at the beginning or near the end of the joint range. Some muscles have a much greater stabilizing force than angular force throughout the range, and therefore are more effective at stabilizing the joint than moving it. The coracobrachialis of the shoulder joint is a good example (see Fig. 10-19). Its line of pull is mostly vertical and quite close to the axis of the shoulder joint. Therefore, the coracobrachalis has a very short moment arm, which makes this muscle more effective at stabilizing the head of the humerus in the shoulder joint than at moving the shoulder joint.

The angular force of the quadriceps muscle is increased by the presence of the patella. The patella, a sesamoid bone encapsulated in the tendon, increases the moment arm of the quadriceps muscle by holding the tendon out and away from the femur. This changes the angle of pull, allowing the muscle to have a greater angular force (Fig. 8-12A). Without a patella, the moment arm is smaller, making the muscle's line of pull more vertical, and much of the force of the quadriceps is directed back into the joint (Fig. 8-12B). Although this is good for stability, it is not effective for motion. To have effective knee motion, it is vital that the quadriceps muscle provides a strong angular force.

In summary, if the moment arm is greater, then the angular force (torque) is also greater. Moment arm is determined by measuring the perpendicular distance between the joint axis and the muscle's line of pull. If the joint angle is near 0 degrees (almost straight), the moment arm is small and the force is a stabilizing action that moves the two bones of the joint together. If the joint angle is nearer 180 degrees (completely bent), the moment arm is small and the force is dislocating, pulling the two bones away from each other. If the joint angle is in the midrange of motion, the moment arm is greatest, and the ability to move the joint is strongest. Moment arm, size of the muscle, and contractile strength of the muscle all determine how effective a muscle is in causing joint motion.

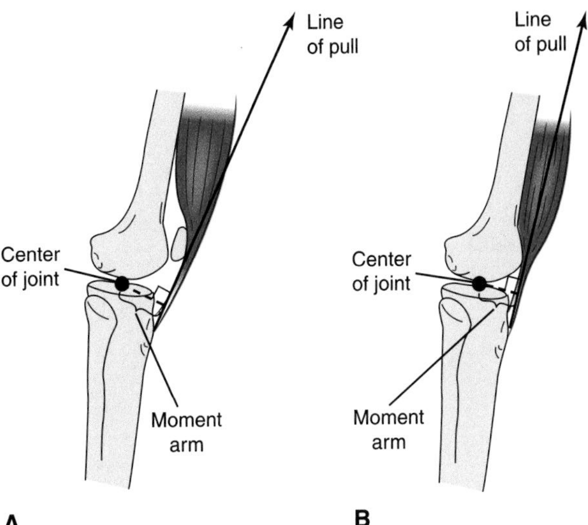

Figure 8-12. Moment arm of quadriceps muscle **(A)** with a patella and **(B)** without a patella.

Stability

When an object is balanced, all torques acting on it are even, and it is in a **state of equilibrium.** How secure or precarious this state of equilibrium is depends primarily on the relationship between the object's center of gravity and its base of support. To understand the principles of stability, certain terms must be defined. **Gravity** is the mutual attraction between the earth and an object. **Gravitational force** is always directed vertically downward, toward the center of the earth. Practically speaking, gravitational force is always directed toward the ground. **Center of gravity (COG)** is the balance point of an object at which torque on all sides is equal. It is also the point at which the planes of the body intersect, as shown in Figure 8-13.

In the human body, the COG is located in the midline at about the level of, though slightly anterior to, the

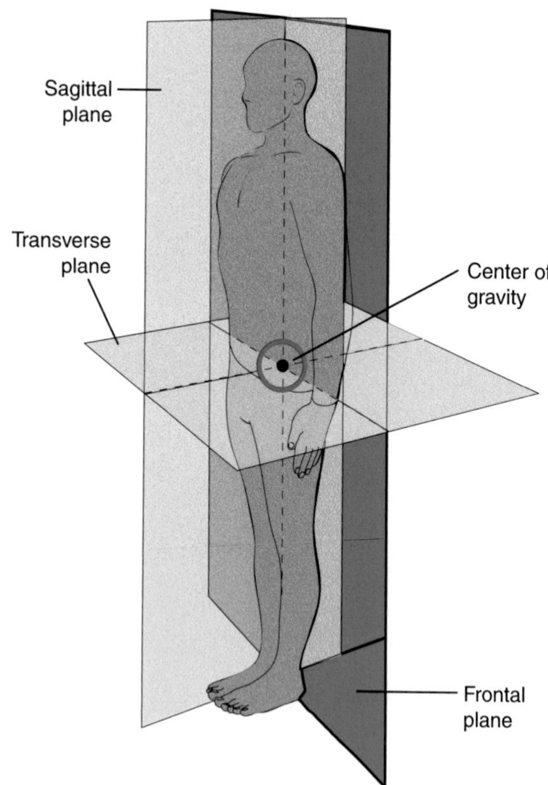

Figure 8-13. The center of gravity is the point at which the three cardinal planes intersect.

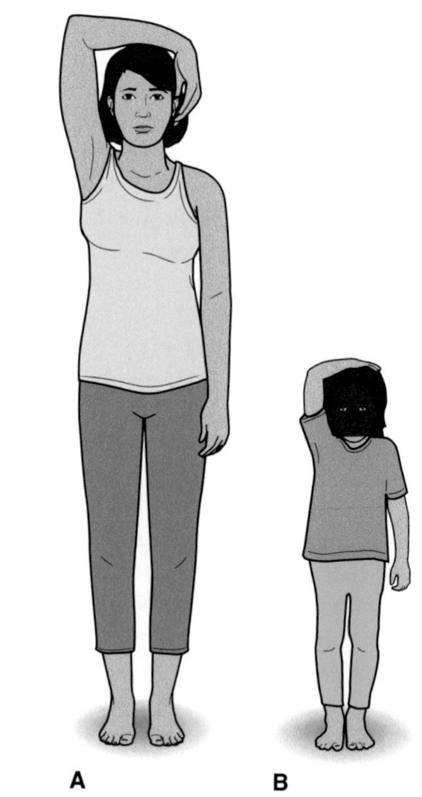

Figure 8-14. Body proportions change as a person grows. (A) Adult can reach over top of head to touch opposite ear. (B) Child can reach over head only part way.

second sacral vertebra of an adult. Because body proportions change with age, the COG of a child is higher than that of an adult. To demonstrate this, move your right arm up over your head and touch your left ear (Fig. 8-14A). Now, ask a 3-year-old to do the same. You will notice that although you can easily touch your ear, the child's hand reaches only to about the top of the head (Fig. 8-14B). The child's head is much larger in proportion to the arms and rest of the body.

As a point of interest, height-arm span is a body proportion made famous by the illustration of Leonardo da Vinci. The length of an adult's outstretched arms is equal to his or her height (Fig. 8-15).

Base of support (BOS) is that part of a body that is in contact with the supporting surface. If you outlined the surface of the body in contact with the ground, you would have identified the BOS. **Line of gravity** (LOG) is an imaginary vertical line passing through the COG toward the center of the earth. These are shown in Figure 8-16.

There are basically three states of equilibrium (Fig. 8-17). **Stable equilibrium** occurs when an object is in a position where disturbing it would require its COG to be raised. A simple example is that of a brick.

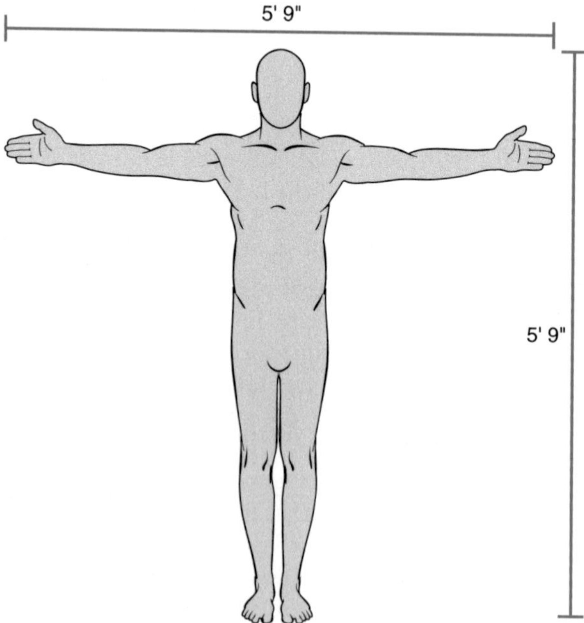

Figure 8-15. In an adult, arm span and body height are equal.

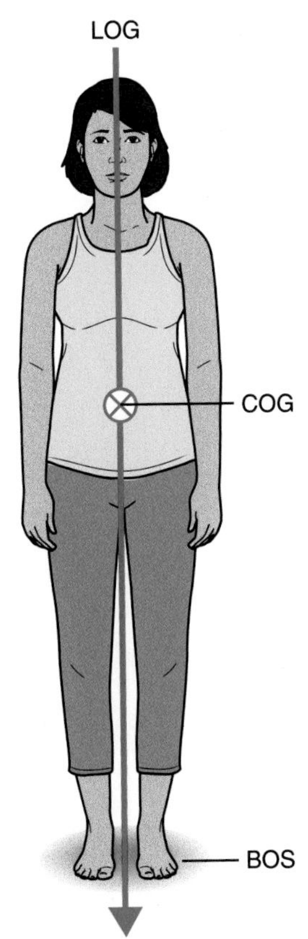

Figure 8-16. Center of gravity (COG), line of gravity (LOG), and base of support (BOS).

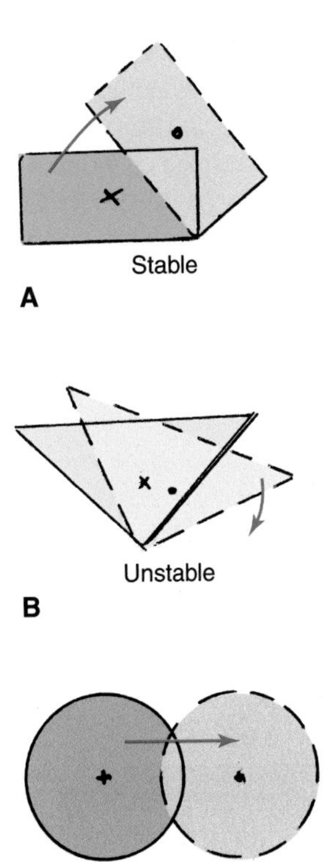

Figure 8-17. Three states of equilibrium: **(A)** stable, **(B)** unstable, and **(C)** neutral.

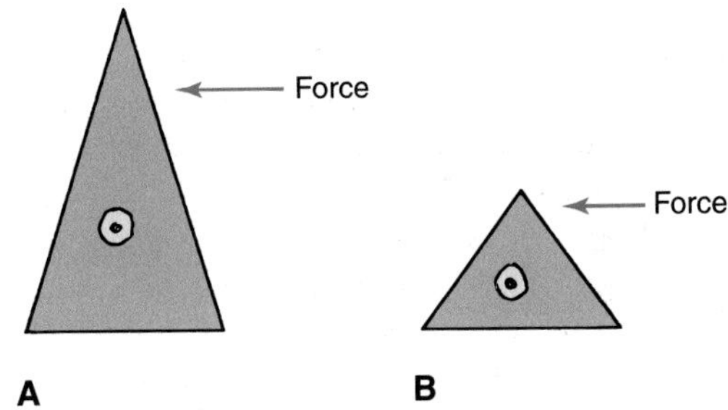

Figure 8-18. Relationship of height of center of gravity to stability. **(A)** Higher COG is less stable. **(B)** Lower COG is more stable.

When the widest part of the brick is in contact with the surface (BOS), it is quite stable (Fig. 8-17A). To disturb it, the brick would have to be tipped up in any direction, thus raising its COG. The same could be said of a person lying flat on the floor. **Unstable equilibrium** occurs when only a slight force is needed to disturb an object. Balancing a pencil on its pointed end is a good example. A similar example is that of a person standing on one leg. Once balanced, it takes very little force to knock over the pencil or person (Fig. 8-17B). **Neutral equilibrium** exists when an object's COG is neither raised nor lowered when it is disturbed. A good example is a ball. As the ball rolls across the floor, its COG remains the same (Fig. 8-17C). A person moving across the room while seated in a wheelchair demonstrates neutral equilibrium.

The following principles demonstrate the relationships between balance, stability, and motion:

1. The lower the COG, the more stable the object. In Figure 8-18, both triangles have the same base of support. However, the triangle on the left is taller, has a higher COG, and thus is more unstable than the triangle on the right. It would take less force to disturb the taller triangle.
2. The COG and LOG must remain within the BOS for an object to remain stable. (Keep in mind that the LOG passes through the COG. Therefore, what can be said of one can be said of the other. For the purpose of clarity, from this point forward, only the term COG will be used.) The wider the BOS, the more stable the object. In the example in Figure 8-19A, the book is resting entirely on its BOS (tabletop) and is quite stable.

As you push the book off the edge (Fig. 8-19B), it becomes less stable. When its COG is no longer over its BOS (Fig. 8-19C), the book will fall.

Another example is a woman standing upright on both feet (Fig. 8-20A). Her COG lies at or near the center of the base of support. As she leans to the side (Fig. 8-20B), her COG moves toward the border of her BOS. As soon as her COG passes beyond the BOS, she becomes unstable, and if her posture is not corrected or if her BOS is not widened, she will fall. To lean farther without losing her balance, she could either raise her opposite arm or widen her stance. In either case, her COG would move back over her BOS.

3. Stability increases as the BOS is widened in the direction of the force. A person standing at a bus stop on a very windy day would be more stable when facing into the wind and placing one foot behind the other, thus widening the BOS in the direction of the wind (Fig. 8-21).
4. The greater the mass of an object, the greater its stability. This concept is observed by looking at the size of players on a football team. Linebackers are traditionally heavier, and thus harder to push over, but they are not particularly fast. Halfbacks, whose job is to run with the ball, are much lighter (and easier to push over). It can be said that what is gained in stability is lost in speed and vice versa.
5. The greater the friction between the supporting surface and the BOS, the more stable the body will be. Walking on an icy sidewalk is a slippery experience because there is essentially no friction between the ice and the shoe. Sanding the sidewalk increases the friction of the icy surface, thus improving traction. Having a surface with a great deal of friction is not always desirable. Pushing a wheelchair across a hardwood floor is much easier than pushing one across a carpeted floor. The carpet creates more friction, making it harder to push the wheelchair.

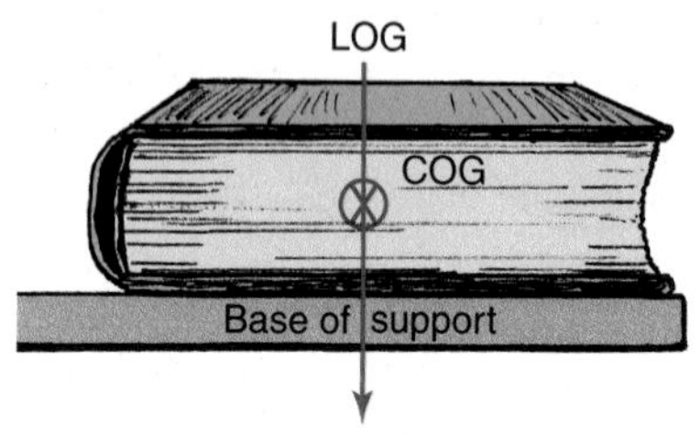

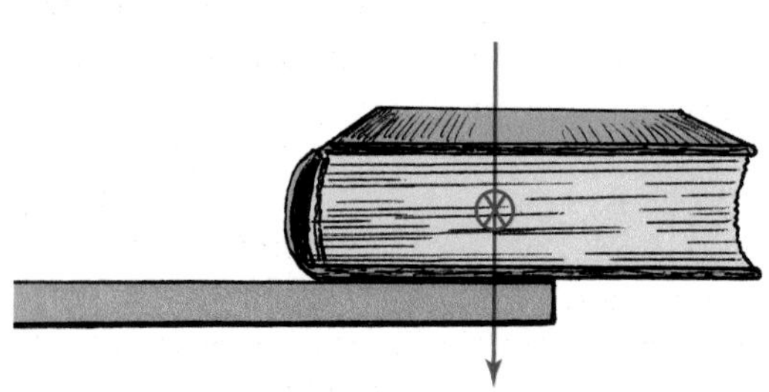

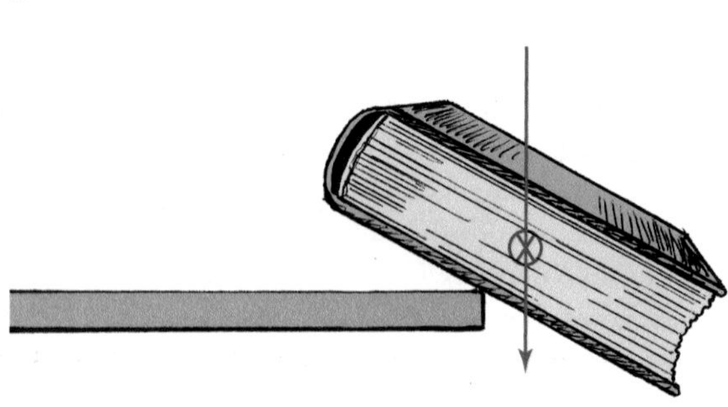

Figure 8-19. Relationship of COG to BOS. **(A)** The book is very stable because its COG is in the middle of its BOS. **(B)** The book is less stable because its COG is near the edge of its BOS. **(C)** The book is unstable and will fall because its COG is beyond its BOS.

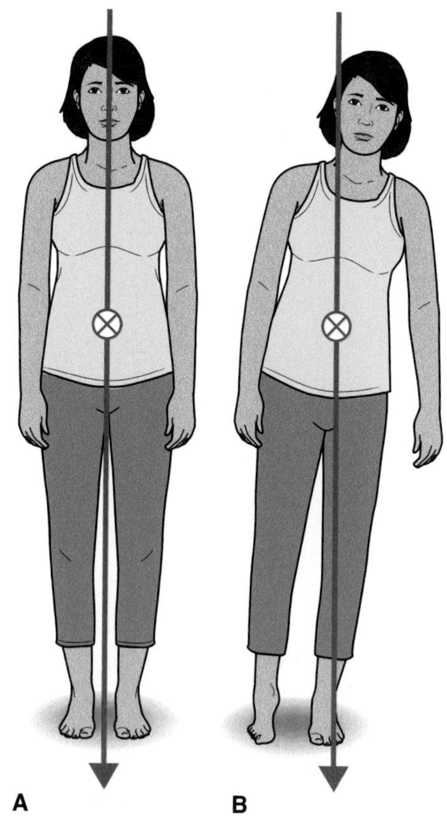

Figure 8-20. Relationship of COG to BOS. **(A)** She is stable—her COG is in the middle of her BOS. **(B)** She is less stable because her COG is near the edge of her BOS.

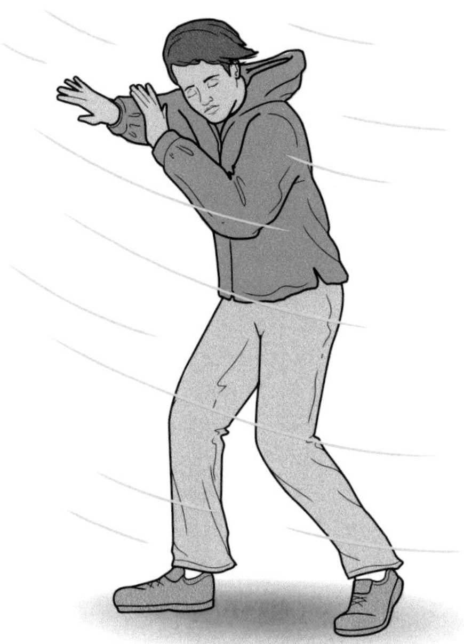

Figure 8-21. Wider base of support in direction of force increases stability.

6. People have better balance while moving if they focus on a stationary object rather than on a moving object. Therefore, people learning to walk with crutches will be more stable if they focus on an object down the hall rather than looking down at their moving feet or the crutches.

Simple Machines

In engineering, various machines are used to change the magnitude or direction of a force. The four simple machines are the lever, the pulley, the wheel and axle, and the inclined plane. Examples of each of these machines, except for the inclined plane, can be found in the human body. The lever, the wheel and axle, and the inclined plane allow a person to exert a force greater than could be exerted by using muscle power alone; the pulley allows force to be applied more efficiently. This increase in force is usually at the expense of speed and can be expressed in terms of mechanical advantage, which will be described later.

Levers

There are three classes of levers, each with a different purpose and a different mechanical advantage. We use levers daily to help us accomplish various activities. Usually a lever will favor either power or distance (range of motion), but not both. However, the basic rule of all simple machines is that the advantage gained in power is lost in distance. Sometimes, a great deal of power is needed, such as moving a heavy rock. Other times, distance (range of motion) is needed, such as swinging a tennis racket. Wheelbarrows, crowbars, manual can openers, scissors, golf clubs, and playground seesaws are but a few examples of levers. Different types of levers can also be found in the human body. Each type of lever will favor power or distance, but not both.

To understand the structure and function of levers, you should be familiar with certain terms. A **lever** is rigid and can rotate around a fixed point when a force is applied. A bone is an example of a lever in the human body. The fixed point around which the lever rotates is the **axis (A),** sometimes referred to as the *fulcrum.* In the body, the joint is the axis. The **force (F),** sometimes called the *effort,* which causes the lever to move, is usually muscular. The **resistance (R),** sometimes called the *load,* that must be overcome for motion to occur can include the weight of the part being moved (arm, leg, etc.), the pull of gravity on the part, or an external weight being moved by the body part. When determining a muscle's role (force or resistance), it is important to use the point of attachment to the bone, not the muscle belly, as the point of reference. When determining the resistance of the part, use its COG.

The **force arm (FA)** is the distance between the force and the axis, whereas the **resistance arm (RA)** is the distance between the resistance and the axis (Fig. 8-22). The arrangement of the axis *(A)* in relation to the force *(F)* and the resistance *(R)* determines the type of lever. The longer the FA, the easier it is to move the part. Conversely, the longer the RA, the harder it is to move the part. Remember, there is always a trade-off. With the longer FA, the part will be easier to move, but the FA will have to move a greater distance. When the RA is longer, it won't have to move as far, but it will be harder to move.

Classes of Levers

In a **first-class lever,** the axis is located between the force and the resistance:

First-class lever F ———————— R
A

If the axis is close to the resistance, the RA will be shorter and the FA will be longer. Therefore, it will be easy to

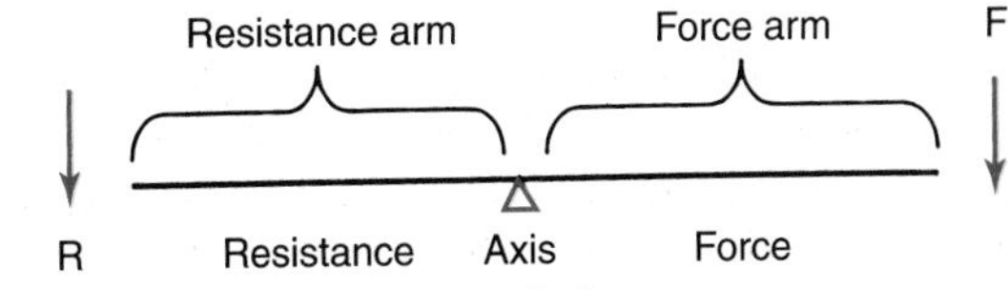

Figure 8-22. Components of a lever.

move the resistance. If the axis is close to the force, just the opposite will occur; it will be hard to move the resistance.

Try this with a pencil (axis), a ruler (force), and a fairly heavy book (resistance). Something small that doesn't roll easily would make a better axis; otherwise, have someone hold the pencil in place. The ruler—or even another long pencil—can be used, but it must be a rigid bar. Place the ruler about 2 inches under the book so it will stay under the book as the book is raised. Place the pencil perpendicularly under the ruler near the book (Fig. 8-23A). You have created a long FA and a short RA. Push down on the outer end of the ruler and notice two things: (1) how easy it is to raise the book, and (2) how far down you have to push the ruler. Next, move the pencil (axis) out toward the other end of the ruler, and push down on the ruler (Fig. 8-23B). This time you should notice that it is harder to raise the book, but you didn't have to push the ruler down very far. You have just demonstrated that with a longer FA (or a shorter RA),

1. It is easy to move the resistance (book),
2. The resistance is moved only a short distance, and
3. The force has to be applied through a long distance.

However, with a shorter FA (or a longer RA),

1. It is harder to move the resistance,
2. The resistance moves a longer distance, and
3. The force is applied through a short distance.

This is an example of a first-class lever because the axis is in the middle, with the force on one side and resistance on the other. By placing the axis close to the resistance, you have a lever that favors force. By placing the axis close to the force, you have a lever that favors distance (range of motion) and speed. If you place the axis midway between the force and the resistance (assuming they are the same weight), the lever favors balance.

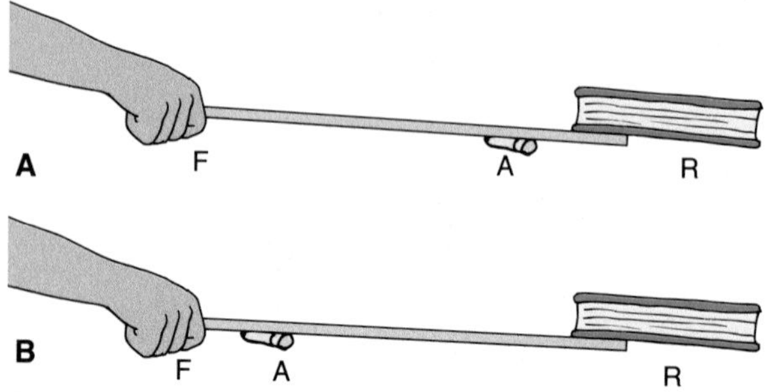

Figure 8-23. First-class lever. FAR (*F* = force; *A* = axis; *R* = resistance). **(A)** *A* is closer to *R*. **(B)** *A* is closer to *F*.

Figure 8-24 shows a worker carrying two bundles of hay. Each bundle (one is force and the other is resistance) is approximately the same weight and distance from the axis. The shoulder is the axis. If one bundle is heavier, it would have to be moved closer to the axis to keep the overall load balanced.

An example of a first-class lever in the human body is the head sitting on the first cervical vertebra, moving up and down in cervical flexion and hyperextension. The vertebra is the axis, the resistance is the weight on one side of the head, and the force is the muscle pulling down on the opposite side of the head. The force and resistance will change places, depending on which way the head is tipped. For example, as shown in Figure 8-25A, if your head is tipped toward your chest and you want to return to the upright position, your posterior neck muscles (force) must contract to pull the weight of your head up against gravity (resistance). If you look up to the sky, your head would rock back and you would use your anterior neck muscles to pull your head into the upright position (Fig. 8-25B). Although force and resistance may change places, depending on the motion, the axis is always in the middle of a first-class lever.

In a **second-class lever,** the resistance is in the middle, with the axis at one end and the force at the other end:

Second-class lever —— R —— F (A below left end)

The wheelbarrow is an example of a second-class lever (Fig. 8-26). The wheel at the front end is the axis, the wheelbarrow contents are the resistance, and the person pushing the wheelbarrow is the force. If we assume that the wheelbarrow is carrying a load of heavy bricks, we can

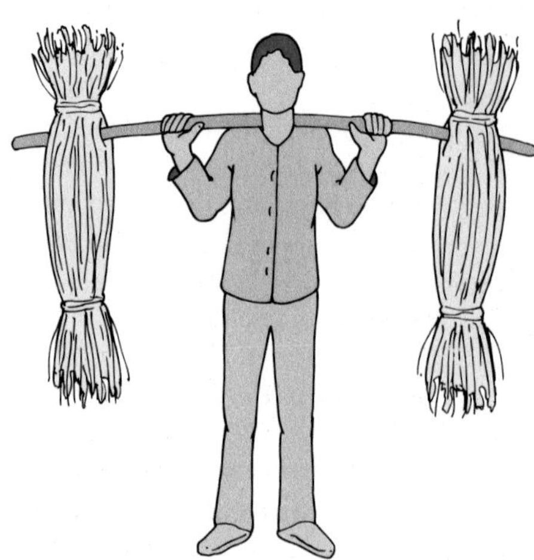

Figure 8-24. First-class lever. The two loads (*F* and *R*) are balanced on the shoulders.

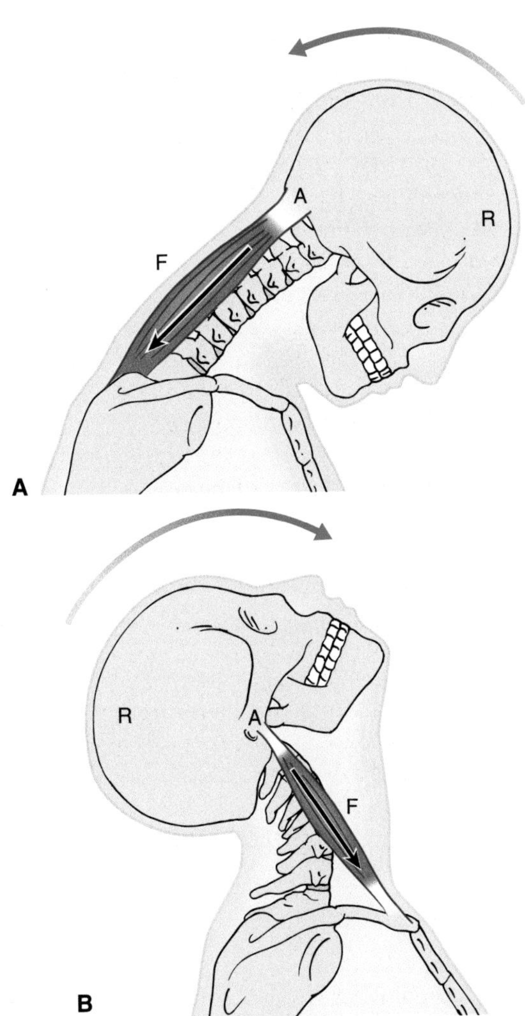

Figure 8-25. Head moving on neck demonstrates a first-class lever. In **(A),** the axis is the head posteriorly moving on the vertebral column and is located between force (extensor muscles) and resistance (weight of the head itself). In **(B),** the axis is the head moving anteriorly on the vertebral column and is located between the force (flexor muscles) and the resistance (weight of head).

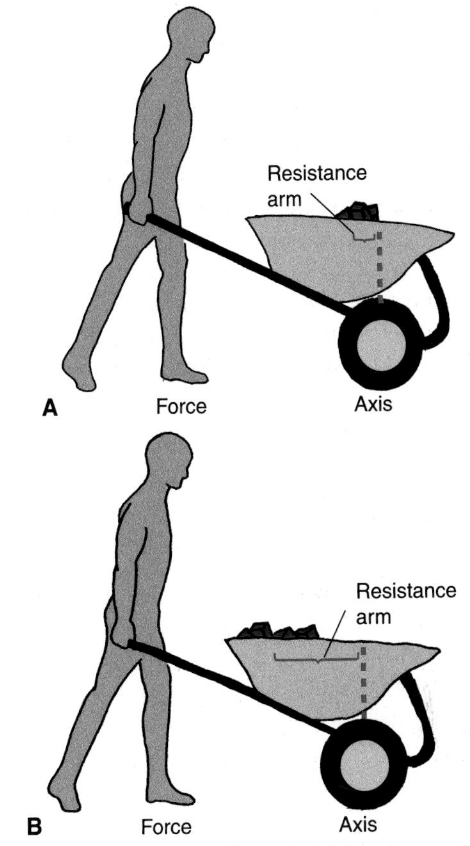

Figure 8-26. Second-class lever. **(A)** *RA* is shorter. **(B)** *RA* is longer.

apply the earlier statement that *the longer the FA, the easier it is to move the part* and *the longer the RA, the harder it is to move the part.* If we put all the bricks as close to the wheel as possible (Fig. 8-26A), we now have a long FA and a short RA. The wheelbarrow should be fairly easy to move. However, if we move the bricks to the other end of the wheelbarrow (Fig. 8-26B), the FA remains the same length, but the RA is longer. The wheelbarrow is now harder to move because we have lengthened the RA.

There are relatively few examples of second-class levers in the body; however, the action of the ankle plantar flexor muscles when a person stands on tiptoe is one (Fig. 8-27). In this case, the axis is the metatarsophalangeal (MTP) joints in the foot, the resistance is the

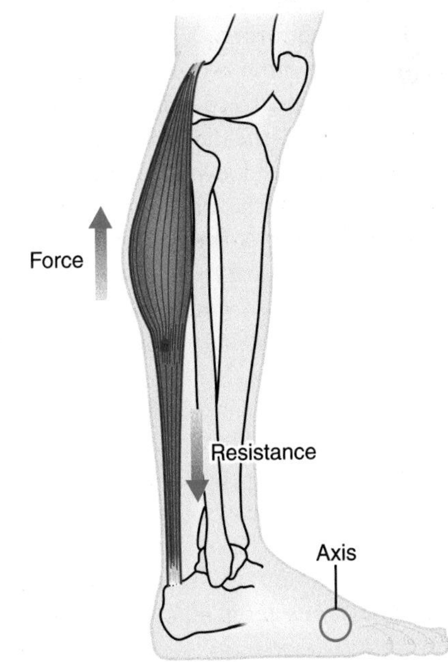

Figure 8-27. Plantar flexors lifting body weight demonstrates a second-class lever.

tibia and the rest of the body weight above it, and the force is provided by the ankle plantar flexors. Therefore, the resistance (body weight) is between the axis (MTP joint) and the force (plantar flexors). The RA is only slightly shorter than the FA. A second-class lever favors power because a relatively small force (the muscle) can move a large resistance (the body). However, the body can be raised only a fairly short distance. This again proves the basic rule of simple machines–what is gained in power (raising the body weight) is lost in distance (the body can't be raised very far).

A **third-class lever** has force in the middle, with resistance and the axis at the opposite ends:

Third-class lever ——F——R—— (A at left end)

An example of this type of lever is a person moving one end of a boat either toward or away from a dock (Fig. 8-28). The axis is the front of the boat tied to the dock. The force is the person pushing on the boat, and the resistance is the weight of the boat. If the person pushes close to the front of the boat as in Figure 8-28A, it will be harder to move the boat, but the back of the boat will swing farther away from the dock. Conversely, if the person pushes farther back on the boat as in Figure 8-28B, the boat stern won't swing away from the dock as far, but it will be easier to move. In this case, the RA doesn't change, but the FA does. When the FA is shorter, the boat is harder to push but moves a greater distance. When the FA is lengthened, the boat is easier to push but doesn't move as far. In other words, any gain in distance is lost in power.

The advantage of the third-class lever is speed and distance. This is, by far, the most common lever in the body. In the example of elbow flexion (Fig. 8-29), the axis is the elbow joint, the biceps muscle exerts the force, and the resistance is the weight of the forearm and hand. For the hand to be truly functional, it must be able to move through a wide range of motion. The resistance, in this case, will vary depending on what, if anything, is in the hand.

Why are there so many third-class levers (which favor speed and distance) and so few second-class levers (which favor power) in the body? Probably because the advantage gained from increased speed and distance is more important than the advantage gained from increased power. Examine the roles of the biceps and the brachioradialis muscles in elbow flexion (Fig. 8-30). They both cross the elbow but attach to the radius at very different places. The biceps muscle attaches to the

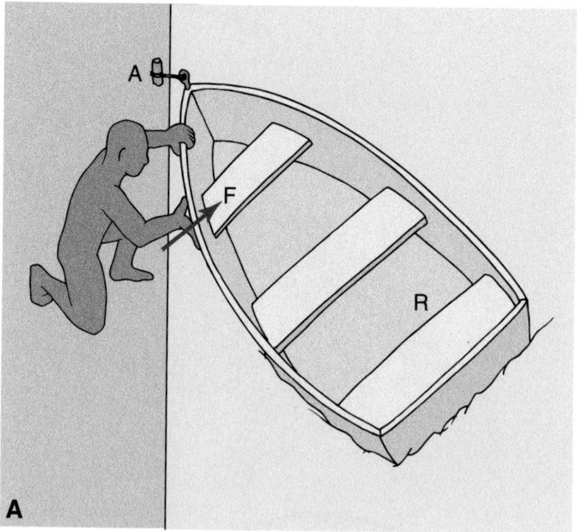

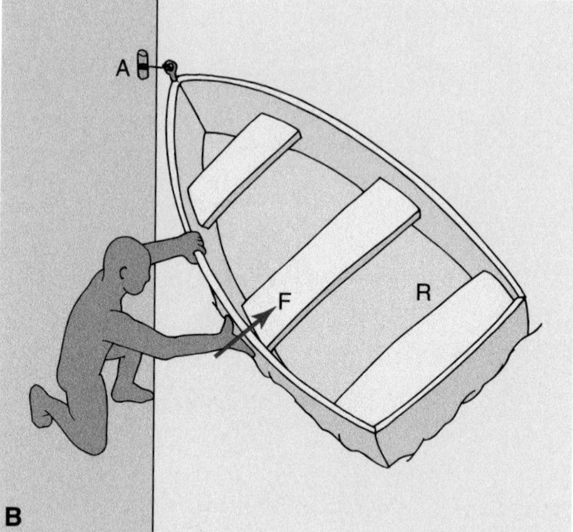

Figure 8-28. Moving boat tied to dock demonstrates a third-class lever (axis, force, resistance). *A* is the point where the boat is held against the dock. *F* is where the person pushes (or pulls) the boat away (toward) the dock, and *R* is the weight of the boat. In **(A)**, it will be harder to move the boat, whereas in **(B)** it will be easier.

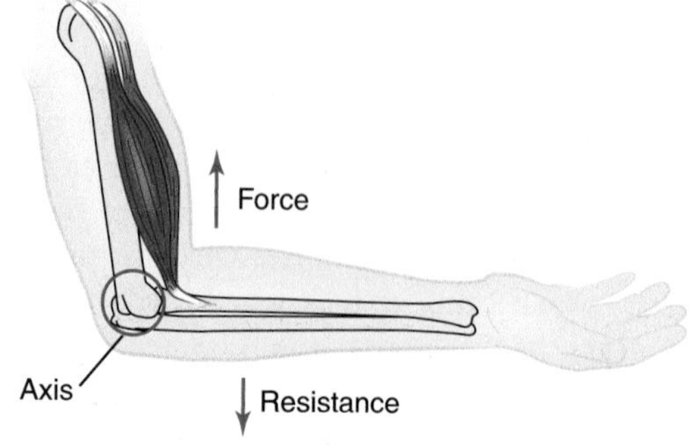

Figure 8-29. Biceps demonstrating a third-class lever.

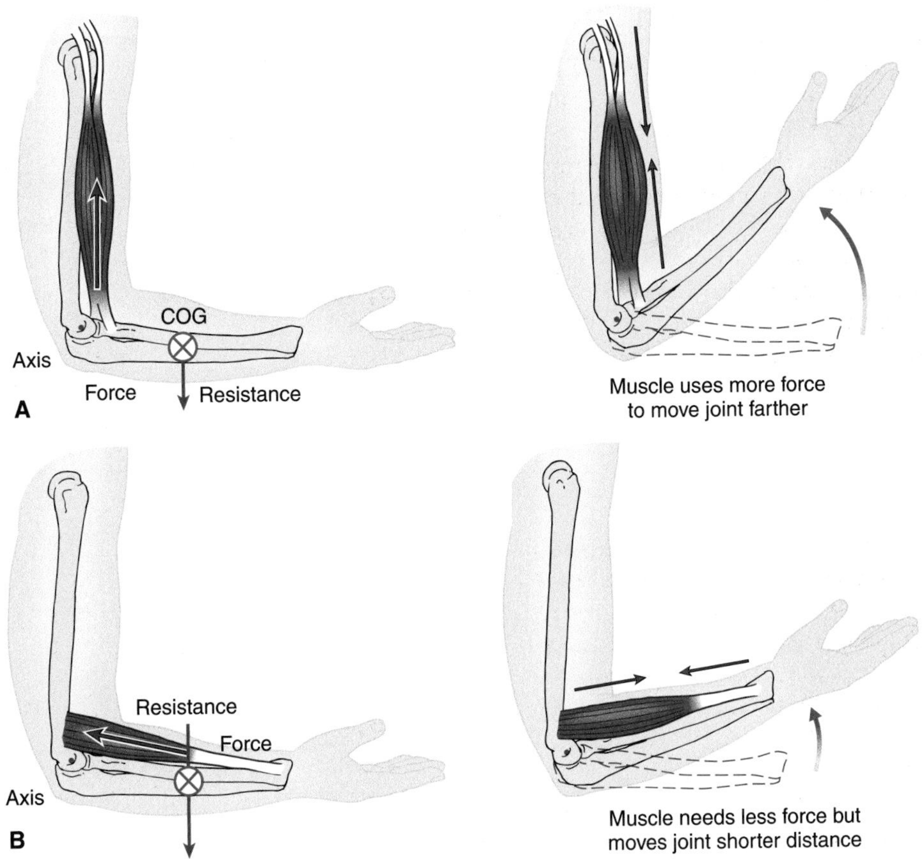

Figure 8-30. **(A)** Third-class levers favor distance, and **(B)** second-class levers favor force.

proximal end of the radius, whereas the brachioradialis muscle attaches to the distal end. The biceps muscle acts as the force in a third-class lever because it attaches between the axis (elbow) and the resistance (COG of forearm/hand; Fig. 8-30A). The brachioradialis muscle is the force in a second-class lever (Fig. 8-30B) because it attaches at the end of the forearm, putting the resistance (COG of forearm/hand) in the middle. For example, say that each muscle is capable of contracting approximately 4 inches. Remember that a muscle can shorten to half of its resting length. Therefore, the brachioradialis muscle will be able to move the distal end of the forearm and, subsequently, the hand approximately 4 inches, because the brachioradialis attachment is near the distal end. The biceps muscle, with its attachment at the proximal end, will move the proximal end of the forearm approximately 4 inches, which will move the hand at the distal end much farther, say 12 inches. Because the main function of the upper extremity is to allow the hand to move through a wide range, it makes sense that most muscles act as third-class levers, favoring range of motion.

Factors That Change Class

Under certain conditions, a muscle may change from a second-class (axis-resistance-force) to a third-class lever (axis-force-resistance), and vice versa. For example, the brachioradialis has been described as a second-class lever, with the weight of the forearm and hand being the resistance. Using the middle of the forearm as its COG, the weight of the forearm and hand (R) is located between the axis (elbow joint) and the force (distal muscle attachment), as shown in Figure 8-31A. However, if you put a weight in the hand, the COG of the resistance is now located farther from the axis than the force (muscle), as depicted in Figure 8-31B. Therefore, the brachioradialis is now working as a third-class lever.

The direction of the movement in relation to gravity is another factor that will affect lever class. For example, the biceps illustrated in Figure 8-32A is a third-class lever because it contracts concentrically to flex the elbow. The muscle is the force and the forearm is the resistance. The force is between the axis and the resistance; therefore, it is a third-class lever. If

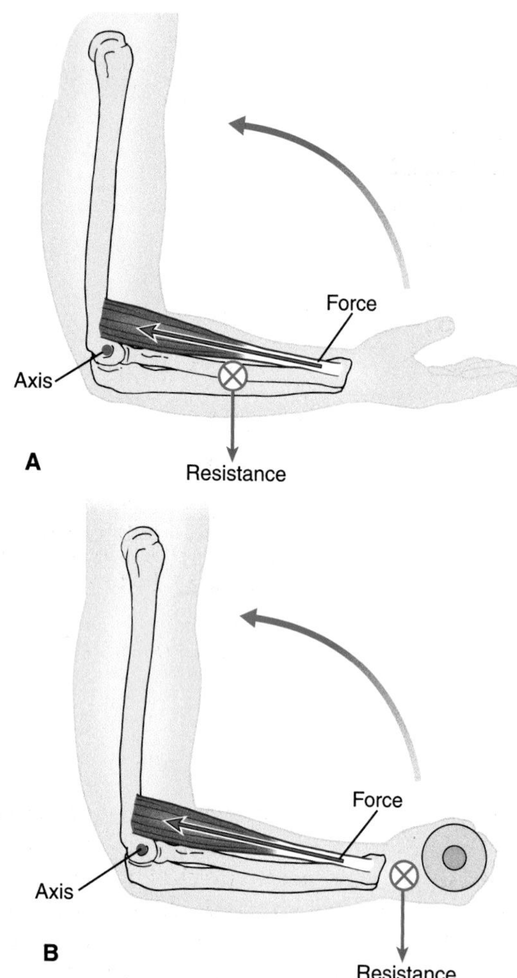

Figure 8-31. **(A)** The brachioradialis as a second-class lever. **(B)** It becomes a third-class lever when a weight is placed in the hand.

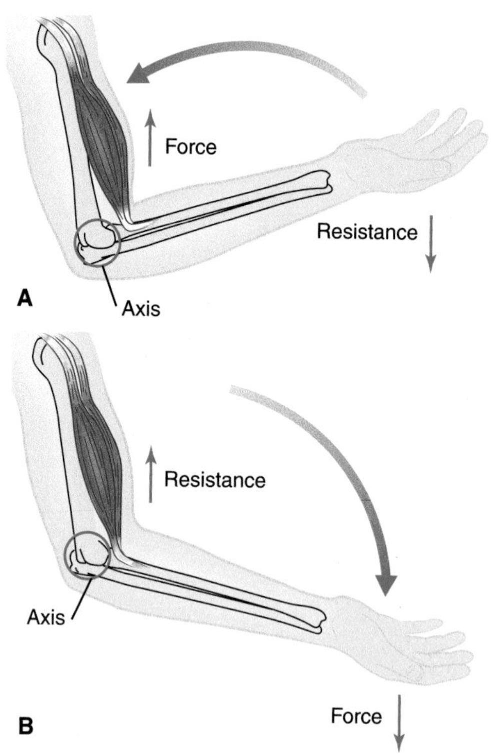

Figure 8-32. **(A)** The biceps acts as a third-class lever when contracting concentrically and **(B)** a second-class lever when contracting eccentrically.

you put a weight in the hand, it will still be a third-class lever. However, if the muscle contracts eccentrically, it will become a second-class lever. What has changed? As the elbow extends, moving the same direction as the pull of gravity, the biceps must contract eccentrically to slow the pull of gravity. Gravity and its pull on the forearm become the force. The biceps becomes the resistance slowing elbow extension (Fig. 8-32B). With the resistance now in the middle between the force and the axis, the biceps becomes a second-class lever.

There are many applications of leverage in rehabilitation. The importance of levers can be seen in such things as saving energy or making tasks possible when strength is limited. To summarize, less force is required if you put the resistance as close to the axis as possible and apply the force as far from the axis as possible.

Pulleys

A **pulley** consists of a grooved wheel that turns on an axle with a rope or cable riding in the groove. Its purpose is to either change the direction of a force or to increase or decrease its magnitude. A **fixed pulley** is a simple pulley attached to a beam. It acts as a first-class lever with *F* on one side of the pulley (axis) and *R* on the other. The fixed pulley is used only to change direction. Clinical examples of this can be found in overhead and wall pulleys (Fig. 8-33) and in home cervical traction units. In the body, the lateral malleolus of the fibula acts as a pulley for the tendon of the fibularis longus and changes its direction of pull (Fig. 8-34). Another example of a pulley is a Velcro strap on a shoe. The strap passes through a slot and folds over on itself.

A **movable pulley** has one end of the rope attached to a beam; the rope runs through the pulley to the other end where the force is applied. The load (resistance) is suspended from the movable pulley (Fig. 8-35). The purpose of this type of pulley is to increase the mechanical advantage of force. **Mechanical advantage** is the number of times a machine multiplies the force. The load is supported by both segments of the rope on

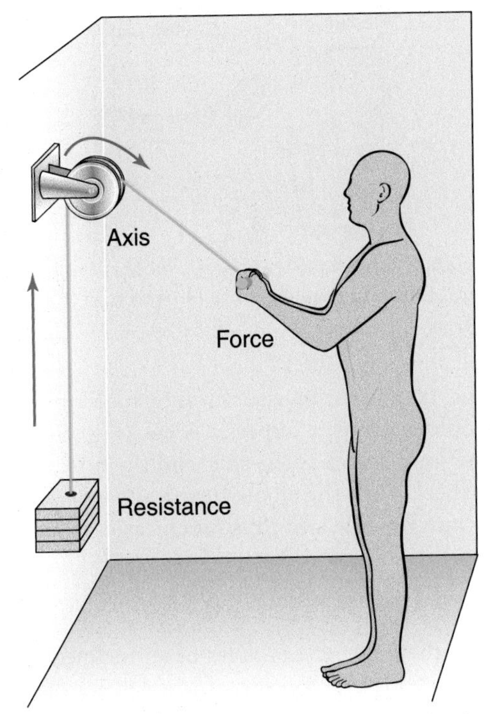

Figure 8-33. Fixed pulley. Its purpose is to change direction.

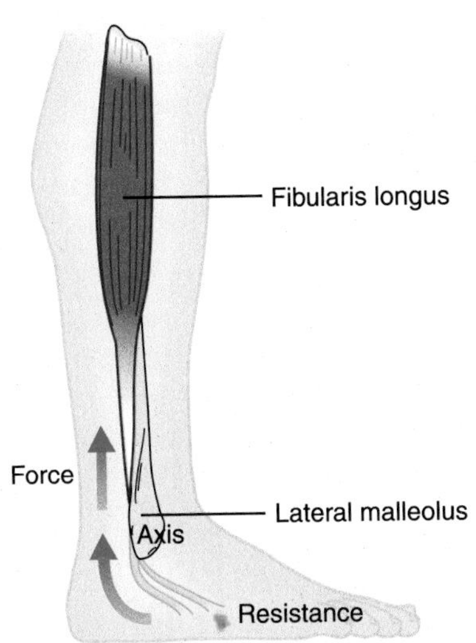

Figure 8-34. The lateral malleolus acts as a pulley, allowing the fibularis longus to change its direction of pull.

either side of the pulley so it has a mechanical advantage of 2. It will require only half as much force to lift the load because the amount of force gained has doubled. Although only half of the force is needed to lift the load, the rope must be pulled twice as far. In other words, it is easier to pull the rope, but the rope must be pulled a much farther distance. The human body has no examples of a movable pulley.

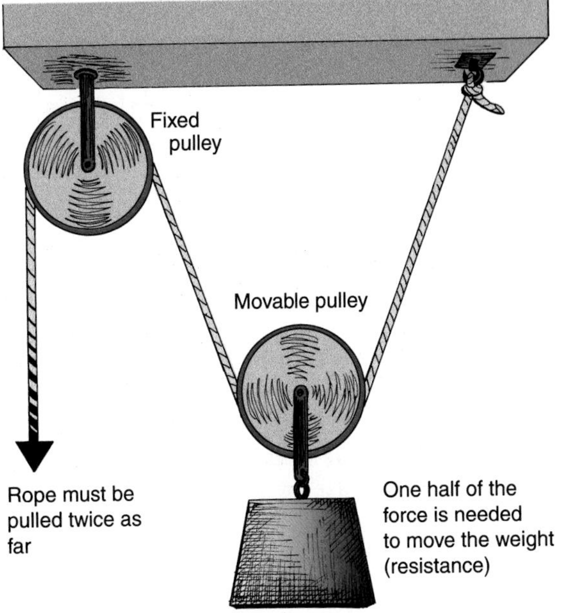

Figure 8-35. A movable pulley has a mechanical advantage for force.

Wheel and Axle

The **wheel and axle** is another type of simple machine. It is actually a lever in disguise. The wheel and axle consists of a wheel, or crank, attached to and turning together with an axle. In other words, it is a large wheel connected to a smaller wheel and typically is used to increase the force exerted. Turning around a larger wheel or handle requires less force, whereas turning around a smaller axle requires a greater force. An example of a wheel and axle is a faucet handle (Fig. 8-36). The

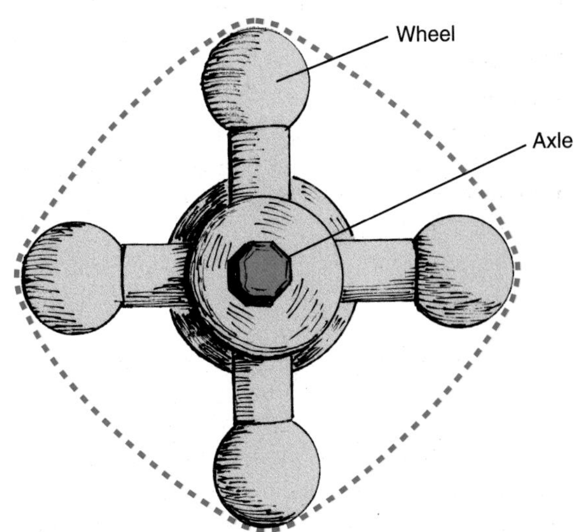

Figure 8-36. A faucet handle demonstrates a wheel and axle.

handle is the wheel, and the stem is the axle. Turning the faucet requires a certain amount of force made easier by a longer force arm (wheel radius; Fig. 8-37A). However, take off the handle and you are left with only the axle (Fig. 8-37B). Try turning the axle and you will realize that a great deal more strength is needed to do so. Simply stated, the larger the wheel (handle) in relation to the axle, the easier it is to turn the object. Just like the lever—in which the longer the FA, the greater the force—the wheel and axle provides greater force with a larger wheel.

Assume that you are treating a person who has severe arthritis in the hands and is unable to turn faucet handles easily. If you replace the handle (Fig. 8-38A) with a long, lever-type handle (Fig. 8-38B), you still have a wheel and axle. Visualize the handle as one spoke of the wheel with the rest of the spokes missing. The longer faucet handle is easier to turn (force advantage), but the handle must be turned a greater distance.

To give an example of a wheel and axle in the human body, think of performing passive shoulder rotation on a patient. It can best be visualized by looking down on the shoulder from a superior view (Fig. 8-39). The shoulder joint serves as the axle, and the forearm serves as the wheel. With the elbow flexed, the wheel is much longer than the axle and thus much easier to turn.

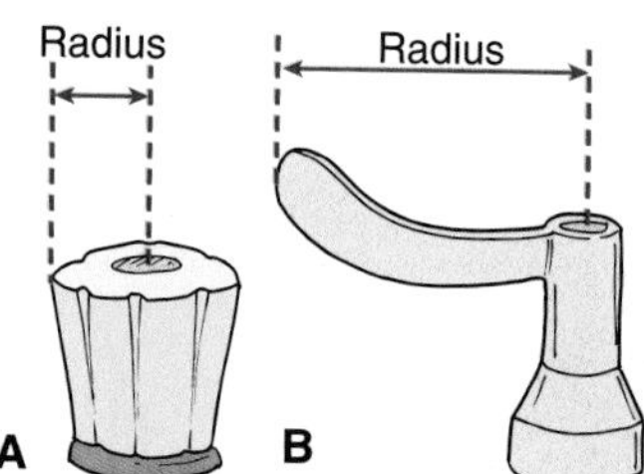

Figure 8-38. Typical faucet handles. Note that **(A)** has a shorter radius and requires more force to turn the wheel than **(B)**.

Inclined Plane

Although there are no examples of an inclined plane in the human body, the concept of wheelchair accessibility often depends on this type of simple machine. An **inclined plane** is a flat surface that slants. It exchanges increased distance for less effort. The longer the length of a wheelchair ramp, the greater the distance the wheelchair must travel; however, it requires less effort to propel the chair up the ramp because the ramp's incline is less. For example, if a porch is 2 feet from the ground and the ramp is 24 feet long, it would be fairly easy to propel the wheelchair up this long ramp (Fig. 8-40A). If the ramp is

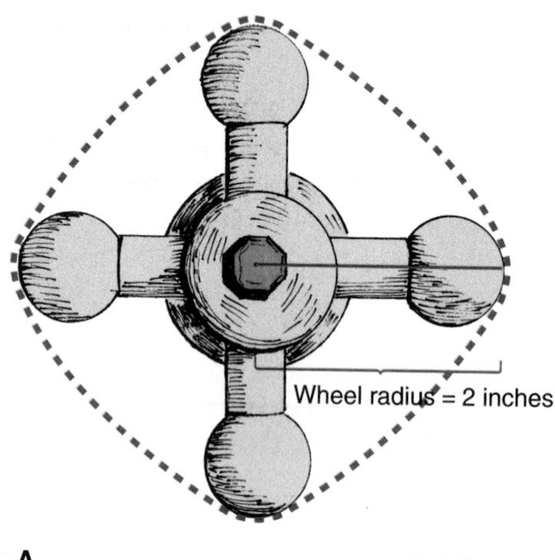

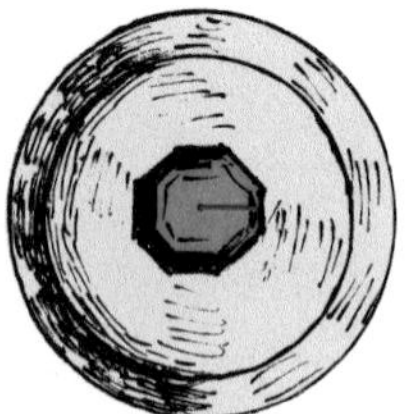

Figure 8-37. The wheel of the faucet handle **(A)** has a longer radius than the axle **(B)**. Therefore, the larger wheel is easier to turn than the smaller axle.

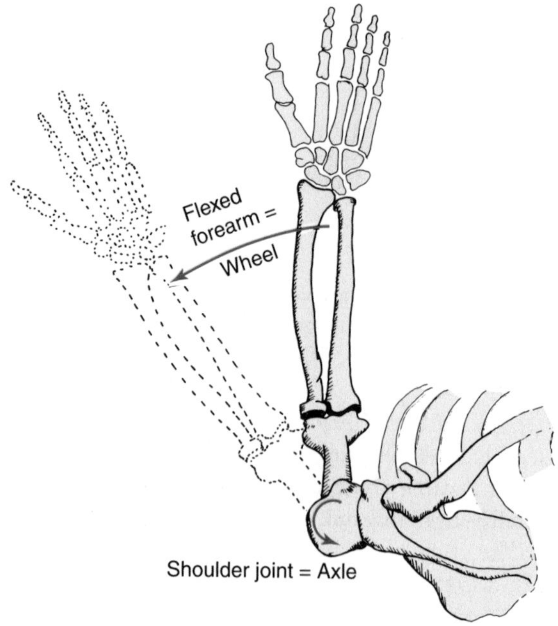

Figure 8-39. Upper extremity acting as a wheel and axle.

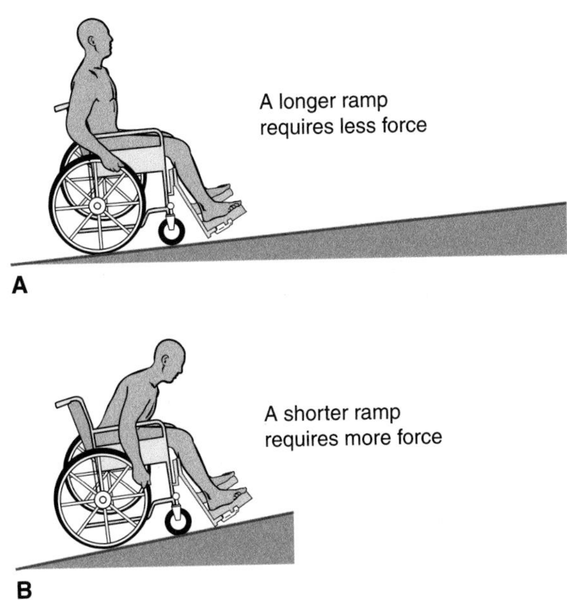
A longer ramp
requires less force
A
A shorter ramp
requires more force
B

Figure 8-40. Inclined plane as a wheelchair ramp. A longer ramp **(A)** requires less force but greater distance to reach a certain height. A shorter ramp **(B)** requires more force but less distance to reach same height.

only 12 feet long, it would be much steeper. The person would not have to propel the wheelchair as far but would have to use more force to do so (Fig. 8-40B). Repeating the basic rule of simple machines: the advantage gained in force (decreased effort needed) is lost in distance (longer ramp needed).

Points to Remember

- The effect of forces can be linear, parallel, or concurrent.
- A force couple occurs when forces act together but in different, often opposite, directions to create rotation around a single axis.
- A scalar quantity describes magnitude, whereas a vector also includes direction.
- Forces can be stabilizing, angular, or dislocating.
- Gravity has an effect on all objects, and its force is always downward.
- Stability is affected by an object's COG and BOS.
- The three classes of levers have different purposes and mechanical advantages, depending on the relationship of the axis, the force, and the resistance.
- Changing the length of the FA or RA will make the part easier or harder to move.
- Fixed pulleys in the human body change the direction of a muscle's force.
- The wheel and axle, much like the lever, can decrease the force required to cause motion.
- Inclined planes can exchange increased distance for decreased effort.

Review Questions

1. Putting a weight cuff in which position would require more effort at the shoulder joint to move the weight cuff through shoulder range of motion? Explain your answer.
   a. Cuff positioned at the wrist
   b. Cuff positioned at the elbow
2. Two people have the same weight and BOS, but one is on stilts. Which person is more stable? Why?
   a. The person on stilts
   b. The person not on stilts
3. What is the resultant force of the following muscles?
   a. Two heads of the gastrocnemius (Fig. 8-41A)

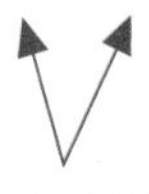

Figure 8-41A.

   b. Sternal and clavicular portions of the pectoralis major (Fig. 8-41B)

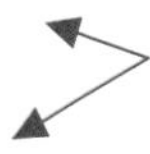

Figure 8-41B.

4. You are given two different sets of instructions. The first instruction tells you to run 5 miles, and the second instruction tells you to walk 30 feet to the north. Circle the correct answer.
   a. Running 5 miles is a vector/scalar quantity.
   b. Walking 30 feet to the north is a vector/scalar quantity.

(continued on next page)

Review Questions—cont'd

5. A delivery person has several boxes stacked on a hand truck. Would the person have to use more force to push the hand truck when the hand truck is more horizontal or more vertical? Why?
6. Compare the push rims of a standard wheelchair and a racing wheelchair. Note that the racing wheelchair has much smaller push rims. What is the advantage of smaller push rims to a wheelchair racer?
7. Label the BOS, COG, and LOG for the object shown in Figure 8-42. The object is of uniform density throughout its shape. Can this object remain upright without support? Why?

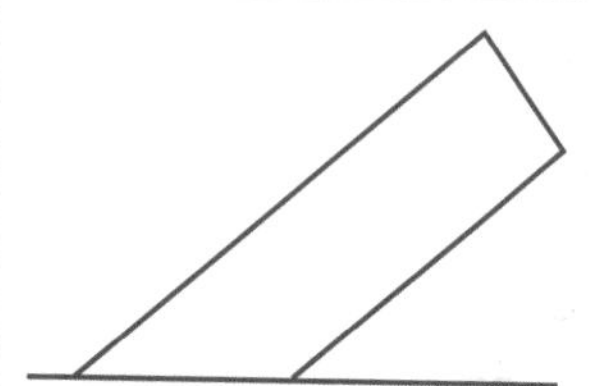

Figure 8-42.

8. In terms of BOS, why is it more difficult for a person in a wheelchair to balance on only the back wheels ("wheelie") rather than on all four wheels?
9. Two people are standing on the same side of a patient's bed. They plan to move the patient toward them by pulling on the draw sheet. This move would be what type of force: linear, parallel, concurrent, or force couple?
10. Before moving the patient, what can the people do to increase their own stability?
11. When cracking an almond with a nutcracker, will the almond be easier to crack if it is closer to the axis or closer to the end of the handles? Why?
12. Does Figure 8-43 represent forces that are linear, parallel, or concurrent? Why?

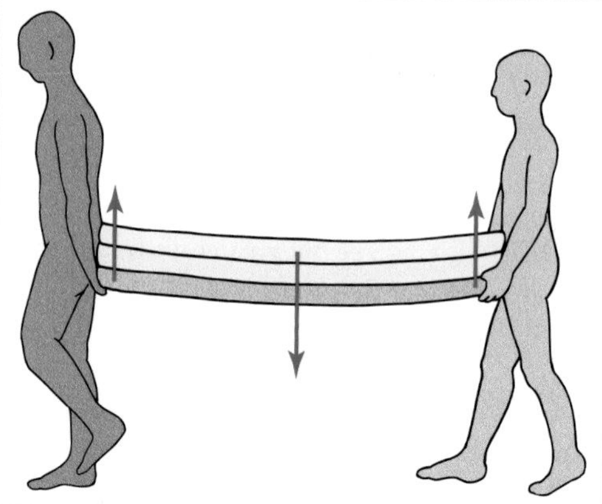

Figure 8-43.

13. Give an example of bony structures at the knee acting as a pulley to increase the angle of pull.
14. Explain why a person leans to the right when carrying a heavy suitcase in the left hand. If the suitcase was very heavy, what might the person do with her right arm? Why?
15. Why are rubber tips put on the ends of crutches?

Review Questions—cont'd

16. Looking at Figure 8-44, answer the following questions:
    a. In Figure 8-44A, identify the force, resistance, and axis.
    b. Identify the approximate center of gravity (COG) of the resistance in parts **(A)** and **(B).**
    c. Identify the FA and RA in parts **(A)** and **(B).**
    d. In which figure is the resistance arm the longest?
    e. In which figure is the force arm the longest?
    f. Is the luggage in **(A)** or **(B)** easier to pull? Why?

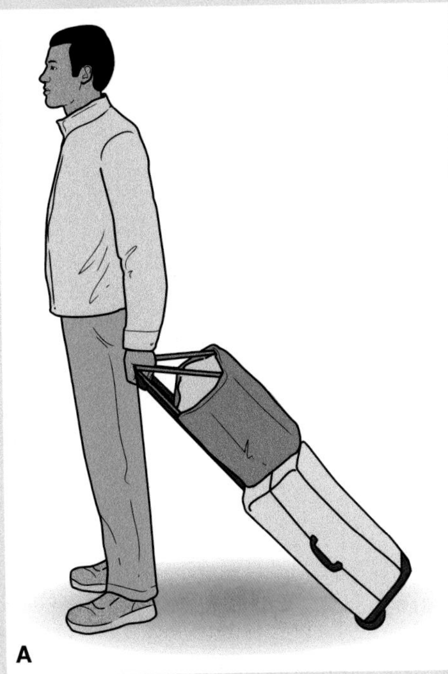

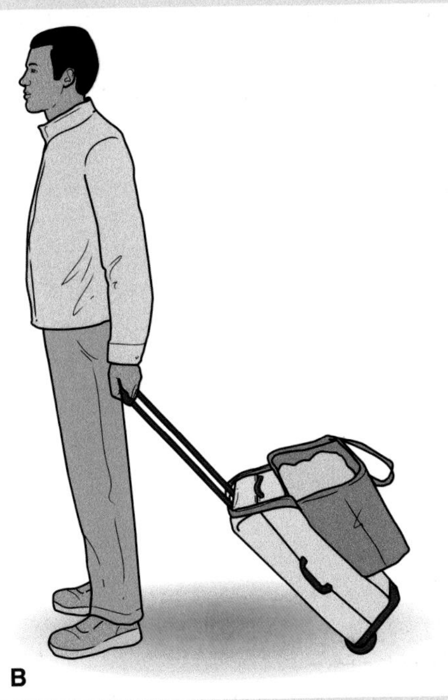

Figure 8-44.

PART II

Clinical Kinesiology and Anatomy of the Upper Extremities

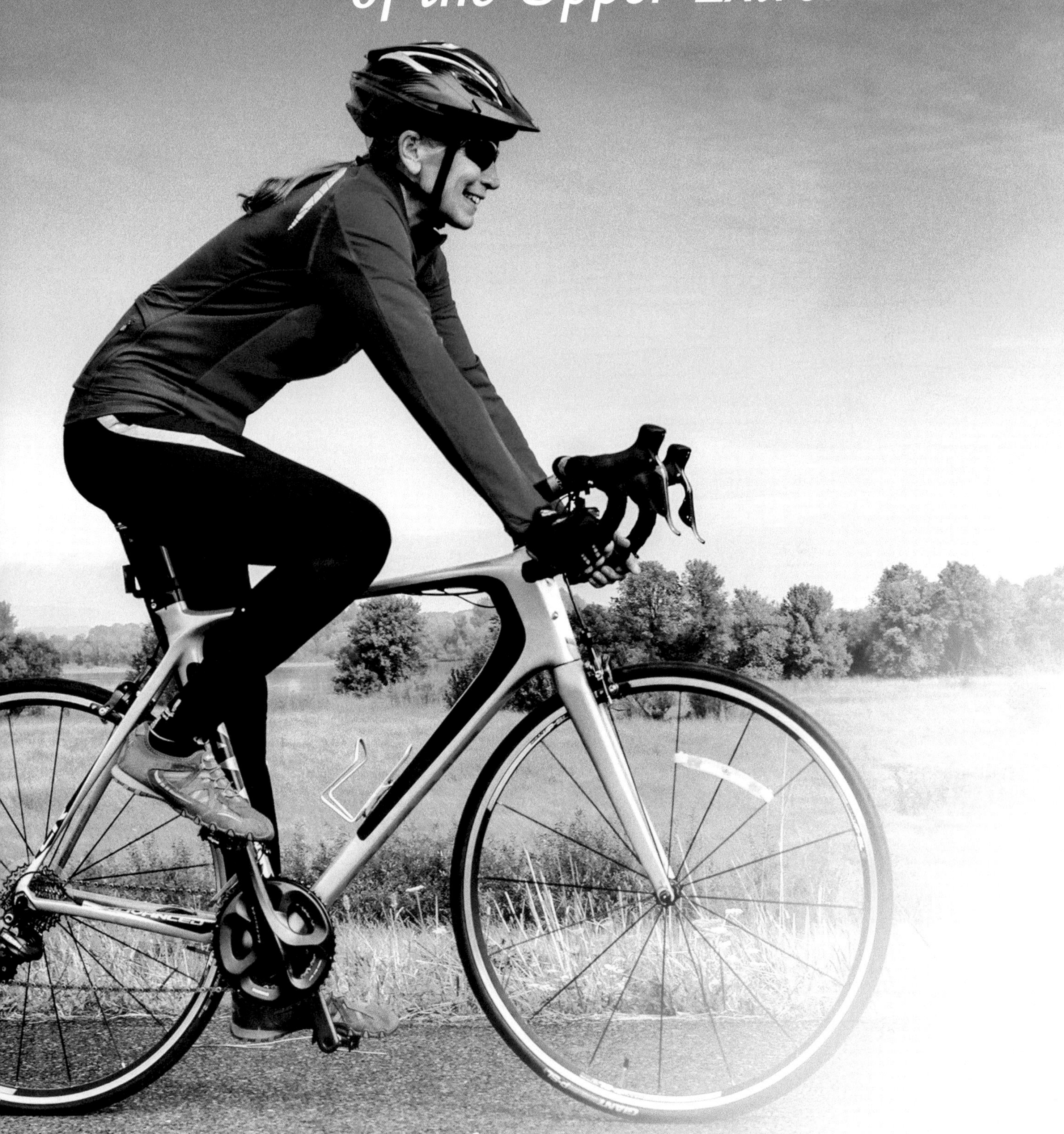

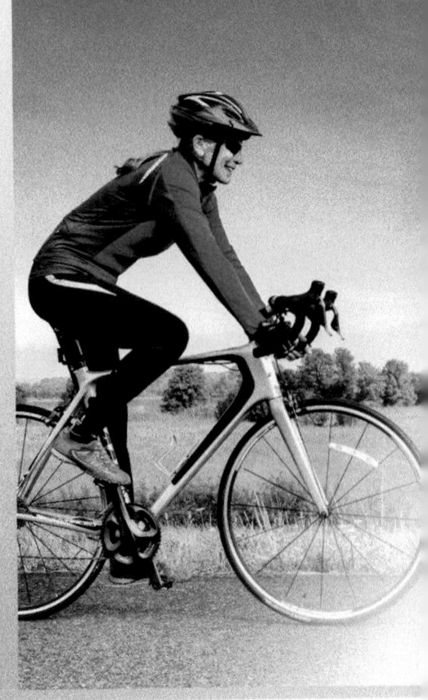

CHAPTER 9
Shoulder Girdle

Clarification of Terms
Bones and Landmarks
Important Bony Landmarks of the Scapula
Important Bony Landmarks of the Clavicle
Important Bony Landmarks of the Sternum
Joints and Ligaments
Joint Motions
Companion Motions of the Shoulder Joint and Shoulder Girdle
Scapulohumeral Rhythm
Muscles of the Shoulder Girdle
Muscle Descriptions
Anatomical Relationships
Force Couples
Reverse Muscle Action
Summary of Muscle Innervation
Common Shoulder Girdle Pathologies
Points to Remember
Review Questions
General Anatomy Questions
Functional Activity Questions
Clinical Exercise Questions

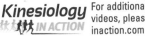

Clarification of Terms

The purpose of the shoulder and the entire upper extremity is to allow the hand to be placed in various positions to accomplish the multitude of tasks the hand is capable of performing. The shoulder, or glenohumeral joint, is the most mobile joint in the body and is capable of a great deal of motion. However, in talking about shoulder motion, we must recognize that motion also occurs at three other joints, or areas. *Shoulder complex* is a term that is sometimes used to include all of the structures involved with motion of the shoulder. The **shoulder complex** consists of the scapula, clavicle, sternum, humerus, and rib cage, and includes the sternoclavicular joint, acromioclavicular joint, glenohumeral joint, and "scapulothoracic articulation" (Fig. 9-1). In other words, it includes the shoulder girdle (scapula and clavicle) and the shoulder joint (scapula and humerus). The **scapulothoracic articulation** is not a joint in the pure

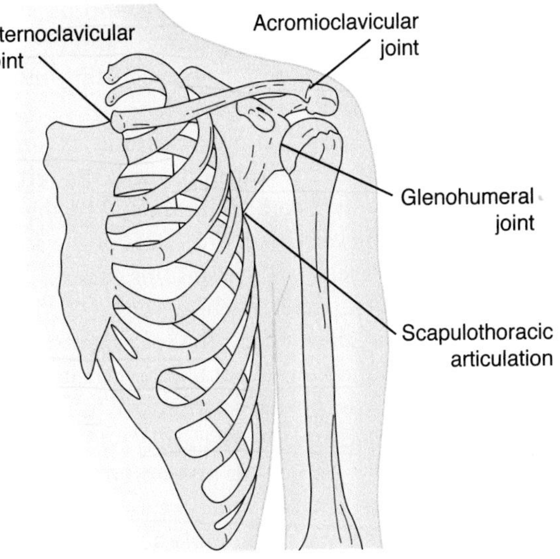

Figure 9-1. Shoulder complex (anterior view).

sense of the word. Although the scapula and thorax do not have a point of fixation, the scapula does move over the rib cage of the thorax. The scapula and thorax are not directly attached but are connected indirectly by the clavicle and by several muscles. The scapulothoracic articulation does provide increased motion to the shoulder complex.

Shoulder girdle is a term often used to discuss the activities of the scapula and clavicle and, to a lesser degree, the sternum and ribs. The sternoclavicular and acromioclavicular joints allow shoulder girdle motions, including elevation and depression, protraction and retraction, and upward and downward rotation. Five muscles attach to the scapula, the clavicle, or both, providing motion of the shoulder girdle.

The **shoulder joint,** also called the *glenohumeral joint,* consists of the scapula and humerus. The motions of the shoulder joint are flexion, extension and hyperextension, abduction and adduction, medial and lateral rotation, and horizontal abduction and adduction. Because the shoulder joint is so mobile, it has few ligaments. The nine muscles that cross the shoulder joint are the prime movers in shoulder joint motion.

Now that the various terms connected with the shoulder complex have been defined, the shoulder girdle will be discussed in more detail. The shoulder joint will be addressed in Chapter 10.

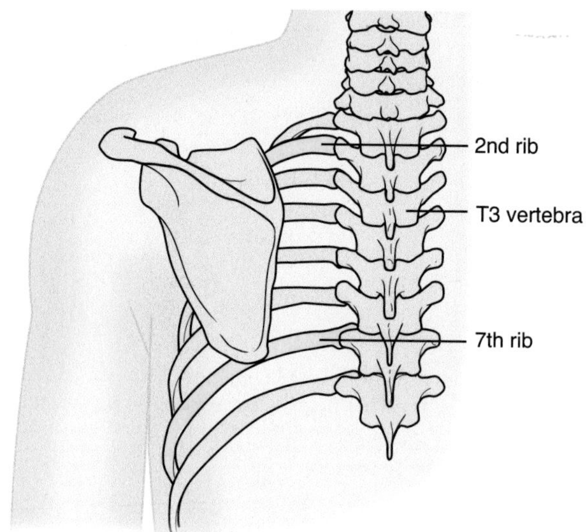

Figure 9-2. Resting position of the scapula on the thorax (posterior view).

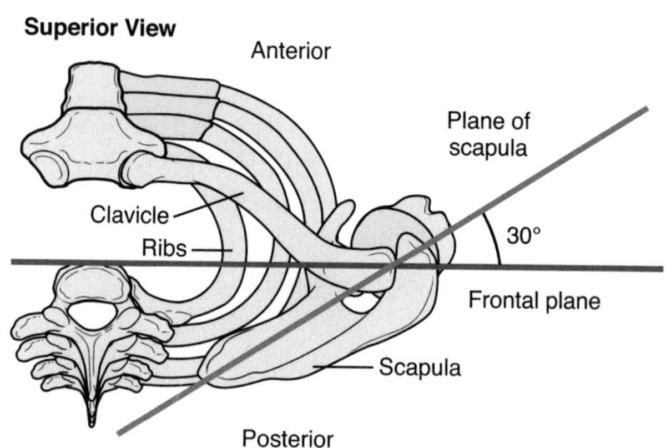

Figure 9-3. Plane of the scapula (superior view)

Bones and Landmarks

The **scapula,** a triangular-shaped bone located superficially on the posterior side of the thorax, and the clavicle make up the shoulder girdle. The scapula attaches to the trunk indirectly through its ligamentous attachment to the clavicle. It is slightly concave anteriorly and glides over the convex posterior rib cage. Many muscles also connect the scapula to the trunk.

In the resting position, the scapula is located between the second and seventh ribs, with the vertebral border approximately 2 to 3 inches lateral to the spinous processes of the vertebrae. The spine of the scapula is approximately level with the spinous process of the third and fourth thoracic vertebrae (Fig. 9-2). Due to the curved shape of the rib cage, the scapula rests about 30 degrees anterior to the frontal plane in its resting position, against the posterior thorax. This is sometimes referred to as the *plane of the scapula* (Fig. 9-3).

Figures 9-1 and 9-2 show the position of the scapula on the body from an anterior and posterior view, respectively. Figure 9-3 shows the scapula's position from a superior view. In terms of shoulder girdle function, the important bony landmarks of the scapula (Fig. 9-4) are the following:

Important Bony Landmarks of the Scapula

Superior Angle

Superior medial aspect, providing attachment for the levator scapula muscle

Inferior Angle

Most inferior point and where vertebral and axillary borders meet. This point determines scapular rotation.

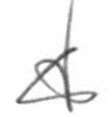

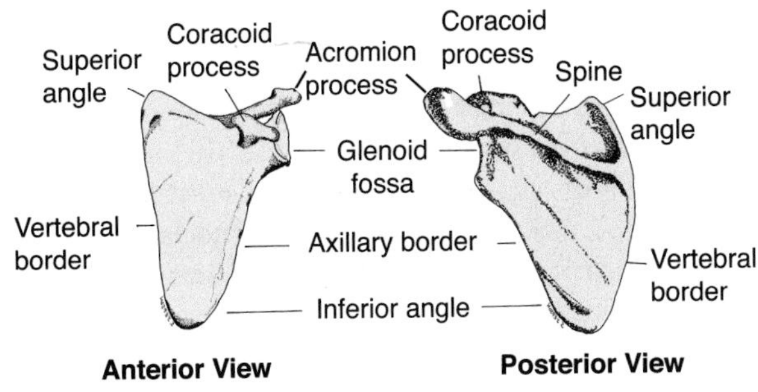

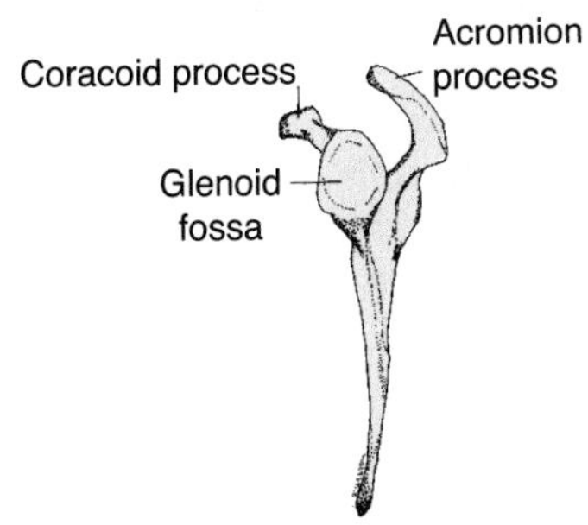

Figure 9-4. Bony landmarks of the left scapula.

Vertebral Border
Between superior and inferior angles medially, and attachment of the rhomboid and serratus anterior muscles

Axillary Border
The lateral side between glenoid fossa and inferior angle

Spine
Projection on posterior surface, running from medial border laterally to the acromion process. It provides attachment for the middle and lower trapezius muscles.

Coracoid Process
Projection on anterior surface, providing attachment for the pectoralis minor muscle

Acromion Process
Broad, flat area on superior lateral aspect, providing attachment for the upper trapezius muscle

Glenoid Fossa
Slightly concave surface that articulates with humerus on superior lateral side above the axillary border and below the acromion process. The fossa is positioned in an anterior, lateral, and upward direction.

The **clavicle** is an S-shaped bone that connects the upper extremity to the axial skeleton at the sternoclavicular joint. Figure 9-1 shows the position of the clavicle in relation to the sternum, scapula, and rib cage. For shoulder girdle function, the important bony landmarks of the clavicle (Fig. 9-5) are as follows:

Important Bony Landmarks of the Clavicle

Sternal End
Attaches medially to sternum

Acromial End
Attaches laterally to scapula and provides attachment for the upper trapezius muscle

Body
Area between the two ends

The **sternum** is a flat bone located in the midline of the anterior thorax (Fig. 9-6). The position of the sternum in relation to the rib cage and the clavicles is shown in Figure 9-1. At its superior end, the sternum provides attachment for the clavicle, followed beneath by attachments for the costal cartilages of the ribs. It is divided into three parts.

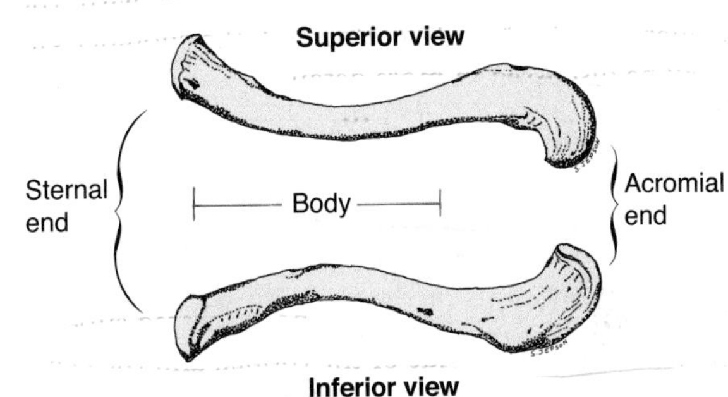

Figure 9-5. Left clavicle.

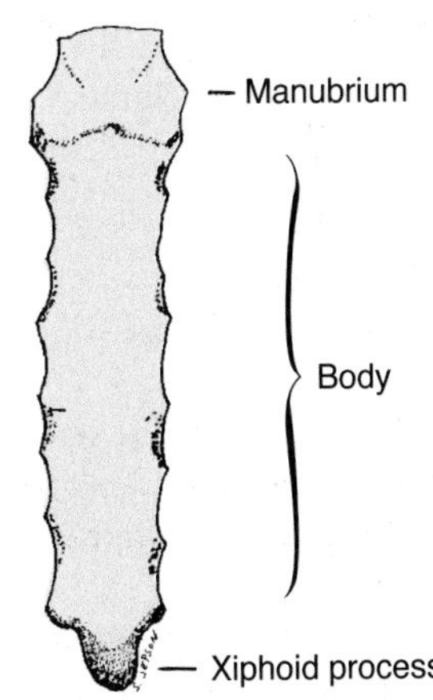

Figure 9-6. Sternum (anterior view).

Important Bony Landmarks of the Sternum

Manubrium
The superior end, providing attachment for the clavicle and the first rib

Body
The middle two-thirds of the sternum, providing attachment for the remaining ribs

Xiphoid Process
Meaning "sword-shaped," the inferior tip

Joints and Ligaments

Sternoclavicular Joint

The **sternoclavicular (SC) joint** (Fig. 9-7) is formed by the articulation between the manubrium of the sternum and the medial (sternal) end of the clavicle. This synovial joint provides the shoulder girdle with its only direct attachment to the trunk. The shape classification of the sternoclavicular joint is not commonly agreed upon among authors. It has been described as a modified ball-and-socket joint, as an incongruent saddle joint, or as a plane-shaped double gliding joint. However, there is consensus that it functions as a triaxial joint, with three degrees of freedom, allowing movement in three planes of motion.

Of the two bones that make up this joint, it is clear that the clavicle is more movable than the sternum. For this reason, motions of the SC joint will be described based on the direction in which the clavicle is moving. Sternoclavicular joint motions include elevation and depression in the frontal plane as well as protraction and retraction in the transverse plane, and rotation occurs along the longitudinal axis of the bone (the clavicle spins on the sternum). Basically, the clavicle moves while the sternum remains stationary.

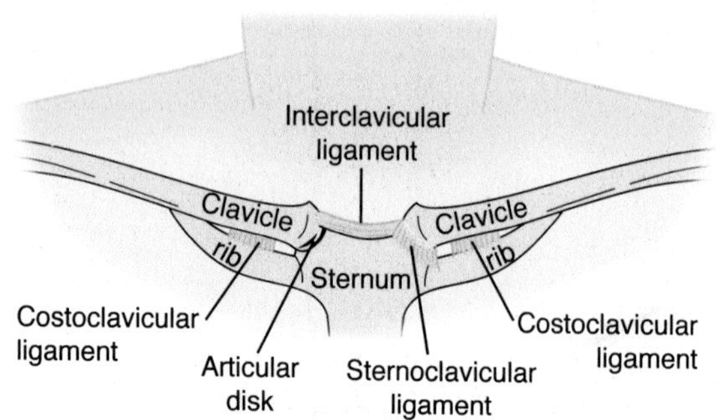

Figure 9-7. Ligaments of the sternoclavicular joint (left side cut away to show the disk; anterior view).

Being a synovial joint, the sternoclavicular joint has a joint capsule. It also has three major ligaments and a joint disk. The articular disk serves as a shock absorber, especially from forces generated by falls on the outstretched hand. The joint capsule surrounds the joint and is reinforced by the anterior and posterior sternoclavicular ligaments. The disk and its ligamentous support are so effective that dislocation at the sternoclavicular joint is rare.

The articular disk has a unique attachment that contributes to the motion of this joint. The upper part of the disk is attached to the posterior superior part of the clavicle, while the lower part is attached to the manubrium and first costal cartilage. This double attachment is much like that of the double hinge found on doors that swing in both directions. During shoulder girdle elevation and depression, the convex surface of the clavicle slides inferiorly and superiorly on the concave manubrium as the clavicle's lateral end moves up and down, respectively. This motion occurs between the clavicle and the disk. During protraction and retraction, the concave portion of the clavicle slides anteriorly and posteriorly on the convex costal cartilage, respectively as the clavicle's lateral end moves forward and backward. This motion occurs between the disk and the sternum. To summarize the double-hinge arrangement of this joint, during elevation and depression, motion occurs between the clavicle and disk, whereas during protraction and retraction, motion occurs between the disk and the sternum.

The three major ligaments supporting this joint are the sternoclavicular, costoclavicular, and interclavicular ligaments. The **sternoclavicular ligament** connects the clavicle to the sternum on both the anterior and posterior surfaces and is therefore divided into the anterior and posterior sternoclavicular ligaments. These ligaments limit anterior-posterior movement of the clavicle's medial end. The posterior sternoclavicular ligament limits anterior motion, and the anterior sternoclavicular ligament limits posterior motion. They both reinforce the joint capsule. The **costoclavicular ligament** is a short, flat, rhomboid-shaped ligament that connects the clavicle's inferior surface to the superior surface of the costal cartilage of the first rib. The primary purpose of this ligament is to limit the amount of clavicular elevation. The **interclavicular ligament** is located on top of the manubrium, connecting the superior sternal ends of the clavicles. Its purpose is to limit the amount of clavicular depression.

Acromioclavicular Joint

The **acromioclavicular (AC) joint** (Fig. 9-8) connects the acromion process of the scapula and the lateral (acromial) end of the clavicle. It is a plane-shaped

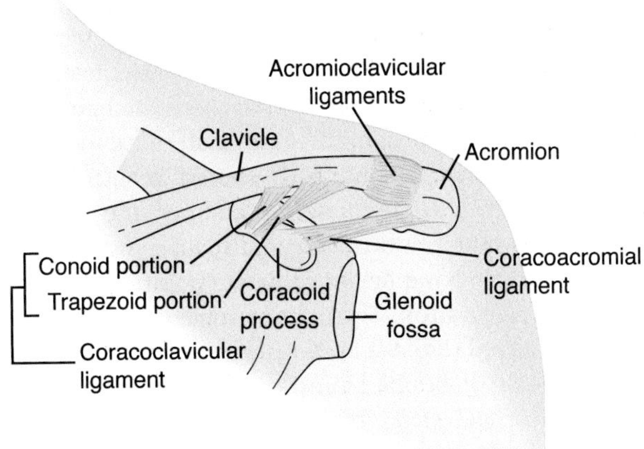

Figure 9-8. Ligaments of the acromioclavicular joint (anterior view).

synovial joint that allows a gliding motion to occur, contributing toward movement in three planes of motion.

Unlike the sternoclavicular joint, which allows much clavicular motion, the AC joint allows subtle movements of the scapula. These motions are minimal but allow continuity between the scapula and thorax during scapular motions. The primary motions at the AC joint are upward and downward rotation in the plane of the scapula (see Fig. 9-3). Because of the curved shape of the rib cage, these motions occur more in the plane of the scapula than in the pure frontal plane. The scapular plane is oriented approximately 30 degrees forward of the frontal plane. The AC joint can also contribute toward scapular tilt in the sagittal plane, and when present, scapular winging in the transverse plane.

The joint capsule surrounds the articular borders of the joint. It is reinforced above and below by the superior and inferior **acromioclavicular ligaments.** These ligaments support the joint by holding the acromion process to the clavicle, thus helping to prevent dislocation of the clavicle. Despite this reinforcement, the joint capsule is quite weak. This capsular weakness leaves the AC joint very susceptible to injury, especially with a fall on the outstretched hand or a blow to the outside of the shoulder.

The coracoclavicular ligament and coracoacromial ligaments are two accessory ligaments of the AC joint. Although the **coracoclavicular ligament** is not directly located at the joint, it does provide stability to that joint and allows the scapula to be suspended from the clavicle. It connects the scapula to the clavicle by attaching to the inferior surface of the clavicle's lateral end and to the superior surface of the scapula's coracoid process (Fig. 9-8). The ligament is divided into a lateral trapezoid portion and the deeper medial conoid portion. Together they prevent backward motion of the scapula, and individually they limit the rotation of the scapula.

The **coracoacromial ligament** does not actually cross the AC joint, but rather forms a roof over the head of the humerus and serves as a protective arch, providing support to the head when an upward force is transmitted along the humerus (Fig. 9-9). It attaches laterally on the superior surface of the coracoid process and runs up and out to the inferior surface of the acromion process.

Scapulothoracic Articulation

The **scapulothoracic articulation,** as mentioned earlier, is not a joint in the pure sense of the word as there is no direct union between the bones, and there is no joint capsule. It consists of the slightly concave anterior surface of the scapula resting on the convex posterior aspect of the rib cage. With the lack of a true joint structure to support the scapula in its normal resting position, stability comes from an indirect link to the trunk through the clavicle and several surrounding muscles. The scapulothoracic articulation provides motion necessary for normal function of the scapula.

Joint Motions

As mentioned previously, the motions of the shoulder girdle are elevation and depression, protraction and retraction, and upward and downward rotation

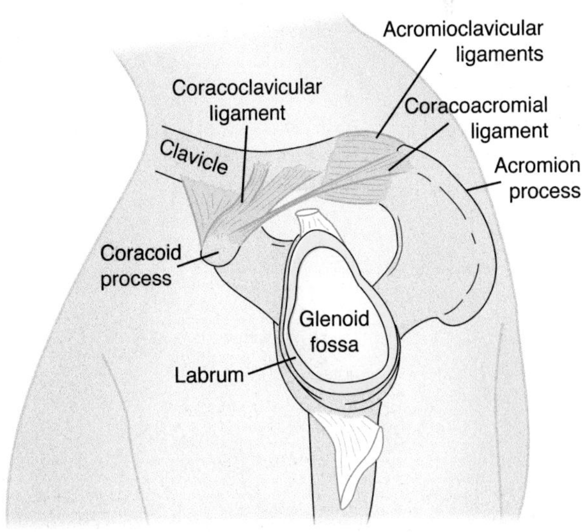

Figure 9-9. The coracoacromial ligament forms a roof over the shoulder joint.

(Fig. 9-10). Because these motions can be seen best by looking at the scapula, they are commonly described as either *shoulder girdle* or *scapular motion.* At this joint, protraction and abduction are synonymous terms, as are retraction and adduction. For example, *shoulder girdle protraction and retraction* is synonymous with *scapular abduction and adduction*. Scapular rotation is the same as shoulder girdle rotation.

Scapular elevation/depression and protraction/retraction are essentially linear motions. All points of the scapula move up and down along the thorax and away from and toward the vertebral column in parallel lines. **Scapular elevation** occurs when the scapula moves in a superior direction, while **scapular depression** occurs when the scapula moves inferiorly. **Scapular protraction** (scapular abduction) occurs when the scapula moves away from the posterior midline, and **scapular retraction** (scapular adduction) occurs when the scapula moves back toward the posterior midline.

The shoulder girdle also performs several angular motions including scapular upward/downward rotation and scapular tilt. Because of the scapula's triangular shape, one side moves one way while another side moves in an opposite or different direction. During **scapular upward rotation**, the inferior angle of the scapula rotates up and away from the vertebral column, whereas **scapular downward rotation** is the return to the resting anatomical position from the upwardly rotated position. The scapula does not move past anatomical position toward the vertebral column. It should be noted that when the inferior angle rotates up and out, the superior angle moves down, and the glenoid fossa moves up and in. Therefore, it is important to have a point of reference to define this rotation. The inferior angle is the reference point used here (Fig. 9-11). **Scapular tilt** (see Fig. 9-10) occurs when the shoulder joint goes into hyperextension. The superior end of the scapula tilts anteriorly, and the inferior end tilts posteriorly. Examples of these combined motions are the "windup" or prerelease phase of a softball pitch, a bowling delivery, or a racing dive in swimming.

Because of the complexity of joint shapes and joint interaction in the shoulder complex, some very subtle motions occur that are beyond the scope of this book. One such movement is worthy of mention so as to clarify normal versus abnormal motion. **Scapular winging** is the posterior lateral movement of the vertebral border of the scapula in the transverse plane. In other words, the vertebral border of the scapula moves away from the rib cage. This motion occurs primarily at the AC joint but is observed most often at the scapulothoracic articulation. This can be demonstrated by asking a

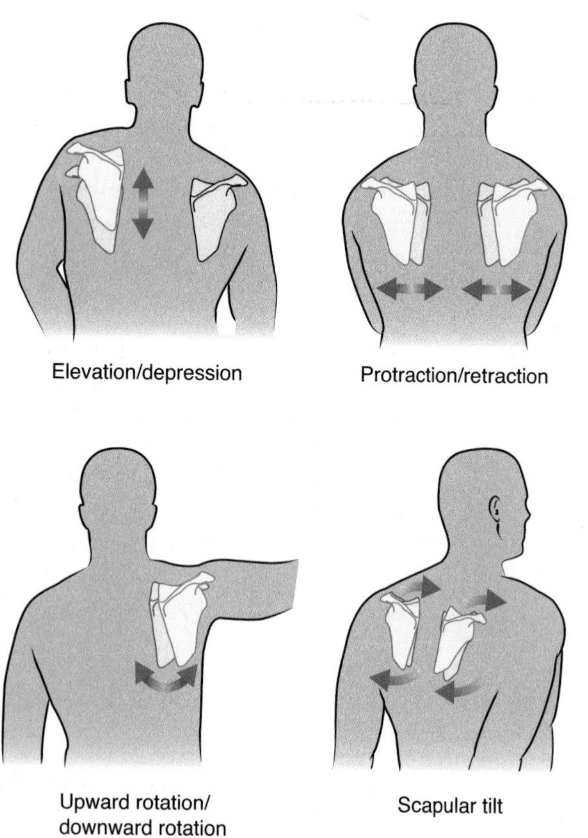

Figure 9-10. Shoulder girdle motions (posterior view).

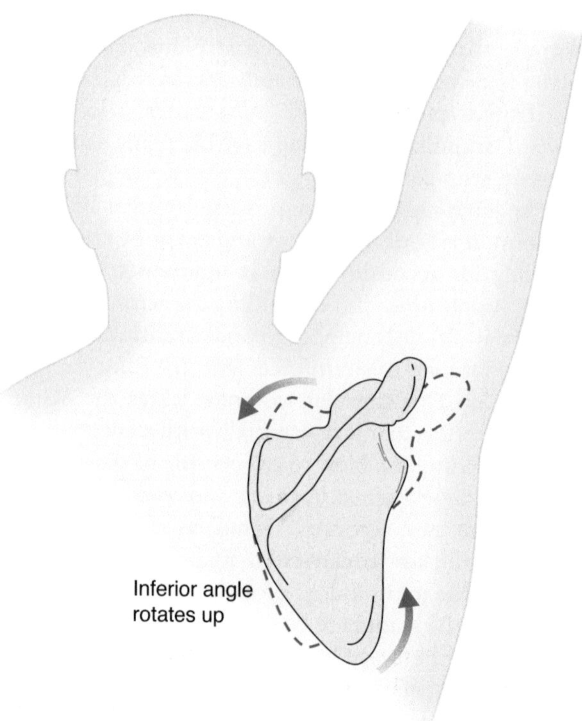

Figure 9-11. Scapular motion during upward rotation.

person with a "normal" shoulder to place his or her hand on the small of the back. The vertebral border of the scapula lifts away from the rib cage. This motion can only be done in combination with several other motions. However, pathological "winging of the scapula" also occurs when the stabilizing muscles around the scapula are weak or paralyzed. Serratus anterior weakness or paralysis is a dramatic example. When a person with that condition pushes against a wall with an outstretched hand (Fig. 9-12), the involved scapula will rise away from the rib cage, standing out like a small wing. Excessive winging is considered abnormal.

Companion Motions of the Shoulder Joint and Shoulder Girdle

During the linear movements of scapular elevation/depression and scapular protraction/retraction, it is possible to move the shoulder girdle (clavicle and scapula) up, down, forward, or backward without moving the humerus. However, shoulder joint motions must accompany the angular motions of scapular upward/downward rotation, and scapular tilt. To rotate the scapula upward, you must also flex or abduct the shoulder joint. Stated another way, when there is flexion or abduction of the shoulder joint, the scapula must also rotate upward. When there is extension or adduction of the shoulder joint, the scapula returns to anatomical position by rotating downward. Scapular tilt can only happen when the shoulder joint goes into hyperextension. Because of the complex and interrelated activities of the shoulder girdle and the shoulder joint, it is difficult to discuss the function of one without discussing activities of the other. Impairment at one joint will also impair function at the other. The following list summarizes the shoulder girdle motions that must occur during various shoulder joint motions:

Shoulder Joint	Shoulder Girdle
Flexion	Upward rotation; protraction
Extension	Downward rotation; retraction
Hyperextension	Scapular tilt
Abduction	Upward rotation
Adduction	Downward rotation
Medial rotation	Protraction
Lateral rotation	Retraction
Horizontal abduction	Retraction
Horizontal adduction	Protraction

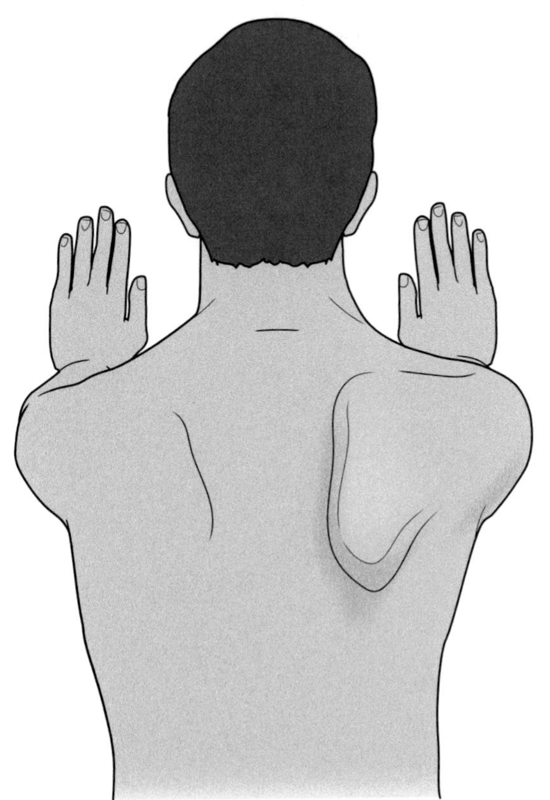

Figure 9-12. Winging of the scapula (posterior view). This person's right serratus anterior muscle is paralyzed. When pushing against the wall with both hands, the right scapula rises away from the rib cage, standing out like a small wing.

Scapulohumeral Rhythm

Scapulohumeral rhythm is a concept that further describes the movement relationship between the shoulder girdle and the shoulder joint. The first 30 degrees of shoulder joint motion is pure shoulder joint motion. However, after that, for every 2 degrees of shoulder flexion or abduction that occurs, the scapula must upwardly rotate 1 degree. This 2:1 ratio is known as *scapulohumeral rhythm*.

It is possible to demonstrate that the first part of shoulder joint motion occurs only at the shoulder joint, but further motion must be accompanied by shoulder girdle motion. With a person in the anatomical position, stabilize the scapula by putting the heel of your hand against the axillary border to prevent rotation of the scapula. Instruct the person to abduct the shoulder joint. Notice that the individual is able to abduct only a short distance before shoulder joint motion is impaired.

Muscles of The Shoulder Girdle

As discussed in Chapter 5, several factors determine the role that a muscle will play in a particular joint motion. Determining whether a muscle has a major role (prime mover), a minor role (assisting mover), or no role at all will depend on such factors as its size, the line of pull, the joint motions possible, and the location of the muscle in relation to the joint axis. Line of pull is usually a major factor because most muscles pull at a diagonal. As discussed in Chapter 8 regarding torque, most muscles have a diagonal line of pull. That diagonal line of pull is the resultant force of a vertical force and a horizontal force. In the case of the shoulder girdle, muscles with a greater vertical line of pull will be effective in pulling the scapula up or down (elevating or depressing the scapula). Muscles with a greater horizontal pull will be more effective in pulling the scapula in or out (protracting or retracting). Muscles with a more equal horizontal and vertical pull will have a role in both motions (see Fig. 5-23). For example, the levator scapula has a stronger vertical component, the middle trapezius has a stronger horizontal component, and the rhomboids have a more equal pull in both directions. As you will see when these muscles are described later in this chapter, the levator scapula is a prime mover in scapular elevation, the middle trapezius is a prime mover in retraction, and the rhomboids are a prime mover in both elevation and retraction.

Muscle Descriptions

There are five muscles primarily responsible for moving the scapula. Each muscle will be discussed with particular emphasis on its location and function. This will be followed by a summary of its proximal attachment origin shown in blue **(O)**, its distal attachment insertion shown in green **(I)**, and its joint motions in which it is a prime mover action **(A)**. This listing is given for clarity and is not intended to be the only description. You are encouraged to visualize the attachments and describe them using proper terminology instead of memorizing these listings. The nerve **(N)** that innervates the muscle, as well as the spinal cord level of that innervation, is also given.

The muscles of the shoulder girdle are the following:

- Trapezius
- Levator scapula
- Rhomboids
- Serratus anterior
- Pectoralis minor

Trapezius

The **trapezius muscle** (Fig. 9-13) is a large, superficial muscle that appears diamond-shaped when looking at both right and left sides. Anatomically it is one muscle,

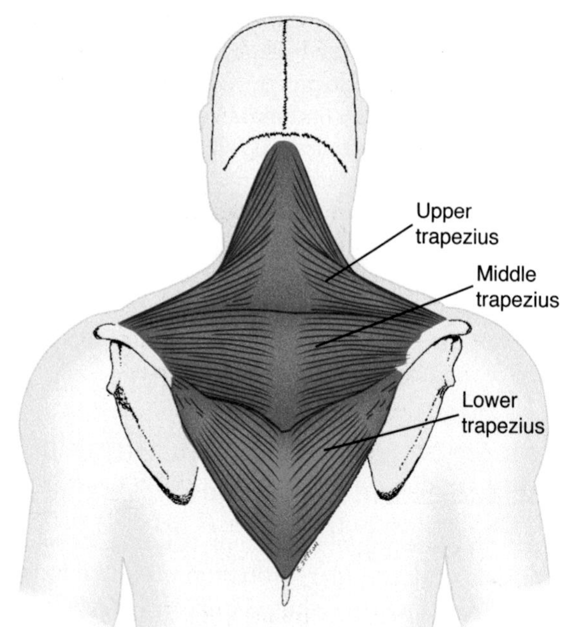

Figure 9-13. Three parts of the trapezius muscle (posterior view).

but functionally, it is usually divided into three parts: upper, middle, and lower. The reason for this separation is that there are three different lines of pull (upward, inward, downward) resulting in different muscle actions.

The **upper trapezius muscle** (Fig. 9-14) originates from the occipital protuberance and the nuchal ligament

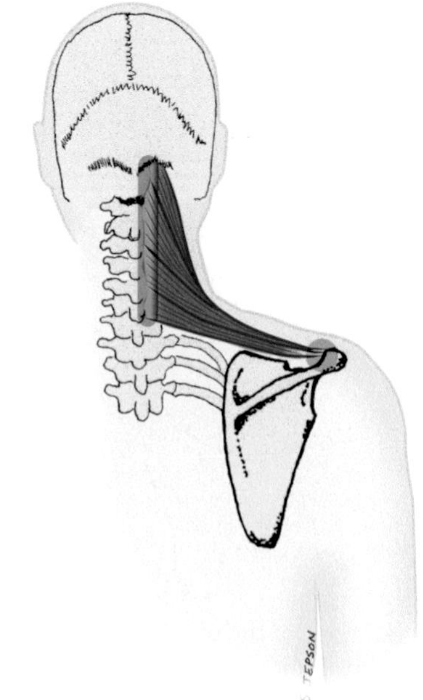

Figure 9-14. Upper trapezius muscle (posterior view).

of the upper cervical vertebrae. The nuchal ligament attaches to the spinous processes of the cervical vertebrae (see Fig. 15-14). The upper trapezius inserts on the lateral end of the clavicle and acromion process. Because its line of pull is more vertical (upward) than horizontal (inward), it is a prime mover in scapular elevation and upward rotation and is only an assisting mover in scapular retraction.

Upper Trapezius Muscle

O	Occipital bone, nuchal ligament on upper cervical spinous processes
I	Outer third of clavicle, acromion process
A	Scapular elevation and upward rotation
N	Spinal accessory (cranial nerve XI), C3 and C4 sensory component

The **middle trapezius muscle** (Fig. 9-15) originates from the nuchal ligament of the lower cervical vertebrae and spinous processes of C7 and the upper thoracic vertebrae as well as the supraspinal ligament in that area. The supraspinal ligament attaches on the posterior tips of spinous processes from C7 to the sacrum (see Figs. 15-13 and 15-14). It inserts on the medial aspect of the acromion process and along the scapular spine. Its line of pull is horizontal, which makes it very effective at scapular retraction. Because the line of pull passes just above the axis for upward rotation, its role in scapular upward rotation is only assistive.

Middle Trapezius Muscle

O	Spinous processes of C7 through T3
I	Scapular spine
A	Scapular retraction
N	Spinal accessory (cranial nerve XI), C3 and C4 sensory component

The **lower trapezius muscle** (Fig. 9-16) originates from the spinous processes and supraspinal ligament of the middle and lower thoracic vertebrae and inserts on the base of the scapular spine. Its diagonal line of pull is more downward (vertical) than inward (horizontal), making it a prime mover in depression and upward rotation of the scapula and only an assisting mover in retraction.

Lower Trapezius Muscle

O	Spinous processes of middle and lower thoracic vertebrae
I	Base of the scapular spine
A	Scapular depression and upward rotation
N	Spinal accessory (cranial nerve XI), C3 and C4 sensory component

All three parts of the trapezius muscle work together (synergists) to retract the scapula. Remember, however, that the middle trapezius muscle is the prime

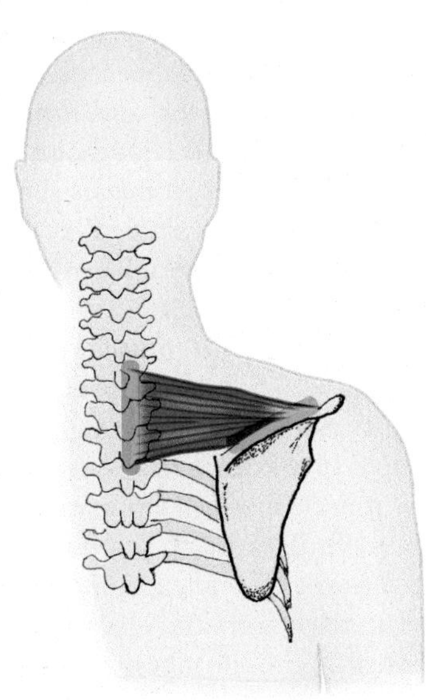

Figure 9-15. Middle trapezius muscle (posterior view).

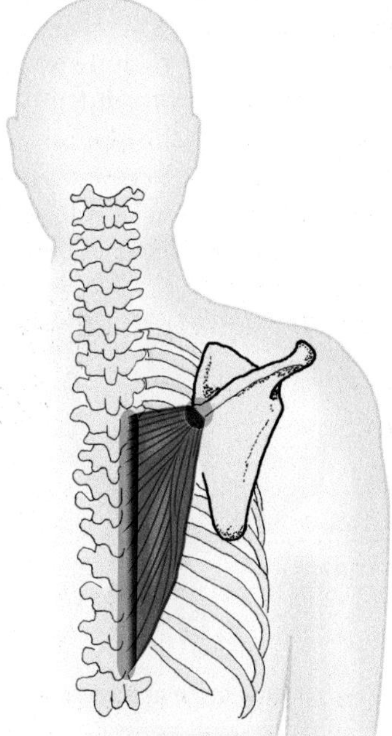

Figure 9-16. Lower trapezius muscle (posterior view).

mover and that the upper and lower trapezius muscles can only assist. The upper and lower trapezius muscles are antagonistic to each other in elevation/depression and are agonistic in upward rotation. To visualize the upward rotation component of these muscles, think of the scapula as a steering wheel (Fig. 9-17). In this example, a right scapula is used. Tie a ribbon at the bottom of the wheel to represent the inferior angle of the scapula. Put your right hand at the two o'clock position, representing the upper trapezius attachment; put your left hand at the ten o'clock position, representing the lower trapezius attachment. Turn the wheel to the left and note that the ribbon moves upward toward the right. In the case of the scapula, the upper trapezius muscle (right hand) moves up and in while the lower trapezius muscle (left hand) moves down and in. This combined effort causes the inferior angle to move up and out (upward rotation).

The **levator scapula muscle** is named for its function of scapular elevation. It is covered entirely by the trapezius muscle. It arises from the transverse processes of C1 through C4 and attaches on the vertebral border of the scapula between the superior angle and the spine (Fig. 9-18). Its diagonal line of pull is mostly vertical. Therefore, it is a prime mover in scapular elevation and only an assisting mover in retraction. Pulling upward on the superior angle also allows the levator scapula to be a prime mover in downward rotation. Visualize the steering wheel with your left hand in the ten o'clock position. Pull up (turning the wheel to the right) and notice that the inferior angle (ribbon) moves to the left (downward rotation). Keep in mind that downward rotation is the return to anatomical position from an upwardly rotated position.

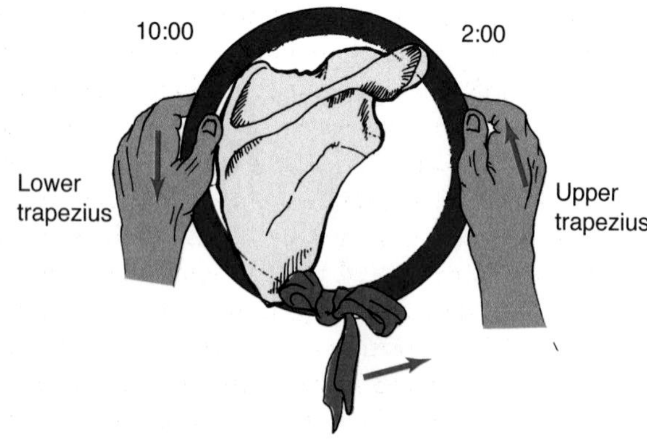

Figure 9-17. Rotational movement of the right scapula.

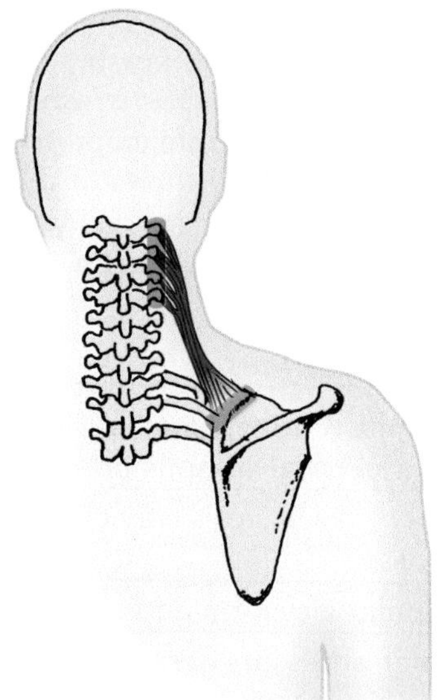

Figure 9-18. Levator scapula muscle (posterior view).

Levator Scapula Muscle

O	Transverse processes of first four cervical vertebrae
I	Vertebral border of scapula between the superior angle and spine
A	Scapular elevation and downward rotation
N	Third and fourth cervical nerves and dorsal scapular nerve (C5)

The **rhomboids** are actually two muscles: rhomboid major and rhomboid minor. They are commonly considered together as one muscle, because it is anatomically difficult to separate them, and functionally they have the same actions. The rhomboids derive their name from their shape. This geometric shape is basically a rectangle that has been skewed so that the sides have oblique angles instead of right angles. The rhomboid muscles lie under the trapezius muscle and can be palpated when the trapezius muscle is relaxed. They originate from the nuchal and supraspinal ligaments and spinous processes of C7 through T5, and they insert on the vertebral border of the scapula below the levator scapula muscle between the spine and the inferior angle (Fig. 9-19). Because their oblique line of pull has good horizontal and vertical components, they are a prime mover in retraction and elevation. Like the levator scapula muscle, the rhomboids rotate the scapula downward.

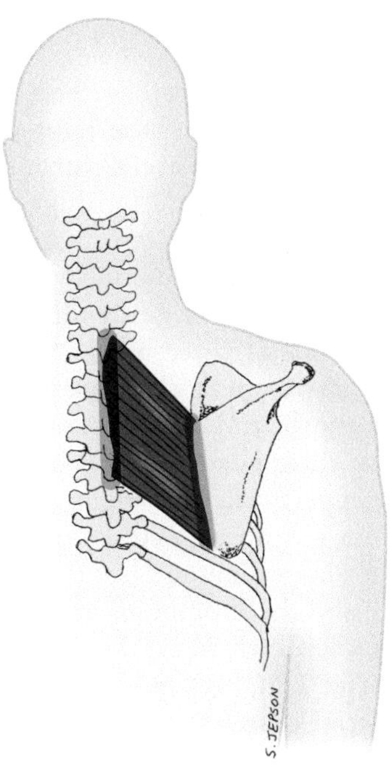

Figure 9-19. Rhomboid muscle (posterior view).

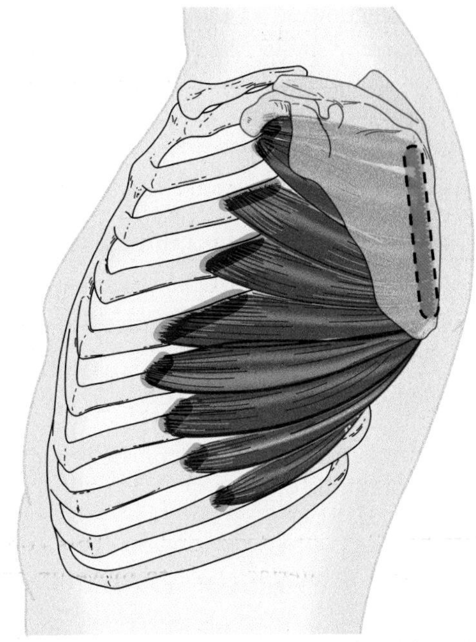

Figure 9-20. Serratus anterior muscle (lateral view).

Rhomboid Muscles

O	Spinous processes of C7 through T5
I	Vertebral border of scapula between the spine and inferior angle
A	Scapular retraction, elevation, and downward rotation
N	Dorsal scapular nerve (C5)

Serratus Anterior Muscle

O	Lateral surface of the upper eight ribs
I	Vertebral border of the scapula, anterior surface
A	Scapular protraction and upward rotation
N	Long thoracic nerve (C5, C6, C7)

It is impossible to raise your arm above your head without the action of the **serratus anterior muscle.** This muscle gets its name from the serrated, or saw-tooth, pattern of attachment on the anterior, lateral side of the thorax. It is superficial at this point and can be palpated when the arm is overhead. The muscle runs posteriorly to pass between the scapula and the rib cage. It attaches on the anterior surface of the scapula along the vertebral border between the superior and inferior angles (Fig. 9-20). Because it has a nearly horizontal line of pull outward, it is a prime mover in scapular protraction. Its lower fibers pulling outward on the lower part of the scapula are effective in rotating the scapula upward. These fibers join with the upper and lower trapezius muscles to form a force couple that rotates the scapula upward. Another function of the serratus anterior muscle is to keep the vertebral border of the scapula against the rib cage. Without this muscle, the vertebral border lifts away from the rib cage, which is called "winging of the scapula" (see Fig. 9-12).

The **pectoralis minor muscle** lies deep to the pectoralis major muscle and is the only shoulder girdle muscle located entirely on the anterior surface of the body. It arises from the anterior surface of the third through fifth ribs near the costal cartilages, and it runs upward to its attachment on the coracoid process of the scapula (Fig. 9-21). Its downward diagonal line of pull is mostly vertical, making it a prime mover in scapular depression, downward rotation, and scapular tilt. Although it is rather easy to see the depression action, the downward rotation is less obvious because the muscle is on the anterior surface while the scapula moves on the posterior surface. Visualize the steering wheel again with the ribbon (inferior angle of the scapula) rotated up to the right. Place your right hand in the two o'clock position (coracoid process) and pull down. Notice that the ribbon (inferior angle) moves downward toward the left (downward rotation). Because the pectoralis minor attaches on the anterior superior surface (coracoid process) of the scapula and moves vertically downward toward its attachment on the ribs, one can visualize the top part of the scapula being pulled down and forward, causing the bottom (inferior angle) to tip "out." In other words, the pectoralis minor causes scapular tilt.

Pectoralis Minor Muscle

O	Anterior surface, third through fifth ribs
I	Coracoid process of the scapula
A	Scapular depression, protraction, downward rotation, and tilt
N	Medial pectoral nerve (C8, T1)

Table 9-1 summarizes the actions of the prime movers of the shoulder girdle.

Table 9-1 Prime Movers of the Shoulder Girdle

Action	Muscles
Retraction	Middle trapezius, rhomboids
Protraction	Serratus anterior, pectoralis minor
Elevation	Upper trapezius, levator scapula, rhomboids
Depression	Lower trapezius, pectoralis minor
Upward rotation	Upper and lower trapezius Serratus anterior (lower fibers)
Downward rotation	Rhomboids, levator scapula, pectoralis minor
Scapular tilt	Pectoralis minor

Clinical Application 9-1

Postural Influences

With rounding of the shoulders, the scapula is pulled into a protracted position (see Fig. 5-17). This places the rhomboids and middle trapezius (scapular retractors) in a chronically stretched position, and as dictated by the length-tension relationship, these muscles become *weak and overstretched.* The pectoralis minor, however, is placed on slack as the coracoid moves anteriorly toward the ribs, and over time it adaptively shortens (adopts a shorter resting length).

Anatomical Relationships

The shoulder girdle muscles have been described by their attachments to bones, the joint motions that can occur because of these attachments, and their lines of pull. However, the relationships between muscles, whether superficial or deep, anterior or posterior, and so on, must also be described (Figs. 9-21, 9-22, and 9-23). All five shoulder girdle muscles have their origins on the trunk; three are located posteriorly (trapezius, levator scapula, rhomboids), one laterally (serratus anterior), and one anteriorly (pectoralis minor). Of the three posterior muscles, the trapezius is the most superficial. The right and left upper, middle, and lower trapezius covers most of the back in the form of a large diamond (see Fig. 9-13). Remove the trapezius, and the rhomboids and levator scapula lay directly underneath (see Fig. 9-22). As you view Figures 9-22 and 9-24, keep in mind that the left side shows superficial muscles, and the right side shows deeper lying muscles. Darkly colored muscles denote shoulder girdle muscles, whereas lighter colored muscles are muscles of other, mostly adjacent, joints. This color-coding will be consistent throughout Chapters 9 through 20 when showing the anatomical relationships of muscles.

The pectoralis minor is on the anterior side of the body but deep to the pectoralis major muscle (see Fig. 9-23). The serratus anterior originates anteriorly

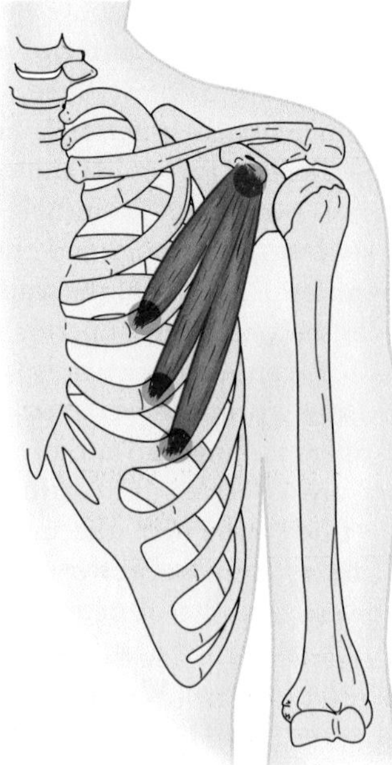

Figure 9-21. Pectoralis minor muscle (anterior view).

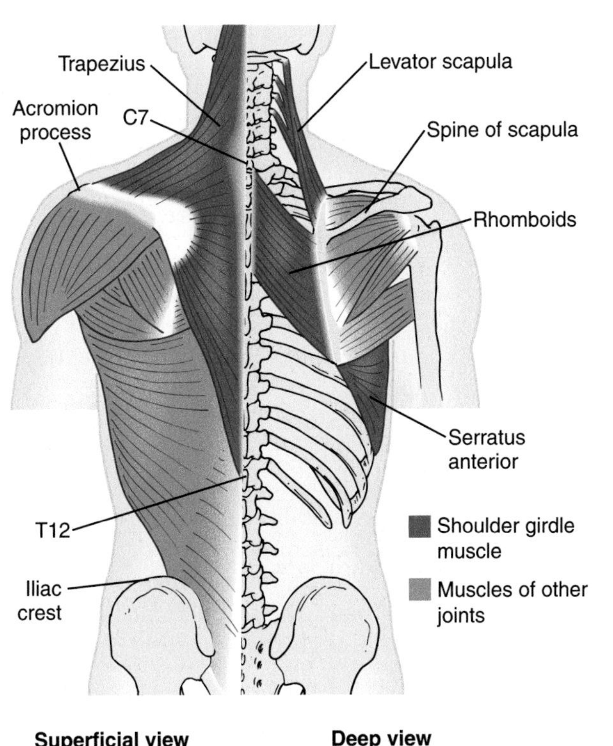

Figure 9-22. Muscles of the posterior shoulder girdle.

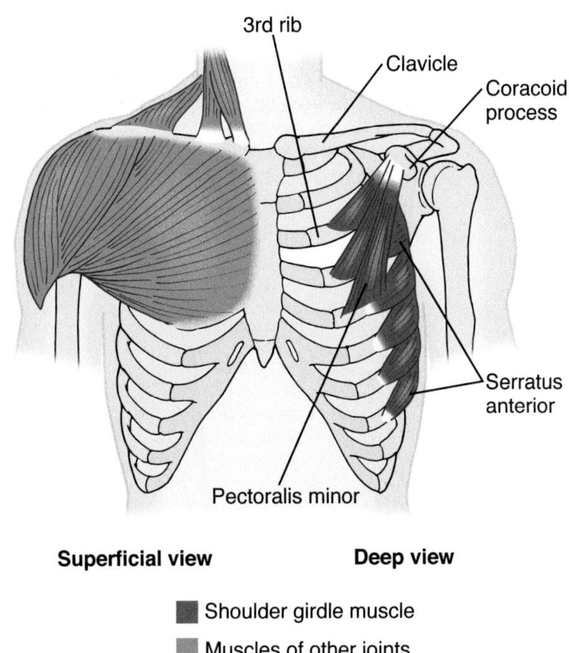

Figure 9-23. Muscles of the anterior shoulder girdle.

and runs posteriorly. As it crosses the lateral chest wall in a horizontal direction, it can be seen between the latissimus dorsi (posteriorly) and the pectoralis major and external oblique (anteriorly), as shown in Figure 9-24.

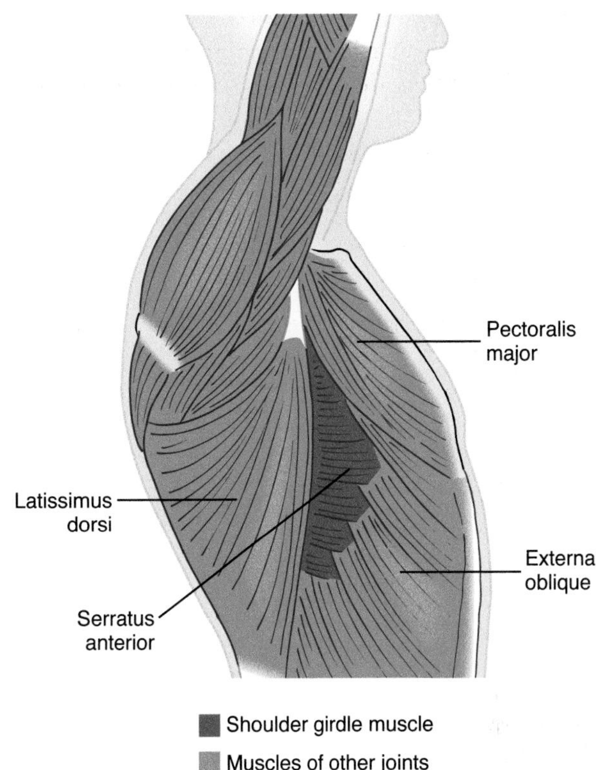

Figure 9-24. Muscles of the lateral shoulder girdle.

Force Couples

A **force couple** is defined as muscles pulling in different directions to accomplish the same motion. In the case of the shoulder girdle, the upper trapezius muscle pulls up, the lower trapezius muscle pulls down, and the lower fibers of the serratus anterior muscle pull outward in a horizontal direction. The net effect is that the scapula rotates upward (Fig. 9-25).

Downward rotation is another example of a force couple. The combined effects of the pectoralis minor muscle pulling down, the rhomboid muscles pulling in, and the levator scapula muscle pulling up is downward rotation of the scapula (Fig. 9-26). This motion is accomplished when the shoulder joint is forcefully extended, as when chopping wood, paddling a canoe, or pulling down on an overhead exercise machine. Downward rotation of the scapula must accompany extension of the shoulder joint.

Reverse Muscle Action

The actions of the shoulder girdle muscles have been described as moving the insertion toward the origin. However, if the insertion is stabilized, the origin will move. As discussed in Chapter 5, this is called **reverse muscle action.** It allows some of the shoulder girdle

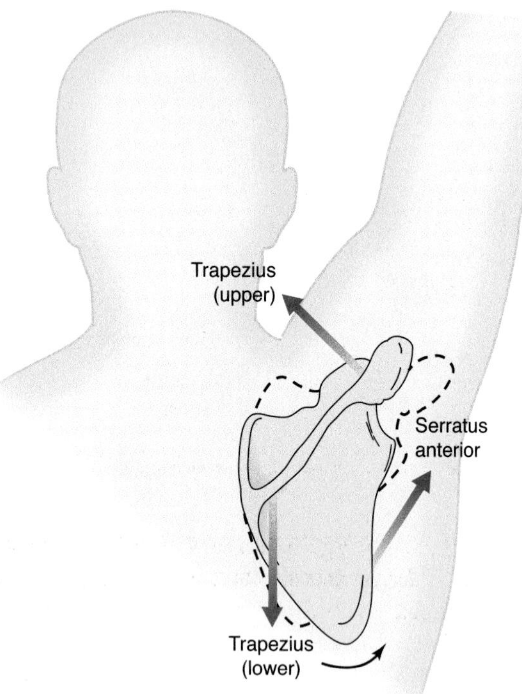

Figure 9-25. The muscular force couple produces upward rotation of the scapula (posterior view).

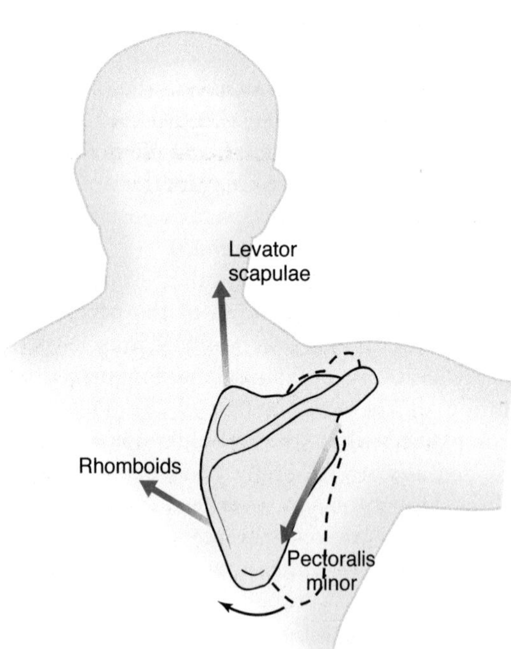

Figure 9-26. The muscular force couple produces downward rotation of the scapula (posterior view).

muscles to have assistive roles in other joints, primarily the head and neck.

Because of its attachment on the occiput and cervical vertebrae, the upper trapezius can play a role in moving the head and neck. When the shoulder girdle is stabilized, bilateral contaction of the upper trapezius muscles can assist in extending the head and neck. When the upper trapezius is contracting unilaterally it can laterally bend the head and neck to the same side (ipsilateral) and rotate it to the opposite side (contralateral).

With the shoulder girdle stabilized, the lower trapezius and pectoralis minor can reverse their actions and assist in elevating the trunk. This is particularly useful during crutch walking. With the crutches planted on the floor and the hands bearing weight on the crutches, the scapula becomes stabilized, preventing the lower trapezius and pectoralis minor from depressing the scapula when they contract. Instead, their origins move the body upward toward the scapula, thus raising the body as it swings through the crutches (Fig. 9-27). A

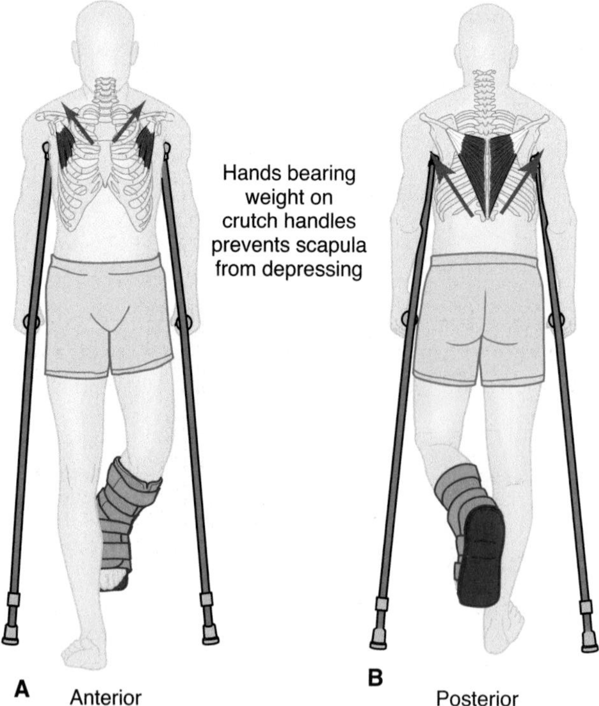

Figure 9-27. Reverse muscle action during crutch walking with hands bearing weight on crutch handles to prevent scapula and rib cage from depressing. The pectoralis minor **(A)** is pulling up on the rib cage while the lower trapezius **(B)** pulls up on the vertebral column and pelvis to elevate the body, allowing it to swing through the crutches.

similar role is played by the latissimus dorsi, which will be discussed in Chapter 10.

When the scapula is stabilized, the levator scapula can move the neck. It can assist the splenius cervicis, a neck muscle, in rotating and laterally bending the neck ipsilaterally.

Summary of Muscle Innervation

The shoulder girdle gets its innervation fairly high off the spinal cord from a variety of sources proximal to the terminal nerves of the brachial plexus. The 11th cranial (spinal accessory) nerve innervates the trapezius muscle with sensory innervation from C3 and C4. The third and fourth cervical nerves innervate the levator scapula muscle with partial innervation by the dorsal scapular nerve coming from C5. The serratus anterior muscle is innervated by the long thoracic nerve, which is made up of branches of C5 through C7, and the rhomboid muscles are innervated by the dorsal scapular nerve, a branch of the anterior ramus to C5. The pectoralis minor muscle receives innervation from the medial pectoral nerve, which branches off the medial cord of the brachial plexus. Table 9-2 summarizes the innervation of these muscles, and Table 9-3 gives the spinal cord level of innervation for each muscle.

Common Shoulder Girdle Pathologies

Acromioclavicular separation is the term commonly used to describe the various amounts of ligament injury at the AC joint. In a *first-degree sprain,* the acromioclavicular ligament (see Fig. 9-8) is stretched. In a *second-degree sprain,* the acromioclavicular ligament is ruptured, and the coracoclavicular ligament (see Fig. 9-8) is stretched. In a *third-degree sprain,* both the acromioclavicular and coracoclavicular ligaments are ruptured.

Clavicular fractures account for the most frequently broken bone in children. They usually result from a fall on the lateral aspect of the shoulder or on the outstretched hand. The clavicle usually breaks in its midportion.

Table 9-2 Innervation of the Muscles of the Shoulder Girdle

Muscle	Nerve	Spinal Segment
Trapezius*	Cranial nerve XI	C3, C4 (sensory)
Levator scapula	Dorsal scapular	C3, C4, C5
Rhomboids	Dorsal scapular	C5
Serratus anterior	Long thoracic	C5, C6, C7
Pectoralis minor	Medial pectoral	C8, T1

*The 11th cranial nerve provides motor innervation. C3 and C4 are sensory.

Table 9-3 Segmental Innervation of Shoulder Girdle Muscles

Spinal Cord Level	C3	C4	C5	C6	C7	C8	T1
Trapezius*	X	X					
Levator scapula	X	X	X				
Rhomboids			X				
Serratus anterior		X	X	X			
Pectoralis minor					X	X	

*The 11th cranial nerve provides motor innervation. C3 and C4 are sensory.

Points to Remember

- The shoulder girdle has both linear and angular motions.
- The inferior angle is the point of reference for scapular rotation.
- Certain shoulder girdle and shoulder joint motions are connected.
- Scapulohumeral rhythm is shoulder girdle and shoulder combined motions of the joints.
- In the shoulder girdle there are force couples for both upward and downward rotation where muscles pulling in different directions help to accomplish the same motion.
- Concentric and eccentric are accelerating and decelerating activities. With isometric activity there is no joint motion.
- Kinetic chain movement depends on whether the distal segment is fixed (closed) or free to move (open).

Review Questions

General Anatomy Questions

1. Identify the structures that make up the shoulder girdle, the shoulder joint, and the shoulder complex.
2. Given that the scapula is shaped somewhat like a triangle,
   a. what landmark is commonly used to determine the direction the scapula is rotating?
   b. what direction is the landmark moving if the scapula is rotating upwardly?
3. Which shoulder girdle motions are mostly linear?
4. Which shoulder girdle motions are mostly angular?
5. Which type of scapular motion can only happen in conjunction with glenohumeral joint motions?
6. What scapular motion is always needed to allow for any overhead reaching activity at the glenohumeral joint?
7. What is scapulohumeral rhythm?
8. How is shoulder joint motion affected by the absence of scapulohumeral rhythm?
9. The trapezius muscle is usually referred to and described as consisting of three different muscles. The two rhomboid muscles (major and minor) are referred to and described as one. From a functional perspective,
   a. why is the trapezius muscle separated into three muscles?
   b. why are the rhomboid muscles described as one muscle?
10. Raising your hand over your head requires the combined action of which three shoulder girdle muscles?
11. Name and define the biomechanical term used to describe the combined action in question 10.
12. Which joints of the shoulder complex produce movement when your hand is reached over your head?
13. Starting at the inferior angle and going clockwise, name the shoulder girdle muscles that attach to the posterior surface of the right scapula.
14. The pectoralis minor muscle is deep to what muscle?
15. As you look at the lateral chest wall, the serratus anterior is deep to what two muscles?

Functional Activity Questions

Identify the shoulder girdle motions that occur with the following actions. Accompanying shoulder joint motions have been provided in parentheses.

1. Closing a window by pulling down
   Shoulder girdle motion ____________________
   (Shoulder extension)
2. Opening a window by pulling up
   Shoulder girdle motion ____________________
   (Shoulder flexion)
3. Carrying a heavy suitcase
   Shoulder girdle motion ____________________
   (No shoulder motion)
4. Combing your hair in the back
   Shoulder girdle motion ____________________
   (Shoulder flexion, lateral rotation)
5. Reaching across the table
   Shoulder girdle motion ____________________
   (Shoulder flexion)
6. In questions 1 to 5, what type of contraction occurs at the shoulder girdle?

Clinical Exercise Questions

1. Lie prone on a table with your right arm hanging over the side of the table and holding a weight in your right hand (Fig. 9-28). Using only shoulder girdle motion and no shoulder joint motion, pull the weight straight up from the floor.
   a. What joint motion is occurring at the shoulder girdle?

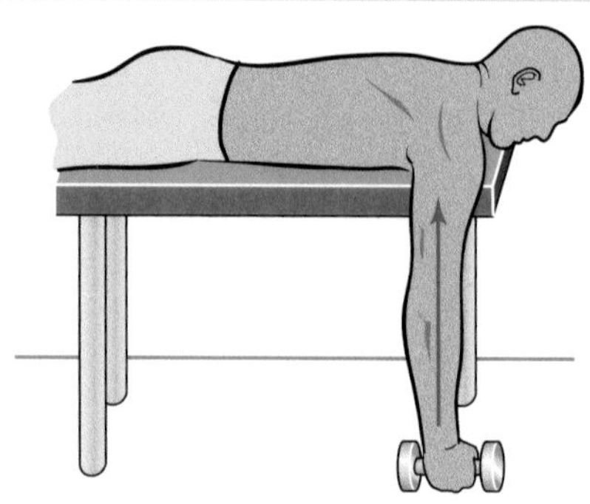

Figure 9-28. Starting position.

Review Questions—cont'd

b. What muscles are prime movers of this shoulder girdle action?
c. Is this an open-chain or closed-chain activity?

2. Lie prone on a table with your right arm hanging over the side of the table and holding a weight in your right hand (Fig. 9-28). Move your arm up and out by doing shoulder horizontal abduction.
   a. What shoulder girdle motion is accompanying shoulder horizontal abduction?
   b. What muscles are prime movers in this shoulder girdle motion?
   c. Is this a concentric, eccentric, or isometric contraction?
3. Sit in a chair that has arms; place your hands on the armrests in a position that puts your shoulders in hyperextension. Push down on the armrests and raise your buttocks off the seat of the chair.
   a. What shoulder girdle motion is accompanying the shoulder flexion action (from hyperextension to neutral)?
   b. What muscles are prime movers in this shoulder girdle motion?
   c. Is this a concentric or eccentric activity?
4. Lie in a prone position with your legs together, hands on the table next to your shoulders, with your fingers pointing forward (Fig. 9-29). Push up with your hands as far as you can while straightening your elbows, bending your knees, and keeping your back straight.
   a. What shoulder girdle motion is occurring?
   b. What muscles are prime movers in this shoulder girdle motion?
   c. Is this an open-chain or closed-chain activity?

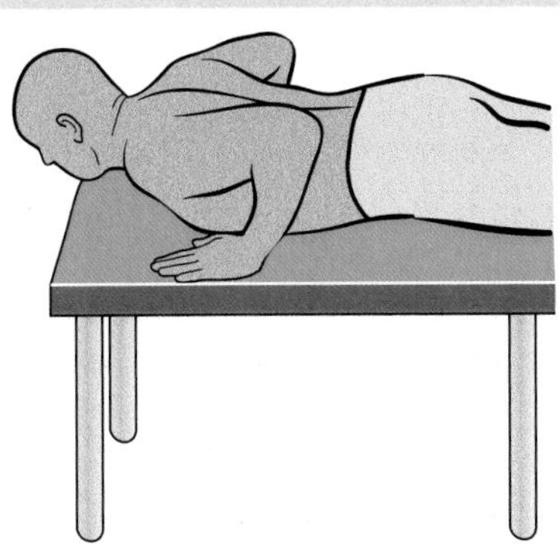

Figure 9-29. Starting position.

5. Using a lat pull-down machine of the Universal Gym (or some other comparable apparatus), reach up and grasp the handles. Pull down while keeping your arms moving in the frontal plane.
   a. What shoulder girdle motions are accompanying shoulder adduction and lateral rotation?
   b. What muscles are prime movers in these shoulder girdle motions?
   c. Is this a concentric or eccentric activity?
6. While standing, grasp some light weights in your hands and perform a shoulder shrug.
   a. What muscle(s) contract to perform this motion, and what type of contraction are they performing?
   b. Next, lower down from the shrug position. What muscle(s) contract to perform this motion, and what type of contraction are they performing?
7. A person has scapular winging. What muscle is involved?

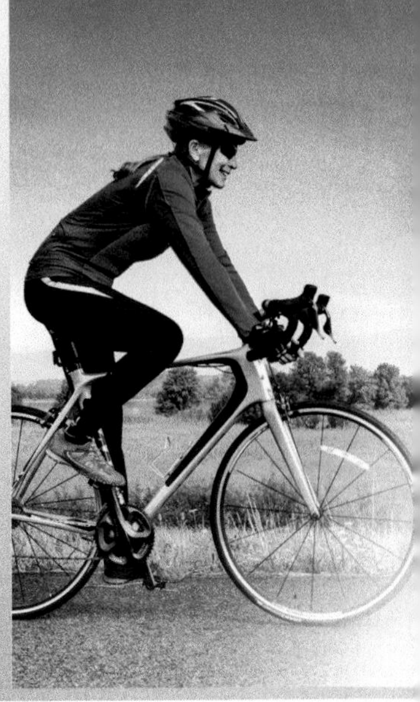

CHAPTER 10
Shoulder Joint

Joint Motions
Bones and Landmarks
Important Bony Landmarks of the Scapula
Important Bony Landmarks of the Humerus
Ligaments and Other Structures
Muscles of the Shoulder Joint
Anatomical Relationships
Glenohumeral Movement
Summary of Muscle Action
Summary of Muscle Innervation
Common Shoulder Pathologies
Points to Remember
Review Questions
General Anatomy Questions
Functional Activity Questions
Clinical Exercise Questions

Kinesiology IN ACTION For additional practice activities and videos, please visit www.kinesiologyinaction.com

The **shoulder joint** is a ball-and-socket joint with movement in all three planes and around all three axes (Fig. 10-1). Therefore, the joint has three degrees of freedom. The humeral head articulating with the glenoid fossa of the scapula makes up the shoulder joint. It is one of the most movable joints in the body, and consequently, one of the least stable.

Joint Motions

There are four groups of motions possible at the shoulder joint (Fig. 10-2): (1) flexion, extension, and hyperextension; (2) abduction and adduction; (3) medial and lateral rotation; and (4) horizontal abduction and adduction. Flexion, extension, and hyperextension

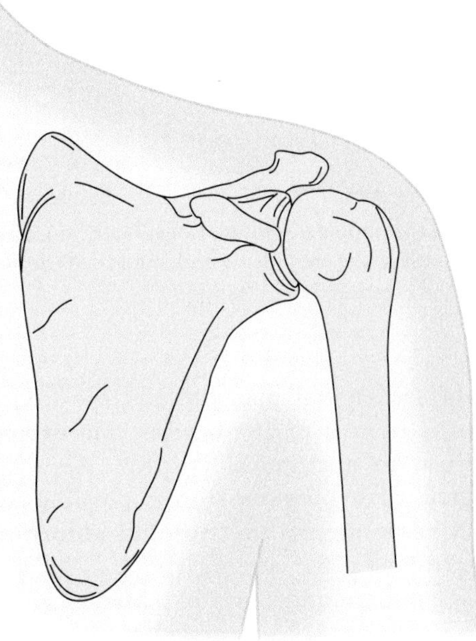

Figure 10-1. Shoulder joint (anterior view).

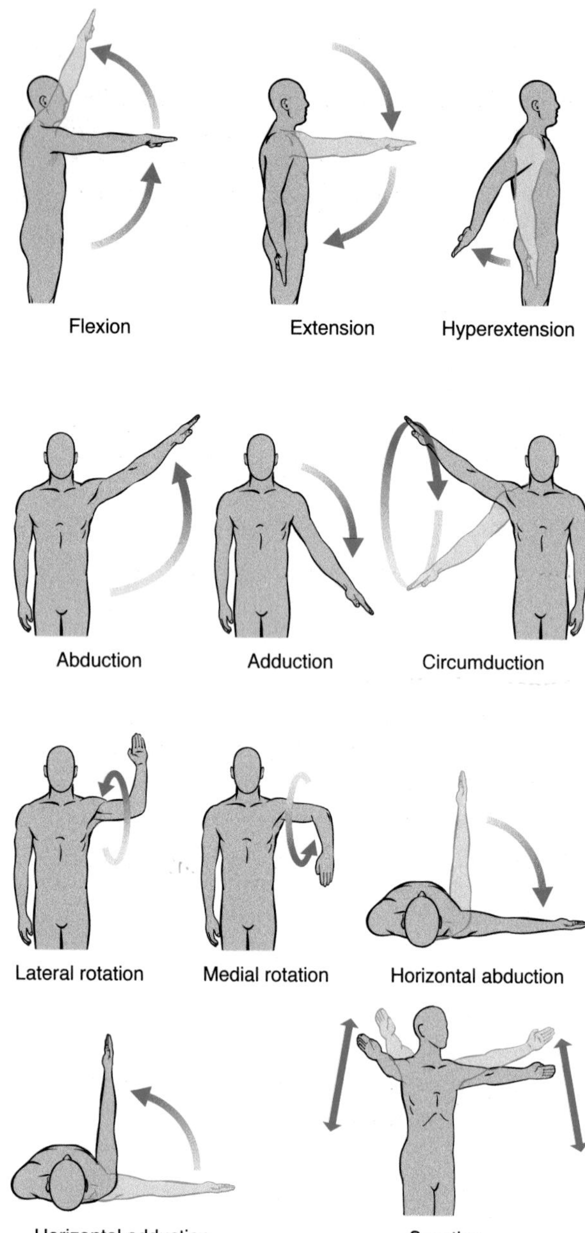

Figure 10-2. Shoulder joint motions. Note: In lateral and medial rotation, the shoulder is abducted to 90 degrees only to show the rotation more clearly.

occur in the sagittal plane around the frontal axis. **Flexion** is from 0 to 180 degrees, and **extension** is the return to anatomical position. Approximately 45 degrees of **hyperextension** is possible from the anatomical position. **Abduction** and **adduction** occur in the frontal plane around the sagittal axis, with 180 degrees of motion possible. **Medial** and **lateral rotation** occur in the transverse plane around the vertical axis. Sometimes the terms *internal* and *external* are used in place of *medial* and *lateral,* respectively. From a neutral position, it is possible to move 90 degrees in each direction. **Horizontal abduction** and **horizontal adduction** also occur in the transverse plane around the vertical axis. From an arbitrary starting position for these motions of 90 degrees of shoulder abduction, there would be approximately 30 degrees of horizontal abduction (backward motion) and approximately 120 degrees of horizontal adduction (forward motion). *Circumduction* is a term used to describe the arc or circle of motion possible at the shoulder. Because it is really only a combination of all the shoulder motions, this term will not be used here.

Another term frequently seen in the literature, especially regarding therapeutic exercise for shoulder conditions, is **scaption.** This motion is similar to flexion or abduction but occurs in the **scapular plane** as opposed to the sagittal or frontal plane (see Fig. 9-3). The scapular plane is approximately 30 degrees forward of the frontal plane. It is not quite midway between flexion and abduction. With scaption of the shoulder, 180 degrees of up and down motion is possible. Most common functional activities occur in the scapular plane.

The normal end feel for all shoulder joint motions is **firm.** This is due to tension from various ligaments and muscles and from the joint capsule. Reviewing its description from Chapter 4, end feel is the feel at the end of a joint's passive range of motion when slight pressure is applied.

Arthrokinematic Motion

At the glenohumeral joint, the convex humeral head moves within the concave glenoid fossa. As stated by the convex-concave rule, this convex joint surface (humeral head) glides in a direction opposite to the movement of the distal end of the moving bone (the humerus). Therefore, when the shoulder joint flexes (Fig. 10-3) or abducts, the humeral head glides posteriorly or inferiorly, respectively. This keeps the head of the humerus articulating with the glenoid fossa. In extension and adduction, the humeral head glides anteriorly or superiorly, respectively. With medial rotation, the humeral head glides posteriorly. With lateral rotation, the opposite motions occur. The head rolls glides anteriorly.

The greatest amount of arthrokinematic motion is possible when the glenohumeral joint is in the open packed position of 55 degrees abduction and 30 degrees horizontal adduction. A mobilizing force that glides the humeral head into the direction of restriction can help restore movement between the joint surfaces and lengthen fibers of the joint capsule.

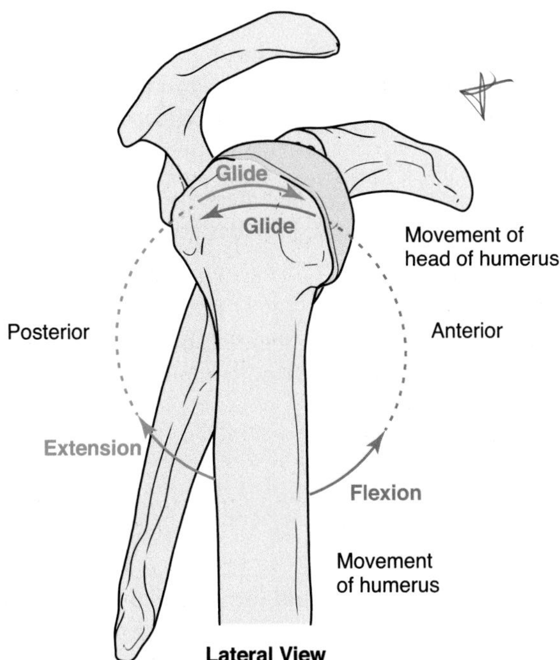

Figure 10-3. Arthrokinematic motions during shoulder flexion and extension. When the shoulder joint flexes, the humeral head glides posteriorly. During extension, the humeral head glides anteriorly.

Clinical Application 10-1

Linking Osteokinematics & Arthrokinematics

Arthrokinematic motion coupled with osteokinematic motion creates normal joint motion. When pathology such as capsular tightness interferes with joint motion, use of arthrokinematic motion can assist in restoring that motion by stretching the joint capsule. Take adhesive capsulitis as an example. With adhesive capsulitis, the following capsular pattern of range of motion loss may be seen: Severe loss of lateral rotation, moderate loss of abduction, and slight loss of medial rotation. Use of arthrokinematic motions (in the form of joint mobilizations) are often used to restore range of motion. For example, gliding the head of the humerus in the direction of restriction to stretch a particular part of the capsule, or by performing a long axis distraction where the head of the humerus is gently pulled away from the glenoid fossa, produces an effective stretch to the joint capsule as a whole. Specific application of these arthrokinematic motions in the use of joint mobilization is beyond the scope of this book.

Bones and Landmarks

The **scapula** and many of its landmarks were described in the chapter on the shoulder girdle. The following are landmarks of the scapula that you should know when talking about the shoulder joint (Fig. 10-4).

Important Bony Landmarks of the Scapula

Glenoid Fossa
A shallow, somewhat egg-shaped socket on the superior end, lateral side; articulates with the humerus

Glenoid Labrum
Fibrocartilaginous ring attached to the rim of the glenoid fossa, which deepens the articular cavity

Subscapular Fossa
Includes most of the area on the anterior (costal) surface, providing attachment for the subscapularis muscle

Infraspinous Fossa
Below the spine, providing attachment for the infraspinatus muscle

Supraspinous Fossa
Above the spine, providing attachment for the supraspinatus muscle

Axillary Border
Providing attachment for the teres major and teres minor muscles

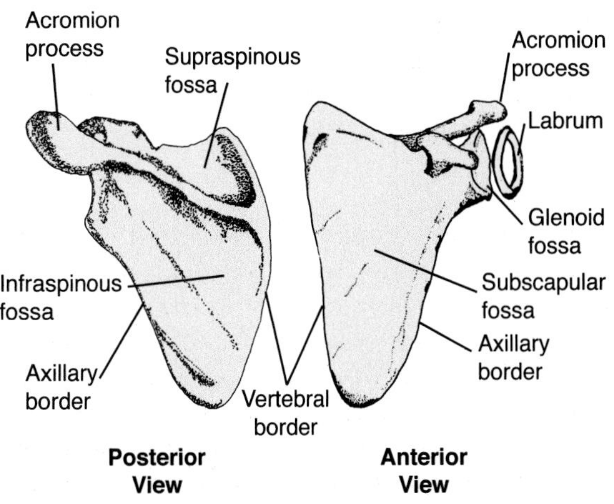

Figure 10-4. Left scapula.

Acromion Process
Broad, flat area on the superior lateral aspect, providing attachment for the middle deltoid muscle

The **humerus** is the longest and largest bone of the upper extremity (Fig. 10-5). The position of the humerus with the scapula is shown in an anterior view in Figure 10-1. The important landmarks are listed.

Important Bony Landmarks of the Humerus

Head
Semirounded proximal end; articulates with the scapula

Surgical Neck
Slightly constricted area just below tubercles where the head meets the body

Anatomical Neck
Circumferential groove separating the head from the tubercle

Shaft
Or "body"; the area between the surgical neck proximally and the wider distal end

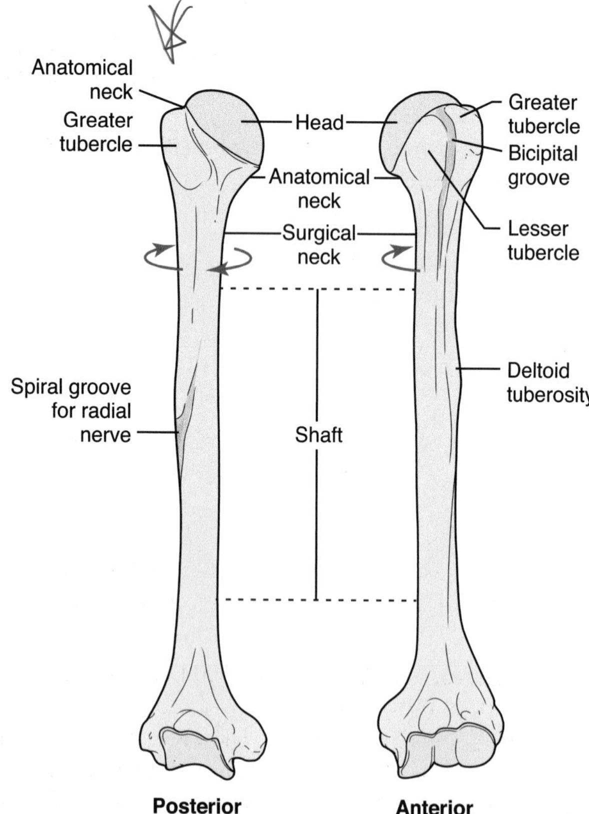

Figure 10-5. Left humerus.

Greater Tubercle
Large projection lateral to head and lesser tubercle; provides attachment for the supraspinatus, infraspinatus, and teres minor muscles

Lesser Tubercle
Smaller projection on the anterior surface, medial to the greater tubercle; provides attachment for the subscapularis muscle

Deltoid Tuberosity
On the lateral side near the midpoint of the shaft; not usually a well-defined landmark

Bicipital Groove
Also called the "intertubercular groove"; the longitudinal groove between the tubercles, containing the tendon of the long head of the biceps

Bicipital Ridges
Also called the lateral and medial lips of the bicipital groove, or the crests of the greater and lesser tubercles, respectively. The lateral lip (crest of the greater tubercle) provides attachment for the pectoralis major, and the medial lip (crest of the lesser tubercle) provides attachment for the latissimus dorsi and teres major.

Ligaments and Other Structures

The **joint capsule** is a thin-walled, spacious container that attaches around the rim of the glenoid fossa of the scapula and the anatomical neck of the humerus (Figs. 10-6 and 10-7). The joint capsule is formed by an outer fibrous membrane and an inner synovial membrane. With the arm hanging at the side, the superior portion of the capsule is taut, and the inferior part is slack. When the shoulder is abducted, the opposite occurs: The inferior portion is taut, and the superior part is slack. The superior, middle, and inferior **glenohumeral ligaments** (see Fig. 10-6) reinforce the anterior portion of the capsule. These are not well-defined ligaments but actually pleated folds of the capsule.

The **coracohumeral ligament** attaches from the lateral side of the coracoid process and spans the joint anteriorly to the medial side of the greater tubercle (see Figs. 10-6 and 10-7). It strengthens the upper part of the joint capsule.

The **glenoid labrum** is a fibrous ring that surrounds the rim of the glenoid fossa (see Figs. 10-4 and 10-8). Its function is to deepen the articular cavity.

There are several **bursae** in the shoulder joint area. The subdeltoid bursa is large and located between the

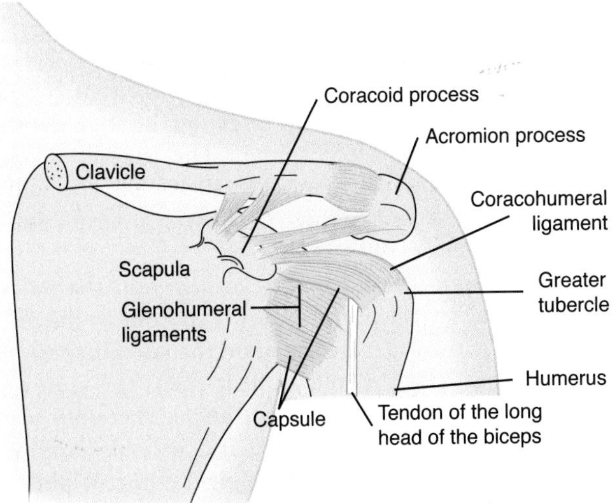

Figure 10-6. Shoulder joint capsule and the ligaments that reinforce it (anterior view).

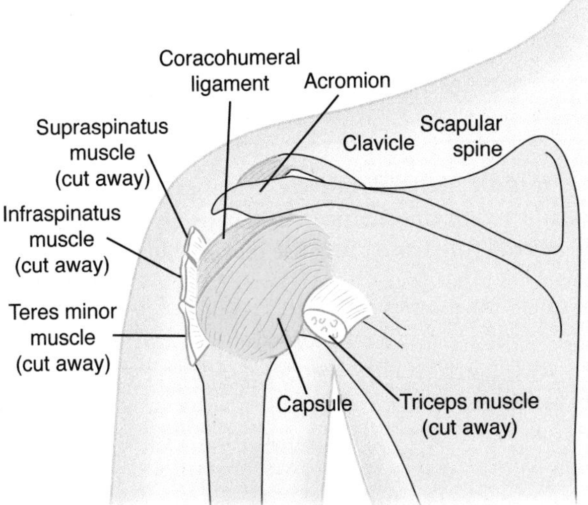

Figure 10-7. Left shoulder joint capsule and coracohumeral ligament (posterior view, muscles cut away).

deltoid muscle and the joint capsule. The subacromial bursa lies below the acromion and coracoacromial ligament, between them and the joint capsule, and it is frequently continuous with the subdeltoid bursa.

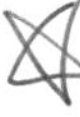

The **rotator cuff** is the tendinous band formed by the blending together of the tendinous insertions of the subscapularis, supraspinatus, infraspinatus, and teres minor muscles (Fig. 10-9). These muscles help to keep the head of the humerus against the glenoid fossa during joint motion. This rotating motion is what inspired the term *rotator cuff*, not the muscular action of medial or lateral rotation.

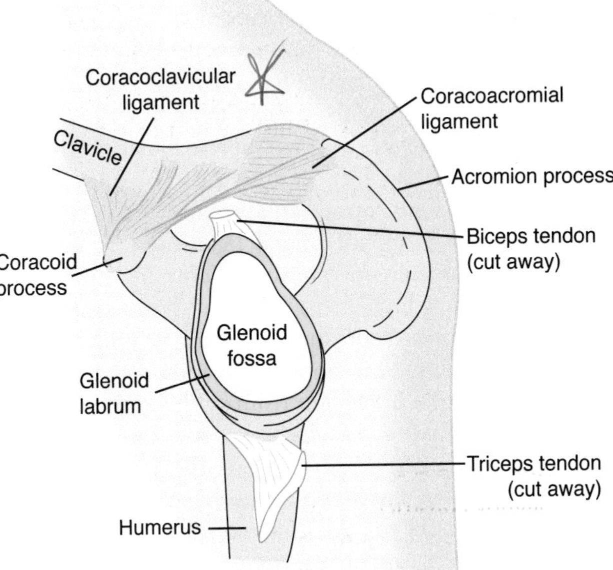

Figure 10-8. Glenoid labrum, lateral view.

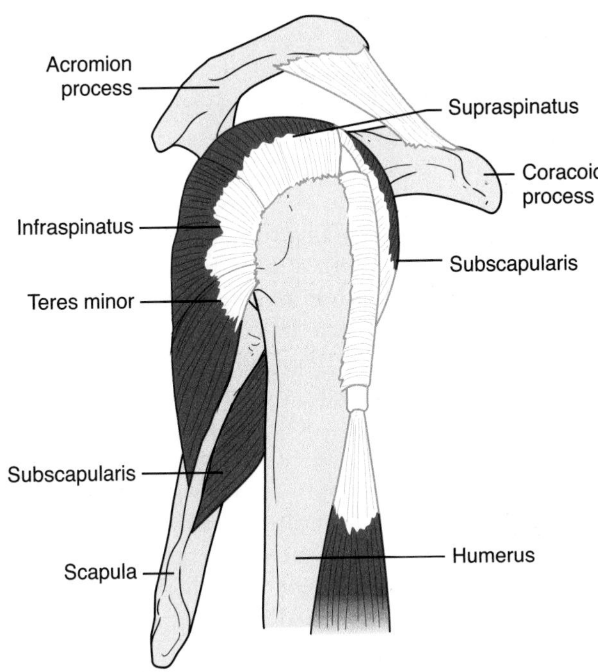

Figure 10-9. Rotator cuff showing the proximal tendinous portion of the SITS muscles blending together to form a "cuff."

The **thoracolumbar fascia** (lumbar aponeurosis) (see Fig. 10-21) is a superficial fibrous sheet that attaches to the spinous processes of the lower thoracic and lumbar vertebrae, the supraspinal ligament, and the posterior part of the iliac crest, covering the sacrospinalis muscle. It provides a very broad attachment for the latissimus dorsi muscle.

As mentioned, the shoulder joint allows a great deal of motion, making it rather unstable. Several features contribute to whatever stability this joint does have. The fairly shallow glenoid fossa is made deeper by the glenoid labrum. The fossa faces in an anterior, lateral, and upward direction. This upward-facing direction provides some stability to the joint. The joint is held intact by the joint capsule and is reinforced by the coracohumeral and glenohumeral ligaments. Because the capsule completely surrounds the joint, it creates a partial vacuum, which helps hold the head against the fossa. The rotator cuff muscles hold the joint surfaces together during joint motion. It is mostly the shoulder muscles that keep the joint from subluxing, or partially dislocating. An individual who has had a stroke and has muscle weakness or paralysis in the involved upper extremity often develops a subluxed shoulder. The lack of a deep socket for the humeral head to fit into, the loss of muscle tone, the weight of the extremity, and gravity all contribute to joint subluxation.

Muscles of the Shoulder Joint

Most shoulder muscles have their origin somewhere on the scapula, clavicle, or rib cage and will insert on the humerus. Because these muscles cross the glenohumeral joint, they are able to create movement at that joint. Muscles crossing the anterior aspect of the glenohumeral joint with a more vertical line of pull will flex the joint, whereas a muscle crossing the joint posteriorly with a vertical line of pull will extend the joint. Muscles with a more horizontal line of pull crossing the anterior aspect of the joint will tend to either create medial rotation and/or horizontal adduction, whereas those muscles crossing the posterior aspect of the joint horizontally will tend to create either lateral rotation and/or horizontal abduction. Muscles crossing the superior/lateral aspect of the glenohumeral joint will tend to abduct, and muscles that cross the inferior/medial aspect of the glenohumeral joint will tend to adduct.

The muscles that span the shoulder joint are as follows:

Deltoid
Pectoralis major
Latissimus dorsi
Teres major
Supraspinatus
Infraspinatus
Teres minor
Subscapularis
Coracobrachialis
Biceps brachii
Triceps brachii, long head

The **deltoid muscle** is a superficial muscle that covers the shoulder joint on three sides, giving the shoulder its characteristic rounded shape. The name *deltoid* describes its triangular shape (Fig. 10-10). Functionally, this muscle is separated into three parts: anterior, middle, and posterior.

The **anterior deltoid muscle** attaches on the outer third of the clavicle and runs down and out to the deltoid tuberosity, which is located on the lateral aspect of the humerus near the midpoint. It spans the joint on the anterior surface at an oblique angle. Therefore, it is effective in abduction, flexion, and medial rotation. When the arm is at shoulder level, the line of pull is mostly horizontal and, therefore, it is an effective horizontal adductor.

Anterior Deltoid Muscle

O	Lateral third of the clavicle
I	Deltoid tuberosity
A	Shoulder abduction, flexion, medial rotation, and horizontal adduction
N	Axillary nerve (C5, C6)

The **middle deltoid muscle** attaches on the lateral side of the acromion process and runs directly down to the deltoid tuberosity. Because its vertical line of pull is

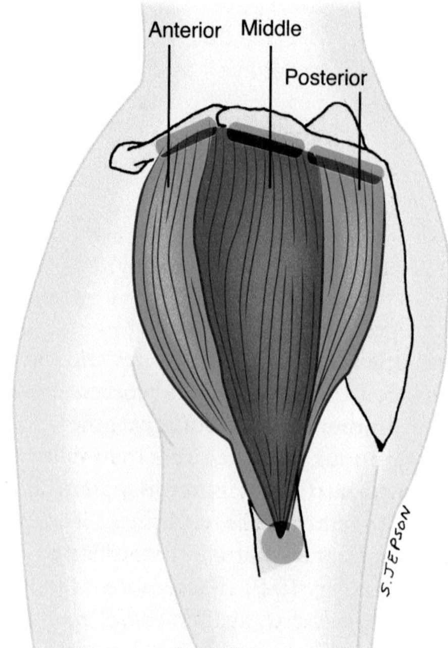

Figure 10-10. Three parts of the deltoid muscle (lateral view).

lateral to the joint axis, it is most effective in abducting the shoulder joint.

Middle Deltoid Muscle	
O	Acromion process
I	Deltoid tuberosity (same as anterior deltoid muscle)
A	Shoulder abduction
N	Axillary nerve (C5, C6)

The **posterior deltoid muscle** attaches to the spine of the scapula and runs obliquely down and lateral to its attachment with the anterior and middle fibers on the deltoid tuberosity. Because its oblique line of pull is posterior to the joint axis, it is strong in shoulder abduction, extension, hyperextension, and lateral rotation. When the arm is at shoulder level, the line of pull is mostly horizontal, making it effective in horizontal abduction.

Posterior Deltoid Muscle	
O	Spine of scapula
I	Deltoid tuberosity (same as anterior deltoid muscle)
A	Shoulder abduction, extension, hyperextension, lateral rotation, horizontal abduction
N	Axillary nerve (C5, C6)

The "inchworm effect" is a concept that describes the action of the shoulder girdle and the deltoid muscles, especially the middle deltoid muscle, during shoulder abduction. The deltoid muscle is at optimal length when the arm is at the side. If the humerus is the only bone that moved during abduction, the middle deltoid muscle would quickly shorten beyond optimal length and run out of contractile power as it approached 90 degrees. However, the middle deltoid muscle is effective throughout the entire range. Remember that for every 2 degrees the shoulder joint abducts, the shoulder girdle upwardly rotates 1 degree (scapulohumeral rhythm; see Chapter 9). With this upward rotation of the scapula, the origin of the deltoid muscle (the acromion process, the lateral end of the clavicle, and the scapular spine) moves away from the insertion on the humerus. This motion lengthens the muscle, restoring its contractile potential (optimal length-tension relationship), and allows it to continue to effectively contract throughout its entire range.

The **pectoralis major muscle** (Fig. 10-11) is a large muscle of the chest, as its name implies (*pectus* means "breast" or "chest"). It is superficial except for its distal attachment lying under the deltoid muscle. This muscle crosses the joint on the anterior surface in a horizontal

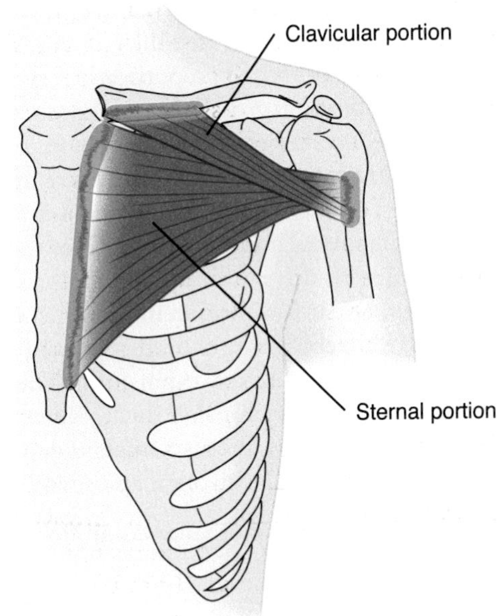

Figure 10-11. Two parts of the pectoralis major muscle (anterior view).

direction, creating a medial pull on the humerus. This makes it effective in adduction, medial rotation, and when elevated to 90 degrees, horizontal adduction of the shoulder joint.

The pectoralis major muscle, because of its proximal attachments and different lines of pull, is often separated into a clavicular and sternal portion. The **clavicular portion** of the pectoralis major attaches to the medial third of the clavicle. The clavicular portion has a more vertical line of pull when the shoulder is extended, making it very effective at flexing the shoulder during the first part of the range. As the shoulder approaches the midpoint of the range (shoulder level), the line of pull changes from vertical to more horizontal; thus, this portion of the pectoralis major muscle is no longer effective in flexing the shoulder. It is most effective in the early portion of the range (0 to 30 degrees) and becomes much less effective as it approaches the midpoint of the range (90 degrees). Therefore, it is safe to say that the clavicular portion of the pectoralis major acts as a prime mover in the first part (approximately 60 degrees) of shoulder flexion.

The **sternal portion** attaches to the sternum and costal cartilages of the first six ribs. It has a more vertical line of pull when the shoulder is in full flexion and loses effectiveness as the shoulder approaches the midrange of extension. Similar to the clavicular portion but in the opposite direction, the sternal portion is most effective in the early part of shoulder extension. It becomes less effective as it approaches the midpoint of the range (90 degrees). Therefore, it is safe to say that the sternal portion of the pectoralis major acts as a prime mover in the first part of shoulder extension (approximately 60 degrees). As an anatomical note, there is a twisting of the tendinous fibers of these two portions of muscle as they insert on the bicipital groove. The lower sternal portion inserts higher on the groove while the more superior clavicular portion inserts below it. This feature increases the vertical line of pull of the clavicular portion as a shoulder flexor and the sternal portion as a shoulder extensor.

Both portions of the pectoralis major muscle are effective in the first parts of motion in the sagittal plane (clavicular portion performing shoulder flexion, sternal portion performing shoulder extension). Therefore, they are antagonistic to each other in shoulder flexion and extension, but they are agonists in shoulder adduction, medial rotation, and horizontal adduction.

Pectoralis Major Muscle, Clavicular Portion

O	Medial third of clavicle
I	Lateral lip of bicipital groove of humerus (inferior to the sternal portion)
A	Shoulder flexion—first 60 degrees

Pectoralis Major Muscle, Sternal Portion

O	Sternum, costal cartilage of first six ribs
I	Lateral lip of bicipital groove of humerus (superior to the clavicular portion)
A	Shoulder extension—first 60 degrees (from 180 degrees to 120 degrees)

Pectoralis Major Muscle, Clavicular and Sternal Portions

O	Medial third of clavicle, sternum, and costal cartilage of ribs 1 to 6
I	Lateral lip of the bicipital groove of humerus
A	Shoulder adduction, medial rotation, and horizontal adduction
N	Lateral and medial pectoral nerves (C5, C6, C7, C8, T1)

As its name implies, the **latissimus dorsi muscle** (Fig. 10-12) is a broad, sheetlike muscle located on the back (in Latin, *latissimus* means "widest" and *dorsi* means "back" or "posterior"). It is mostly superficial except for a small portion covered posteriorly by the lower trapezius muscle and covered distally as it passes through the axilla to attach on the floor of the bicipital groove just anterior to the insertion of the teres major. This groove is on the proximal, anterior surface of the humerus.

The latissimus dorsi muscle is a strong agonist in extension, hyperextension, adduction, and medial rotation of the shoulder because it crosses the shoulder joint inferior and medial to the joint axis.

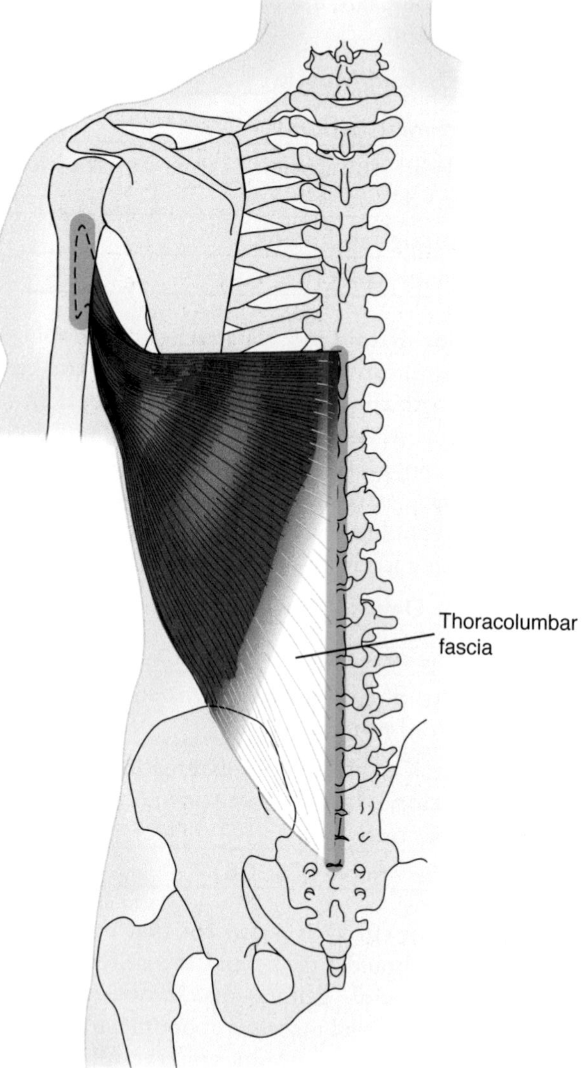

Figure 10-12. Latissimus dorsi muscle (posterior view). Note that the humeral attachment is on the anterior surface, as indicated by the dotted line.

Latissimus Dorsi Muscle

O	Spinous processes of T7 through L5 (via **thoracolumbar** fascia), posterior surface of sacrum, iliac crest, and lower three ribs
I	Medial floor of bicipital groove of humerus
A	Shoulder extension, adduction, medial rotation, hyperextension
N	Thoracodorsal nerve (C6, C7, C8)

Clinical Application 10-2

Reverse Muscle Action During Crutch Walking

As described in Chapter 9, the pectoralis minor and lower trapezius can elevate the pelvis when the arms are stabilized (see Fig. 9-27). This action occurs during crutch walking, when the arms are stabilized on the crutch handles. The pectoralis major and latissimus dorsi (see figure below) perform much like the pectoralis minor and lower trapezius in elevating the rib cage, sternum, and pelvis and allowing the body to swing through the crutches. This closed-chain activity is a good example of "reverse muscle action," where the origin moves toward the insertion instead of the more common insertion moving toward the origin.

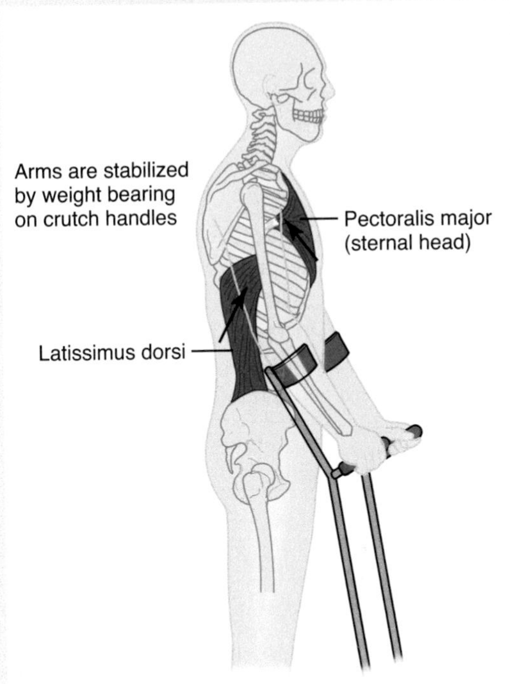

Reverse action of pectoralis major and latissimus dorsi elevates axial skeleton during crutch walking

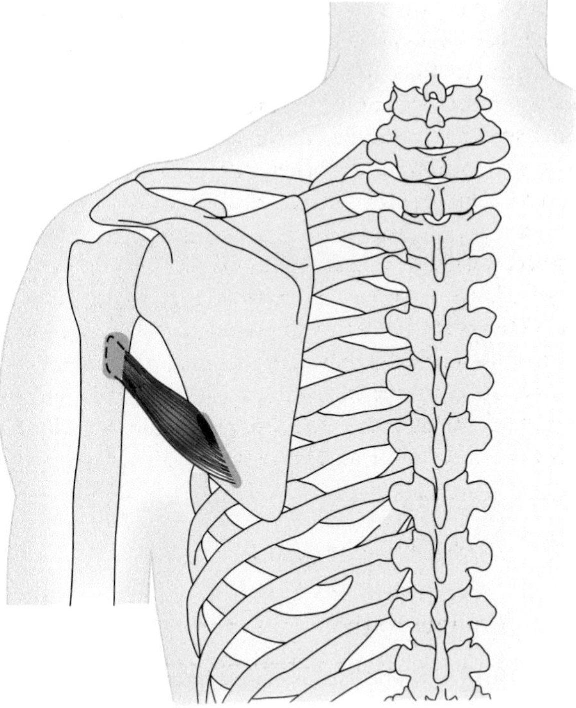

Figure 10-13. Teres major muscle (posterior view). Note that the humeral attachment is on the anterior surface, as indicated by the dotted line.

The **teres major muscle** (Fig. 10-13) has its proximal attachment on the axillary border of the scapula, just below the teres minor muscle. In Latin, *teres* means "long and round." Both muscles are superficial at this point. The teres major muscle travels with the latissimus dorsi muscle through the axilla to the point where they attach close together. The teres major attaches on the medial lip of the bicipital groove of the humerus. It is often referred to as the "little helper" of the latissimus dorsi muscle because it is much smaller in size and it does everything that the latissimus dorsi muscle does except hyperextension (its origin is not oriented far enough posteriorly to extend the shoulder beyond neutral). Although the teres major muscle is a prime mover in extension, adduction, and medial rotation, its much smaller size makes it less effective than the latissimus dorsi.

Teres Major Muscle

O	Inferior axillary border of scapula near the inferior angle
I	Medial lip of bicipital groove on the anterior surface of the humerus
A	Shoulder extension, adduction, and medial rotation
N	Lower subscapular nerve (C5, C6, C7)

The **supraspinatus muscle** (Fig. 10-14) originates above the spine of the scapula in the supraspinous fossa of the scapula. It passes underneath the acromion process, crossing the superior aspect of the shoulder joint to attach on the greater tubercle of the humerus. It is deep to the trapezius muscle above and to the deltoid muscle laterally. It pulls the greater tubercle up and in toward the supraspinous fossa, producing abduction at

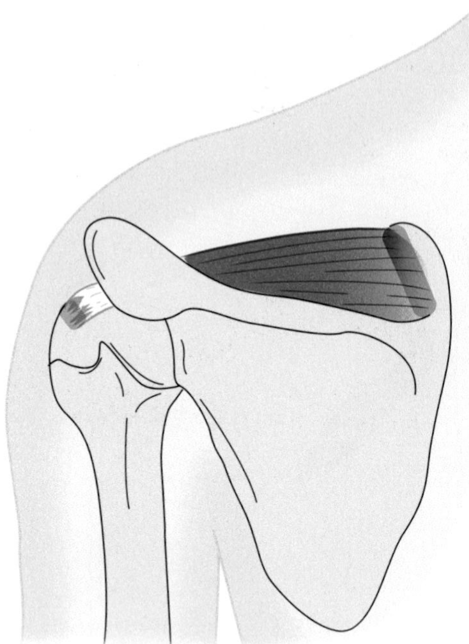

Figure 10-14. Supraspinatus muscle (posterior view).

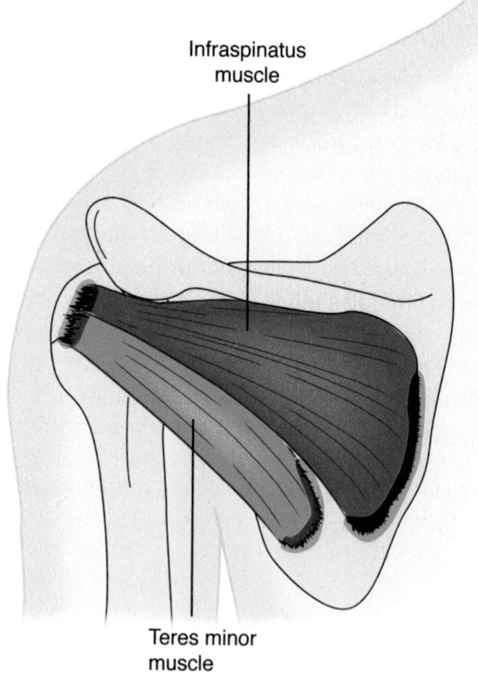

Figure 10-15. Infraspinatus and teres minor muscles (posterior view).

the glenohumeral joint. Early kinesiology studies suggested that the supraspinatus muscle was most effective in only initiating shoulder abduction. However, electromyography studies have since shown that while the deltoid does become more powerful later in the abduction range, the supraspinatus remains active throughout the full range of abduction.

In addition to its joint movement function, the supraspinatus muscle is very important in stabilizing the head of the humerus against the glenoid fossa. This is due to the horizontal orientation of its muscle fibers, which pull the head of the humerus into the glenoid fossa.

Supraspinatus Muscle

O	Supraspinous fossa of the scapula
I	Greater tubercle of the humerus
A	Shoulder abduction
N	Suprascapular nerve (C5, C6)

The **infraspinatus muscle** (Fig. 10-15) lies below the spine of the scapula in the infraspinous fossa. Most of the muscle is superficial; however, the trapezius and deltoid muscles cover portions of it. The distal attachment of the infraspinatus muscle is just inferior to the attachment of the supraspinatus muscle on the greater tubercle of the humerus. Given its more horizontal line of pull passing posterior to the joint, it creates lateral rotation, or if the shoulder is elevated to 90 degrees, horizontal abduction. Like the supraspinatus, it also plays an important role in stabilizing the head of the humerus against the glenoid fossa. Although some authors refer to the infraspinatus muscle's ability to extend the shoulder joint, its more horizontal line of pull must be recognized. Therefore, its extension action is assistive at best.

Infraspinatus Muscle

O	Infraspinous fossa of scapula
I	Greater tubercle of humerus
A	Shoulder lateral rotation, horizontal abduction
N	Suprascapular nerve (C5, C6)

The **teres minor muscle** (see Fig. 10-15) is closely related to the infraspinatus muscle in both anatomical location and function. Both muscles are mostly superficial, with portions covered by the trapezius and the deltoid muscles. Both the teres major and teres minor muscles attach along the axillary border of the scapula with the teres minor attaching above the teres major. They run obliquely up and outward to attach on the humerus. The teres minor muscle attaches posteriorly on the greater tubercle of the humerus just inferior to the infraspinatus, whereas the teres major muscle passes through the axilla to attach anteriorly on the medial lip of the humerus. In the axilla they are separated by the long head of the triceps muscle passing between them (Fig. 10-16). As one of the SITS muscles described in the next paragraph, it has an important role in stabilizing the head of the humerus against the glenoid fossa as the shoulder joint moves in various directions.

Teres Minor Muscle	
O	Axillary border of scapula
I	Greater tubercle of humerus
A	Shoulder lateral rotation, horizontal abduction
N	Axillary nerve (C5, C6)

If you observe the distal attachments of the supraspinatus, infraspinatus, and teres minor muscles on the greater tubercle of the humerus, you will notice that they are essentially in a line (Fig. 10-17). For this reason, they are collectively referred to as the *SIT muscles,* taking the first letter from each muscle. These three muscles plus the subscapularis are referred to as the *rotator cuff,* or *SITS, muscles.*

The **subscapularis** muscle (Fig. 10-18) gets its name from its location, which can be slightly misleading. In Latin, *sub* means "under." The subscapularis muscle is located deep on the "underside" of the scapula, lying next to the rib cage. This underside is actually the anterior, or costal, surface of the scapula. From this attachment on the anterior surface, the subscapularis muscle runs laterally to cross the shoulder joint anteriorly and it attaches on the lesser tubercle of the humerus. This distal attachment blends into a common tendinous sheath with the other rotator cuff muscles to cover the humeral head and hold the head against the glenoid fossa. Because the subscapularis crosses the anterior side of the joint and has a horizontal line of pull, it pulls the lesser tubercle medially. This makes it a prime mover in medial rotation and assists in adduction of the shoulder joint.

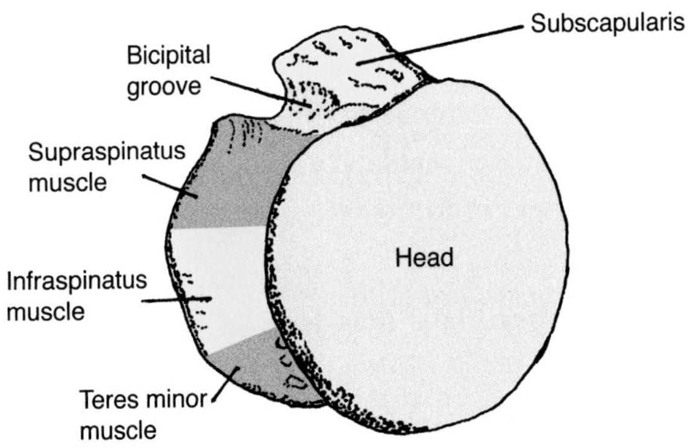

Figure 10-17. This superior view of the proximal end of the left humerus shows the attachments of the rotator cuff muscles.

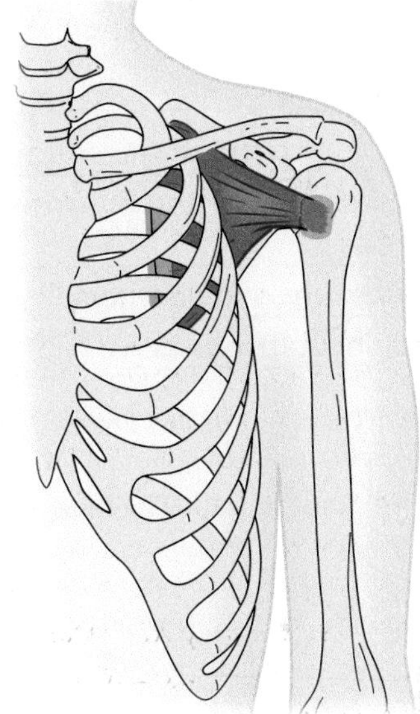

Figure 10-18. Subscapularis muscle (anterior view).

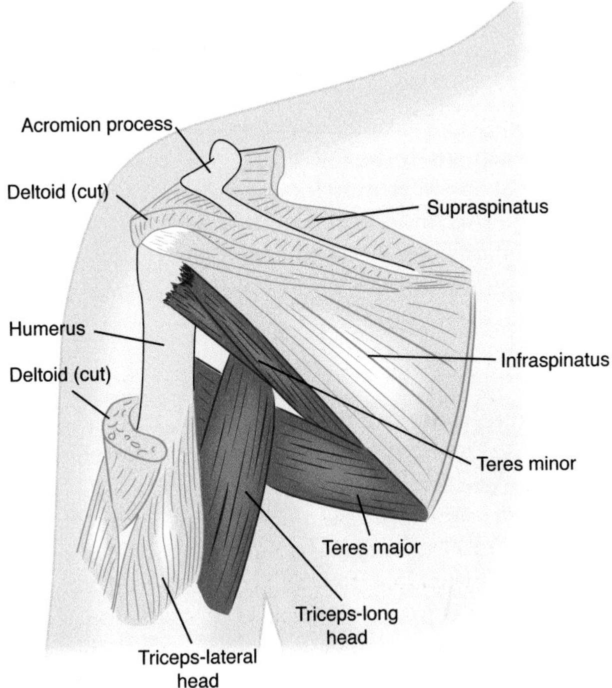

Figure 10-16. The long head of the triceps muscle separates the teres major and teres minor muscles at the axilla (posterior view).

Subscapularis Muscle

O	Subscapular fossa of the scapula
I	Lesser tubercle of the humerus
A	Shoulder medial rotation
N	Upper and lower subscapular nerves (C5, C6)

The **coracobrachialis muscle** (Fig. 10-19) derives its name from its attachments on the coracoid process of the scapula and on the humerus, or arm (in Latin, *brachium*). It has an almost vertical line of pull quite close to the joint axis. Therefore, most of its force is directed back into the joint, stabilizing the head against the glenoid fossa. Some authors refer to this muscle's ability to flex and adduct the shoulder. However, because its vertical line of pull is so close to the joint axes, these actions are assistive at best.

Coracobrachialis Muscle

O	Coracoid process of the scapula
I	Medial surface of the humerus near the midpoint
A	Stabilizes the shoulder joint
N	Musculocutaneous nerve (C5, C6, C7)

The biceps and triceps muscles are two-joint muscles that cross both the shoulder and the elbow. Both muscles have vertical lines of pull. The **biceps** originates by two heads (see Fig.11-15) on the scapula (supraglenoid tubercle and coracoid process), crosses the shoulder and elbow joints anteriorly to insert on the radius (radial tuberosity). The **triceps** has three heads (see Fig. 11-18), but only the long head crosses the shoulder joint. It originates on the scapula (infraglenoid tubercle), crosses both the shoulder and elbow joints posteriorly, and joins the other two heads to insert on the ulna (olecranon process). Because the biceps crosses the shoulder joint anteriorly, it can flex that joint. As the long head of the triceps crosses the shoulder joint posteriorly, it can extend that joint. Their actions at the shoulder joint are assistive at best. Because their major roles are at the elbow joint, where they are both powerful muscles, they will be discussed in more detail in Chapter 11. At the shoulder joint their roles are assistive movers not prime movers.

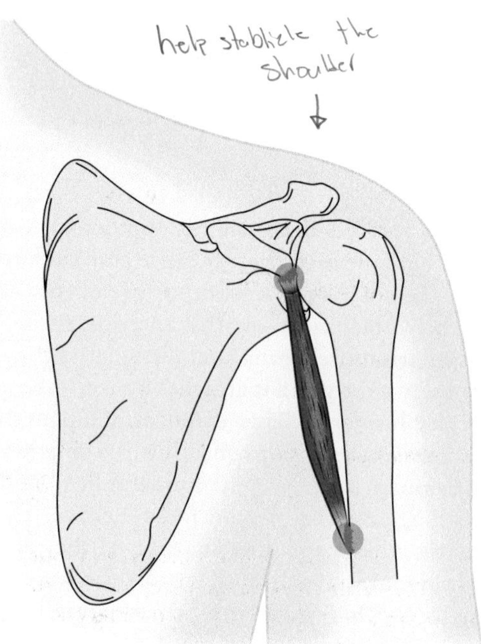

Figure 10-19. Coracobrachialis muscle (anterior view).

Anatomical Relationships

The relationship between the shoulder girdle and shoulder joint muscles is logical. Shoulder girdle muscles originate on the trunk and insert on the scapula, causing either movement or stabilization of the scapula. Shoulder joint muscles tend to originate on the scapula or trunk and insert on the humerus (or forearm in the case of the biceps and triceps), causing movement of the shoulder joint.

The deltoid forms a superficial cap over the anterior, lateral, and posterior sides of the shoulder (see Fig. 10-10). Anteriorly, the pectoralis major covers most of the superficial chest wall, whereas the biceps brachii (Fig. 10-20) and triceps brachii cover most of the anterior and posterior arm, respectively (see Fig. 11-24).

Several shoulder muscles can be seen posteriorly if the trapezius muscle is removed (Fig. 10-21). The supraspinatus lies deep to the trapezius above the

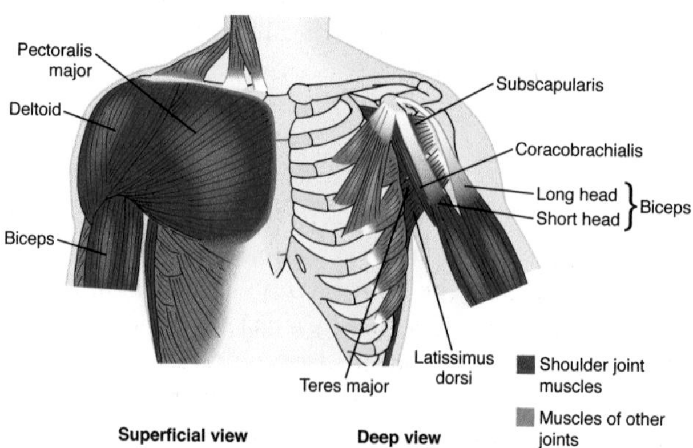

Figure 10-20. Anterior shoulder muscles. Right side shows the superficial layer. Left side has that layer removed.

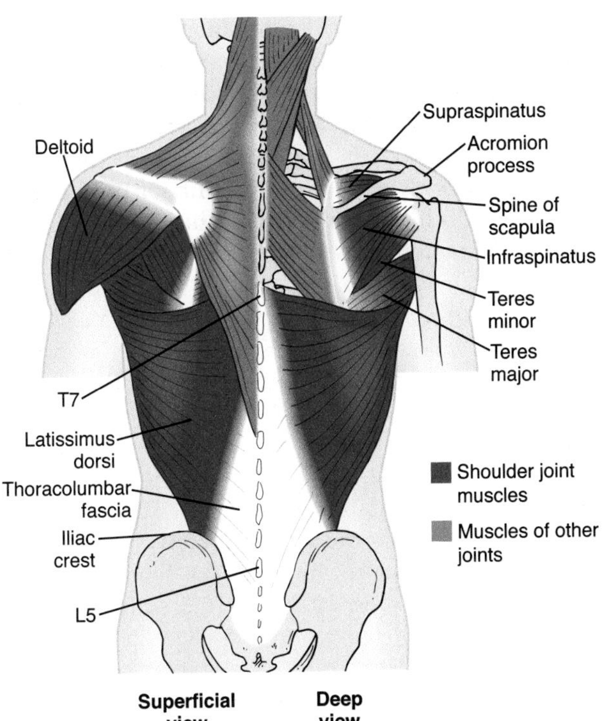

Figure 10-21. Posterior shoulder muscles. Left side shows the superficial layer. Right side has that layer (trapezius) removed.

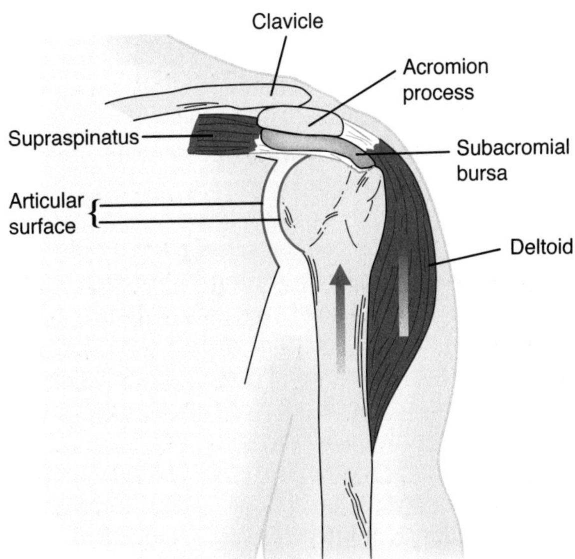

Figure 10-22. The articular surfaces of the glenohumeral joint and the vertical pull of the deltoid muscle (anterior view). If the deltoid muscle acted alone, it would pull the humeral head upward and impinge it under the coracoacromial arch.

scapular spine. In descending order, the infraspinatus, teres minor, and teres major lie below the scapular spine. The latissimus dorsi covers the lumbar and lower thoracic regions of the back.

Viewed anteriorly, the coracobrachialis lies deep to the pectoralis major and anterior deltoid and lies medial to the short head of the biceps (see Fig. 10-20). The subscapularis is truly a deep muscle. With the pectoralis major and deltoid muscles removed (Fig. 10-20, right side) and with the arm slightly abducted, the subscapularis can be seen as it passes between the rib cage and the scapula, and it runs horizontally through the axilla to the proximal end of the anterior humerus.

Glenohumeral Movement

The movement of the humeral head on the glenoid fossa must be given some additional attention. Note that the articular surface of the humeral head is greater than that of the glenoid fossa (Fig. 10-22). If the humeral head simply rotated in the glenoid fossa, it would run out of articular surface before much abduction occurred. Also, the vertical pull of the deltoid muscle would pull the head upward, impinging the supraspinatus and subacromial bursae against the acromion process.

It is the arthrokinematic motions of glide, spin, and roll (see Chapter 4 for a detailed description of these terms) that keep the head of the humerus articulating with the glenoid fossa. As abduction occurs, the humeral head rolls superiorly across the glenoid fossa. At the same time, the head glides inferiorly, keeping the head of the humerus articulating with the glenoid fossa. This is accomplished by the rotator cuff muscles (Fig. 10-23). In addition to abducting the shoulder joint, the supraspinatus muscle pulls the humeral head into the glenoid fossa.

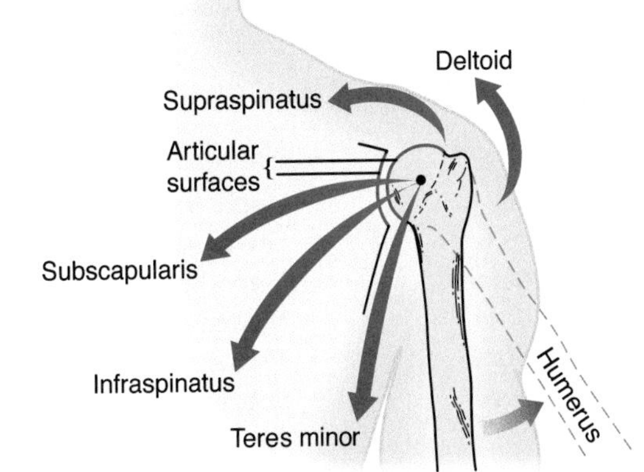

Figure 10-23. Force couple of the deltoid and rotator cuff muscles (SITS). While the deltoid pulls upward on the humerus, the rotator cuff muscles pull the humeral head down and into the glenoid fossa, allowing it to rotate in place during shoulder abduction.

The other rotator cuff muscles (subscapularis, infraspinatus, and teres minor) pull the head in and downward against the glenoid fossa, counteracting the upward pull the deltoids would have otherwise imposed. The glenoid labrum serves to slightly deepen the glenoid fossa, making the joint surfaces more congruent.

Another feature of shoulder abduction is that complete range of motion can be accomplished only if the shoulder joint is also laterally rotated. Try this on yourself. Start with your arm at your side (shoulder adduction) and in medial rotation; abduct your shoulder, keeping your thumb pointed down. This is referred to as the "empty can" position. Notice how much motion you can comfortably achieve.

Next, repeat the motion with your shoulder in a neutral position between medial and lateral rotation and with your thumb pointed forward. Notice how much motion you can comfortably accomplish. Finally, repeat the motion with your shoulder in a laterally rotated position, keeping your thumb pointed up in the hitchhiking position. This is referred to as the "full can" position. It is this laterally rotated position that should allow the most comfortable shoulder motion, because the greater tubercle is being rotated from under the acromion process, allowing full abduction. The greater tubercle in the medially rotated or neutral position runs into the acromion process overhead.

Summary of Muscle Action

Table 10-1 summarizes the prime mover actions of the shoulder joint muscles.

Summary of Muscle Innervation

Muscles of the shoulder joint receive innervation from various branches high on the brachial plexus (see Fig. 6-22). Tables 10-2 and 10-3 summarize the

Table 10-1 Prime Mover Muscles of the Shoulder Joint

Action	Muscles
Flexion, major	Anterior deltoid, pectoralis (clavicular)*
Extension	Posterior deltoid, latissimus dorsi, teres major, pectoralis major (sternal)†
Hyperextension	Latissimus dorsi, posterior deltoid
Abduction	Deltoid, supraspinatus
Adduction	Pectoralis major, teres major, latissimus dorsi
Horizontal, abduction	Posterior deltoid, infraspinatus, teres minor
Horizontal, adduction	Pectoralis major, anterior deltoid
Lateral rotation	Infraspinatus, teres minor, posterior deltoid
Medial rotation	Latissimus dorsi, teres major, subscapularis, pectoralis major, anterior deltoid

*To approximately 60 degrees
†To approximately 120 degrees

Table 10-2 Innervation of the Muscles of the Shoulder Joint

Muscle	Nerve	Plexus Portion	Segment
Subscapularis	Upper and lower subscapular	Posterior cord	C5, C6
Teres major	Lower subscapular	Posterior cord	C5, C6, C7
Pectoralis major	Lateral pectoral	Lateral cord	C5, C6, C7
	Medial pectoral	Medial cord	C8, T1
Latissimus dorsi	Thoracodorsal	Posterior cord	C6, C7, C8
Supraspinatus	Suprascapular	Superior trunk	C5, C6
Infraspinatus	Suprascapular	Superior trunk	C5, C6
Deltoid	Axillary		C5, C6
Teres minor	Axillary		C5, C6
Coracobrachialis	Musculocutaneous		C5, C6, C7
Biceps	Musculocutaneous		C5, C6
Triceps	Radial		C7, C8

Table 10-3 Segmental Innervation of Shoulder Joint

Spinal Cord Level	C4	C5	C6	C7	C8	T1
Supraspinatus		X	X			
Infraspinatus		X	X			
Teres minor		X	X			
Subscapularis		X	X			
Teres major		X	X	X		
Deltoid		X	X			
Biceps		X	X			
Pectoralis major		X	X	X	X	X
Coracobrachialis		X	X	X		
Latissimus dorsi			X	X	X	
Triceps				X	X	

muscle innervation and the segmental innervation of the shoulder joint, respectively. There is some discrepancy among various sources regarding the spinal cord level of innervation.

Common Shoulder Pathologies

A **humeral neck fracture** is another injury caused by a fall on the outstretched hand. It is common in the elderly and usually results in an impacted fracture. **Midhumeral fractures** are often caused by a direct blow or a twisting force. Spiral fractures in this region increase the risk of a **radial nerve injury,** as the nerve passes next to the bone in the spiral groove. **Pathological fractures** of the humerus may be caused by benign tumors or metastatic carcinoma from primary sites such as the lung, breast, kidney, and prostate.

One of the most common joint dislocations involves the shoulder, and most of those are **anterior shoulder dislocations.** A forced shoulder abduction and lateral rotation tends to be the dislocating motion causing the humeral head to slide anteriorly out of the glenoid fossa. **Glenohumeral subluxation** is commonly seen in individuals who have hemiplegia, usually from a cerebrovascular accident (stroke). Paralysis of the shoulder muscles leaves them no longer able to hold the head of the humerus in the glenoid fossa. This paralysis, combined with the pull of gravity and the weight of the arm, over time causes this partial dislocation.

Impingement syndrome is an overuse condition that involves compression between the acromial arch, the humeral head, and soft tissue structures. These soft tissues include the coracoacromial ligament, rotator cuff muscles, long head of the biceps, and subacromial bursa. A type of impingement known as *swimmer's shoulder* is common with swimmers specializing in freestyle, butterfly, and backstroke. **Adhesive capsulitis** refers to the inflammation and fibrosis of the shoulder joint capsule, which leads to pain and loss of shoulder range of motion. It is also known as *frozen shoulder.* A **torn rotator cuff** involves the distal tendinous insertion of the supraspinatus, infraspinatus, teres minor, and subscapularis on the greater/lesser tubercle area of the humerus. Tears can be the result of acute trauma or gradual degeneration. A **labral tear** involves damage to the glenoid labrum. It can have a degenerative or traumatic etiology and results in pain and limited motion in the shoulder joint.

Chronic inflammation of the supraspinatus tendon can lead to an accumulation of mineral deposits and can result in **calcific tendonitis,** which may be asymptomatic or quite painful. **Bicipital tendonitis** usually involves the long head of the biceps proximally as it crosses the humeral head, changes direction, and descends into the bicipital groove. A rupture of the biceps long head tendon commonly occurs during repetitive or forceful overhead positions. Irritation as it slides in the groove can lead to **subluxing of the biceps tendon** (long head). Overloading the muscle in an abducted and laterally rotated position tends to be the force subluxing the tendon out of the bicipital groove.

Clinical Application 10-3

Postural Influence on Latissimus Dorsi

With a slouched posture, the latissimus dorsi can become adaptively shortened. Two things happen at the glenohumeral joint when you slouch: (1) The humerus medially rotates slightly, and (2) the trunk flexes. These positional changes move the origin and insertion of the latissimus dorsi closer together, placing the muscle on slack. Over time this muscle will adaptively shorten, leading to muscle tightness and limited shoulder flexion. Passively moving the shoulder into flexion stretches the latissimus dorsi, which can help restore normal upper body posture. Before the stretch is performed, the thoracolumbar fascia (part of the muscle origin) must be stabilized so it does not move upward during the stretch. This can be achieved by lying supine with the knees flexed and feet flat on the floor.

Points to Remember

- The shoulder is a triaxial ball-and-socket joint.
- Scaption is a specific type of glenohumeral joint elevation that happens in the plane of the scapula (30 degrees anterior to the frontal plane).
- The glenohumeral joint demonstrates convex on concave joint surface motion where the head of the humerus moves in the opposite direction from the distal end of the humerus.
- The rotator cuff and deltoid muscles form a force couple that allows them to pull in different directions to achieve the same motion.
- In addition to their individual motions, the rotator cuff muscles work collectively to stabilize the head of the humerus by holding it against the glenoid fossa.
- Most shoulders dislocate in an anterior direction.

Review Questions

General Anatomy Questions

1. There are four sets of motions that occur at the shoulder joint. Which motions occur
   a. in the frontal plane around the sagittal axis?
   b. in the transverse plane around the vertical axis?
   c. in the sagittal plane around the frontal axis?
2. Describe circumduction and the shoulder joint motions involved.
3. Which fossa is located on the anterior surface of the scapula?
4. The spine of the scapula divides the posterior surface into which two fossae?
5. What landmarks can be used to determine whether a model of an unattached bone is a right or left humerus?
6. What are the SITS muscles, and why are they called *rotator cuff muscles?*
7. Name the shoulder joint muscles attaching on the anterior surface of the scapula.
8. Name the shoulder joint muscles attaching on the posterior surface of the scapula.
9. Which shoulder joint muscles do not attach on the scapula?
10. Regarding the pectoralis major:
    a. Which portion of it is effective in shoulder flexion?
    b. In what part of the range is it more effective?
    c. Why?
11. Name two reasons why the anterior deltoid is a stronger flexor than the coracobrachialis.

Functional Activity Questions — All

Identify the shoulder joint motions and the accompanying shoulder girdle motions in the following actions.

1. Putting your billfold in your left back pocket with your left hand
   a. Shoulder joint motion ________________
   b. Shoulder girdle motion ________________
2. Reaching up to get hold of your seat belt (driver's side with left hand)
   a. Shoulder joint motion ________________
   b. Shoulder girdle motion ________________

Review Questions—cont'd

3. Fastening your seat belt with your left hand
   a. Shoulder joint motion ________________
   b. Shoulder girdle motion ________________
4. Placing a book on the upper bookshelf
   a. Shoulder joint motion ________________
   b. Shoulder girdle motion ________________
5. Tucking and holding a book under your arm
   a. Shoulder joint motion ________________
   b. Shoulder girdle motion ________________
6. Reaching over top of head to touch the lobe of the contralateral ear
   a. Shoulder joint motion ________________
   b. Shoulder girdle motion ________________
7. The backstroke in swimming involves what collective joint motion at the shoulder joint?

Clinical Exercise Questions

1. Lie prone on a table with your arm over the edge and with your shoulder flexed 90 degrees, elbow extended, and a weight in your hand (Fig. 10-24A). Lift the weight away from the table in a sideward motion (Fig. 10-24B).
   a. What is the shoulder joint motion?
   b. What type of contraction (isometric, concentric, eccentric) is occurring?
   c. What muscles are prime movers in this shoulder joint motion?
2. Repeat the exercise in Question 1, except flex the elbow to 90 degrees as you lift the weight up.
   a. Does flexing the elbow shorten the force arm?
   b. Does flexing the elbow shorten the resistance arm?
   c. Why is this exercise easier than the one in Question 1?

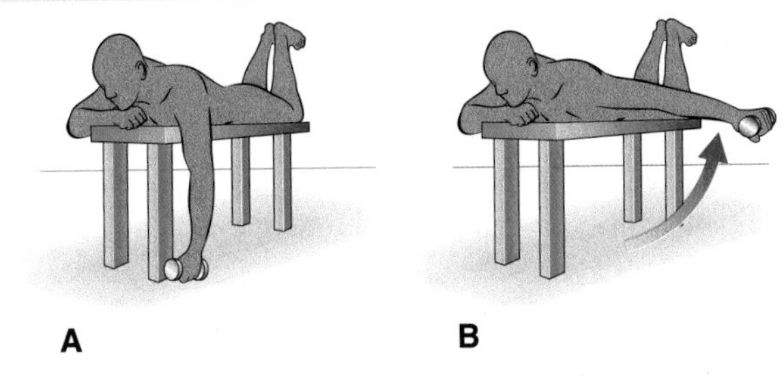

Figure 10-24. **(A)** Starting position. **(B)** Ending position.

3. Lie prone as shown in Figure 10-24, except with the starting position of the arm in anatomical position. Move arm to 90 degrees in the sagittal plane.
   a. What is the joint motion?
   b. What type of contraction is occurring?
   c. Name the prime movers of this motion.
   d. About which axis is this motion occurring?
4. Stand with your arm adducted at the side of your body, elbow flexed to 90 degrees, and hold a loop of elastic tubing whose other end is anchored in front of you at the same level as your hand. In a sawing motion (back and forth motion like you are sawing wood), pull back on the tubing.
   a. What is the shoulder joint motion?
   b. What type of contraction (isometric, concentric, eccentric) is occurring?
   c. What muscles are prime movers in this shoulder joint motion?
5. Return to the starting position of the exercise in Question 3.
   a. What is the shoulder joint motion?
   b. What type of contraction (isometric, concentric, eccentric) is occurring?
   c. What muscles are prime movers in this shoulder joint motion?
6. Stand and hold a cane or weight bar in both hands.
   a. With your hands approximately 12 inches apart and elbows extended, raise the bar. What shoulder motion is occurring?
   b. With your arms as far apart as possible and elbows extended, raise the bar. What predominant shoulder motion is occurring?
   c. In what plane is the motion in part (b) occurring? (Hint: It is not sagittal, frontal, or transverse.)
7. Lie on your right side with your left elbow flexed to 90 degrees and holding a weight in your hand. Keep your left elbow resting on the left side of your body.

   First part: Roll the weight up toward the ceiling.
   a. What is the shoulder joint motion?
   b. What type of contraction (isometric, concentric, eccentric) is occurring?
   c. What muscles are prime movers in this shoulder joint motion?

(continued on next page)

Review Questions—cont'd

Second part: Hold for the count of five.
a. What is the shoulder joint motion?
b. What type of contraction (isometric, concentric, eccentric) is occurring?
c. What muscles are prime movers in this shoulder joint motion?

Third part: Slowly return to the starting position.
a. What is the shoulder joint motion?
b. What type of contraction (isometric, concentric, eccentric) is occurring?
c. What muscles are prime movers in this shoulder joint motion?

8. The ability of this gymnast (Fig. 10-25) to hold the position in this iron cross maneuver may be limited by the strength of which group of shoulder joint muscles?

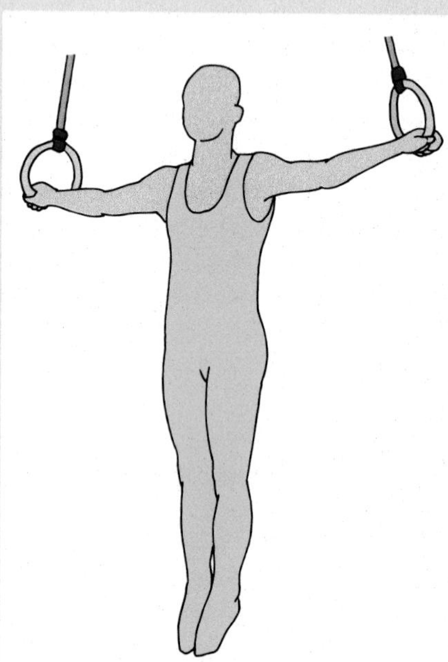

Figure 10-25. Iron cross.

9. As a person performs a sliding board transfer (Fig. 10-26):
   a. Identify the *shoulder joint* muscles that must contract to lift the body up off the supporting surface.
   b. Are these muscles performing a normal contraction or reverse muscle action?
   c. Identify the *shoulder girdle* muscles that must contract to lift the body up off the supporting surface. Are these muscles performing a normal contraction or working through reverse muscle action?

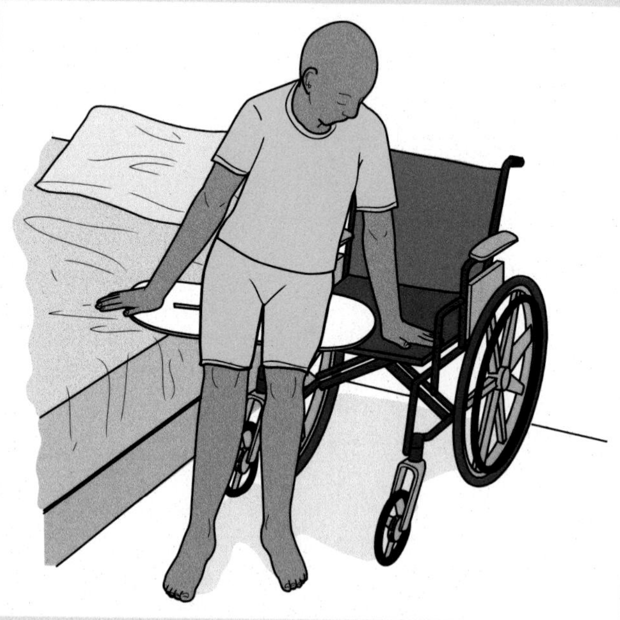

Figure 10-26. Sliding board transfer.

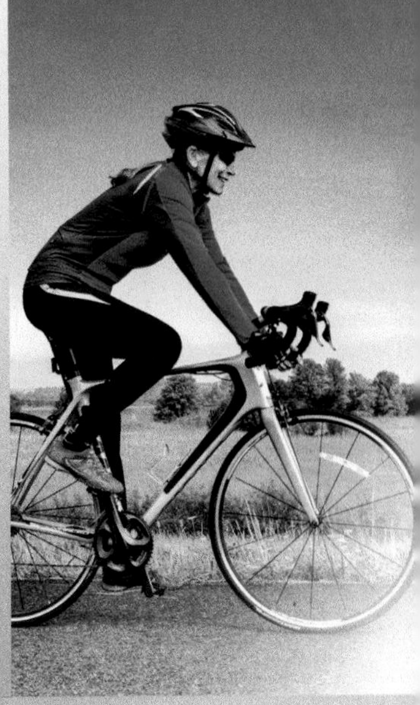

CHAPTER 11
Elbow Joint

Joint Structure and Motions
Carrying Angle
End Feel
Bones and Landmarks
Important Bony Landmarks of the Scapula
Important Bony Landmarks of the Humerus
Important Bony Landmarks of the Ulna
Important Bony Landmarks of the Radius
Ligaments and Other Structures
Muscles of the Elbow and Forearm
Anatomical Relationships
Summary of Muscle Action
Summary of Muscle Innervation
Common Elbow Pathologies
Points to Remember
Review Questions
General Anatomy Questions
Functional Activity Questions
Clinical Exercise Questions

Joint Structure and Motions

The elbow complex includes three bones, three ligaments, two joints, and one capsule. The articulation of the humerus with the ulna and radius is commonly called the **elbow joint** (Fig. 11-1). On the humerus, the trochlea articulates with the trochlear notch of the ulna, and the capitulum articulates with the head of the radius. These articulations are sometimes referred to as the humeroulnar and humeroradial articulations, respectively. However, they move together to produce the same joint motion; therefore, they are collectively called the elbow joint.

The elbow is a uniaxial hinge joint that allows only **flexion** and **extension,** which occurs in the sagittal plane around the frontal axis (Fig. 11-2). Measured from anatomical position (the 0-degree position of extension), the joint has approximately 145 degrees of flexion. Extension is the return to anatomical position from flexion.

Unlike the shoulder joint, the elbow has no active hyperextension. This motion is blocked by the olecranon

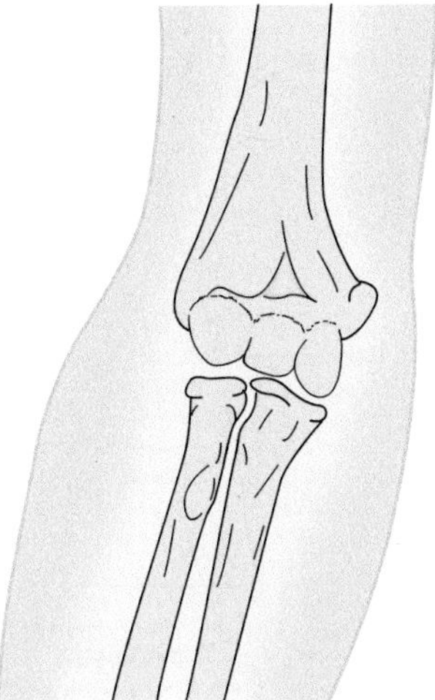

Figure 11-1. Right elbow joint (anterior view).

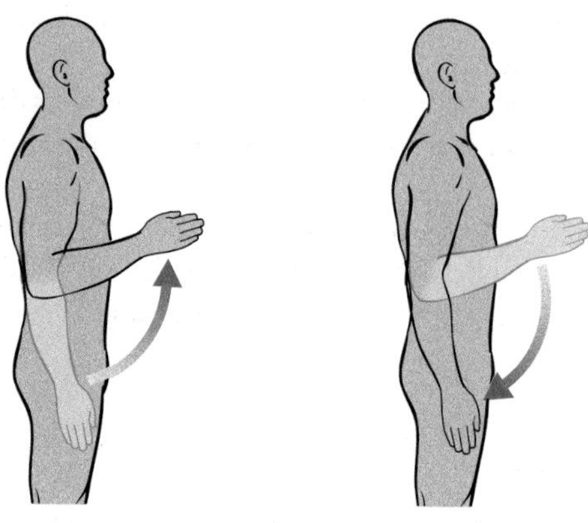

Figure 11-2. Elbow motions.

process of the ulna making bone-on-bone contact as it fits into the olecranon fossa of the humerus. Some individuals may be able to hyperextend a few degrees, but this is due to a laxity of ligaments rather than bony structure.

The second joint of the elbow complex involves articulations between the radius and ulna. This is known as the **radioulnar joint** (Fig. 11-3) and involves each bone articulating with the other at both ends of the forearm. At the proximal end, the head of the radius pivots within the radial notch of the ulna, forming the superior or **proximal radioulnar joint.** Due to the shape of the radius, the distal end of the radius rotates around the distal end of the ulna, forming the inferior or **distal radioulnar joint.** Functionally, they are considered one joint as they move together to produce the same motions.

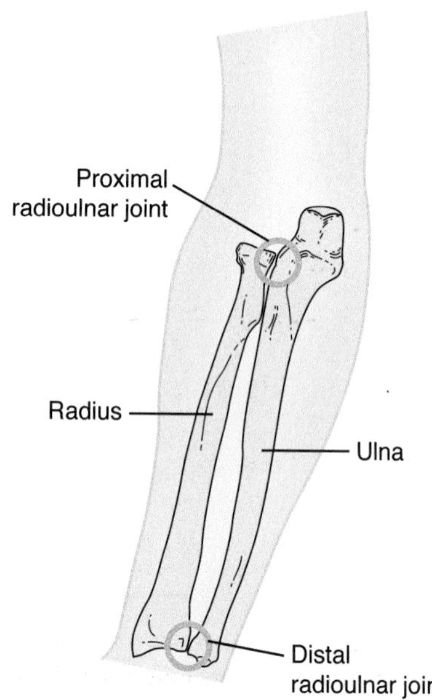

Figure 11-3. Radioulnar joints (anterior view).

The radioulnar joint is a uniaxial pivot joint, allowing only **pronation** and **supination** of the forearm (Fig. 11-4). These motions occur in the transverse plane around the vertical axis. When the upper extremity is in anatomical position, the forearm is supinated. When the palm is turned so that it faces posteriorly, the forearm is pronated. Measured from the neutral or midposition, there are approximately 90 degrees of supination and 80 degrees of pronation.

When pronation and supination occur, the radius moves around the ulna (Fig. 11-5). The ulna does not rotate, as it is locked in place by its bony shape at the proximal end. You can confirm this on your own elbow. With your elbow flexed, place the fingers of your opposite hand on either side of the olecranon process and then pronate and supinate your forearm. Note that the olecranon process does not move. If you put your fingers on the shaft of the ulna, you again will notice that the ulna does not move. Remember this when figuring

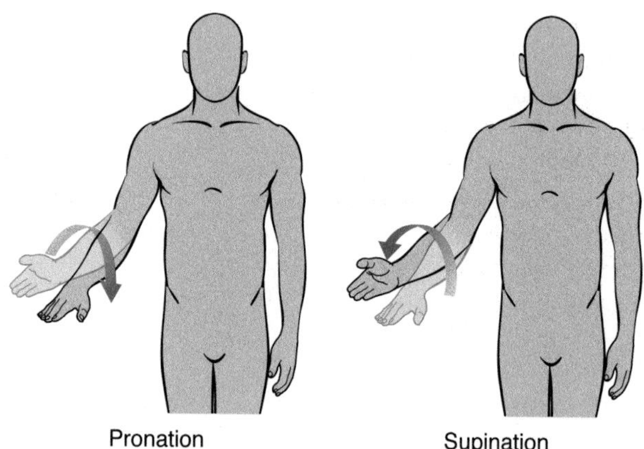

Figure 11-4. Forearm motions.

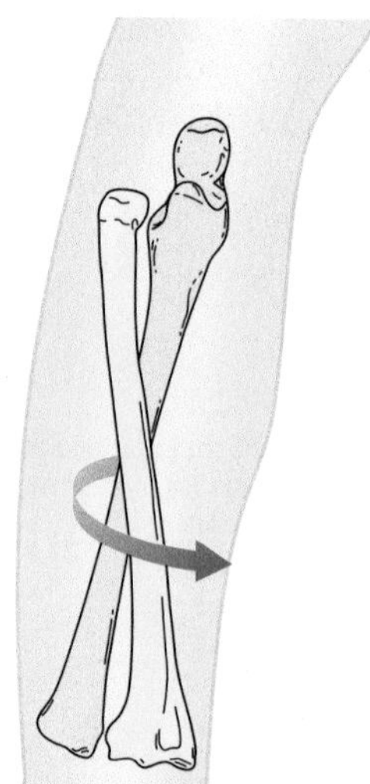
Figure 11-5. Radius moves around the ulna (anterior view).

out muscle action. The radius moves and the ulna does not. Therefore, a muscle must attach on the radius to be able to pronate or supinate the forearm.

The elbow functions to shorten or lengthen the upper extremity and to place the hand in space.

It allows the forearm to move the hand closer or farther from the body.

Carrying Angle

In the anatomical position, the longitudinal axes of the humerus and forearm form an angle called the **carrying angle** (Fig. 11-6). This angle tends to be greater in women than in men. Normal carrying angle measures approximately 5 degrees in males and between 10 and 15 degrees in females. This angle occurs because the distal end of the humerus is not level. The medial side (trochlea) is lower than the lateral side (capitulum). Therefore, as the ulna and radius move around the trochlea and capitulum of the humerus, they do not move in a straight line like a typical hinge joint, in which the long axis of the lower segment is in line with the long axis of the upper segment. The effect of this carrying angle can be seen if a line is drawn along the long axis of the humerus and extended down the forearm. You will notice that during elbow extension, the hand is on the outside of that imaginary line. When the elbow is flexed, the hand moves to the inside of the imaginary line. This angle is quite functional in getting your hand to your mouth.

End Feel

There are two distinctly different end feels at the elbow joint. With flexion, the end feel is **soft** because the muscle bulk of the arm and forearm compresses together and limits further motion.

The end feel for extension is just the opposite. It is described as hard due to bone-on-bone contact as the olecranon process of the ulna moves into the olecranon fossa of the humerus, limiting further motion. This is called a **bony end feel.**

The end feels at the forearm are not quite as distinct. In supination, the end feel is **firm** because of muscle and ligament tension.

Pronation has a bony end feel due to the bony contact between the radius and ulna. This bony end feel is more subtle than that felt during elbow extension.

Arthrokinematics

Joint surface movement is analyzed separately at the elbow and forearm. The distal end of the humerus has two convex areas: the trochlea articulating with the ulna and the capitulum articulating with the radius (see Fig. 11-1). The concave trochlear notch is at the proximal end of the ulna, and the concave radial head is at the proximal end of the radius. With open-chain activities, both of these joint surfaces glide on the humerus in the same direction as the motion of the forearm as dictated by the convex-concave rule. Therefore, the trochlear notch and radial head glide anteriorly during flexion and posteriorly during extension (Fig. 11-7).

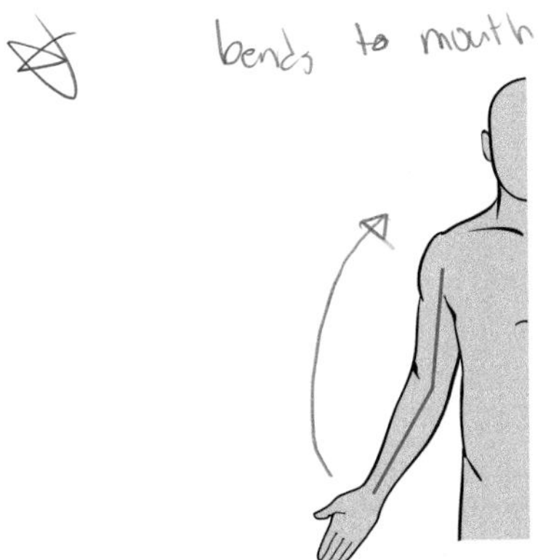

Figure 11-6. Carrying angle (anterior view).

Bones and Landmarks

Some bony landmarks of the **scapula** were covered in Chapters 9 and 10, but those important to elbow function are listed below (Fig. 11-8).

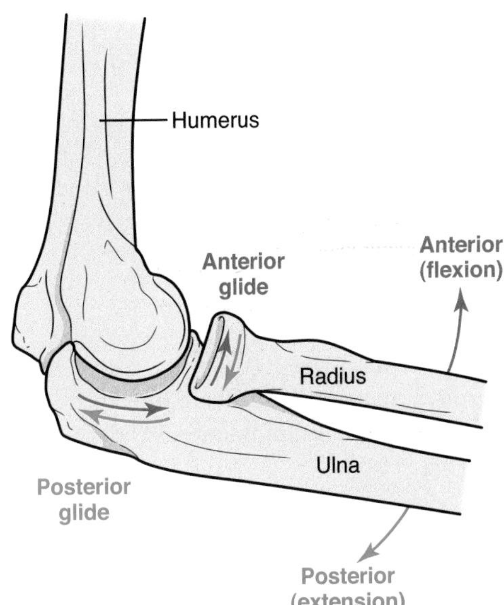

Figure 11-7. Concave articular surfaces of radius and ulna gliding on convex humerus during elbow flexion and extension.

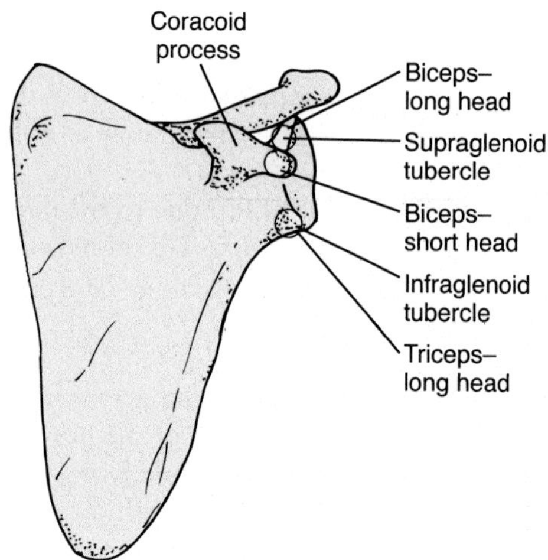

Figure 11-8. Attachments for the biceps and triceps muscles (anterior view).

Important Bony Landmarks of the Scapula

Infraglenoid Tubercle
Raised portion on the inferior lip of the glenoid fossa that provides attachment of the long head of the triceps muscle

Supraglenoid Tubercle
Raised portion on the superior lip of the glenoid fossa that provides attachment for the long head of the biceps muscle

Coracoid Process
Projection on the anterior surface that provides attachment for the short head of the biceps muscle (described in Chapter 9)

The distal end of the **humerus** (Fig. 11-9) provides the bony landmarks important to elbow function.

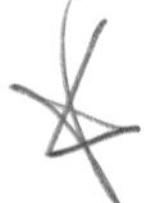

Important Bony Landmarks of the Humerus

Spiral Groove
The groove that the radial nerve runs through as it spirals around the midhumerus (hence its name) (see Fig. 10-5)

Trochlea
Located on the medial side of the distal end; articulates with the ulna

Capitulum
On the lateral side, next to the trochlea; articulates with head of radius

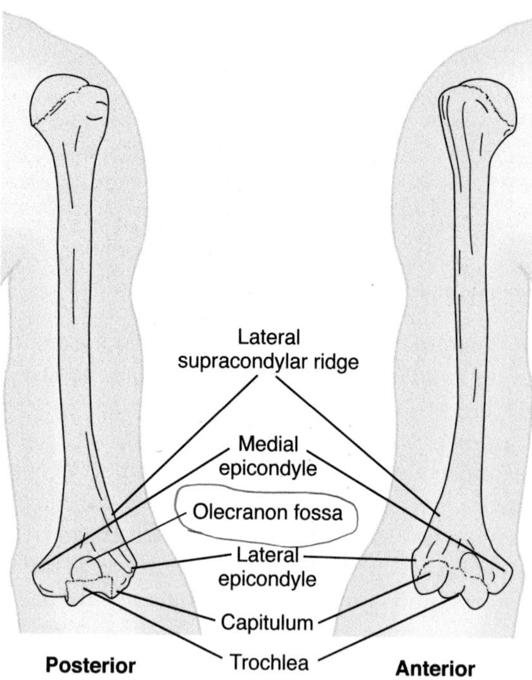

Figure 11-9. Right humerus.

Medial Epicondyle
Located on the medial side of the distal end, above the trochlea; larger and more prominent than the lateral epicondyle. It provides attachment for the pronator teres muscle.

Lateral Epicondyle
Located on the lateral side of the distal end, above the capitulum; provides attachment for the anconeus and supinator muscles

Lateral Supracondylar Ridge
Located above the lateral epicondyle; provides attachment for the brachioradialis muscle

Olecranon Fossa
Located on the posterior surface between the medial and lateral epicondyles; articulates with the olecranon process of the ulna

The **ulna** is the medial bone of the forearm lying parallel to the radius. The bony landmarks important to elbow function are listed below (Fig. 11-10).

Important Bony Landmarks of the Ulna

Olecranon Process
Located at the proximal end of the ulna, on the posterior surface; forms the prominent point of the elbow and provides attachment for the triceps muscle

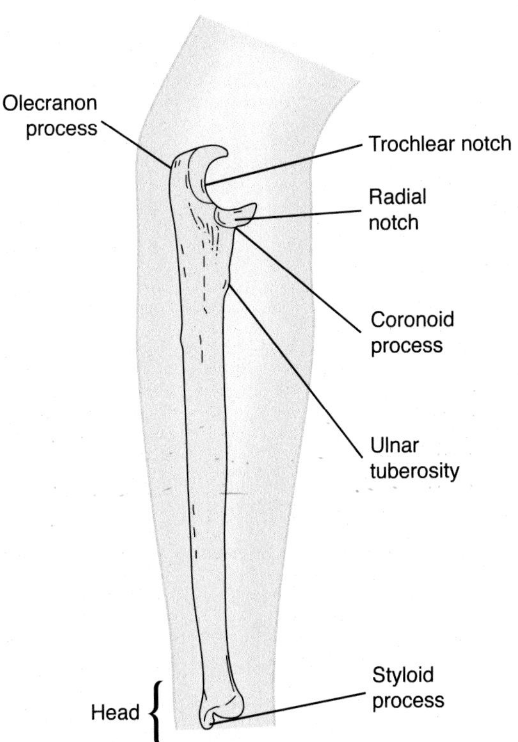

Figure 11-10. Right ulna, lateral view.

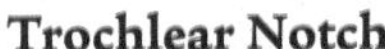

Trochlear Notch
Also called the *semilunar notch;* articulates with the trochlea of the humerus; makes up the anterior surface at the proximal end

Coronoid Process
Located just below the trochlear notch; with the ulnar tuberosity, provides attachment for the brachialis muscle

Radial Notch
Located at the proximal end on the lateral side, just distal to the trochlear notch; articulation point for the head of the radius

Ulnar Tuberosity
Located below the coronoid process; provides attachment for the brachialis muscle

Styloid Process
At the distal end, on the posterior medial surface

Head
At the distal end, on the lateral surface; the ulnar notch of the radius pivots around it during pronation and supination.

The **radius,** located lateral to the ulna, provides many important bony landmarks for elbow function (Fig. 11-11).

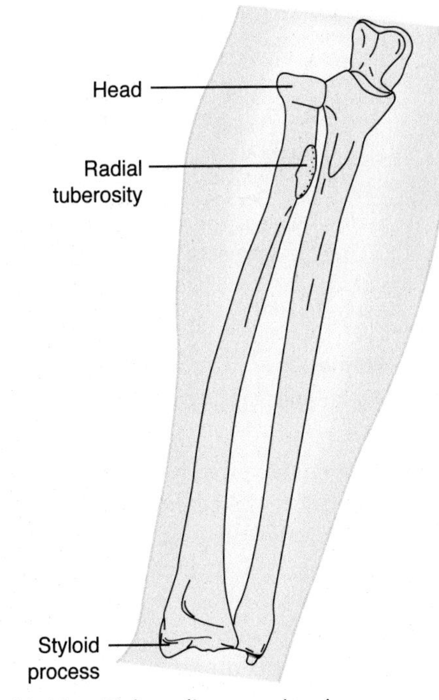

Figure 11-11. Right radius, anterior view.

Important Bony Landmarks of the Radius

Head
Proximal end; has a cylinder shape with a depression in the superior surface where it articulates with the capitulum of the humerus

Radial Tuberosity
Located on the medial side, near the proximal end; provides attachment for the biceps muscle

Styloid Process
Located on the posterior lateral side of the radius, at the distal end; provides attachment for the brachioradialis muscle

Ligaments and Other Structures

The three ligaments of the elbow are the medial and lateral collateral ligaments and the annular ligament (Fig. 11-12). The **medial collateral ligament** is triangular and spans the medial side of the elbow. It attaches on the medial epicondyle of the humerus and runs obliquely to the medial sides of the coronoid process and olecranon process of the ulna. The **lateral collateral ligament** is also triangular. It attaches proximally on the lateral epicondyle of the humerus and distally on the annular ligament and the lateral side of the

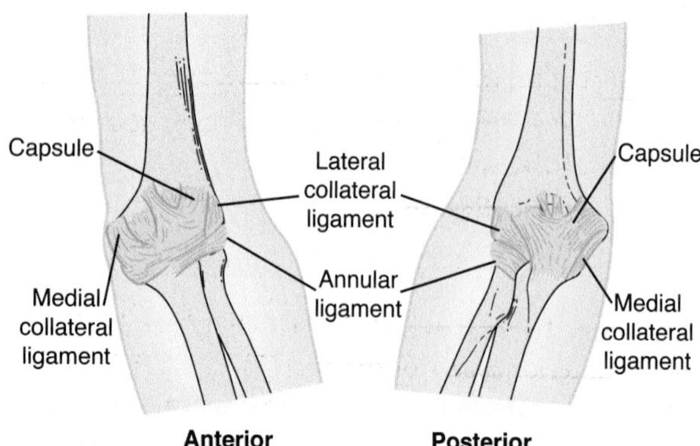

Figure 11-12. Elbow joint capsule and ligaments.

ulna. These two ligaments provide a great deal of medial and lateral stability to the elbow. The **annular ligament** attaches anteriorly and posteriorly to the radial notch of the ulna, encompassing the head of the radius and holding it against the ulna.

The **joint capsule** attaches around the distal end of the humerus and encompasses the trochlea and capitulum and the fossas located above them. It attaches around the proximal end of the ulna, under the radial notch and coronoid process, and around the trochlear notch. It attaches around the radius, just under the head. The capsule is strengthened anteriorly and somewhat posteriorly by the annular ligament. The collateral ligaments reinforce the capsule on the sides of the joint.

During elbow flexion, the joint capsule becomes taut over the posterior aspect of the joint, while it is slack over the anterior aspect of the elbow joint. Conversely, elbow extension causes the anterior aspect of the joint capsule to become taut, while the posterior aspect is placed on a slack.

In addition to the annular ligament, the radioulnar articulations are held together by the **interosseous membrane** (Fig. 11-13). This broad, flat membrane is located between the radius and the ulna for most of their length. The interosseous membrane keeps the two bones from separating and provides more surface area for attachment of the forearm and wrist muscles.

The cubital fossa is a shallow, somewhat triangular depression on the anterior elbow. It is bordered laterally by the brachioradialis, medially by the pronator teres, and superiorly by an imaginary line between the medial and lateral epicondyles. This line corresponds closely to the skin crease in the bend of the elbow. The floor is formed by the brachialis and supinator muscles. From lateral to medial, the main vertical structures within the fossa are the biceps tendon, the brachial artery, and the median nerve. The radial nerve lies between the biceps tendon and the brachioradialis muscles but is not usually considered to be within the fossa. The brachial artery divides into the radial (superficial) and ulnar (deeper) arteries near the inferior apex of the fossa. Superficial to the fossa, and not considered part of it, are the three superficial veins: median cubital, cephalic, and basilic veins. The brachial pulse can be palpated in the cubital fossa, and during blood pressure measurements, the stethoscope is placed over the brachial artery in this location.

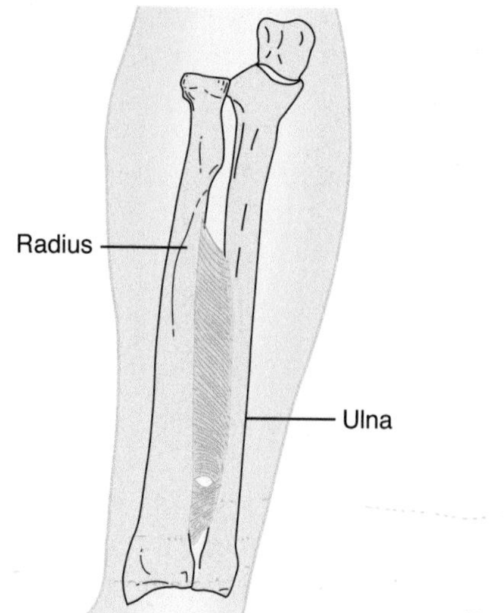

Figure 11-13. Interosseous membrane (anterior view).

Muscles of the Elbow and Forearm

The line of pull of a muscle will play a major role in determining the action of a muscle. Muscles of the elbow and forearm originate on the humerus, and sometimes the scapula, and insert on the radius or ulna. Some generalizations can be made about muscle line of pull affecting muscle action when muscles contract:

- Muscles crossing the anterior aspect of the elbow joint bring the anterior surfaces of the arm and forearm closer together, producing flexion.
- Muscles crossing the posterior aspect of the elbow joint bring the posterior surfaces of the arm and forearm closer together, producing extension.
- Muscles that originate medially, crossing the anterior aspect of the joint to insert on the radius, will pull the forearm into pronation.
- Muscles that originate posteriorly, crossing the lateral side of the forearm to insert on the radius, will pull the forearm into supination.

The muscles of the elbow and forearm are as follows:

Brachialis
Brachioradialis
Biceps
Supinator
Triceps
Anconeus
Pronator teres
Pronator quadratus

The **brachialis muscle** (Fig. 11-14) gets its name from its location (Latin for "arm"). It attaches to the distal half of the humerus on the anterior surface and spans the elbow joint anteriorly to attach on the coronoid process and ulnar tuberosity of the ulna. It lies deep to the biceps muscle. Because the brachialis muscle has no attachment on the radius, it has no role in pronation or supination. However, this muscle is a very strong elbow flexor, regardless of the forearm's position, and is sometimes called the "workhorse of the elbow joint."

Brachialis Muscle

O	Distal half of humerus, anterior surface
I	Coronoid process and ulnar tuberosity of the ulna
A	Elbow flexion
N	Musculocutaneous nerve (C5, C6)

The **biceps brachii muscle** has two heads and is located on the anterior aspect of the arm (Fig. 11-15). This muscle is commonly referred to simply as the *biceps.* Both heads attach on the scapula. The **long head** arises from the supraglenoid tubercle, runs over the head of the humerus and out the joint capsule to descend through the intertubercular (bicipital) groove, and joins with the **short head** that comes from the coracoid process. Because tendons of both heads cross the shoulder joint anteriorly, the biceps assists in shoulder flexion. However, its main function is at the elbow. After joining, the two heads form a common muscle belly that covers the anterior surface of the arm. The biceps muscle tendon crosses the elbow joint to attach on the radial tuberosity. It is the superficial muscle of the anterior arm. Because the biceps muscle spans the elbow joint anteriorly and has a vertical

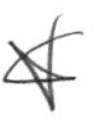

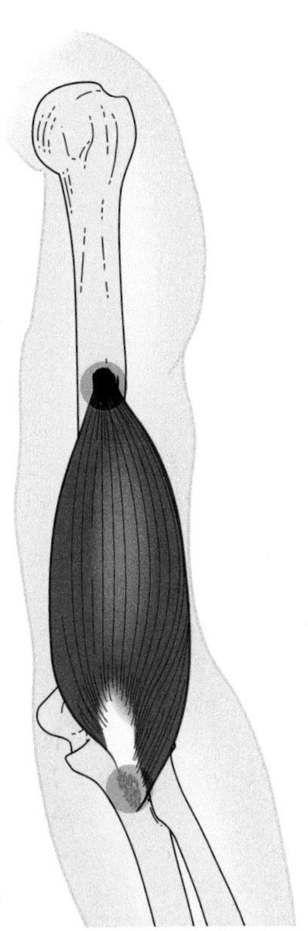

Figure 11-14. Brachialis muscle (anterior view).

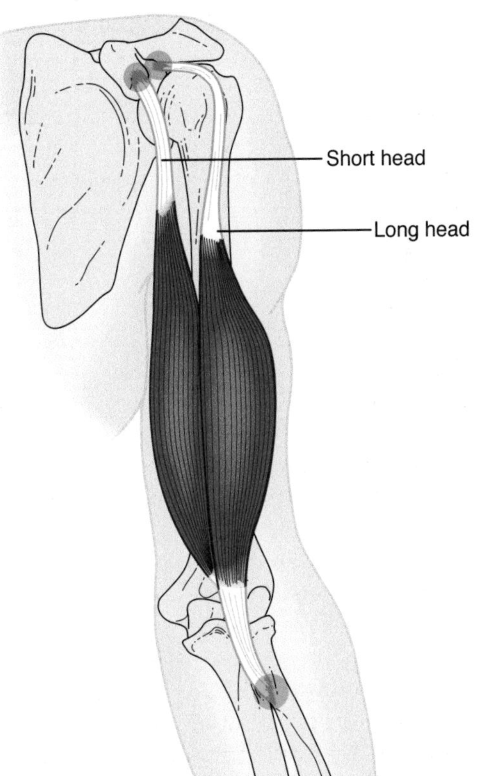

Figure 11-15. Biceps brachii muscle, commonly referred to as the *biceps,* has two heads (anterior view).

line of pull, it is a strong elbow flexor, especially in the midrange. Because it attaches obliquely on the radius, it contributes to supination of the forearm.

To understand the supination component of the biceps muscle, think of it as a corkscrew. The tendon crosses the elbow joint anteriorly to attach medially on the radial tuberosity. When the forearm is in pronation, the radial tuberosity rotates farther medially toward the posterior side. In effect, the tendon of the biceps muscle wraps partially around the radius in the pronated position. During supination, the biceps muscle contracts and essentially "unwraps" or "untwists" the forearm (Fig. 11-16). It is most effective in supination when the elbow is in approximately 90 degrees of flexion, and it loses its effectiveness as the elbow is extended. This is because the muscle's moment arm is greatest at 90 degrees; therefore, its angular force is also greatest. As the elbow is extended, the moment arm decreases, as does angular force, while the stabilizing force increases. (See Figs. 8-10 and 8-11 and Chapter 8 for a discussion on torque.)

Biceps Muscle

O	Long head: Supraglenoid tubercle of scapula Short head: Coracoid process of scapula
I	Radial tuberosity of radius
A	Elbow flexion, forearm supination
N	Musculocutaneous nerve (C5, C6)

The **brachioradialis muscle** gets its name from its two attachments: one on the humerus (brachii) and the other on the radius (Fig. 11-17). Proximally, it is attached on the supracondylar ridge, which is slightly above the lateral epicondyle of the humerus. The brachioradialis crosses the elbow anteriorly and laterally to attach distally near the styloid process of the radius. It is a superficial muscle and is easy to identify. Place your hand in your lap in a neutral position between supination and pronation and then give resistance to elbow flexion. The brachioradialis muscle should be quite prominent on the top of your forearm near the elbow. Because of its vertical line of pull over the anterior elbow, it is an effective elbow flexor. Regardless of the starting position, contracting this muscle will also pull the forearm into a neutral position. In other words, it assists in returning the forearm to the mid-position from the extremes of either pronation or supination. With the elbow joint at 90 degrees and the forearm supinated, have someone give resistance at the distal forearm as you pronate. You will see the brachioradialis muscle contract from the fully supinated position until the forearm reaches neutral, but not beyond the midrange into pronation. Repeat the same activity with the forearm pronated and moving into supination. You will see the brachioradialis contracting from the starting position of pronation until the forearm reaches neutral, but not beyond into supination. This demonstrates that the brachioradialis has

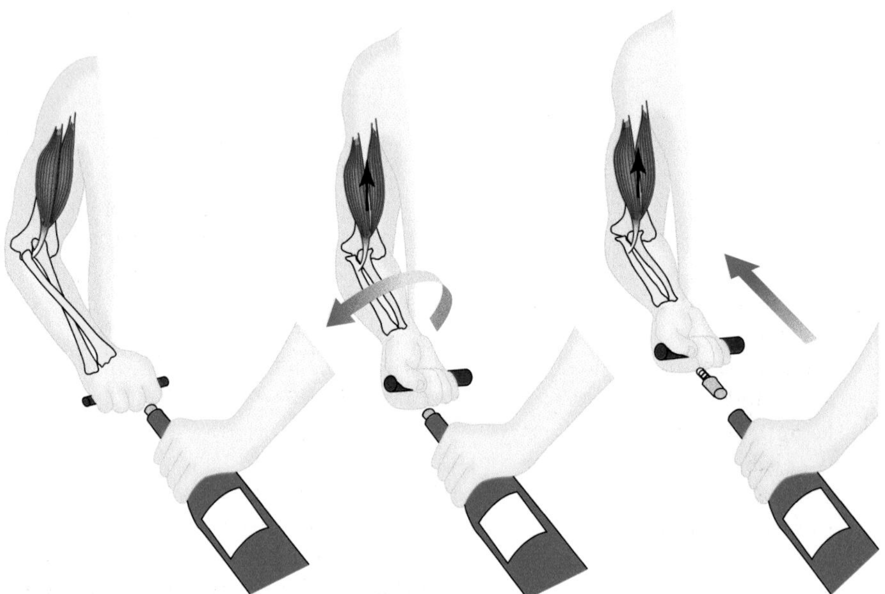

Figure 11-16. Supination action of biceps (anterior view). The action of the biceps as a forearm supinator and elbow flexor is used when pulling a cork out of a bottle with a corkscrew. First, it unscrews the cork (supination); then it pulls on the cork (flexion).

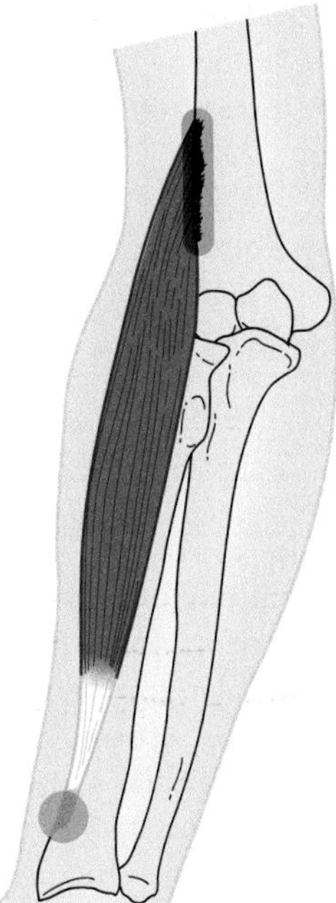

Figure 11-17. Brachioradialis muscle (anterior view).

an assistive role in pronation and supination only through part of the joint range.

Brachioradialis Muscle

O	Lateral supracondylar ridge on the humerus
I	Styloid process of the radius
A	Elbow flexion
N	Radial nerve (C5, C6)

The **triceps brachii muscle,** commonly called the **triceps,** derives its name from its three heads. This muscle is located posteriorly and makes up the entire muscle mass of the posterior arm (Fig. 11-18). The **long head** comes from the inferior rim of the glenoid fossa of the scapula (infraglenoid tubercle) and descends between the teres minor and teres major muscles to join the other two heads. The **lateral head** originates laterally on the posterior surface of the humerus below the greater tubercle, yet above the spiral groove. The **medial head** lies deep to the long and lateral heads and originates on most of the posterior surface below the spiral groove. The three heads come together to form the muscle belly. The triceps tendon distal to the muscle belly crosses the elbow posteriorly to attach to the olecranon process of the ulna. It spans the elbow quite vertically and is very effective in elbow extension. Because it has no attachment on the radius, it can play no role in pronation or supination.

Clinical Application 11-1

Elbow Flexion Strength Testing

The forearm is placed in different positions when testing strength generated by the various elbow flexors. Due to their insertions on the radius, the biceps and brachioradialis can move both the elbow and the forearm and must be allowed to perform actions at both joints simultaneously. Before testing elbow flexion, the forearm is positioned according to the supination/pronation action of that muscle. When testing biceps strength, the forearm is placed in supination, and when testing brachioradialis strength, the forearm is placed in a neutral position (midposition). These positions allow the muscles to direct their strength toward elbow flexion rather than rotating the forearm while also allowing the radial insertion points to "face" their respective origins, giving the muscles a straight line of pull for elbow flexion. Testing brachialis strength is performed with the forearm in the pronated position, not because it favors this position, but because the pronated position of the forearm puts the other two flexors (biceps and brachioradialis) at a disadvantage, thus isolating the effect of the brachialis to the greatest extent possible.

Triceps Muscle

O	Long head: Infraglenoid tubercle of scapula Lateral head: Inferior to greater tubercle on posterior humerus Medial head: Posterior surface of humerus
I	Olecranon process of ulna
A	Elbow extension
N	Radial nerve (C6, C7, C8)

The **anconeus muscle** is a very small muscle that attaches next to the much larger triceps muscle (Fig. 11-19). It attaches proximally to the posterior surface of the lateral epicondyle and then spans the elbow posteriorly to attach laterally and inferior to the olecranon process. The anconeus is a small muscle in comparison with the triceps and therefore does not

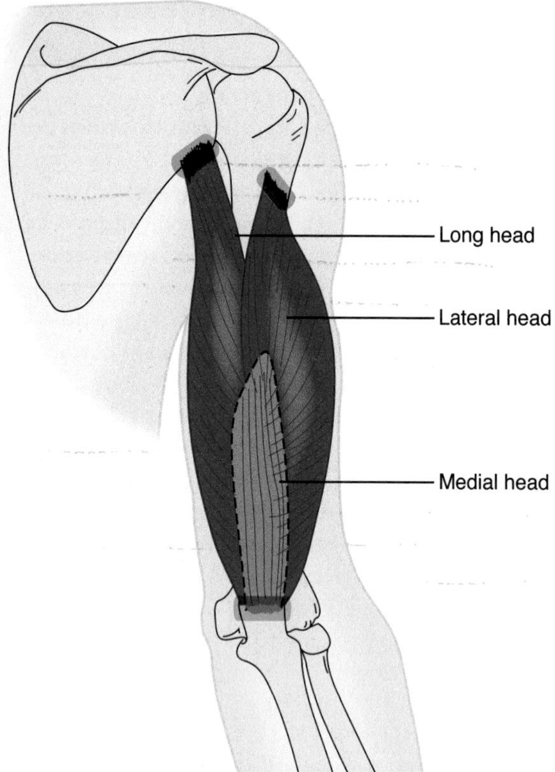

Figure 11-18. The triceps brachii muscle, commonly referred to as the *triceps,* has three heads (posterior view). The dotted line indicates the portion of the muscle that lies deep.

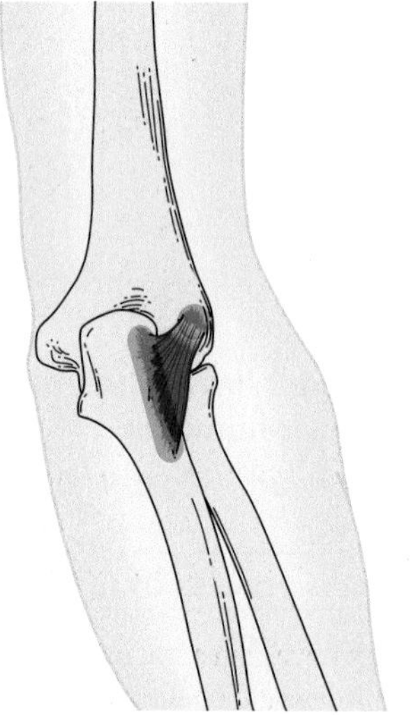

Figure 11-19. Anconeus muscle (posterior view).

play a significant role in elbow extension. This muscle lies on top of the annular ligament and attaches to part of it. The annular ligament has some fibers attaching to the joint capsule. Therefore, when the anconeus contracts, it pulls on the annular ligament and indirectly on the joint capsule. This action keeps the joint capsule from being pinched in the olecranon fossa during elbow extension.

Anconeus Muscle

O	Lateral epicondyle of humerus
I	Lateral and inferior to olecranon process of ulna
A	Not a prime mover in any joint action; assists in elbow extension
N	Radial nerve (C6, C7, C8)

The **pronator teres muscle** (Fig. 11-20) gets its name partially from its action (pronation) and partially from its shape (*teres,* Latin for "long and round"). It is a superficial muscle as it crosses the elbow, but it is covered by the brachioradialis muscle at its distal attachment. Proximally, it attaches on the medial epicondyle of the humerus and the medial aspect of the coronoid process of the ulna. It crosses the anterior surface of the elbow, running diagonally to attach distally on the lateral surface of the radius at about the midpoint. Because it crosses the elbow anteriorly, it has the ability to flex the elbow. This muscle's role in elbow flexion is only assistive because of its smaller size compared with the other flexors and its diagonal (not vertical) line of pull. It is effective as a pronator because it pulls the radial insertion medially across the ulna.

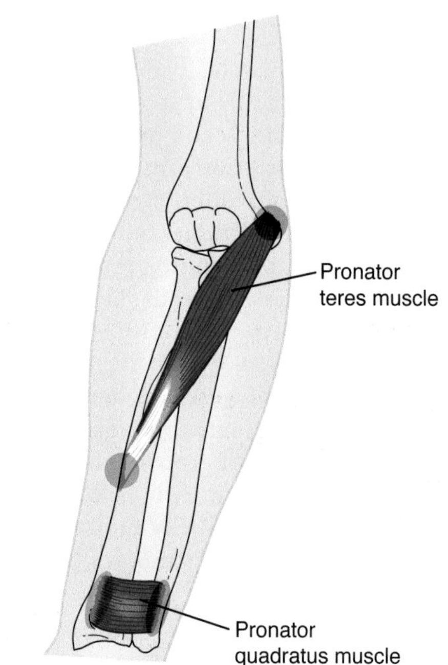

Figure 11-20. Pronator muscles (anterior view).

Clinical Application 11-2

Mechanics of Pushing and Pulling

Shoulder flexors and extensors work synergistically with the biceps and triceps to exert great force at the elbow during pushing and pulling activities. The shoulder muscles (see Table 10-1) are one-joint muscles acting only on the shoulder. The biceps and triceps, being two-joint muscles, can exert force at both joints. They are assistive at the shoulder and very strong at the elbow. As with all multijoint muscles, they simultaneously *lengthen* over one joint (shoulder) while *shortening* over the other (elbow) to maintain an optimal length-tension relationship and exert a constant contractile force throughout the activity. So, while the shoulder muscles are strongest at moving the shoulder joint, the biceps and triceps are strongest at moving the elbow. The figure below shows each person's starting position for the activity. The person on the left is preparing to push. The shoulder flexors and elbow extensors are lengthened, preparing to contract (shorten). The person on the right is in the opposite position, preparing to pull. As each person moves through the motion, the shoulder muscles are performing their respective action while the biceps and triceps are able to exert a strong elbow contraction (shortening) by simultaneously being lengthened over the shoulder. In summary, the biceps and triceps are able to exert a strong force at the elbow because the shoulder muscles are exerting a strong force at the shoulder. The respective motion at the shoulders lengthens the biceps and triceps.

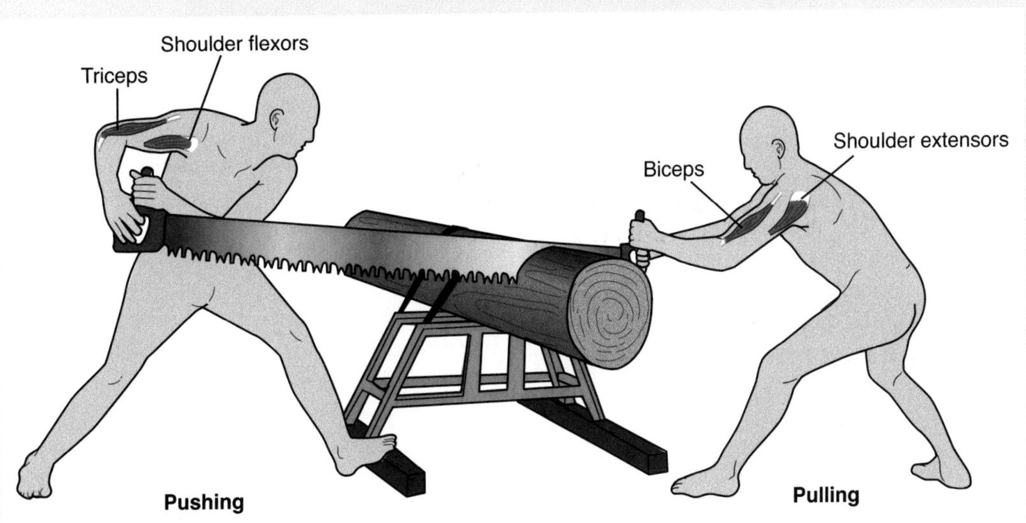

Starting position for push-pull activity.

Pronator Teres Muscle

O	Medial epicondyle of humerus and coronoid process of ulna
I	Lateral aspect of radius at its midpoint
A	Forearm pronation, assistive in elbow flexion
N	Median nerve (C6, C7)

The **pronator quadratus muscle** (see Fig. 11-20) also gets its name from its action (pronation) and partially from its shape (quadratus). It is a small, flat, quadrilateral muscle located deep on the anterior surface of the distal forearm; therefore, it cannot be palpated. It attaches from the distal one-fourth of the ulna to the distal one-fourth of the radius. It has a horizontal line of pull from the distal ulna to the distal radius. Because the radius rotates around the ulna, this line of pull makes the pronator quadratus an effective forearm pronator. It pulls on the radius distally while the pronator teres pulls on the radius more proximally, and together they pronate the forearm.

Pronator Quadratus Muscle

O	Distal one-fourth of ulna
I	Distal one-fourth of radius
A	Forearm pronation
N	Median nerve (C8, T1)

The **supinator muscle** (Fig. 11-21) is a deep muscle that wraps around the elbow joint laterally from the posterior surface to the anterior surface. It originates posteriorly on the lateral epicondyle and adjacent surface of the ulna. It crosses the elbow joint laterally to wrap around the proximal end of the radius and inserts on the proximal anterior surface of the radius. When the forearm is pronated, the insertion of the supinator is facing medially (away from the origin). Contraction of the supinator pulls the radius laterally, bringing the radial insertion point back to an anterior orientation (supination). It combines with the biceps muscle as a prime mover in forearm supination (Fig. 11-22).

Supinator Muscle

O	Lateral epicondyle of humerus and adjacent ulna
I	Anterior surface of the proximal radius
A	Forearm supination
N	Radial nerve (C6)

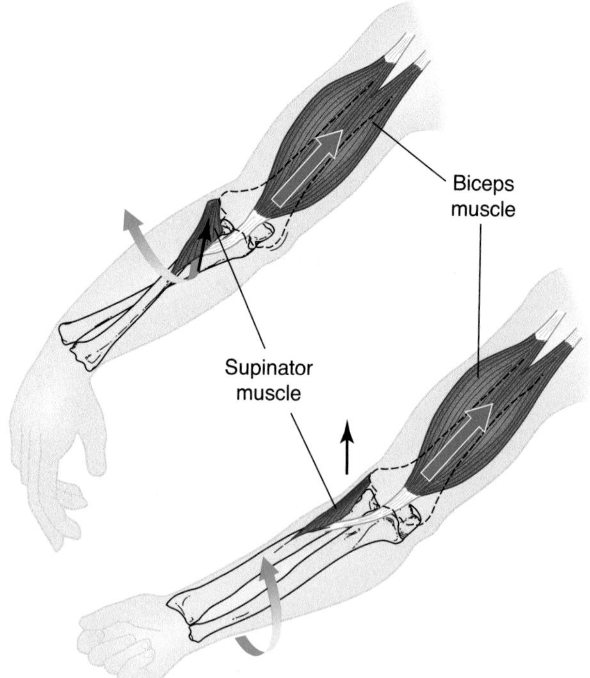

Figure 11-22. The supinator and biceps muscles combine in a force couple action to move the radius around the ulna from a pronated forearm to a supinated forearm (anterior view).

Anatomical Relationships

The muscle bellies of the biceps, brachialis, and triceps are proximal to the joint, whereas the muscle bellies of the brachioradialis, pronator teres, pronator quadratus, and supinator are at or distal to the elbow. Figure 11-23 shows the anterior muscles. You can feel the biceps if you put your hand on the anterior surface of your arm. Lying directly underneath the biceps is the brachialis. The dotted lines in Figure 11-23 indicate that the brachialis lies beneath the biceps, except at the distal humerus, where it can be palpated on either side of the biceps tendon. The brachioradialis is the most superficial muscle on the lateral side of the forearm. The pronator teres is also superficial, but it has its proximal attachment on the medial side, along with the wrist flexors and palmaris longus. The pronator quadratus is located deep to several wrist and hand tendons at the distal end of the anterior forearm.

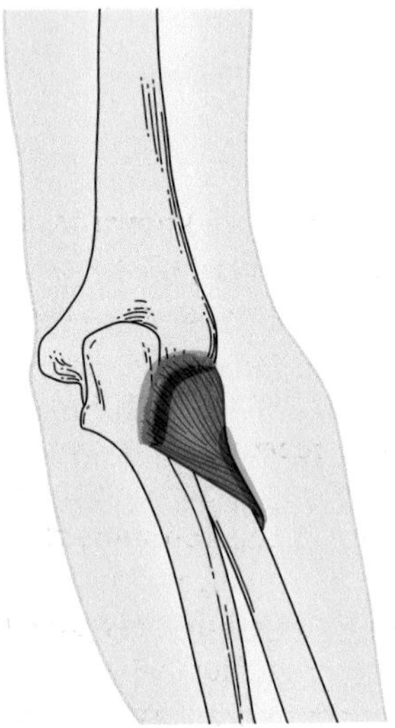

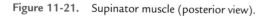

Figure 11-21. Supinator muscle (posterior view).

Figure 11-24 shows the posterior muscles. The triceps makes up the entire posterior arm. The long and lateral heads are superficial, and the medial head is deep. The medial head is almost the same shape as the triceps distal tendon and lies deep to it (as indicated by the dotted lines in Fig. 11-24). The anconeus is a very small muscle located superficially on the posterior elbow, just distal to the triceps insertion. The supinator lies deep to the wrist extensors and the brachioradialis near their origins (Fig. 11-25).

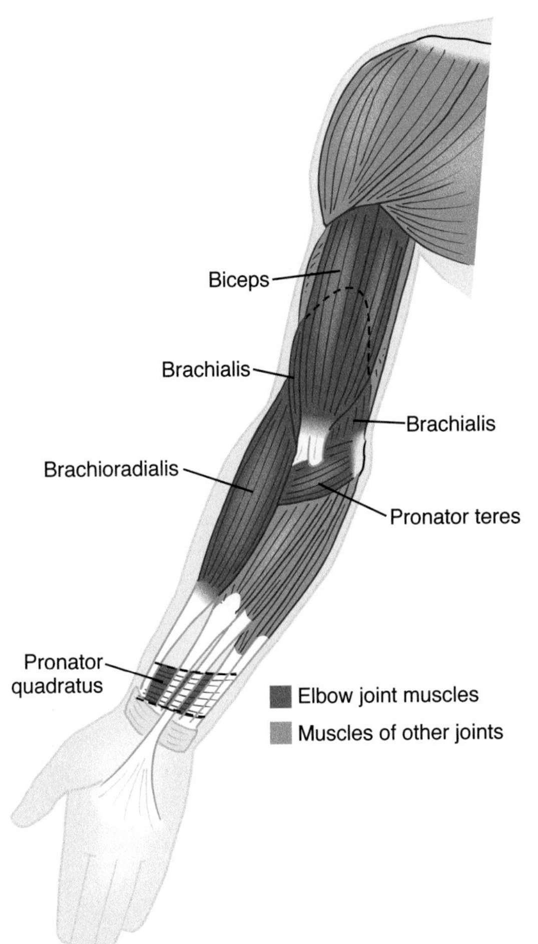

Figure 11-23. Anterior elbow muscles. Note that dotted lines indicate the brachialis muscle lying underneath the biceps.

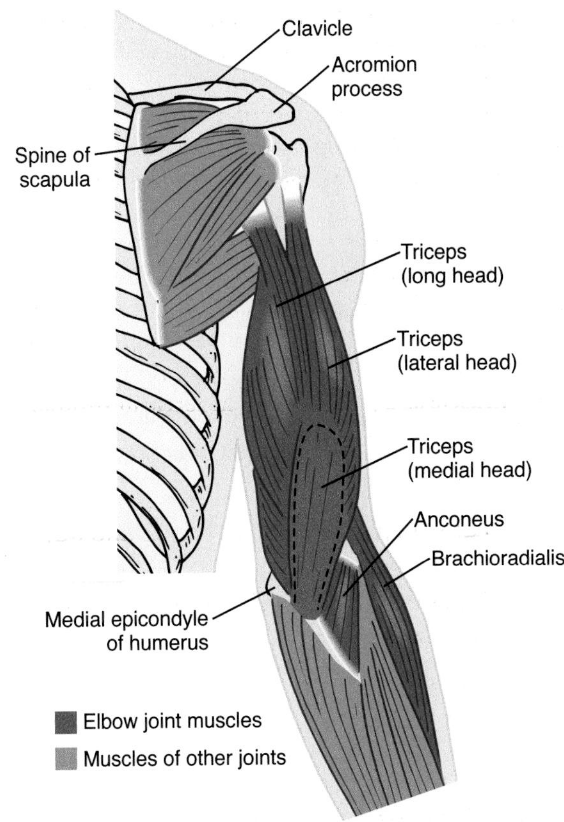

Figure 11-24. Posterior elbow muscles. Note the dotted lines indicating the portion of the muscle that lies deep.

Summary of Muscle Action

Table 11-1 summarizes the muscle actions of the prime movers of the elbow and forearm.

Summary of Muscle Innervation

Terminal nerves of the brachial plexus innervate all muscles of the elbow. The musculocutaneous nerve innervates muscles of the anterior arm involved with elbow flexion. The radial nerve travels through the axilla and around the middle portion of the humerus to innervate the posterior surface of the arm, forearm, and hand. It is responsible for all elbow extension. The median nerve descends the arm anteriorly, sending branches to the pronator muscles. Table 11-2 summarizes the innervation of elbow joint musculature. Table 11-3 summarizes the segmental innervation. Please note that there is some discrepancy among various sources regarding the spinal cord level of innervation.

Common Elbow Pathologies

Lateral epicondylitis, also known as **tennis elbow,** is a very common overuse condition that affects the common extensor tendon where it inserts into the lateral epicondyle of the humerus. The extensor carpi radialis brevis is particularly affected. It is common in racquet sports and other repetitive wrist extension activities. **Medial epicondylitis,** also known as **golfer's elbow,** is an inflammation of the common flexor tendon that inserts into the medial epicondyle. It is an overuse condition that results in tenderness over the medial epicondyle and pain on resisted wrist flexion.

Little League elbow is an overuse injury of the medial epicondyle, usually caused by a repetitive throwing

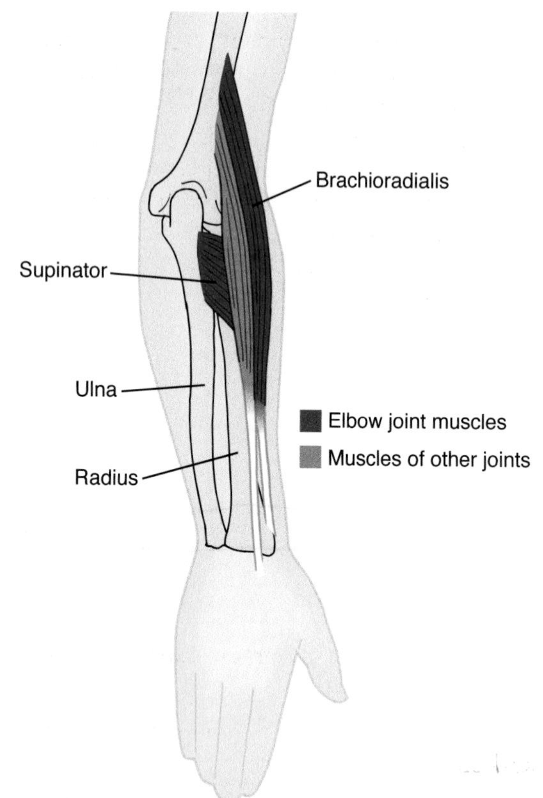

Figure 11-25. Supinator, a deep muscle, in relation to surrounding muscles. Note that most of the extensor muscles of the wrist and hand that lie over the supinator have not been included.

Table 11-1 Prime Movers of the Elbow and Forearm

Action	Muscle
Elbow flexion	Biceps
	Brachialis
	Brachioradialis
Elbow extension	Triceps
Forearm pronation	Pronator teres
	Pronator quadratus
Forearm supination	Biceps
	Supinator

motion. It is seen in young baseball players who have not reached skeletal maturity. The throwing motion places a valgus stress on the elbow, causing lateral compression and medial distraction on the joint. **Pulled elbow,** or **nursemaid's elbow,** is seen in young children under the age of 5 years who have experienced a sudden strong traction force on the arm. This often occurs when an adult suddenly pulls on the child's arm, or the child falls

Table 11-2 Innervation of the Muscles of the Elbow Joint

Muscle	Nerve	Spinal Segment
Brachialis	Musculocutaneous	C5, C6
Biceps	Musculocutaneous	C5, C6
Brachioradialis	Radial	C5, C6
Triceps	Radial	C6, C7, C8
Anconeus	Radial	C6, C7, C8
Pronator teres	Median	C6, C7
Pronator quadratus	Median	C8, T1
Supinator	Radial	C6

Table 11-3 Segmental Innervation of the Elbow Joint

Spinal Cord Level	C5	C6	C7	C8	T1
Biceps	X	X			
Brachialis	X	X			
Brachioradialis	X	X			
Supinator		X			
Pronator teres		X	X		
Triceps		X	X	X	
Anconeus		X	X	X	
Pronator quadratus				X	X

away from an adult while being held by the arm. This force causes the radial head to sublux out from under the annular ligament.

Elbow dislocation is caused when a great deal of force is applied to an elbow that is in a slightly flexed position. This causes the ulna to slide posterior to the distal end of the humerus. **Supracondylar fractures** are among the most common fractures in children and are caused by falling on the outstretched hand. The distal end of the humerus fractures just above the condyles. The great danger of both supracondylar fracture and elbow dislocation is the potential damage to the brachial artery because of its close proximity. This can lead to **Volkmann's ischemic contracture,** a rare but potentially devastating ischemic necrosis of the forearm muscles.

Pain from "hitting the funny bone" does not come from a bone, but from **ulnar nerve compression**. It is very superficial where it crosses the medial elbow between the bony olecranon process and medial epicondyle. Any impact to the nerve can create pain, numbness, and tingling in the medial hand and fourth and fifth fingers innervated by this nerve.

Points to Remember

- Synovial joint shapes can be irregular (plane), hinge, pivot, condyloid, saddle, or ball-and-socket.
- Synovial joints can have zero to three axes.
- When a muscle has contracted (shortened) over all of its joints as far as it can, it has become actively insufficient.
- When a muscle has elongated (stretched) over all of its joints as far as possible, it has become passively insufficient.
- An activity can be an open- or closed-kinetic-chain movement, depending on whether the distal segment is fixed.
- The concave-convex rule has the convex joint surface moving in a direction opposite to the movement of the body segment and the concave joint surfacing moving in the same direction as the body segment.

Review Questions

General Anatomy Questions

1. In terms of the elbow and forearm joints, identify the following:
   a. Names of bones involved:
      Forearm ____________________
      Elbow ____________________
   b. Number of axes:
      Forearm ____________________
      Elbow ____________________
   c. Shape classification of joint:
      Forearm ____________________
      Elbow ____________________
   d. Joint osteokinematic motion allowed:
      Forearm ____________________
      Elbow ____________________
2. If you were handed an unattached model of an ulna, how could you orient landmarks to determine on which side of the body it belonged?
3. Name the ligament that stabilizes:
   a. the lateral side of the elbow
   b. the medial side of the elbow
   c. the radius and allows it to rotate
4. Which muscles of the elbow and/or forearm are two-joint muscles?
5. To which bone must a muscle attach to perform forearm supination or pronation?
6. Which elbow or forearm muscles do not attach to the humerus?
7. Which muscles connect the scapula to the ulna and/or radius?
8. Which muscles connect the humerus and ulna?
9. The only part of the triceps that crosses the shoulder joint is the ______________.
10. To stretch the long head of the triceps, you would place the elbow in ______________ and the shoulder in ______________.
11. In what positions would you put the upper extremity to achieve:
    a. active insufficiency of the biceps?
    b. passive insufficiency of the biceps?
12. In a closed-chain activity, such as a push-up, the humerus is moving on the ulna and radius (forearm) in extending the elbow joint. Does the humeral joint surface move in the same or opposite direction as the forearm? (Hint: Think concave/convex.)
13. a. If you put your hand on the anterior surface of your arm, you would be touching what muscle?
    b. Placing your hand on the posterior surface is over what muscle?
    c. Touching the lateral forearm is touching what muscle?
    d. Is that hand touching the contralateral or ipsilateral arm?

(continued on next page)

Review Questions—cont'd

14. a. The anconeus attaches to what ligament?
    b. It attaches to what other soft tissue structure by way of the ligament named in (a)?
    c. What purpose do the attachments of the anconeus to these structures serve?
15. a. With the elbow partially flexed, forceful supination involves contraction of what prime mover muscles?
    b. The triceps also contracts to maintain this partially flexed position. What is the term used for the role of the triceps? Explain.

Functional Activity Questions

Answer the questions that refer to each of the following functional activities:

1. Place a dinner plate in an upper kitchen cabinet.
   a. Identify the shoulder motion occurring.
   b. What shoulder muscle(s) is/are contracting to create this motion?
   c. Identify the elbow motion occurring.
   d. What elbow muscle is the prime mover for this elbow motion?
   e. Identify the forearm motion occurring.
   f. What forearm muscle(s) is/are contracting?
   g. What is the normal end feel for this motion?
   h. Is this an open- or closed-chain motion?
2. Identify the motions needed to put a piece of chocolate in your mouth.
   a. Elbow ________________
   b. Forearm ________________
3. When answering the telephone, reach for the receiver (Fig. 11-26A).
   a. Identify the elbow motion occurring.
   b. During this elbow motion, the anterior aspect of the joint capsule is ____________, and the posterior aspect of the joint capsule is ____________
   c. What is the normal end feel for this motion?
   d. Identify the forearm motion occurring.
   e. What is the normal end feel for this motion?
   f. What muscle(s) is/are contracting to create this motion?

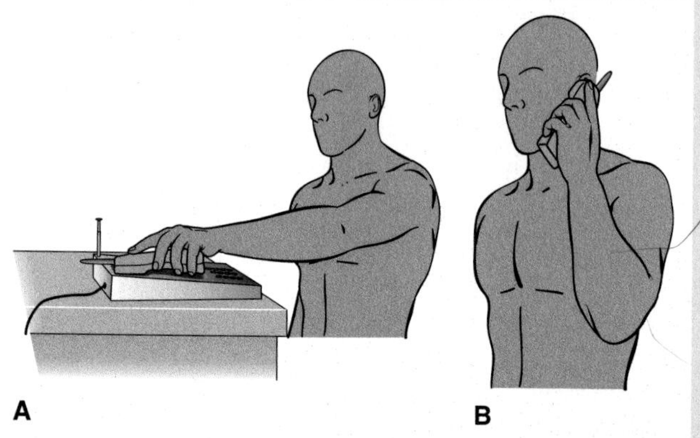

Figure 11-26. Elbow and forearm motion when answering the telephone. **(A)** Starting position. **(B)** Ending position.

4. Next, put the receiver to your ear (Fig. 11-26B).
   a. Is this an open- or closed-chain activity?
   b. Identify the elbow motion occurring.
   c. What is the normal end feel for this motion?
   d. What muscle(s) is/are contracting to create this motion?
   e. Identify the forearm motion occurring.
   f. Identify the joints that are moving in order for this motion to occur. Be specific.
5. With a hammer in your hand, pound on a nail that has been set in the wall.
   a. Identify the elbow motion occurring.
   b. Describe the movement of the joint surfaces compared with the rest of the bone. (Name the bony surfaces and describe their shapes in your answer.)
   c. Identify the position of the forearm during this activity.
   d. Regardless of the starting position of the forearm, name the muscle that will bring the forearm into the position described in (c).

Clinical Exercise Questions

1. In a sitting position, place your right forearm on the table palm down with your elbow flexed as necessary (Fig. 11-27A). Using your left hand, push against the radial side of the right forearm just proximal to the wrist until the right palm is facing up (Fig. 11-27B). The right forearm remains relaxed.
   a. What joint motion is occurring in the right forearm?
   b. What muscles are being stretched?

Review Questions—cont'd

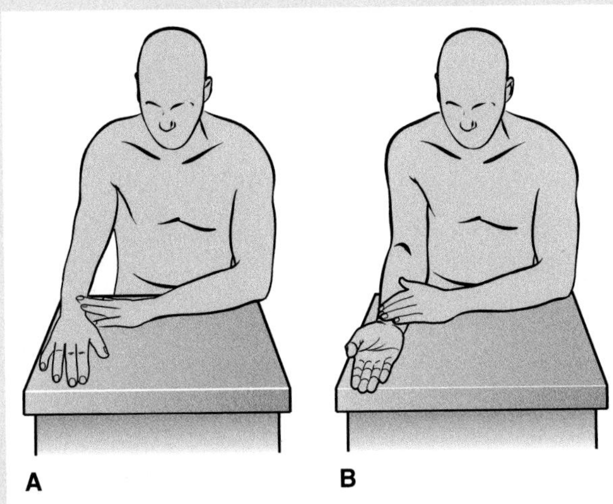

Figure 11-27. Self-stretch at the forearm. **(A)** Starting position. **(B)** Ending position.

2. Sit in a chair that has armrests and place your hands on them. Do a chair push-up, lifting your buttocks off the seat.
   a. What joint motion is occurring at the elbow?
   b. What type of contraction (isometric, concentric, or eccentric) is occurring?
   c. What muscles are being strengthened?
   d. Is this an open- or closed-kinetic-chain activity?
3. Stand with your right arm extended straight up toward the ceiling. Using your left hand, push your right hand down behind your head (Fig. 11-28). Allow your elbow to bend.
   a. What joint motion is occurring in the right elbow?
   b. What muscles are being stretched?

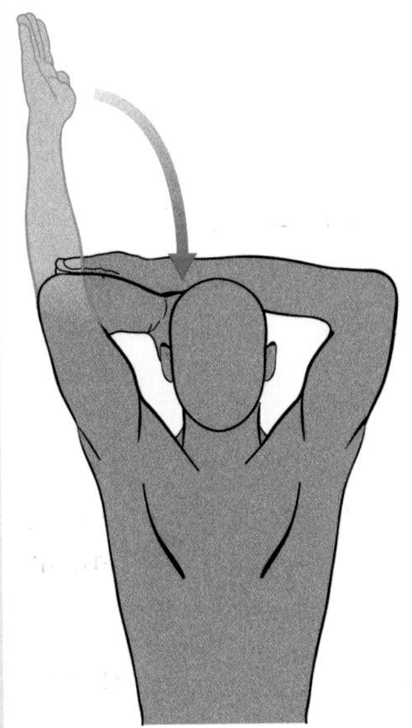

Figure 11-28. Self-stretch at the elbow.

4. In a sitting position, place your hands and forearms on the table. Push on the table as if you are trying to hold it down.
   a. What type of contraction (isometric, concentric, or eccentric) is occurring?
   b. What muscles are being strengthened?
5. Stand with your right hand next to your right shoulder, and hold a small weight. Move your hand to anatomical position.
   a. What joint motion is occurring in the right elbow?
   b. What type of contraction (isometric, concentric, or eccentric) is occurring?
   c. What muscles are being strengthened?
   d. Is this an open- or closed-kinetic-chain activity?
6. Lie prone on the floor and prepare to perform a push-up exercise by placing your hands next to your shoulders.
   a. As you complete the "up" phase of the push-up, you move into the plank position. What elbow motion is occurring?
   b. What muscle(s) is/are contracting, and what type of contraction are they performing?
   c. As you slowly lower yourself back down to the ground, what elbow motion is occurring?
   d. What muscle(s) is/are contracting, and what type of contraction are they performing?
7. While holding the end of a hammer handle in your hand, stand with your elbow flexed to 90 degrees and your forearm in pronation so that the hammer is facing medially.
   a. As you move from pronation to the neutral position of the forearm, which muscles are contracting, and what type of contraction are they performing?
   b. As you continue moving from the neutral position to the fully supinated position, which muscles are contracting, and what type of contraction are they performing?

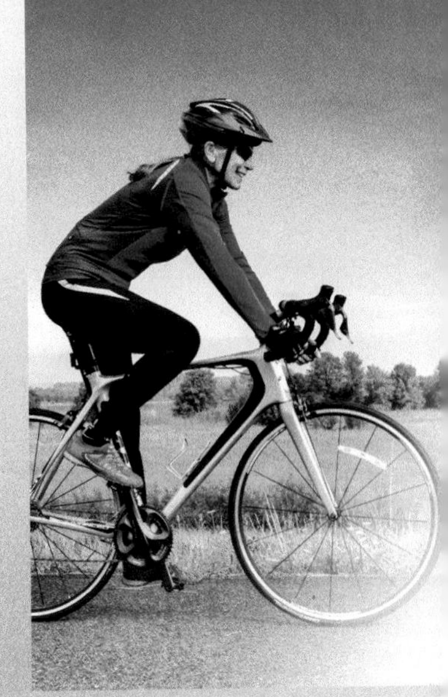

CHAPTER 12
Wrist Joint

Joint Structure
Joint Motions
Bones and Landmarks
Ligaments and Other Structures
Muscles of the Wrist
Anatomical Relationships
Common Wrist Pathologies
Summary of Muscle Action
Summary of Muscle Innervation
Points to Remember
Review Questions
General Anatomy Questions
Functional Activity Questions
Clinical Exercise Questions

Kinesiology IN ACTION For additional practice activities and videos, please visit www.kinesiologyinaction.com

Joint Structure

The wrist joint is perhaps one of the most complex joints of the body. It provides the control and stability required to maintain the hand in a functional position. It is actually made up of two joints: the radiocarpal joint and the midcarpal joint. The **radiocarpal joint** (Fig. 12-1) consists of the distal end of the radius and the radioulnar disk proximally and the scaphoid, lunate, and triquetrum distally. Because an articular disk is located between the ulna and the proximal row of carpals, the ulna is not considered part of this joint. The pisiform, located in the proximal row of carpal bones, does not articulate with the disk because it is more anterior to the triquetrum. Therefore, it is not considered part of this joint either. As a synovial joint, the radiocarpal joint is classified as a biaxial **condyloid**

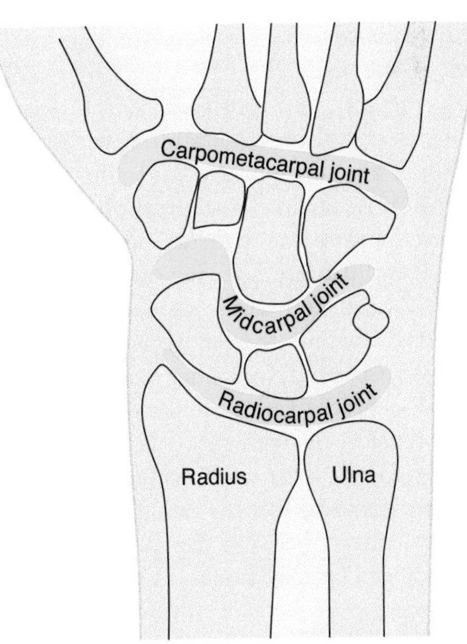

Figure 12-1. Joints of the left wrist (anterior view).

joint allowing flexion and extension, radial deviation, and ulnar deviation. The combination of all four of these motions is called *circumduction*. There is no rotation at the wrist.

The **midcarpal joint** (see Fig. 12-1) is located between the two rows of carpal bones, whereas the **intercarpal joints** are located between the carpal bones in each individual row. The shape of these joints are irregular, and they are classified as nonaxial plane joints. They allow gliding motions, which collectively contribute to motion of the wrist.

The **carpometacarpal (CMC) joints** appear between the distal row of carpal bones and the proximal end of the metacarpal bones (see Fig. 12-1). Because they have a more direct function in the movement of the hand, they will be discussed in more detail in Chapter 13.

Joint Motions

Osteokinematic Motion

When discussing wrist motion, several terms are frequently used. *Wrist flexion* and *palmar flexion* are synonymous, as are *hyperextension* and *dorsiflexion*. Approximately midway between flexion and extension, putting the hand in a straight line with the forearm, is *neutral position*. This is the position of the wrist joint in anatomical position. *Extension* is the return from *flexion*. Movement beyond the neutral position is *hyperextension*. However, the most commonly used terms describing wrist motions are **flexion, extension,** and **hyperextension. Neutral position** is the common term for the extended or the anatomical position of the wrist (Fig. 12-2A). This terminology for joint motion and position will be used here. Nevertheless, you should be familiar with these other terms, which are summarized in Table 12-1. Flexion and extension occur in the sagittal plane around the frontal axis. From the neutral position, there are approximately 90 degrees of flexion and 70 degrees of extension. **Radial** and **ulnar deviation** occur in the frontal plane around the sagittal axis (Fig. 12-2B). There are approximately 25 degrees of radial deviation and 35 degrees of ulnar deviation.

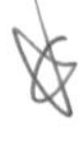

Due to tension of ligaments and the joint capsule, the end feel for all wrist motions, except radial deviation, is firm. The end feel for radial deviation is hard, due to bony contact between the radial styloid process and the scaphoid (carpal) bone.

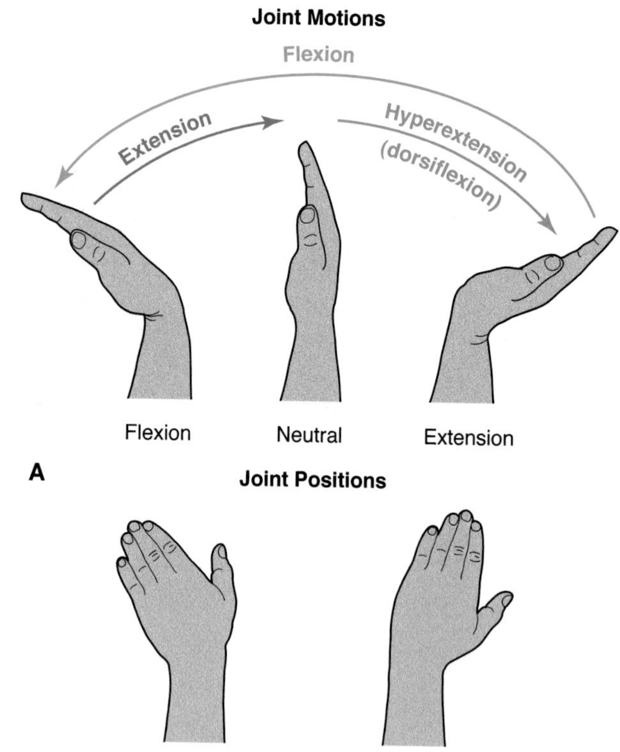

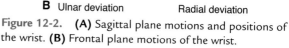

Figure 12-2. **(A)** Sagittal plane motions and positions of the wrist. **(B)** Frontal plane motions of the wrist.

Table 12-1 Comparison of Wrist Joint Terminology*

Preferred Terminology	Alternative Terminology	Motion or Position
Flexion	Palmar flexion	Anterior from anatomical position
Neutral	Extension	Anatomical position
Hyperextension	Extension, dorsiflexion	Posterior from anatomical position
Radial deviation	Abduction	Lateral from anatomical position
Ulnar deviation	Adduction	Medial from anatomical position

*__Bold print__ indicates which terms are used in this book.

Arthrokinematic Motion

The radiocarpal joint has the most joint play when it is in the neutral position with slight ulnar deviation (open-packed position). This joint is a convex-on-concave articulation where the convex-shaped proximal row of carpal bones moves in the opposite direction of the hand motion. Therefore, during wrist flexion, the carpals glide posteriorly on the radius and articular disk. During wrist extension, they glide anteriorly. With radial deviation, they glide in a medial direction, and with ulnar deviation, they glide in the lateral direction (Fig. 12-3).

Joint mobilizations are often performed to restore normal length to the capsule and restore normal movement to the joint. Tightness in the anterior joint capsule will limit wrist extension. An anterior glide of the proximal row of carpals can be performed to restore normal length to the anterior capsule and increase wrist extension.

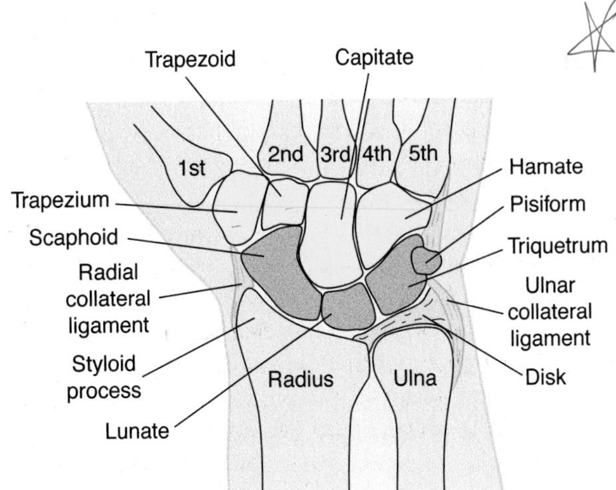

Figure 12-4. Bones of the wrist, (anterior view, left hand).

Bones and Landmarks

The carpal bones consist of two rows of four bones each (Fig. 12-4). Starting on the thumb side of the proximal row are the **scaphoid, lunate, triquetrum,** and **pisiform.** In the distal row, lateral to medial, are the **trapezium, trapezoid, capitate,** and **hamate.** These are short bones arranged in an arch, with the concavity on the anterior (palmar surface) side and the convexity on the posterior side. This arched arrangement contributes greatly to the thumb's ability to oppose.

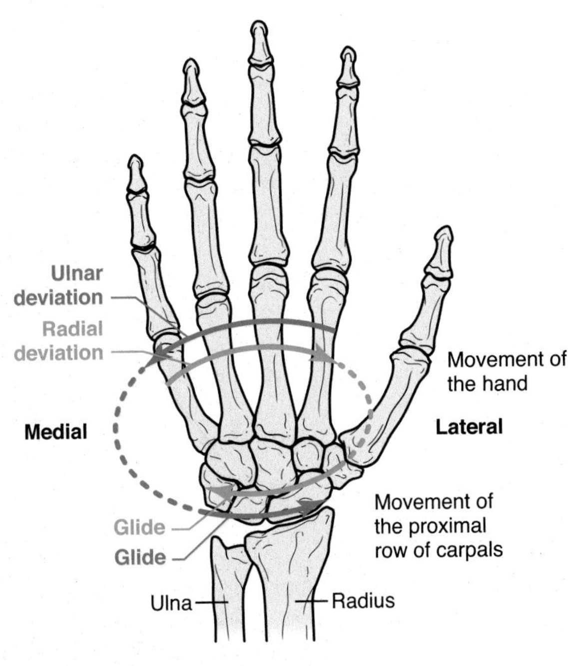

Figure 12-3. Arthrokinematic motions accompanying radial and ulnar deviation.

Bony Landmarks of the Wrist

Styloid Processes

Distal projection on the lateral side of the radius (see Fig. 12-4) and distal medial posterior side of the ulna (see Fig. 11-10), providing attachment for the collateral ligaments

Hook of the Hamate

Projection on the anterior surface of the hamate, providing attachment for the transverse carpal ligament

Medial Epicondyle

Located on the distal medial side of the humerus; attachment for the common flexor tendon (see Fig. 11-9)

Lateral Epicondyle

Located on the distal lateral side of the humerus; attachment for the common extensor tendon (see Fig. 11-9)

Lateral Supracondylar Ridge

Located just proximal to the lateral epicondyle; attachment for the extensor carpi radialis longus muscle (see Fig. 11-9)

Ligaments and Other Structures

There are basically four ligaments of the radiocarpal joint that provide the major support of the wrist. In addition, there are numerous smaller ligaments supporting the intercarpal joints. The **radial collateral ligament** attaches to the styloid process of the radius and to the scaphoid and trapezium bones. The **ulnar collateral ligament** attaches to the styloid process of the ulna and to the pisiform and triquetrum. These ligaments provide lateral and medial support, respectively, to the wrist joint. They are illustrated in Figures 12-4, 12-5, and 12-6.

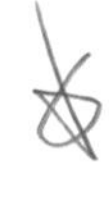

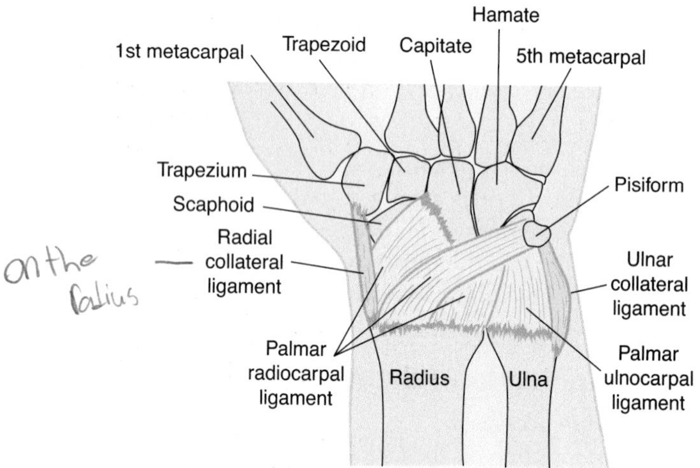

Figure 12-5. Palmar radiocarpal ligament (left hand).

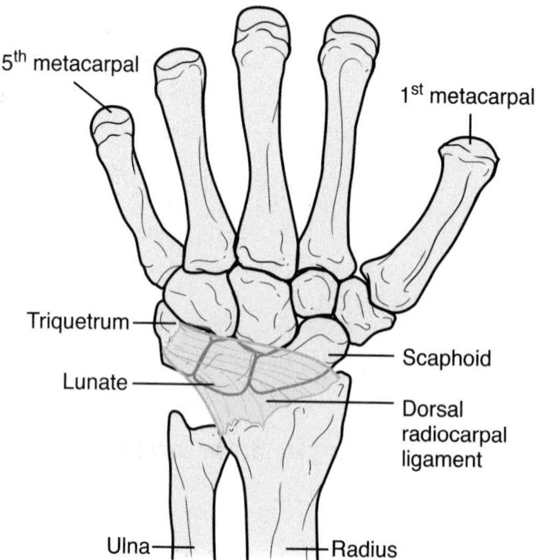

Figure 12-6. Dorsal radiocarpal ligament (left hand). Note that other dorsal ligaments have been removed.

The **palmar radiocarpal ligament** is a thick, tough ligament that becomes taut in extension, thus limiting wrist extension. It is a broad band that attaches from the anterior surface of the distal radius and ulna to the anterior surface of the proximal carpal bones and to the capitate bone in the distal row (see Fig. 12-5). It is perhaps more important to wrist function than its counterpart, the dorsal radiocarpal ligament, because most activities of the hand occur with the wrist extended, as opposed to being flexed. Therefore, the palmar radiocarpal ligament is also more apt to be stretched or sprained. It should be noted that some sources separate the radiocarpal ligament from the ulnocarpal ligament, and some do not. Functionally, they essentially act as one.

The **dorsal radiocarpal ligament** attaches from the posterior surface of the distal radius to the same surface of the scaphoid, lunate, and triquetrum (Fig. 12-6). This ligament becomes taut in flexion, therefore limiting the amount of flexion allowed at the wrist. Because forces causing excessive flexion are not as great as those causing excessive extension, this ligament is not as strong as the palmar radiocarpal ligament.

A **joint capsule,** which encloses the radiocarpal joint, is reinforced by the radial and ulnar collateral ligaments and by the palmar and dorsal radiocarpal ligaments. The **articular disk** (see Fig. 12-4) is located on the distal end of the ulna and articulates with the triquetrum and lunate bones. It acts as a shock absorber and as filler between the distal ulna and its adjacent carpal bones—the triquetrum and lunate. The disk fills the gap created because the ulna and its styloid process do not extend as far distally as the radius and its styloid process.

The **palmar aponeurosis** is a relatively thick, triangular fascia located superficially in the palm of the hand (Fig. 12-7). It covers the tendons of the extrinsic muscles and provides some protection to the structures in the palm. It serves as the distal attachment of the palmaris longus, which blends into this fascia, as does the flexor retinaculum.

Muscles of the Wrist

There are a large number of wrist and hand muscles that originate on the medial and lateral epicondyles of the humerus. These bony landmarks are small and do not have enough surface area to accommodate all of these muscle attachments. This challenge it met by having a single tendon originate from each of these humeral landmarks that splits into multiple different muscle bellies, each belly being identified as a separate muscle.

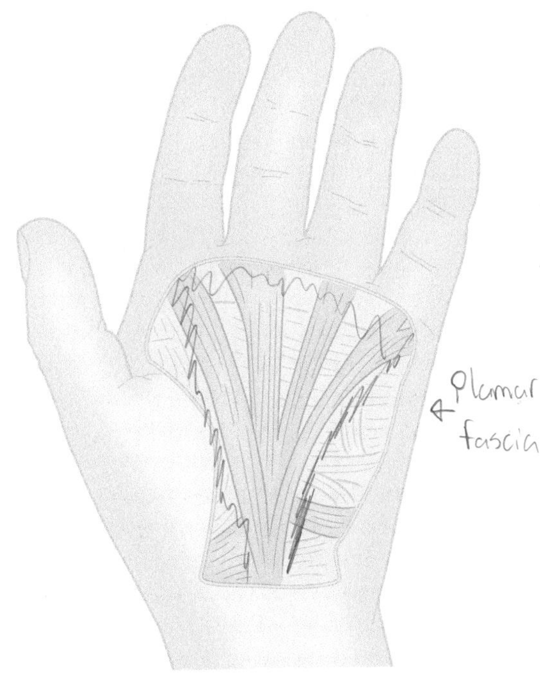

Figure 12-7. Palmar aponeurosis (anterior view).

The **common flexor tendon** is a single tendon that originates on the medial epicondyle of the humerus. It gives rise to many muscles that are prime movers for flexion at either the wrist or the hand, i.e., pronator teres, flexor carpi radialis, palmaris longus, flexor digitorum superficialis, and flexor carpi ulnaris. Similarly, the **common extensor tendon** originates on the lateral epicondyle. This single tendon gives rise to many muscles that are prime movers for either wrist or finger extension, i.e., extensor carpi radialis longus and brevis, extensor carpi ulnaris, extensor digitorum, and extensor digiti minimi.

Wrist muscles have very vertical lines of pull. Therefore, muscle actions can essentially be determined by the joint surfaces that the muscles cross. Any muscle crossing the anterior side of the wrist will draw the anterior surfaces of the forearm and hand together, creating wrist flexion. A muscle that crosses the posterior side of the wrist will create wrist extension by pulling the posterior aspects of the hand and forearm closer together. Muscles crossing or inserting on the medial or lateral aspect of the wrist joint will create ulnar or radial deviation, respectively. Given that all of the prime movers at the wrist have origins on the humerus, they can all be classified as two-joint muscles that cross the elbow and wrist. While their primary actions are at the wrist, some, depending on their line of pull, size, and moment arms, can be said to have assistive functions at the elbow.

The muscles spanning and having a primary function at the wrist will be discussed here; the muscles that cross the wrist but have a more significant function at the thumb or fingers will be discussed in Chapter 13. The following are the muscles to be discussed in this section:

Anterior	Posterior
Flexor carpi ulnaris	Extensor carpi radialis longus
Flexor carpi radialis	Extensor carpi radialis brevis
Palmaris longus	Extensor carpi ulnaris

Some general statements can be made about the proximal muscle attachments of the wrist muscles. First, the flexors originate from the common flexor tendon on the medial epicondyle, and the extensors originate from the common extensor tendon on the lateral epicondyle. It should be noted, however, that the extensor carpi radialis longus is an exception to this rule and originates just above the lateral condyle on the lateral supracondylar ridge. Second, the distal attachment for all the wrist muscles is a metacarpal, except for the palmaris longus muscle. Third, the names of the muscles tell generally what their action is (flexor, extensor), what they act on (*carpi* means "wrist"), and on what side of the wrist the distal attachment is located (*radialis* means "radial"; *ulnaris* means "ulnar"). Their names will also describe whether the muscle functions in ulnar or radial deviation.

The **flexor carpi ulnaris muscle** is a superficial muscle running along the ulnar, slightly anterior, side of the forearm (Fig. 12-8). Its proximal attachment is mostly on the medial epicondyle of the humerus from the common flexor tendon, and its distal attachment is the base of the fifth metacarpal and pisiform bone. It is the only wrist muscle attaching to a carpal bone. It crosses the anterior side of the wrist and inserts on the ulnar side of the hand; therefore it is a prime mover in wrist flexion and ulnar deviation. Given the relative anterior orientation of the common flexor tendon on the medial epicondyle, this muscle crosses just anterior to the axis of rotation for the elbow joint, allowing it to assist with elbow flexion.

Flexor Carpi Ulnaris Muscle

O	Medial epicondyle of humerus
I	Pisiform and base of fifth metacarpal
A	Wrist flexion, ulnar deviation
N	Ulnar nerve (C8, T1)

The **flexor carpi radialis muscle** is also a relatively superficial muscle running from the common flexor tendon on the medial epicondyle diagonally across the

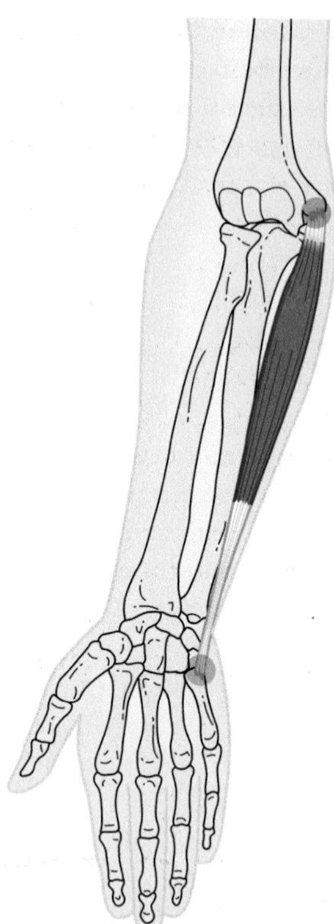

Figure 12-8. Flexor carpi ulnaris muscle (anterior view).

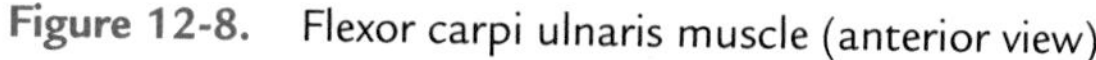

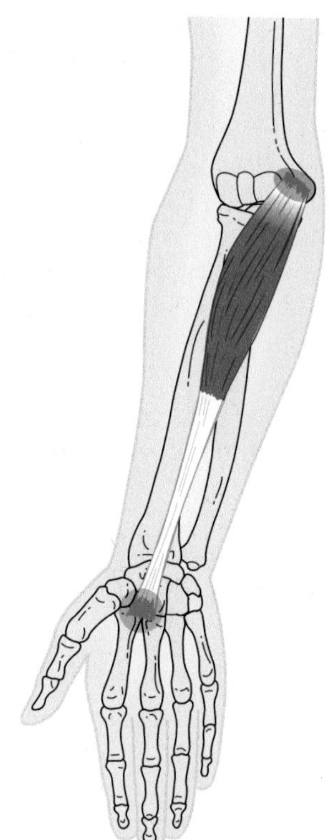

Figure 12-9. Flexor carpi radialis muscle (anterior view).

anterior forearm to attach laterally at the base of the second and third metacarpals (Fig. 12-9). It is a prime mover in wrist flexion and radial deviation. Like the flexor carpi ulnaris, this muscle can assist with elbow flexion.

Flexor Carpi Radialis Muscle	
O	Medial epicondyle of the humerus
I	Base of second and third metacarpals
A	Wrist flexion, radial deviation
N	Median nerve (C6, C7)

The **palmaris longus muscle** is also a superficial muscle running down the anterior surface of the forearm from the common flexor attachment of the medial epicondyle. It attaches in the midline to the palmar aponeurosis (Fig. 12-10). It is easily identified in the midline at the base of the wrist, especially against slight resistance to wrist flexion. This muscle is rather unique because it has only one bony attachment, which is at the proximal end. This muscle is missing in approximately 21% of individuals, either unilaterally or bilaterally (Moore, 1985, p 698). Because the palmaris longus muscle is quite small, its absence does not result in any significant loss of strength. To further

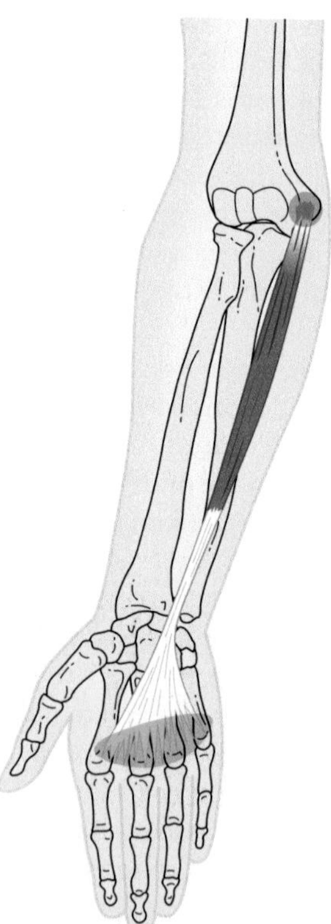

Figure 12-10. Palmaris longus muscle (anterior view).

illustrate its dispensable nature, in cases where a different tendon ruptures in the hand, the palmaris longus (when present) is often used to replace the damaged tendon. Although it is in an ideal position to flex the wrist, it is assistive at best because of its size. Because of its attachment to the palmar aponeurosis, the palmaris longus may have a slight role in cupping the hand. While it crosses the elbow joint anteriorly, its ability to contribute toward elbow flexion is negligible because of its very small size.

Palmaris Longus Muscle

O	Medial epicondyle of humerus
I	Palmar aponeurosis
A	Assistive in wrist flexion
N	Median nerve (C6, C7)

On the posterior side of the wrist is the **extensor carpi radialis longus muscle.** This muscle is mostly superficial (Fig. 12-11). The term "longus" refers to the fact that this muscle originates superior to the rest of the extensor group, hence its longer length. It attaches proximally just above the lateral epicondyle on the lateral supracondylar ridge, making it the only wrist extensor that does not originate from the common extensor tendon. It runs down the lateral posterior side of the forearm, under two tendons that go to the thumb, and under the extensor retinaculum (see Fig. 12-16) to attach at the base of the second metacarpal. Because it crosses the posterior side of the wrist and inserts on the radial side, it is a prime mover in wrist extension and radial deviation. It also crosses the elbow slightly anteriorly, allowing it to assist in elbow flexion. Functionally, its elbow action is unimportant. However, it does become more important when needing to stretch the muscle.

Extensor Carpi Radialis Longus Muscle

O	Supracondylar ridge of humerus
I	Base of second metacarpal
A	Wrist extension, radial deviation
N	Radial nerve (C6, C7)

Because the extensor carpi radialis muscle also has *longus* in its name, this implies that there is a "brevis." The **extensor carpi radialis brevis muscle** lies next to the extensor carpi radialis longus muscle (Fig. 12-12). It

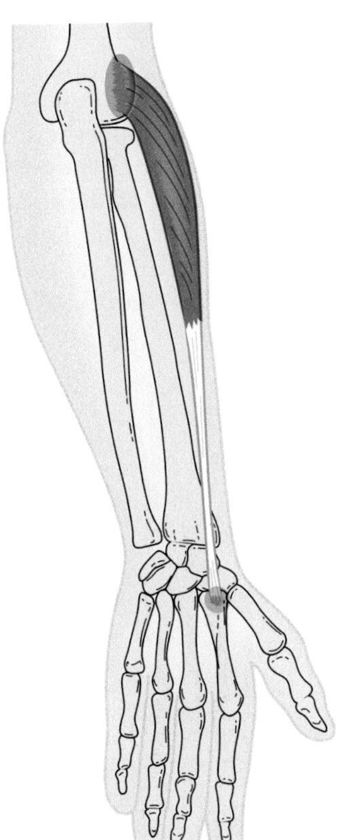

Figure 12-11. Extensor carpi radialis longus muscle (posterior view).

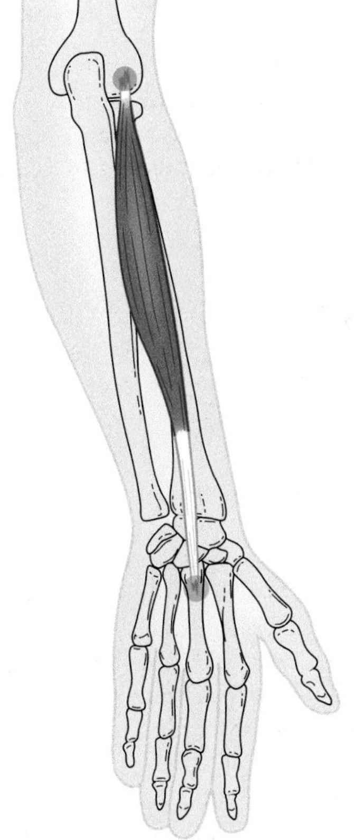

Figure 12-12. Extensor carpi radialis brevis muscle (posterior view).

arises from the common extensor tendon on the lateral epicondyle. Like the "longus," it passes under two tendons that go to the thumb and then under the extensor retinaculum. Its distal attachment is at the base of the third metacarpal. Because its attachment is close to the axis of motion for radial and ulnar deviation, its moment arm for this motion is very short, making it only assistive in radial deviation. However, because it crosses the posterior side of the joint, it is a prime mover in wrist extension. Like the extensor carpi radialis longus, it has an assisting role in elbow extension.

Extensor Carpi Radialis Brevis Muscle

O	Lateral epicondyle of humerus
I	Base of third metacarpal
A	Wrist extension
N	Radial nerve (C6, C7)

The **extensor carpi ulnaris muscle** is also a superficial muscle arising from the common extensor tendon on the lateral epicondyle (Fig. 12-13). It runs down the medial side of the posterior forearm to attach at the base of the fifth metacarpal. It crosses the posterior side of the wrist and inserts on the medial side of the hand, making it a prime mover in wrist extension and ulnar deviation and assistive in elbow extension. Like the extensor carpi radialis longus and brevis, knowing which side of the elbow joint axis the muscle crosses becomes important when stretching this two-joint muscle.

Extensor Carpi Ulnaris Muscle

O	Lateral epicondyle of humerus
I	Base of fifth metacarpal
A	Wrist extension, ulnar deviation
N	Radial nerve (C6, C7, C8)

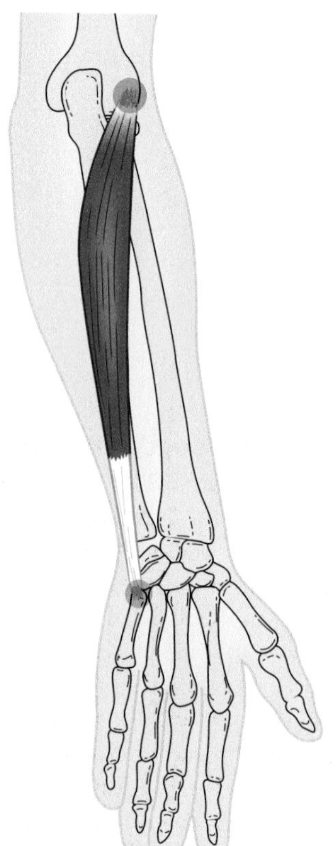

Figure 12-13. Extensor carpi ulnaris muscle (posterior view).

Anatomical Relationships

For the most part, the wrist flexors are relatively superficial, are located on the anterior surface of the forearm, and originate on the medial epicondyle. As shown in Figure 12-14, if you take the index, middle, and ring fingers of your left hand and place them at your right wrist (anterior surface), this represents the location and order of the flexor carpi radialis (index finger), the palmaris longus (middle finger), and the flexor carpi ulnaris (ring finger). These attachments also line up with the second, third, and fifth fingers, respectively. Figure 12-15 shows the three superficial wrist flexors. The brachioradialis is also superficial, but it is an elbow muscle that does not cross the wrist. Beneath the wrist flexors are the flexors of the thumb and hand, which will be described in Chapter 13.

The muscles of the wrist extensor group are also relatively superficial but are on the posterior surface of the

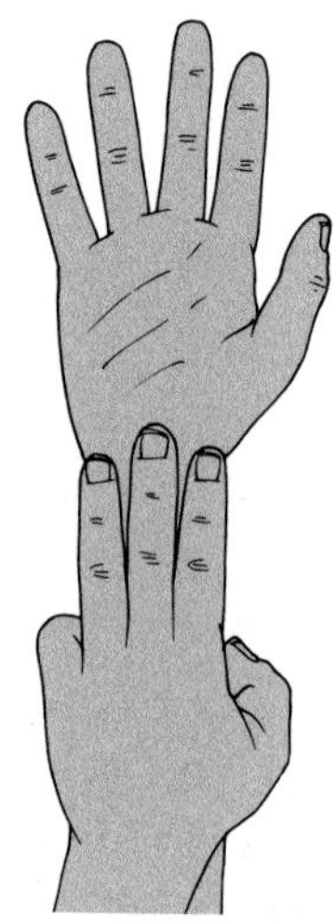

Figure 12-14. Tendon position of anterior wrist muscles.

Clinical Application 12-1

Dual Role of Wrist Muscles

Most wrist muscles have more than one action and therefore are not capable of creating motion in a cardinal plane when they contract alone. For example, the flexor carpi radialis will always pull the wrist obliquely into a combined flexion and radial deviation motion, and cannot, by itself, perform a cardinal plane motion of either flexion or radial deviation (see figure below). When cardinal plane motions are desired, the wrist muscles act as neutralizers to one another and agonists with each other. For example, when flexion is desired, the flexor carpi ulnaris needs to contract along with the flexor carpi radialis. The radial and ulnar deviation actions of these muscles cancel one another out (neutralize), and the muscles work as agonists to create the desired motion of flexion. Similarly, if a pure ulnar deviation motion is needed, the extensor carpi ulnaris will contract at the same time as the flexor carpi ulnaris. The flexion and extension components of these concurrent forces will cancel one another out, and the resultant force will move the wrist into ulnar deviation.

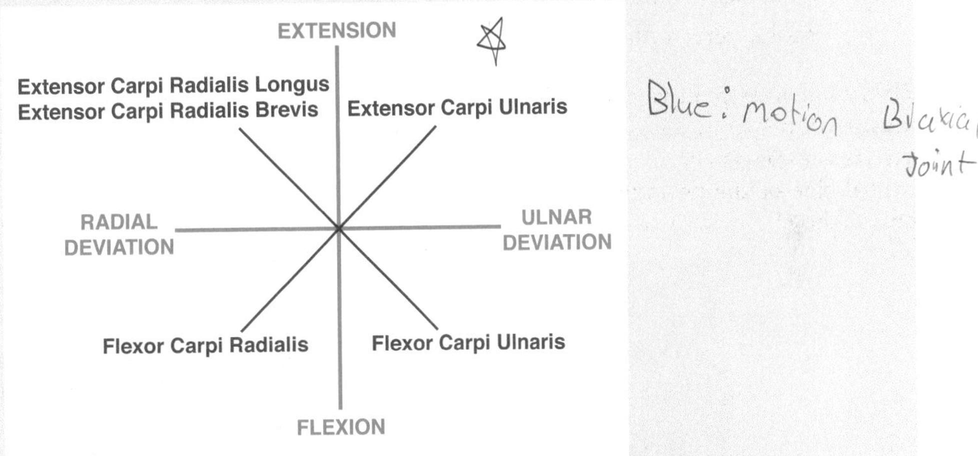

Dual role of wrist muscles. For motion to occur in a cardinal plane (blue lines), muscle actions (red lines) must have their unwanted motions neutralized.

forearm (Fig. 12-16). Their common origin is mostly the lateral epicondyle. Just distal to that landmark, they parallel each other. The extensor carpi radialis longus is most lateral, followed by the extensor carpi radialis brevis. The extensor digitorum and extensor digiti minimi (both hand muscles) lie in the midline. Medial to them and on the ulnar side is the extensor carpi ulnaris. Note that all wrist, hand, and thumb tendons are contained by the **extensor retinaculum** (see Fig. 12-16).

Common Wrist Pathologies

Two of the most common bones fractured at the wrist joint are the scaphoid and the radius. Both types of fractures can happen when falling on the outstretched hand. A **Colles fracture** is a break in the distal radius at the level of the metaphysis and is a common injury in the elderly. This transverse fracture of the distal radius includes a posterior displacement of the distal fragment. In **Smith's fracture,** the distal fragment is displaced anteriorly (reverse Colles) and is caused by a fall on the back of the hand. A **"greenstick" fracture** refers to an incomplete fracture, usually of the radius and more proximal than a Colles fracture. It is more common in children than adults. This fracture is similar to the breaking of a young or new tree limb. If you try to break the limb, you will find that it does not break completely in half like an older, more brittle limb. A **scaphoid fracture** is sometimes associated with damage to the blood vessel that supplies this bone, which can lead to **avascular necrosis,** or death of bone tissue.

A **ganglion cyst** is a benign, fluid-filled cyst commonly seen as a bump on the dorsal surface of the wrist. They can appear, disappear, and change size quickly. Only if

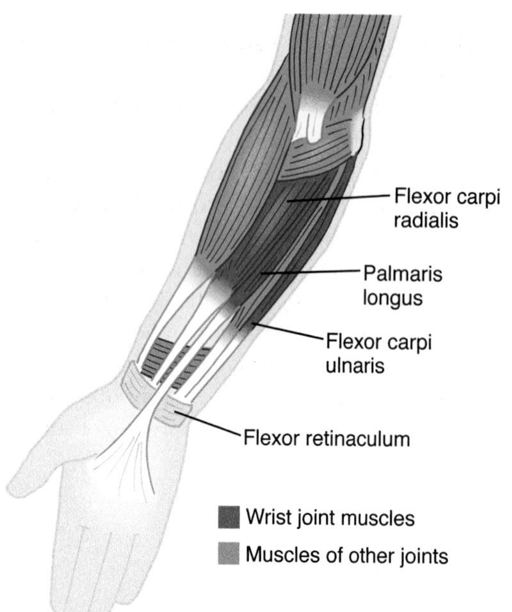

Figure 12-15. Anterior wrist muscles in relation to muscles of hand and thumb.

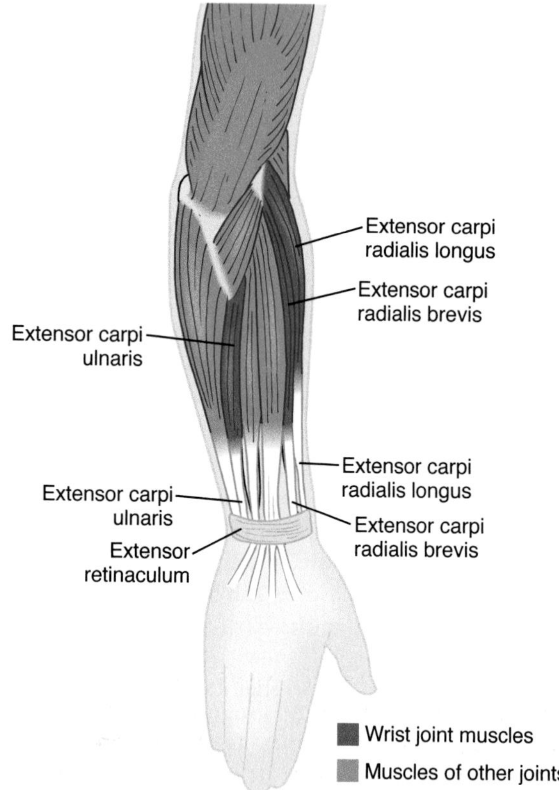

Figure 12-16. Posterior wrist muscles in relation to muscles of hand and thumb.

the cyst is painful or interferes with function is treatment necessary. **Wrist sprains** are common when a person falls on the outstretched hand. The wrist is usually hyperextended when the hand hits the ground. There are many ligaments in the wrist, but the most commonly injured ligament is the scapholunate ligament. As its name implies, it connects the scaphoid with the lunate bones.

Summary of Muscle Action

Table 12-2 summarizes the muscle action of the prime movers of the wrist.

Table 12-2 Muscle Action of the Wrist

Action	Muscles (Prime Movers)
Flexion	Flexor carpi radialis, flexor carpi ulnaris
Extension	Extensor carpi radialis longus and brevis, extensor carpi ulnaris
Radial deviation	Flexor carpi radialis, extensor carpi radialis longus
Ulnar deviation	Flexor carpi ulnaris, extensor carpi ulnaris

Clinical Application 12-2

Joint positioning for Stretching the Wrist Flexors and Extensors

The wrist flexors and extensors are two joint muscles that cross both the wrist and elbow. The wrist flexors all cross anterior to the axis of rotation for the elbow so when they contract (shorten), the elbow and wrist both move into flexion. To stretch (lengthen) these muscles, the elbow and wrist joints must be moved into extension (opposite of the contracting action). The wrist extensors have a slightly more complex arrangement in that the extensor carpi radialis longus and brevis produce elbow flexion and wrist extension, whereas the extensor carpi ulnaris creates wrist and elbow extension when it contracts (shortens). To stretch the extensor carpi radialis longus, the elbow is placed in extension while the wrist is moved into a flexed position. To stretch the extensor carpi ulnaris, the elbow and wrist are both placed in flexion.

Summary of Muscle Innervation

Innervation of the wrist muscles is quite straightforward. The radial nerve innervates the posterior muscles. The median nerve innervates the anterior muscles on the thumb side, and the ulnar nerve innervates muscles on the ulnar side. Tables 12-3 and 12-4 summarize the innervation of the muscles of the wrist. There is some variation among sources regarding segmental innervation.

Points to Remember

- An isometric contraction has relatively no joint motion.
- The muscle attachments move closer together with a concentric contraction.
- An eccentric contraction is a deceleration activity.
- A mnemonic to help remember the order of the wrist bones: "Sally Likes To Push The Toy Car Hard" = scaphoid, lunate, triquetrum, pisiform, trapezium, trapezoid, capitate, and hamate.
- When using a longer resistance arm, more force is needed. Conversely, when using a shorter resistance arm, less force is needed.
- Working against gravity requires more work than working with gravity or with gravity eliminated.

Table 12-3 Innervation of the Muscles of the Wrist

Muscle	Nerve	Spinal Segment
Extensor carpi radialis longus	Radial	C6, C7
Extensor carpi radialis brevis	Radial	C6, C7
Extensor carpi ulnaris	Radial	C6, C7, C8
Flexor carpi radialis	Median	C6, C7
Palmaris longus	Median	C6, C7
Flexor carpi ulnaris	Ulnar	C8, T1

Table 12-4 Segmental Innervation of the Wrist Joint

Spinal Cord Level	C6	C7	C8	T1
Extensor carpi radialis longus	X	X		
Extensor carpi radialis brevis	X	X		
Extensor carpi ulnaris	X	X	X	
Palmaris longus	X	X		
Flexor carpi radialis	X	X		
Flexor carpi ulnaris			X	X

Clinical Application 12-3

Lever Systems at the Wrist

The wrist muscles are set up as a third-class lever system with a very short force arm running from the wrist joint axis to the point where the wrist muscles attach and a resistance arm running to the center of gravity of the hand (Fig. A). With a longer resistance arm and shorter force arm, these muscles are suited to produce large amounts of speed and/or range of motion in response to a small shortening of the muscle, but as a trade-off, the muscle will

continued

Clinical Application 12-3—cont'd

need to produce a relatively large amount of force to create this movement. When holding an object flat in one's hand, such as passing a heavy platter across the dinner table, the center of gravity moves distally due to the weight of the platter (Fig. B). This increase in the resistance arm requires the wrist muscles to produce even more force to maintain the wrist in a neutral position.

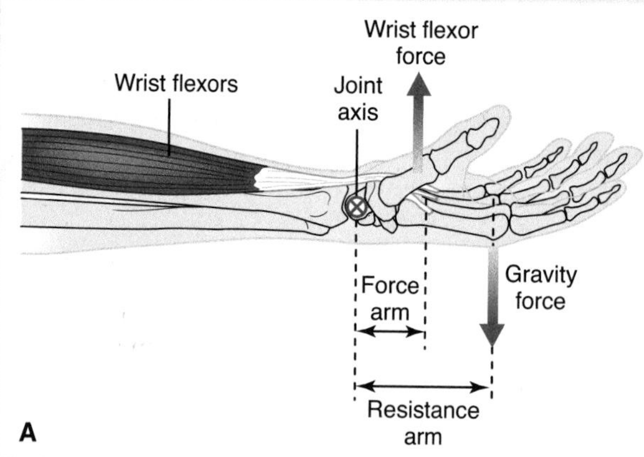

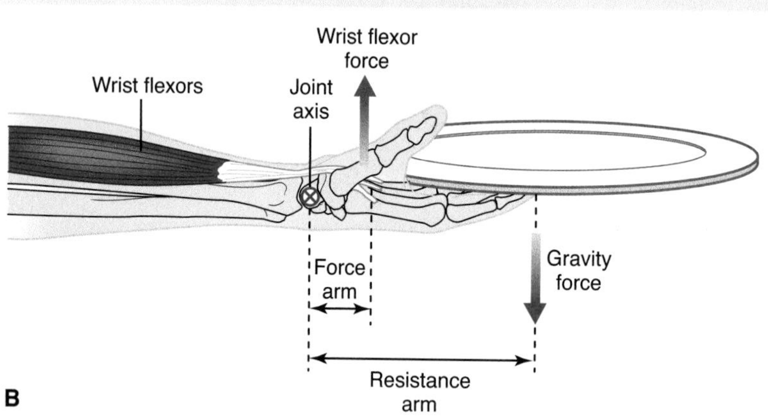

Levers. **(A)** When FA is less than RA, great force in needed to create movement. **(B)** When RA is increased, even greater force is needed (to hold platter).

Review Questions

General Anatomy Questions

1. Name the bones of the wrist joint, starting laterally on the proximal row and going medially. Use the same order for the distal row.
2. Which wrist motions occur in:
   a. the sagittal plane around the frontal axis?
   b. the frontal plane around the sagittal axis?
   c. the transverse plane around the vertical axis?
3. Describe the wrist joints:
   a. Number of axes
      Radiocarpal ____________
      Midcarpal ____________
   b. Shape of joint
      Radiocarpal ____________
      Midcarpal ____________
   c. Joint motion allowed
      Radiocarpal ____________
      Midcarpal ____________

Review Questions—cont'd

4. Which muscles attach on the medial epicondyle of the humerus?
5. Which muscles attach on or close to the lateral epicondyle of the humerus?
6. If you were shown a drawing of only a wrist joint, what landmarks could tell you if the drawing were a posterior or anterior view?
7. Which muscles cross the wrist on the radial side?
8. Which muscles cross the wrist on the ulnar side?
9. Which muscle, if present, is very easy to identify but has little functional importance?
10. Starting on the anterior surface of the ulnar side and moving in the direction of the radial side, name the wrist muscles that cross the wrist. Go completely around the wrist.
11. Why is the ulna not considered part of the wrist joint?
12. Generally speaking, you use wrist muscles when hammering. However, when extra force is needed, you may use elbow or even shoulder muscles. Why does that create greater force?
13. When hammering overhead into the ceiling, why are your wrist ulnar deviators working harder than when hammering a nail into the floor?
14. The wrist motions have what types of end feels?
15. What is the name of the bony landmark just proximal to the lateral epicondyle?

Functional Activity Questions

Many, but not all, functional activities have the wrist in a neutral or slightly hyperextended position. Often an isometric contraction is required to maintain that position. In the following activities, identify the wrist joint position and the muscle group contracting isometrically.

1. Holding a cup of coffee
   a. What wrist motion does gravity want to impose?
   b. Wrist muscles contracting to prevent motion in (a) ________________
   c. What concurrent forces are neutralized when these muscles contract?
2. Typing on a conventional computer keyboard
   a. What wrist motion does gravity want to impose?
   b. Wrist muscles contracting to prevent motion in (a) ________________
   c. What concurrent forces are neutralized when these muscles contract?
3. Brushing long hair with a comb (with right hand brushing on left side; Fig. 12-17)
   a. What wrist motion does the brush want to impose?
   b. Wrist muscles contracting to prevent motion in (a) ________________
   c. What concurrent forces are neutralized when these muscles contract?

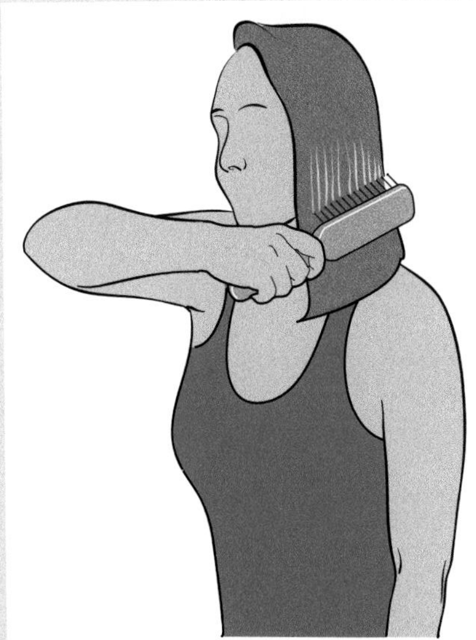

Figure 12-17. Brushing hair.

(continued on next page)

Review Questions—cont'd

4. Holding a box from the bottom (Fig. 12-18)
   a. What wrist motion does gravity want to impose?
   b. Wrist muscles contracting to prevent the motion in (a) ____________________
   c. What concurrent forces are neutralized when these muscles contract?

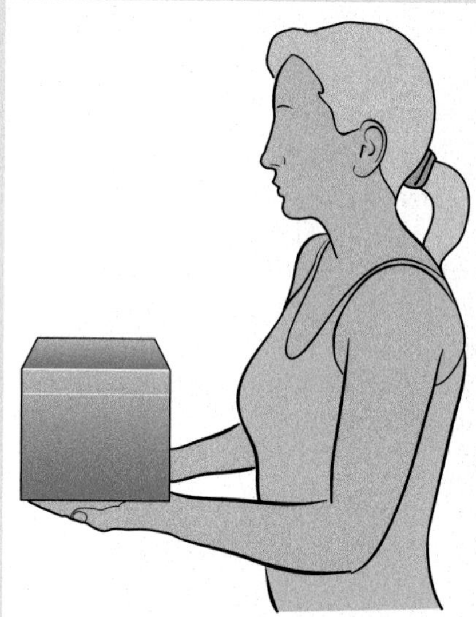

Figure 12-18. Holding a box.

5. Using a walker for ambulation
   a. What motion does the walker want to create at the wrist?
   b. What prime movers are contracting to prevent this motion?

Clinical Exercise Questions

Remember that elastic tubing loses its recoil quickly and is not as effective in the end range of an eccentric contraction. There may be more effective ways to perform eccentric contractions than examples given here. You should be able to recognize an eccentric contraction regardless of an exercise's effectiveness.

1. Sit with your forearm resting on your thigh, palm up, and holding a weight in your hand. Bend your wrist up.
   a. What joint motion is occurring in the wrist?
   b. What type of contraction (isometric, concentric, or eccentric) is occurring?
   c. What muscles are being strengthened?
   d. What portion of the joint capsule is being lengthened at the end range of this motion?
2. Slowly lower the weight to the starting position described in the exercise in Question 1.
   a. What joint motion is occurring in the wrist?
   b. What type of contraction (isometric, concentric, or eccentric) is occurring?
   c. What muscles are being strengthened?
3. Standing with your arm at your side, elbow flexed, palm down, hold on to a loop of elastic tubing that has the other end anchored under your foot. Curl your wrist up.
   a. What joint motion is occurring in the wrist?
   b. What ligament limits this motion at the end range?
   c. What type of contraction (isometric, concentric, or eccentric) is occurring?
   d. What muscles are being strengthened?
4. Slowly lower your wrist to the starting position described in the exercise in Question 3.
   a. What joint motion is occurring in the wrist?
   b. What type of contraction (isometric, concentric, or eccentric) is occurring?
   c. What muscles are being strengthened?
5. Standing with your arm at your side, elbow flexed, forearm in a neutral position, hold on to a loop of elastic tubing that has the other end anchored above your head to some stationary object. Bend your wrist down.
   a. What joint motion is occurring in the wrist?
   b. What type of contraction (isometric, concentric, or eccentric) is occurring?
   c. What muscles are being strengthened?
6. Slowly return to the starting position described in the exercise in Question 5.
   a. What joint motion is occurring in the wrist?
   b. What type of contraction (isometric, concentric, or eccentric) is occurring?
   c. Explain why it is this type of contraction.
   d. What muscles are being strengthened?
7. An individual has tight wrist flexors.
   a. What joint motion will be limited?
   b. During performance of passive stretch to restore this motion and to facilitate normal arthrokinematics at the wrist joint, do the proximal row of carpals need to glide in an anterior or posterior direction?

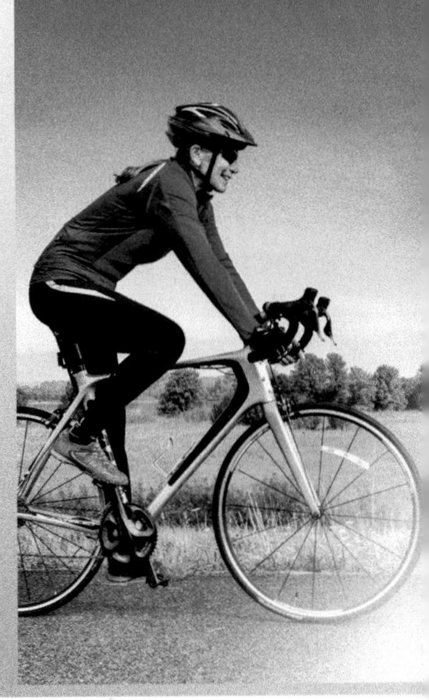

CHAPTER 13 Hand

Joint Structure and Motions of the Thumb
Joint Structure and Motions of the Finger
Bones and Landmarks
Ligaments and Other Structures
Muscles of the Thumb and Fingers
Extrinsic Muscles
Intrinsic Muscles
Anatomical Relationships
Common Wrist and Hand Pathologies
Summary of Muscle Actions
Summary of Muscle Innervation
Hand Function
Grasps
Points to Remember
Review Questions
General Anatomy Questions
Functional Activity Questions
Clinical Exercise Questions

Kinesiology IN ACTION For additional practice activities and videos, please visit www.kinesiologyinaction.com

The hand is the distal end of the upper extremity. It is made up of the thumb and finger metacarpals and phalanges. The hand is the key point of function for the upper extremity. We use our hands to accomplish an inexhaustible number of activities, ranging from very simple to quite complex tasks. The main purpose of the upper extremity's other joints is to place the hand in various positions to accomplish these tasks. Not only is the hand extremely useful and versatile, but it is also quite complex. This chapter will deal only with the hand's more basic structures and functions.

Joint Structure and Motions of the Thumb

The first digit, the thumb, has three joints: the carpometacarpal (CMC) joint, the metacarpophalangeal (MCP) joint, and the interphalangeal (IP) joint (Fig. 13-1).

The Carpometacarpal Joint

The **CMC joint** is made up of the trapezium bone, which articulates with the base of the first metacarpal (Fig. 13-2). Its classification is debated by some, but it is most commonly described as a modified biaxial saddle joint. With both joint surfaces being concave and convex, the shape and relationship of these joint surfaces can be compared with two Pringles potato chips stacked one on top of the other. The shape of the inferior surface of the top chip is similar to the shape of the first metacarpal; the shape of the superior surface of the bottom chip is similar to the trapezium bone. Each surface is concave in one direction and convex in the other.

If you look at your thumb in anatomical position, you will notice that the pad is perpendicular to the palm. When you oppose your thumb, the pad is now facing, or parallel to, the palm. Clearly, rotation has occurred. However, if you try to rotate the thumb without any

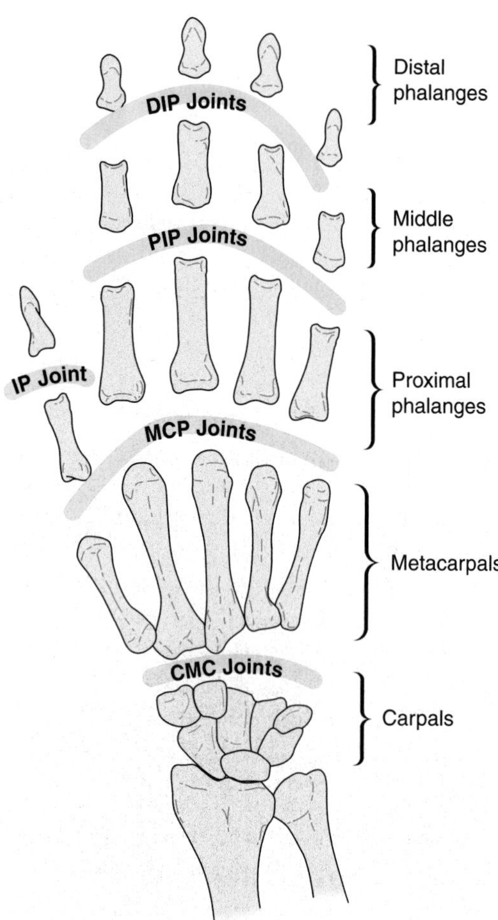

Figure 13-1. Joints and bones of the fingers and thumb (anterior view). Note that each finger has a DIP and PIP joint, whereas the thumb has only an IP joint.

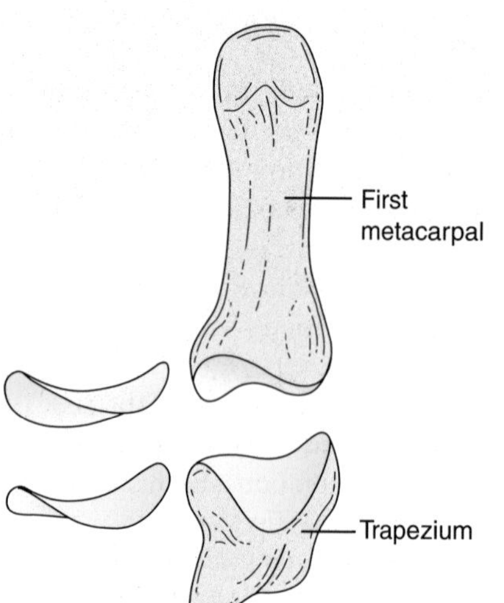

Figure 13-2. The saddle shape of the carpometacarpal (CMC) joint of the thumb can be compared with the shape of two Pringles potato chips.

other joint movement, you will find it impossible to do so. The rotation at the CMC joint is a passive, not voluntary, motion. This rotation occurs as a result of the joint's shape and not by any muscle action. This type of motion is commonly referred to as an **accessory movement** (a movement that accompanies the active movement and is essential to normal motion).

The CMC joint of the thumb allows more mobility than the CMC joints of the other four fingers, yet it also provides as much stability. It is unusual to benefit from stability and mobility at the same time. The joint allows flexion and extension, abduction and adduction, and opposition and reposition (Fig. 13-3). Thumb motions differ from the usual way we name joint motions. **Flexion** and **extension** occur in the frontal plane (a plane *parallel* to the palm). **Abduction** and

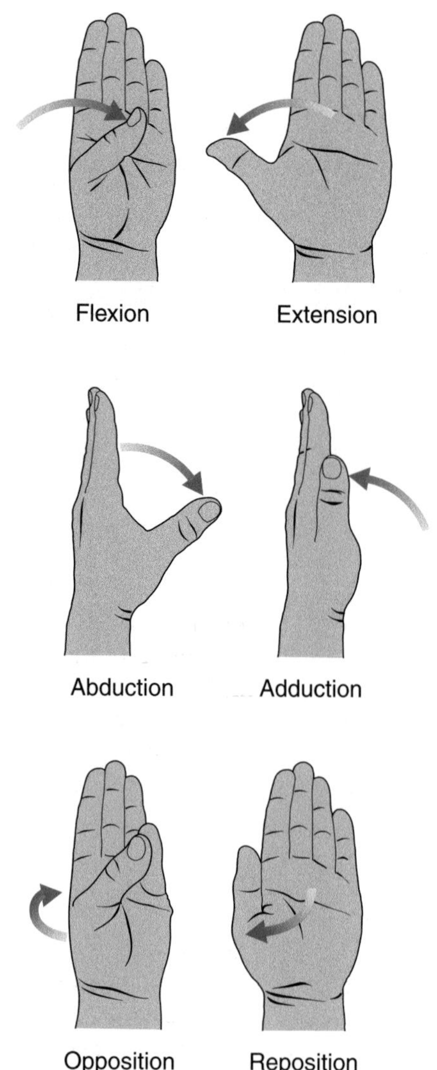

Figure 13-3. Motions of the CMC joint of the thumb.

adduction occur in the sagittal plane (a plane *perpendicular* to the palm). In other words, with the forearm supinated and the palm facing up, the thumb moving side to side across the palm is flexion and extension. The thumb moving up toward the ceiling, away from the palm, is abduction, and its return is adduction. **Opposition** is a combination of flexion and abduction in which the tips of the first and fifth digits move toward one another, with the "built-in" accessory motion of rotation; **reposition,** using a combination of extension, adduction and "rotation," is the return to anatomical position.

Arthrokinematics

From an arthrokinematic perspective, during flexion and extension (frontal plane motion), the concave base of the first metacarpal glides in the same direction as the distal end of the metacarpal (concave-on-convex articulation). When flexion occurs, the base of the metacarpal glides medially while the distal end of the metacarpal also glides medially. During extension, the base glides laterally, along with lateral movement of the distal metacarpal.

When abduction and adduction (sagittal plane motion) occur, the convex base of the first metacarpal glides on the concave trapezium in the opposite direction from the distal end of the metacarpal (convex-on-concave articulation). During abduction, the distal end of the metacarpal moves anteriorly while the base of the metacarpal glides posteriorly, whereas adduction causes posterior movement of the distal end of the metacarpal with an anterior glide of the base.

The Metacarpophalangeal and Interphalangeal Joints

Although the CMC joint of the thumb is quite mobile, the MCP and IP joints are not. The **MCP joint** is a hinge joint that allows only flexion and extension, and is therefore a uniaxial joint. The **IP joint,** the only phalangeal joint of the thumb, also allows only flexion and extension. Note that *phalanx* is singular, and *phalanges* is plural.

Arthrokinematics

Arthrokinematically, both the MCP and IP joints have a concave-on-convex articulation where the concave base on the proximal end of the distal segment articulates with the convex head on the distal end of the proximal segment. This causes the concave joint surface to glide in the same direction as the distal end of the bony segment during movement.

Joint Structure and Motions of the Fingers

The second, third, fourth, and fifth digits, commonly known as the *index, middle, ring,* and *little fingers,* respectively, have four joints each. These joints are the CMC joint, MCP joint, proximal interphalangeal (PIP) joint, and distal interphalangeal (DIP) joint (see Fig. 13-1).

The Carpometacarpal Joints

The **CMC joints** of the fingers (digits 2 to 5) are classified as nonaxial, plane-shaped synovial joints that provide slight gliding motion. Actually, they provide more stability than mobility. The trapezoid articulates with the base of the second metacarpal, the capitate with the base of the third metacarpal, and the hamate with the bases of the fourth and fifth metacarpals (Fig. 13-4). The second and third CMC joints have very little mobility. The fourth CMC joint allows slightly more motion. The fifth CMC joint is the most mobile of the fingers because of its more condyloid shape, which allows for a small amount of **fifth finger opposition.** It does not, however, allow as much opposition as the thumb (the first CMC joint).

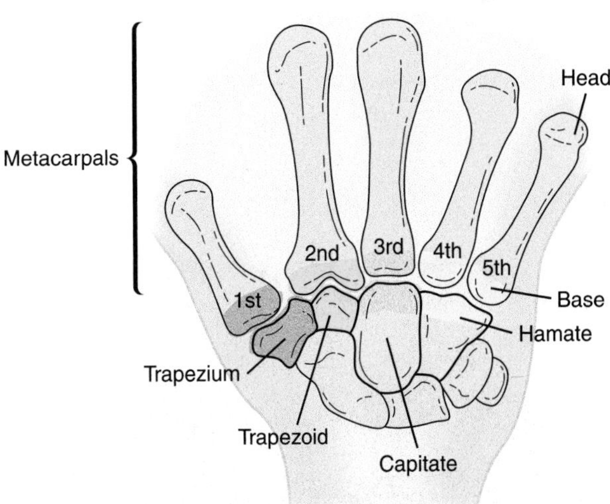

Figure 13-4. Carpometacarpal (CMC) joints of the thumb and fingers (posterior view). Note that the trapezium articulates with the first metacarpal, the trapezoid with the second metacarpal, the capitate with the third metacarpal, and the hamate with the fourth and fifth metacarpals.

This can be demonstrated with your hand in a fist, your forearm supinated and your elbow flexed. Note that with a relaxed fist, the metacarpal heads are essentially in a straight line. When you make a tight fist, the fifth metacarpal moves a great deal, and the fourth metacarpal moves to a lesser extent, while the second and third metacarpals remain stationary. This movement seen at the metacarpals is actually a result of the gliding occurring at the CMC joints.

The Metacarpophalangeal Joints

The **MCP joints** of the fingers are formed by the concave-shaped bases of the proximal phalanges articulating with the convex, rounded heads of the metacarpals (see Figs. 13-1 and 4-6). These are commonly referred to as the "knuckles." They are biaxial condyloid joints with two degrees of freedom, allowing flexion, extension, and hyperextension, plus abduction and adduction (Fig. 13-5). The middle finger is the point of reference for abduction and adduction. **Abduction** occurs when the second, fourth, and fifth fingers move away from the middle (third) finger. **Adduction** is the return from abduction and occurs with the second, fourth, and fifth fingers. There is no adduction of the middle finger, only abduction occurring in either direction.

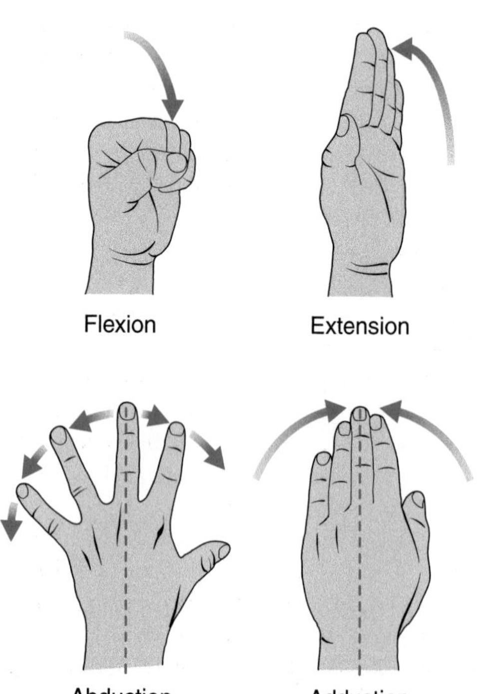

Figure 13-5. Motions of the metacarpophalangeal (MCP) joints and fingers.

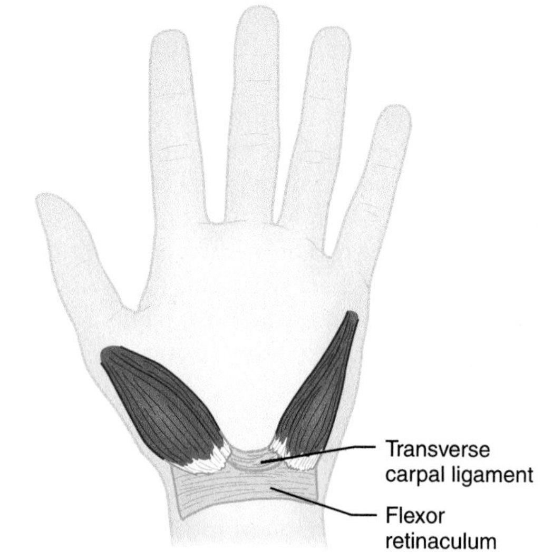

Figure 13-6. The flexor retinaculum is made up of the palmar and transverse carpal ligaments (anterior view).

Arthrokinematics

In analyzing arthrokinematic motion, the MCP joints have a concave-on-convex articulation, in that the concave base of the proximal phalanges will move in the same direction as the distal end of the proximal phalanges during movement. Therefore, the base of the proximal phalanx glides anteriorly during flexion and posteriorly during extension, medially (toward the midline of the hand) during adduction, and laterally (away from the midline of the hand) during abduction, while the distal end of the proximal phalanx moves in the same direction with all of these motions.

The Interphalangeal Joints

There are two **interphalangeal joints** in each finger. The **PIP joint** is the articulation between the base of the middle phalanx and the head of the proximal phalanx. The **DIP joint** is formed by the base of the distal phalanx articulating with the head of the middle phalanx. Both the PIP and DIP joints are uniaxial hinge joints allowing only flexion and extension, which occurs in the sagittal plane. They are all concave-on-convex articulations, with the mechanics of their arthrokinematic movements being identical to that of the IP joint of the thumb. A summary of the joints of the hand can be found in Table 13-1.

Arthrokinematics

Given that the hinge joint structure yields a concave-on-convex articulation at the majority of finger and thumb joints (see Table 13-1), the arthrokinematic movement

Table 13-1 Summary of Joints of the Hand

Joint	Joint Classification	Osteokinematic Movement	Plane of Motion
Nonaxial Joints			
CMC joints (digits 2 to 5)	Plane	Gliding/sliding	
Uniaxial Joints			
MCP joint (digit 1)	Hinge	Flexion/extension	Oblique
IP joint (digit 1)	Hinge	Flexion/extension	Oblique
PIP joints (digits 2 to 5)	Hinge	Flexion/extension	Sagittal
DIP joints (digits 2 to 5)	Hinge	Flexion/extension	Sagittal
Joints			
CMC joint (digit 1)	Saddle	Flexion/extension	Frontal
		Abduction/adduction	Sagittal
MCP joints (digits 2 to 5)	Condyloid	Flexion/extension	Sagittal
		Abduction/adduction	Frontal

is the same for all of these joints. The base of the more distal segment must glide anteriorly during flexion, and posteriorly during extension, moving with the distal end of the bony segment. When joint mobilizations are performed to restore motion that is limited, an anterior glide is performed to increase flexion, and a posterior glide is used to increase extension.

Bones and Landmarks

Although the thumb and fingers have essentially the same bony structure, there is one major difference. The thumb has two phalanges, whereas the fingers each have three. This feature makes the thumb shorter, allowing opposition to be more functional.

Therefore, the hand, made up of the thumb and four fingers, has five metacarpals, five proximal phalanges, and five distal phalanges, but only four middle phalanges (see Fig. 13-1). There are no significant landmarks on these bones other than the bone ends. The proximal end of the metacarpals and phalanges is called the *base,* and the distal end is called the *head.* It should be noted that the bases of all phalanges are concave, and the heads of all phalanges and metacarpals are convex. There is one indistinct landmark on the forearm, the oblique line which is sometimes referred to when describing muscle attachments.

Landmark of the Forearm

Oblique Line

Located on the anterior surface of the radius from below the tuberosity, running diagonally to approximately midradius

Ligaments and Other Structures

Although there are numerous structures in the hand, only a few of those more commonly referred to will be described here. The **flexor retinaculum** is a fibrous band of connective tissue that spans the anterior surface of the wrist in a mediolateral (horizontal) direction (Fig. 13-6). It attaches to the styloid processes of the radius and ulna and crosses over the flexor muscle tendons. Its main function is to hold these tendons close to the wrist, thus preventing the tendons from pulling away from the wrist (bowstringing) when the wrist flexes. It also prevents the two sides of the carpal bones from spreading apart or separating. In the construction world, this horizontal structure is called a "tie beam." Its distal border merges with the transverse carpal ligament.

The **palmar carpal ligament** is more proximal and superficial than the transverse carpal ligament. It attaches to the styloid processes of the radius and ulna and crosses over the flexor muscle tendons.

The **transverse carpal ligament** lies deeper and more distally. It attaches to the pisiform and hook of the hamate on the medial side and to the scaphoid and trapezium bones laterally. It arches over the carpal bones, forming a tunnel through which the median nerve and nine extrinsic flexor tendons of the fingers and thumb pass (four tendons each of the flexor digitorum superficialis and flexor digitorum profundus, and one tendon for the flexor pollicis longus). Figure 13-7 shows the bony floor of the carpal bones and the fibrous ceiling of the transverse carpal ligament. Together they form the tunnel through which the tendons and nerve pass. The figure also shows the area of the hand innervated by the median nerve.

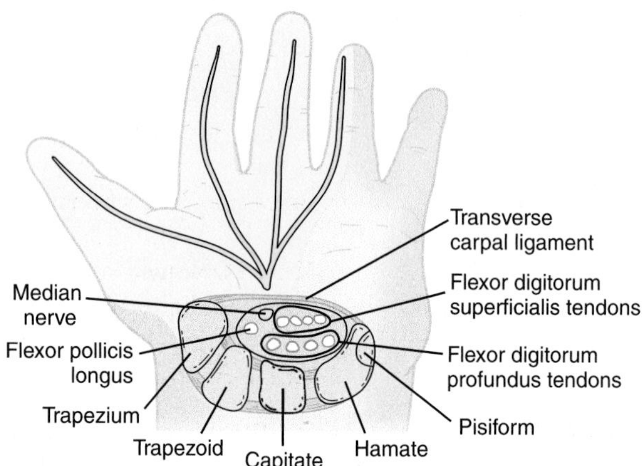

Figure 13-7. Carpal tunnel (anterior superior view): formed by the bony floor of the carpal bones and the fibrous ceiling of the transverse carpal ligament. The scaphoid, providing some lateral attachment of the ligament, is not visible from this view as it is positioned distal to (in this drawing, behind) the trapezium.

The **extensor retinaculum ligament** is a fibrous band traversing the posterior side of the wrist in a horizontal mediolateral direction (Fig. 13-8). It attaches medially to the styloid process of the ulna and to the triquetrum, pisiform, and lateral side of the radius. It holds the extensor tendons close to the wrist, especially during wrist extension.

The **extensor expansion ligament,** also called the *extensor hood* (Fig. 13-9), is a small, triangular, flat aponeurosis covering the dorsum and sides of the proximal phalanx of each finger. The extensor digitorum tendon blends into the expansion. The extensor expansion is wider at its base over the MCP joint, actually wrapping over the sides somewhat. As it approaches the PIP joint, the expansion is joined by tendons of the lumbricals and interosseus muscles. It narrows toward its distal end at the base of the distal phalanx. The extensor digitorum, lumbricals, and interosseus muscles form an attachment to the middle or distal phalanx by way of this expansion. The **extensor hood** area, formed by the extensor expansion proximally, covers the head of the metacarpal and keeps the extensor tendon in the midline.

When the hand is relaxed, the palm assumes a cupped position. This palmar concavity is due to the arrangement of the bony skeleton reinforced by ligaments. There are three arches that are responsible for this shape (Fig. 13-10). The **proximal carpal arch** is formed by the proximal end of the metacarpals (base) and carpal bones and is maintained by the flexor retinaculum (see Fig. 13-6). The shallower **distal carpal arch** is made up of the metacarpal heads. The **longitudinal arch** begins at the wrist and runs the length of the metacarpal and

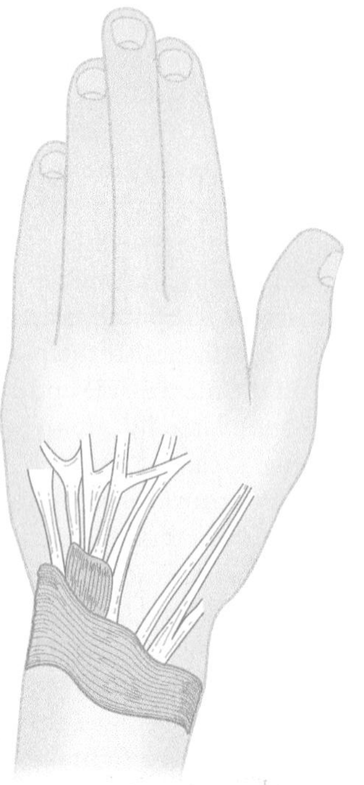

Figure 13-8. Extensor retinaculum (posterior view).

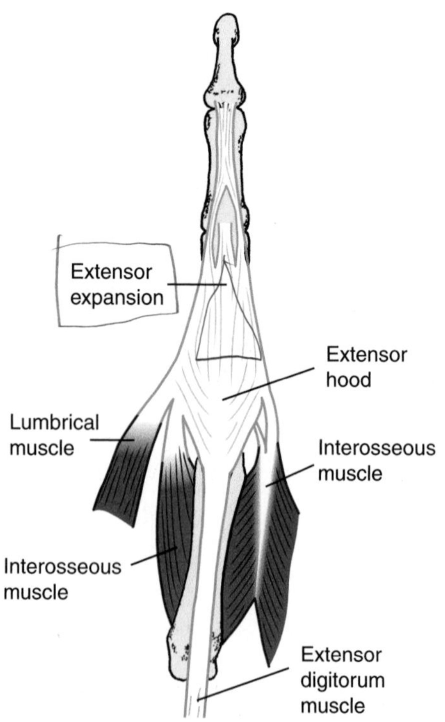

Figure 13-9. The extensor expansion provides an attachment on the middle and/or distal phalanx for several muscles (posterior view).

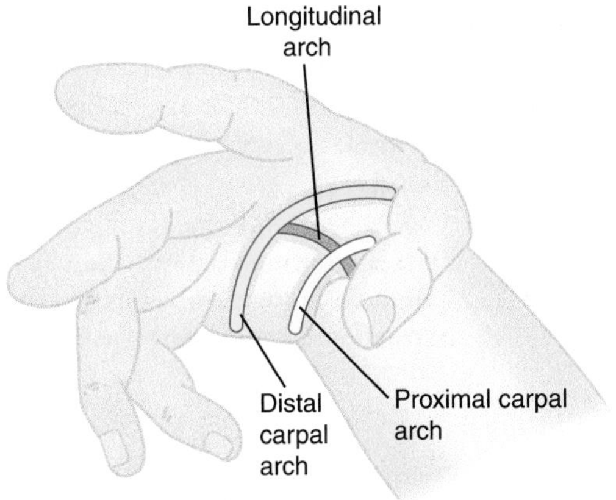

Figure 13-10. Three arches in palm of the hand.

phalanges for each digit. It is perpendicular to the other two arches. These arches contribute to the function of the various grasps described at the end of this chapter.

Muscles of the Thumb and Fingers

Any muscle spanning the anterior aspect of the finger or the anteromedial aspect of the thumb will pull the anterior surfaces together, causing flexion. Muscles crossing the posterior aspect of the fingers or the posterolateral aspect of the thumb will cause extension.

It is helpful to keep some generalizations in mind when learning the muscles of the hand. First, their names give much information about function and location. For example, it is rather easy to distinguish the muscles having a function on the thumb because *pollicis* means "thumb" and *digitorum* means "digits (fingers)" in Latin. Second, if the muscle has "longus" in its name, it implies that there is a counterpart "brevis" muscle. The "longus" muscle either runs out to the distal phalanges or originates more proximally than its "brevis" counterpart. Third, keep in mind that a muscle can only move the joints it crosses. By looking at the specific joints that each hand muscle crosses, we can determine at what joints a muscle will have an action.

Extrinsic Muscles

In addition to the wrist muscles previously described, there are several other muscles that span the wrist and cross the joints in the hand. These muscles are called **extrinsic muscles** of the hand because their proximal attachment is above, or proximal to, the wrist joint. They have an assistive role in wrist function, but their primary function is at the thumb or finger. The extrinsic muscles are as follows:

Anterior	Posterior
Flexor digitorum superficialis	Abductor pollicis longus
Flexor digitorum profundus	Extensor pollicis brevis
Flexor pollicis longus	Extensor pollicis longus
	Extensor digitorum
	Extensor indicis
	Extensor digiti minimi

The **flexor digitorum superficialis** muscle lies deep to the wrist flexors and palmaris longus muscle (Fig. 13-11). Its broad proximal attachment is part of the common flexor tendon on the medial epicondyle of the humerus. It also has an attachment on the coronoid process of the ulna and the oblique line of the radius. It divides into four tendons and crosses the wrist with one tendon going to each finger. Each distal attachment splits into two parts and attaches on each side of the middle phalanx of each finger (Fig. 13-12). Its primary action is to flex the PIP and then MCP joints of the second through fifth fingers. This is an important muscle in the power grip.

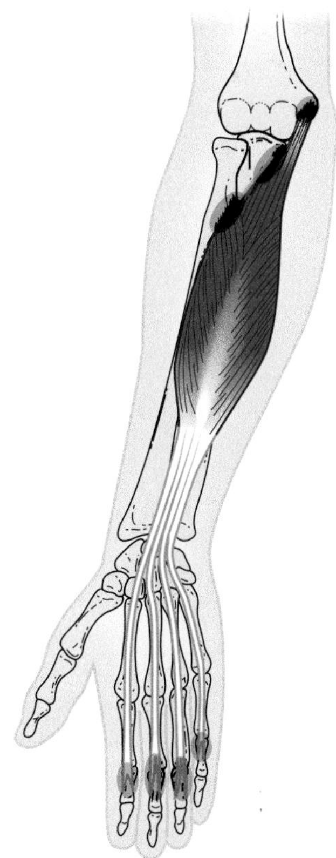

Figure 13-11. Flexor digitorum superficialis muscle (anterior view).

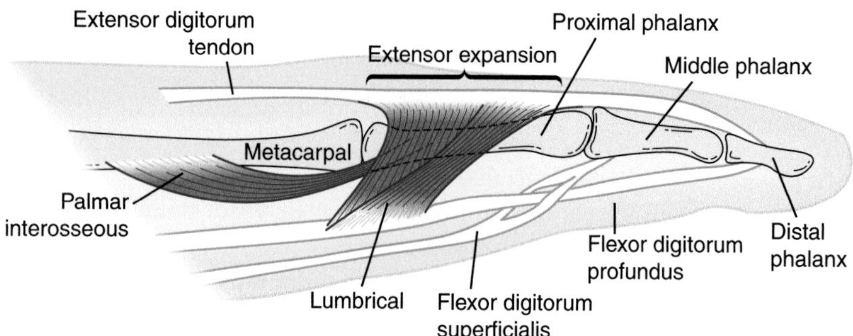

Figure 13-12. Side view of a digit showing tendon relationship of the flexor digitorum superficialis with the flexor digitorum profundus and the two flexor tendons with the extensor digitorum tendon.

Flexor Digitorum Superficialis Muscle

O	Common flexor tendon on the medial epicondyle, coronoid process, and radius
I	Sides of the middle phalanx of the four fingers
A	Flexes the PIP and MCP joints of the fingers
N	Median nerve (C7, C8, T1)

The **flexor digitorum profundus muscle** lies deep to the flexor digitorum superficialis muscle; these two muscles traverse the forearm and hand together (Fig. 13-13).

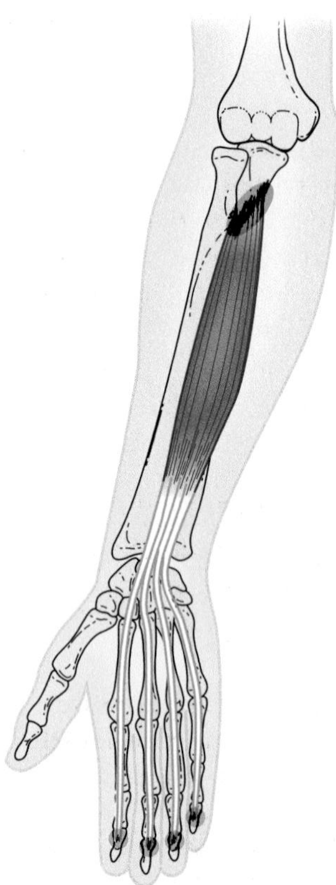

Figure 13-13. Flexor digitorum profundus muscle (anterior view).

The profundus muscle has its proximal attachment on the ulna on the anterior and medial surfaces, from the coronoid process to approximately three-fourths of the way down the ulna. It runs beneath the flexor digitorum superficialis muscle until the superficialis tendon splits into two parts at its distal attachment. The profundus muscle tendon passes through this split and continues distally to attach at the base of the distal phalanx of the second through fifth fingers (see Fig. 13-12). Its action is to flex the DIP, then the PIP and MCP joints of the second through fifth fingers. This is the only muscle that flexes the DIP joints.

Flexor Digitorum Profundus Muscle

O	Upper three-fourths of the ulna
I	Distal phalanx of the four fingers
A	Flexes all three joints of the fingers (DIP, PIP, and MCP)
N	Median and ulnar nerves (C8, T1)

The **flexor pollicis longus muscle** is a deep muscle that has its proximal attachment on the anterior surface of the radius and interosseus membrane and its distal attachment at the base of the thumb's distal phalanx (Fig. 13-14). It is a prime mover in flexion of the IP joint of the thumb. It is the only muscle to do so. It also flexes the MCP and CMC joints of the thumb.

Flexor Pollicis Longus Muscle

O	Radius, anterior surface
I	Distal phalanx of thumb
A	Flexes all three joints of the thumb (IP, MCP, CMC)
N	Median nerve (C8, T1)

The **abductor pollicis longus muscle** is located deep on the posterior forearm (Fig. 13-15). It attaches to the radius just distal to the supinator, the interosseus membrane, and the middle portion of the ulna. It becomes superficial just proximal to crossing the wrist and

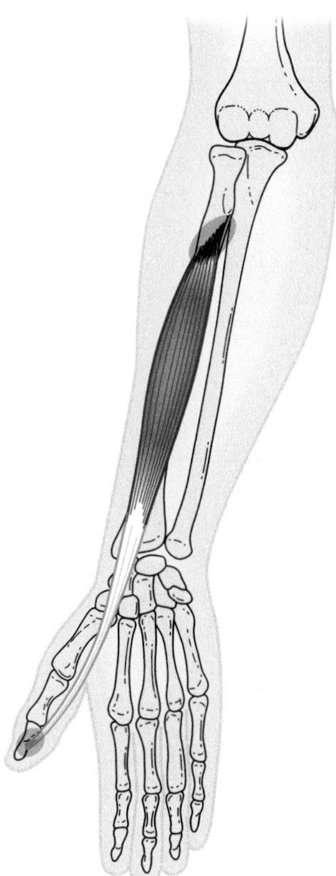

Figure 13-14. Flexor pollicis longus muscle (anterior view).

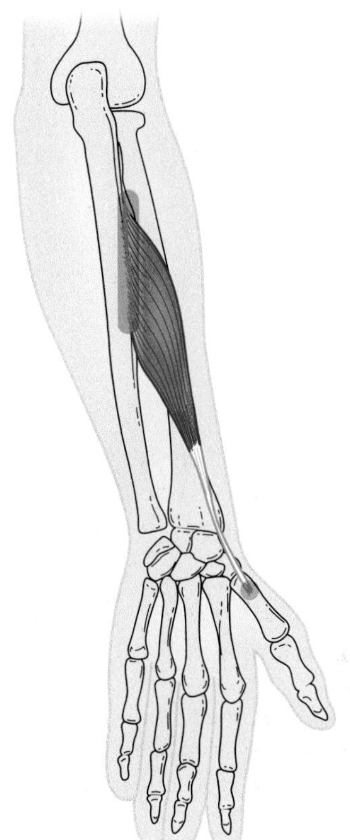

Figure 13-15. Abductor pollicis longus muscle (posterior view).

attaches to the base of the first metacarpal on the radial side. Although the abductor pollicis longus crosses the thumb's MCP joint, it only abducts the CMC joint because the MCP joint allows only flexion/extension. The thumb moves as one unit in the direction of abduction and adduction. Similarly, abduction of the thumb's CMC joint adducts the entire thumb. Therefore, in this text, when referring to thumb abduction, adduction, opposition, and reposition, it is implied that the action occurs at the CMC joint. Without the abductor pollicis longus, the thumb cannot be moved away from the palm. It also has a secondary action of extending the thumb.

Abductor Pollicis Longus Muscle	
O	Posterior radius, interosseus membrane, middle ulna
I	Base of the first metacarpal
A	Abducts thumb (CMC)
N	Radial nerve (C6, C7)

The **extensor pollicis brevis muscle** is also located deep on the posterior forearm and spans the wrist just medial to the abductor pollicis longus muscle. Its proximal attachment is on the posterior radius near the distal end and just below the abductor pollicis longus muscle. Its distal attachment is on the posterior surface at the base of the thumb's proximal phalanx (Fig. 13-16). It functions to extend the MCP and CMC joints of the thumb. Without the function of this muscle, the thumb MCP joint remains in a flexed position.

Extensor Pollicis Brevis Muscle	
O	Posterior distal radius
I	Base of the proximal phalanx of thumb
A	Extends MCP and CMC joints of thumb
N	Radial nerve (C6, C7)

The **extensor pollicis longus muscle** is located near the two previously mentioned muscles, deep on the posterior forearm. Its proximal attachment is on the middle third of the ulna and interosseus membrane (Fig. 13-17). Like the other two muscles, it becomes superficial just before crossing the wrist. Its distal attachment is at the base of the thumb's distal phalanx, on the posterior side. It functions to extend the

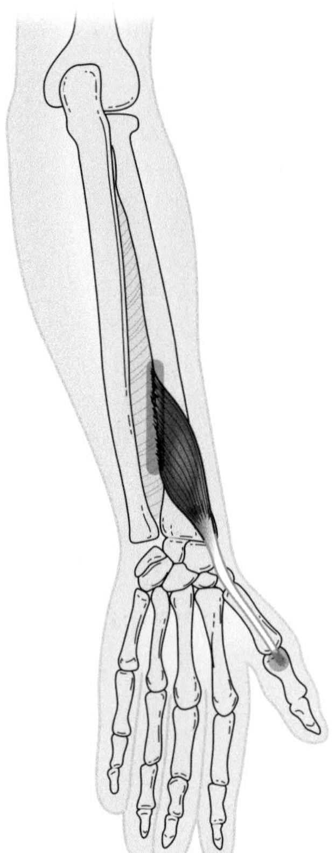

Figure 13-16. Extensor pollicis brevis muscle (posterior view).

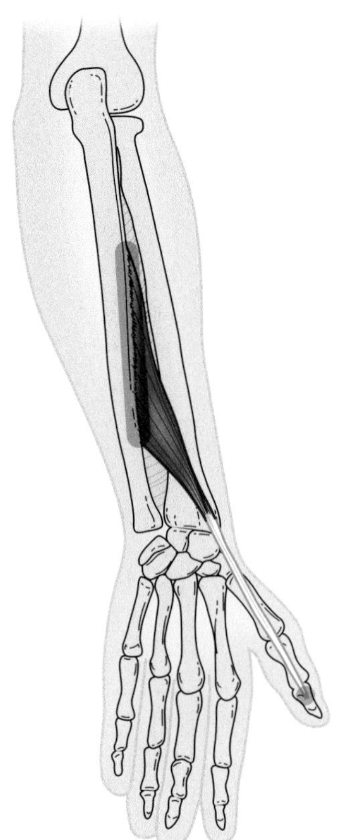

Figure 13-17. Extensor pollicis longus muscle (posterior view).

IP, MCP, and CMC joints of the thumb. We use this muscle to pull the thumb back when a flat and open hand is needed. An example of this is clapping.

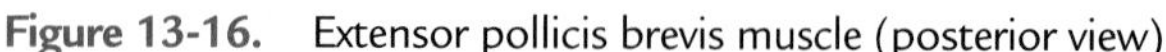

Extensor Pollicis Longus Muscle

O	Middle posterior ulna and interosseus membrane
I	Base of distal phalanx of thumb
A	Extends all three joints of the thumb (IP, MCP, and CMC)
N	Radial nerve (C6, C7, C8)

If you extend your thumb, you will notice that a depression is formed between what appears to be two tendons. Actually, there are three tendons. The abductor pollicis longus and extensor pollicis brevis muscles form the lateral border, and the extensor pollicis longus muscle forms the medial border. This depression is called the **anatomical snuffbox** (Fig. 13-18).

The **extensor digitorum muscle** is a superficial muscle on the posterior forearm and hand (Fig. 13-19). It attaches proximally to the lateral epicondyle of the humerus as part of the common extensor tendon. It passes under the extensor retinaculum to attach distally on the distal phalanx of the second through fifth fingers via the extensor expansion (see Fig. 13-12). In the area of the metacarpals are interconnecting bands joining the four extensor digitorum tendons. These interconnecting bands limit independent finger extension. The extensor digitorum muscle is the only common extensor muscle of the fingers. It extends the DIP, PIP, and MCP joints of the second, third, fourth, and fifth fingers.

Extensor Digitorum Muscle

O	Lateral epicondyle of the humerus
I	Base of distal phalanx of the second through fifth fingers
A	Extends all three joints of the fingers (DIP, PIP, and MCP)
N	Radial nerve (C6, C7, C8)

The **extensor indicis muscle** is a deep muscle that has its proximal attachment on the posterior surface of the distal ulna (Fig. 13-20). It crosses the wrist under the extensor retinaculum medial to the extensor digitorum muscle and attaches into the extensor expansion of the

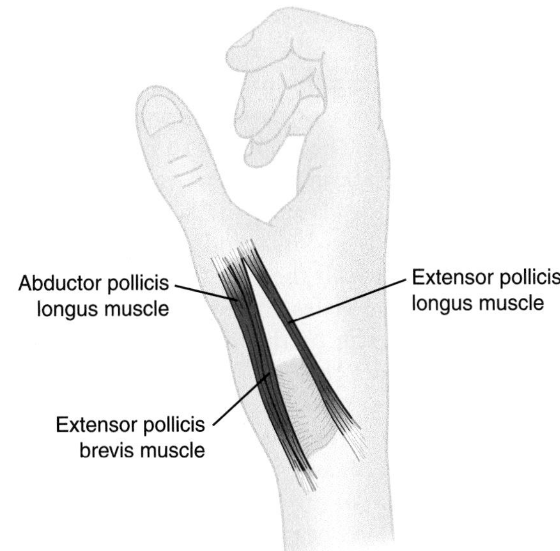

Figure 13-18. The borders of the anatomical snuffbox are defined by the tendon of the extensor pollicis longus muscle on one side and the tendons of the abductor pollicis longus and brevis muscles on the other side (side view).

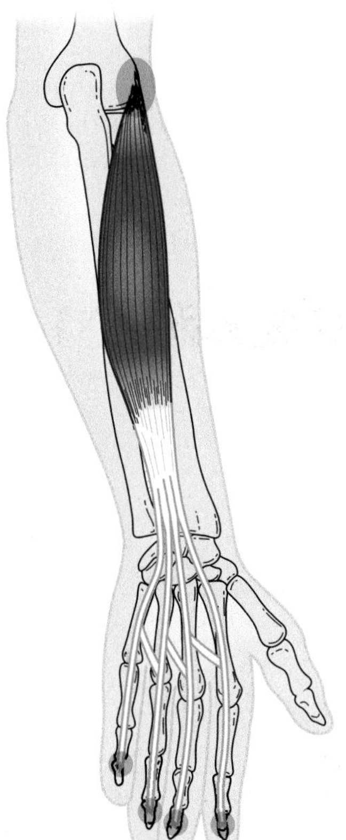

Figure 13-19. Extensor digitorum muscle (posterior view).

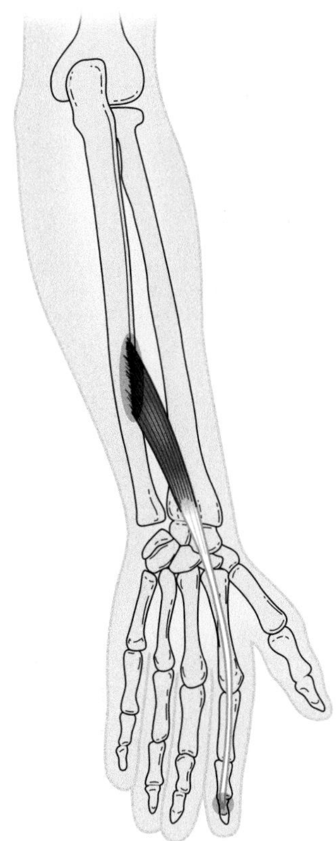

Figure 13-20. Extensor indicis muscle (posterior view).

second finger along with the extensor digitorum muscle. It extends the DIP, PIP, and MCP joints of the index finger. This allows us to point with our index finger while the other fingers are in a fist.

Extensor Indicis Muscle	
O	Distal ulna
I	Base of distal phalanx of the second finger
A	Extends all three joints of the second finger (DIP, PIP, MCP)
N	Radial nerve (C6, C7, C8)

The **extensor digiti minimi muscle** is a long, narrow muscle (Fig. 13-21) that is deep to the extensor digitorum and extensor carpi ulnaris muscles near its proximal attachment. It becomes superficial before crossing the wrist. It comes off the common extensor tendon on the lateral epicondyle of the humerus, crosses the wrist under the extensor retinaculum and attaches to the base of the distal phalanx of the fifth finger via the extensor expansion. It is a prime mover in extending the DIP, PIP, and MCP joints of the fifth finger. It makes possible isolated extension of the fifth finger.

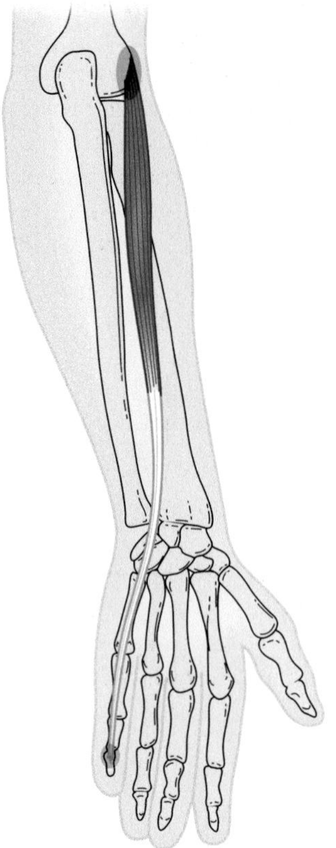

Figure 13-21. Extensor digiti minimi muscle (posterior view).

Extensor Digiti Minimi Muscle

O	Lateral epicondyle of humerus
I	Base of distal phalanx of fifth finger
A	Extends all three joints of fifth finger (DIP, PIP, MCP)
N	Radial nerve (C6, C7, C8)

In review, the extrinsic muscles have their proximal attachment above the wrist and their distal attachment on the hand. Because they cross the wrist, they could have a function there; however, any wrist function is usually assistive at best. The prime function of the extrinsic muscles is in moving the fingers or thumb. Usually the muscle is strongest at the most distal joint it moves.

Intrinsic Muscles

Intrinsic muscles have their proximal attachment at or distal to the carpal bones and have a function on the thumb or fingers. These muscles are responsible for the hand's fine motor control and precision movement. The intrinsic muscles can be further divided into the thenar, hypothenar, and deep palm muscles. The **thenar muscles** are those that function to move the thumb. They form the thenar eminence, or ball of the thumb. The **deep palm muscles** are located deep in the palm of the hand between the thenar and hypothenar muscles. They perform some of the more intricate motions that usually involve multiple muscles. These muscles are the adductor pollicis, the interossei (of which there are four dorsal and three palmar), and the lumbricals (of which there are also four muscles). The **hypothenar muscles,** forming the hypothenar eminence, act primarily on the little finger. Table 13-2 summarizes the three groups of intrinsic muscles.

In the thenar group, the **flexor pollicis brevis muscle** is a relatively superficial muscle. It attaches proximally to the trapezium and the flexor retinaculum and distally to the base of the proximal phalanx of the thumb (Fig. 13-22). Its primary actions are to flex the MCP and CMC joints of the thumb.

Flexor Pollicis Brevis Muscle

O	Trapezium and flexor retinaculum
I	Proximal phalanx of the thumb
A	Flexes the MCP and CMC joints of thumb
N	Median nerve (C6, C7)

The **abductor pollicis brevis muscle** lies just lateral to the flexor pollicis brevis muscle. It attaches proximally to the flexor retinaculum, scaphoid, and trapezium, and distally to the base of the thumb's proximal phalanx (Fig. 13-23). It acts to abduct the CMC joint of the thumb. It also has a secondary role in flexing the thumb at the MCP and CMC joints.

Abductor Pollicis Brevis Muscle

O	Scaphoid, trapezium, and flexor retinaculum
I	Proximal phalanx of the thumb
A	Abducts the thumb (CMC joint)
N	Median nerve (C6, C7)

Table 13-2 Intrinsic Muscles of the Hand

Thenar	Deep Palm	Hypothenar
Flexor pollicis brevis	Adductor pollicis	Flexor digiti minimi
Abductor pollicis brevis	Interossei	Abductor digiti minimi
Opponens pollicis	Lumbricals	Opponens digiti minimi

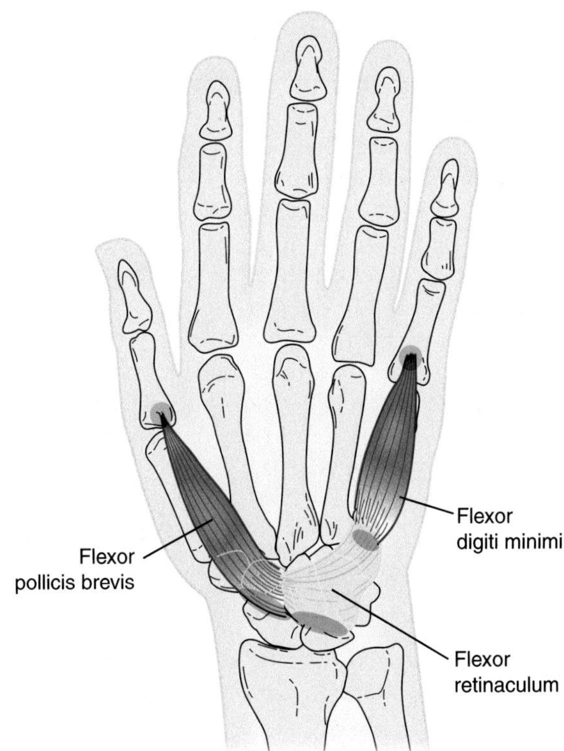

Figure 13-22. Flexor pollicis brevis and flexor digiti minimi muscles (anterior view).

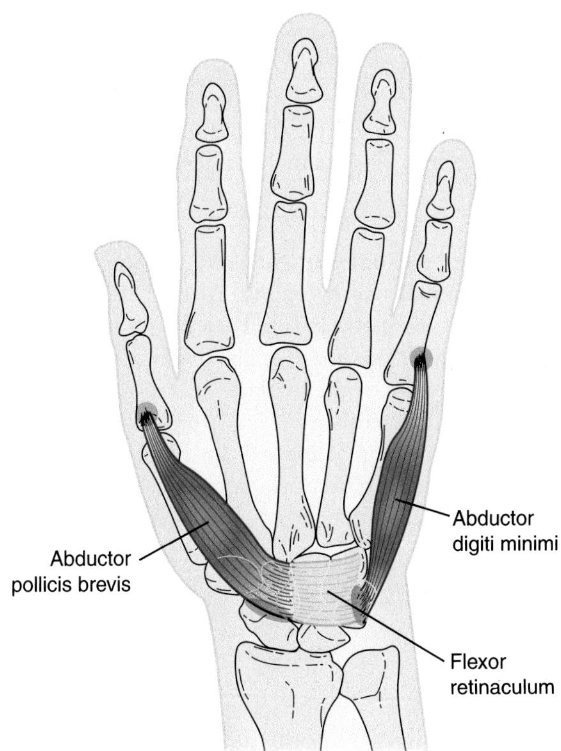

Figure 13-23. Abductor pollicis brevis and abductor digiti minimi muscles (anterior view).

The **opponens pollicis muscle** lies deep to the abductor pollicis brevis muscle. It attaches proximally to the trapezium and flexor retinaculum and distally to the entire lateral surface of the first metacarpal (Fig. 13-24). Its primary function is to oppose the thumb. Remember, this action occurs at the CMC joint. Loss of thumb opposition is caused by damage to the median nerve and is referred to as "ape hand deformity."

Opponens Pollicis Muscle	
O	Trapezium and flexor retinaculum
I	First metacarpal
A	Opposes the thumb (CMC joint)
N	Median nerve (C6, C7)

Thumb opposition is perhaps the most important function of the hand. Because it is a combination of flexion, abduction, and rotation of the thumb, other muscles such as the flexor pollicis brevis and abductor pollicis muscles assist in this function.

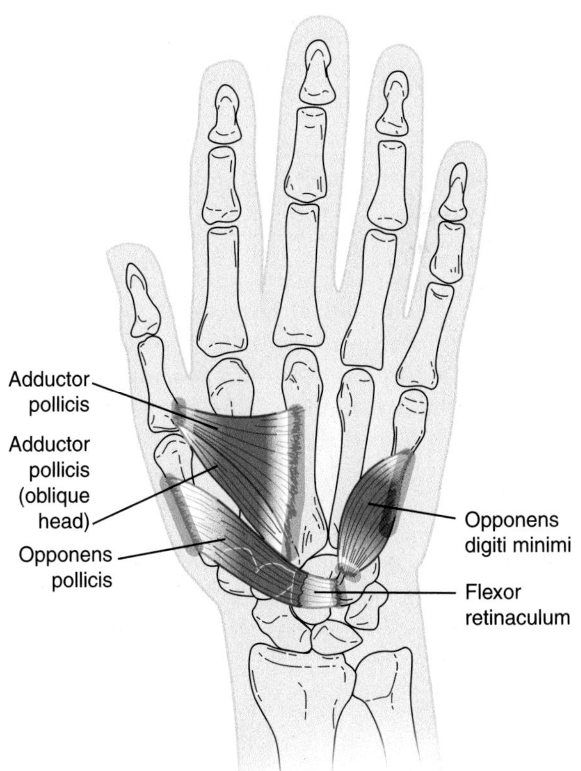

Figure 13-24. Opponens pollicis, adductor pollicis, and opponens digiti minimi muscles (anterior view). Note that the attachments of the oblique head of the adductor pollicis on the bases of the second and third metacarpals and the capitate cannot be seen as they are deep to the opponens pollicis.

The muscles located in the area between the thenar and hypothenar muscle groups are often called the **deep palm group,** or the *intermediate group*. The adductor pollicis muscle is sometimes placed in this group because it is located deep within the palm. Other sources place it with the thenar group because of its action on the thumb. It is placed here in the deep palm group for perhaps no other reason than to discuss the intrinsic muscles in groups of three!

The **adductor pollicis muscle** is a thumb muscle, although it is not usually considered part of the thenar group. This is because it is located deep and does not make up the muscle bulk of the thenar eminence. It actually has two heads. The oblique head has its proximal attachments on the capitate and bases of the second and third metacarpals. The transverse head arises from the distal two-thirds of the palmar surface of the third metacarpal. The fibers of the two heads unite to attach on the ulnar side of the base of the proximal phalanx of the thumb (see Fig. 13-24). As its name implies, its function is to adduct the thumb (at the CMC joint). It gives much power to grasp.

Adductor Pollicis Muscle

O	Capitate, bases of the second and third metacarpal, and distal two-thirds of the palmar surface of the third metacarpal
I	Base of proximal phalanx of thumb
A	Adducts thumb (CMC joint)
N	Ulnar nerve (C8, T1)

There are two sets of interosseus muscles: dorsal and palmar. There are four **dorsal interosseus** muscles. They each attach proximally to two adjacent metacarpals and distally to the base of the proximal phalanx (Fig. 13-25). Table 13-3 summarizes the attachments and actions of each of the dorsal interosseus muscles. Their action is to abduct the second, third, and fourth fingers at the MCP joint. The third digit has two dorsal interosseus muscles, one on either side of the proximal phalanx. This allows the third digit to abduct in either direction. The fifth finger is abducted by the abductor digiti minimi. The ulnar nerve innervates all dorsal interosseus muscles.

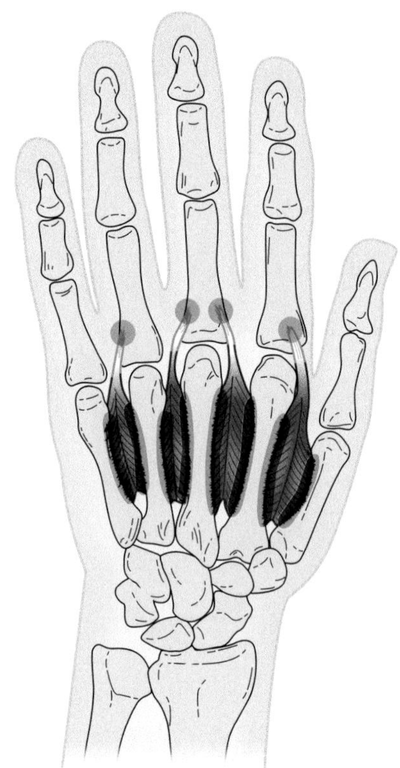

Figure 13-25. Dorsal interosseus muscles. Note that the middle finger has two attachments (posterior view).

Dorsal Interossei

O	Adjacent metacarpals
I	Base of proximal phalanx
A	Abduct fingers at MCP joint
N	Ulnar nerve (C8, T1)

There are three **palmar interosseus** muscles. They attach proximally to the palmar surface of the second, fourth, and fifth metacarpals. They do not attach to, or have a function on, the middle finger. Distally, they attach to the base of the phalanx of the same finger as the proximal attachment (Fig. 13-26). They pull the digits toward the midline of the hand, creating an adduction motion. These attachments are summarized in Table 13-4. Like the dorsal interosseus muscles, the

Table 13-3 Dorsal Interosseus Muscles of the Hand

Muscle	Proximal Attachment	Distal Attachment	Action
First	First and second metacarpals	Lateral side of index finger	Abduct index finger
Second	Second and third metacarpals	Lateral side of middle finger	Abduct middle finger laterally
Third	Third and fourth metacarpals	Medial side of middle finger	Abduct middle finger medially
Fourth	Fourth and fifth metacarpals	Medial side of ring finger	Abduct ring finger

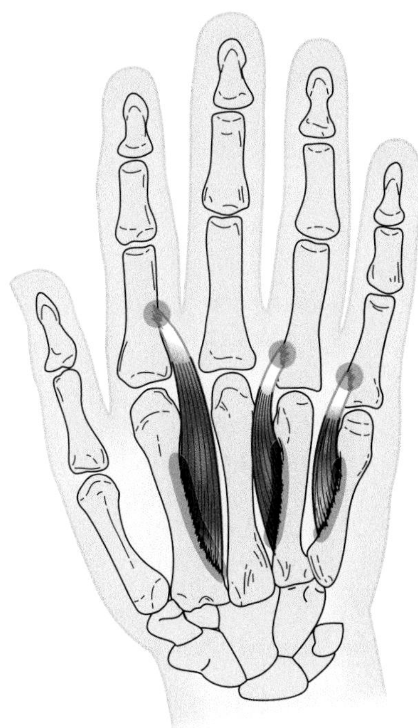

Figure 13-26. Palmar interossei muscles (anterior view). Note that the middle finger has no attachments.

palmar interosseus muscles are innervated by the ulnar nerve. Both the dorsal and palmar interossei play an important role in such activities as typing and playing the piano.

Palmar Interosseus Muscles

O	2nd, 4th, and 5th metacarpals
I	Base of respective proximal phalanx
A	Adduct fingers at MCP joint
N	Ulnar nerve (C8, T1)

As mentioned, the middle finger is the point of reference for abduction and adduction. Movement away from the middle finger is abduction, and movement toward it is adduction. Note that the middle finger abducts in two directions and therefore does not adduct.

The last muscle group to be discussed is rather unique. The **lumbricals,** of which there are four, have no bony attachment. They are located quite deep and attach only to tendons. Proximally, they attach to the tendon of the flexor digitorum profundus muscle, spanning the MCP joint anteriorly (Fig. 13-27). This allows them to flex the MCP joint. They then pass posteriorly at the proximal phalanx to attach to the tendinous expansion of the extensor digitorum muscle (Fig. 13-28). This allows them to extend the PIP and DIP joint. Therefore, their action is to flex the MCP joint and extend the PIP and DIP joints of the second through fifth fingers. This combined motion is referred to as the "tabletop position." Incidentally, the plural of *lumbrical* can be spelled with an "s" or "es."

Loss of lumbrical function will result in "claw hand," characterized by MCP hyperextension and PIP and DIP

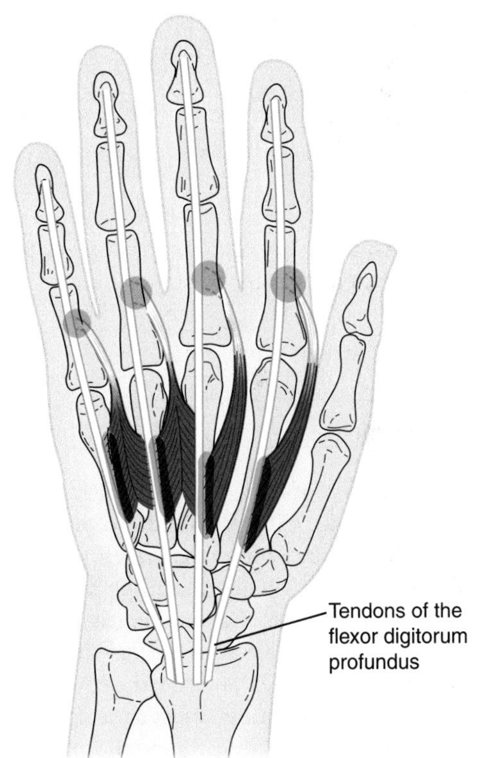

Figure 13-27. Lumbrical muscles (palmar view). Note that the distal attachment on the tendons of the extensor digitorum cannot be seen in this view.

Table 13-4 Palmar Interosseus Muscles

Muscles	Proximal Attachment	Distal Attachment	Action
Second	Second metacarpal	Medial side of index finger	Adduct index finger
Third	Fourth metacarpal	Lateral side of ring finger	Adduct ring finger
Fourth	Fifth metacarpal	Lateral side of little finger	Adduct little finger

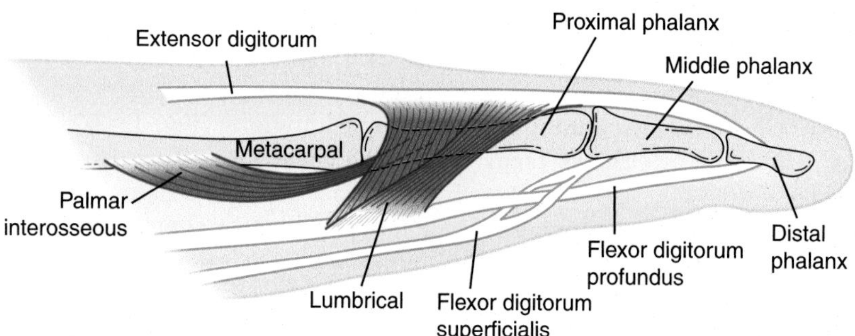

Figure 13-28. Lumbrical muscles (side view).

flexion (opposite positions from the lumbricals' actions). The lumbricals are innervated in part by the median and ulnar nerves. If the median nerve is involved affecting the first and second lumbricals, then only the second and third fingers will be involved. If the ulnar nerve is affected involving the third and fourth lumbricals, then the fourth and fifth fingers will assume this posture.

Lumbrical Muscles

O	Tendon of the flexor digitorum profundus muscle
I	Tendon of the extensor digitorum muscle
A	Flex the MCP joint while extending the PIP and DIP joints
N	First and second lumbricals: median nerve (C8, T1)
	Third and fourth lumbricals: ulnar nerve (C8, T1)

The counterpart to the thenar muscle group is the hypothenar group. The **flexor digiti minimi muscle** serves the same function on the little finger as the flexor pollicis brevis does on the thumb. It is attached proximally to the hook of the hamate and the flexor retinaculum, and distally to the base of the little finger's proximal phalanx (see Fig. 13-22). It flexes the MCP joint of that finger. Remember, although most thumb motion occurs at the CMC joint, most finger motion occurs at the MCP joint.

Flexor Digiti Minimi Muscle

O	Hamate and flexor retinaculum
I	Base of proximal phalanx of the fifth finger
A	Flexes MCP and CMC joints of the fifth finger
N	Ulnar nerve (C8, T1)

The **abductor digiti minimi muscle** lies superficially, just medial to the flexor digiti minimi muscle on the ulnar border of the hypothenar eminence. It attaches proximally to the pisiform and to the tendon of the flexor carpi ulnaris muscle and distally to the base of the proximal phalanx of the fifth finger (see Fig. 13-23). It abducts the MCP joint of that finger. By being able to abduct the fifth digit, one is able to increase one's grasp.

Abductor Digiti Minimi Muscle

O	Pisiform and tendon of flexor carpi ulnaris
I	Proximal phalanx of fifth finger
A	Abducts the MCP joint of the fifth finger
N	Ulnar nerve (C8, T1)

The **opponens digiti minimi muscle** lies deep to the other hypothenar muscles. Its proximal attachments, the hook of the hamate and the flexor retinaculum, are similar to the proximal attachments of the flexor digiti minimi muscle. Distally, it attaches to the ulnar border of the fifth metacarpal (see Fig. 13-24). Its primary action is in opposition of the fifth finger. This action occurs at the CMC joint.

Opponens Digiti Minimi Muscle

O	Hamate and flexor retinaculum
I	Fifth metacarpal
A	Opposes the fifth finger (CMC joint)
N	Ulnar nerve (C8, T1)

Anatomical Relationships

Describing the muscles of the hand in relation to each other is a rather involved process. It is difficult to separate wrist and hand extrinsic muscles. One must consider not only anterior and posterior groups, but also extrinsic and intrinsic muscles. We will start with the extrinsic muscles spanning the wrist anteriorly. The palmaris longus is the most superficial muscle, but it has no significant function. The tendons of the flexor digitorum superficialis are deep to it. The flexor digitorum profundus tendons are deep to both, essentially forming the third layer of extrinsic muscle tendons in the palm. The other extrinsic muscle on the anterior surface is the flexor pollicis longus, which crosses the wrist to attach on the thumb.

In Figure 13-29, remove the palmaris longus and look at the palm. On the fifth finger side and heading toward the thumb, you will see three intrinsic muscles that move the little finger: the opponens digiti minimi, the abductor digiti minimi, and the flexor digiti minimi. In the middle of the palm are the tendons of the flexor digitorum profundus (attaching on the distal phalanx of each finger), beneath the tendons of the flexor digitorum superficialis (attaching to either side of the middle phalanx of each finger). Each muscle has tendons going to the second, third, fourth, and fifth fingers. The flexor digitorum profundus gives rise to the proximal attachments of the lumbricals. Moving toward the thumb side, you will see the muscles that move the thumb–the adductor pollicis, flexor pollicis brevis, abductor pollicis brevis, and opponens pollicis–and the tendon of the flexor pollicis longus. Remove the tendons of the flexor digitorum superficialis and profundus, and you can see the deepest layer, the palmar interossei.

On the lateral and posterior side of the thumb, the extrinsic muscles are, in order of appearance, the abductor pollicis longus, the extensor pollicis brevis, and the extensor pollicis longus, which together make up the anatomical snuffbox (see Figs. 13-18 and 13-30). Next, and most superficial in the middle of the posterior forearm, are the extensor digitorum and extensor digiti minimi muscles (Fig. 13-30). Deep to the extensor digitorum above the wrist is the extensor indicis. The only intrinsic muscles (somewhat on the posterior side) are the dorsal interossei. They are actually located between the metacarpals, slightly more anterior than posterior. They are, however, deep to the extensor digitorum tendons below the wrist.

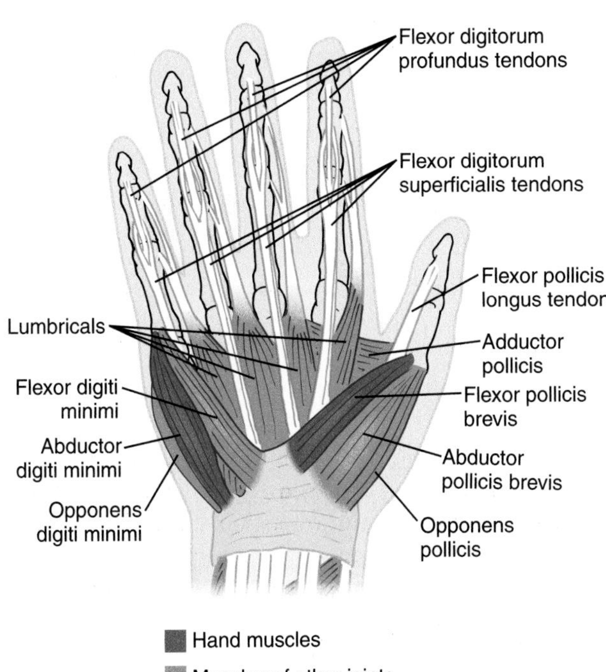

Figure 13-29. Anterior hand muscles.

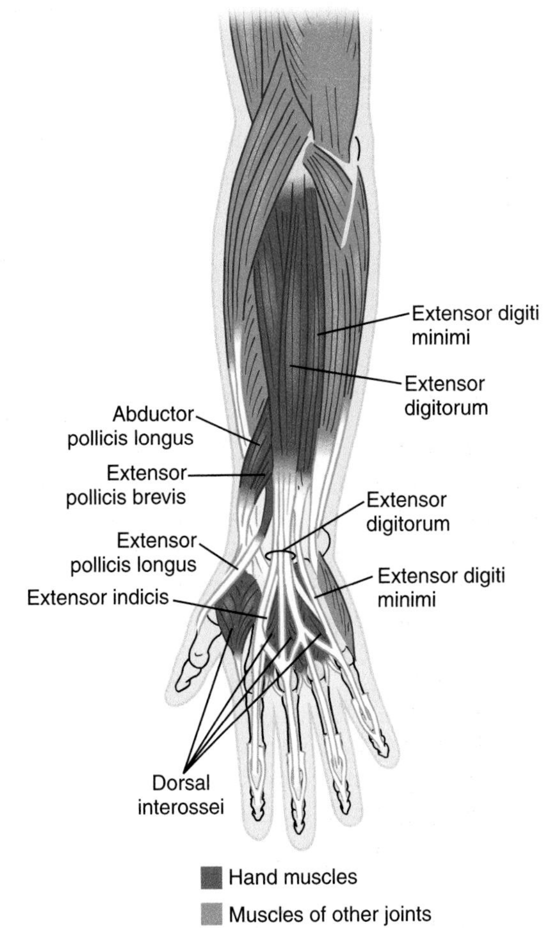

Figure 13-30. Posterior hand muscles.

Common Wrist and Hand Pathologies

Carpal tunnel syndrome is an extremely common condition caused by compression of the median nerve within the carpal tunnel. Symptoms include numbness and tingling in the hand, which often begins at night. Patients often complain of tingling, pain, and weakness in the hand, particularly in the thumb, index, and middle fingers. Tapping over the carpal tunnel often produces symptoms. Some, but not all, fibers of the transverse carpal ligament are often surgically cut to relieve the symptoms. If all fibers were cut, it would allow bowstringing of the extrinsic tendons on the flexor surface. **De Quervain's disease** is caused by an inflammation and thickening of the sheath containing the extensor pollicis brevis and abductor pollicis longus, resulting in pain on the radial side of the wrist. Because it is an inflammation of tendons and their surrounding sheaths, it is called a **tenosynovitis.** Making a fist with your thumb inside and then moving the wrist into ulnar deviation can elicit pain in those tendons and is considered a positive test. Care should be exercised in doing this test because it often causes some discomfort in a normal wrist.

Dupuytren's contracture occurs when the palmar aponeurosis undergoes a nodular thickening. It is most common in the area of the palm in line with the ring and little fingers. Often those fingers will develop flexion contractures. **Stenosing tenosynovitis,** commonly known as **trigger finger,** is a problem with the sliding mechanism of a tendon in its sheath. When a nodule or swelling of the sheath lining or the tendon develops, the tendon can no longer slide in and out smoothly. It may pass into the sheath when the finger flexes, but it becomes stuck as the finger attempts to extend. The finger can become locked in that position, and it must be manually extended. The flexor tendons of the middle and ring fingers are most commonly involved. **Skier's thumb,** a common hand injury among athletes, involves an acute tear of the ulnar collateral ligament of the thumb. **Gamekeeper's thumb** is an old term referring to a stretching injury of this same ligament developed over time by English gamekeepers as they twisted the necks of small game. Most injuries to the ulnar collateral ligament occur with a fall on an outstretched hand.

Swan neck deformity is characterized by flexion of the MCP joint, (hyper)extension of the PIP joint, and flexion of the DIP joint. With a **boutonnière deformity,** the deformity is in the opposite direction—extension of the MCP joint, flexion of the PIP joint, and extension of the DIP joint. **Ulnar drift** results in ulnar deviation of the fingers at the MCP joints. **Mallet finger** is caused by disruption of the extensor mechanism of the DIP joint, either because the tendon was severed or because the portion of bone where the tendon attached has avulsed from the distal phalanx. In either case, the distal phalanx remains in a flexed position and cannot be extended. The scaphoid is the most frequently injured carpal bone. A **scaphoid fracture** usually results from a fall on the outstretched hand of a younger person. Because of a poor vascular supply, it has a high incidence of avascular necrosis. **Kienböck's disease** refers to the necrosis of the lunate, which may develop after trauma.

Summary of Muscle Actions

The actions of the prime movers of the hand are summarized in Table 13-5.

Table 13-5 Prime Movers of the Hand

Action	Joint	Muscle
Thumb		
Flexion	MCP, CMC	Flexor pollicis brevis
	IP (MCP, CMC)	Flexor pollicis longus
Extension	MCP, CMC	Extensor pollicis brevis
	IP (MCP, CMC)	Extensor pollicis longus
Abduction	CMC	Abductor pollicis brevis, abductor pollicis longus
Adduction	CMC	Adductor pollicis
Opposition	CMC	Opponens pollicis
Reposition	CMC	Adductor pollicis, extensor pollicis longus, extensor pollicis brevis
Finger		
Flexion	MCP	Lumbricals, flexor digitorum superficialis, flexor digitorum profundus
	PIP	Flexor digitorum superficialis, flexor digitorum profundus
	DIP	Flexor digitorum profundus
Extension	MCP	Extensor digitorum, extensor indicis, extensor digiti minimi
	DIP and PIP	Lumbricals, extensor digitorum, extensor digiti minimi, extensor indicis
Abduction	MCP	Dorsal interossei, abductor digiti minimi
Adduction	MCP	Palmar interossei
Opposition (fifth)	CMC	Opponens digiti minimi

Summary of Muscle Innervation

Innervation of the hand is almost as straightforward as innervation of the wrist (Fig. 13-31). However, a few exceptions must be discussed. Similar to the wrist, muscles on the posterior surface of the hand are innervated mostly by the radial nerve. Anteriorly, muscles on the thumb side are supplied primarily by the median nerve, and muscles on the little finger side are supplied primarily by the ulnar nerve.

The adductor pollicis muscle appears to be the exception; it is innervated by the ulnar nerve rather than the median nerve like all the other thumb (pollicis) muscles. However, remember that the adductor pollicis muscle attaches in the middle of the palm to the third metacarpal (see Fig. 13-24). It is here that the ulnar nerve changes direction and runs toward the thumb. As it does, it sends branches to the adductor pollicis and dorsal and palmar interosseus muscles (see Fig. 6-27). The flexor digitorum profundus muscle receives its innervation from both the median and ulnar nerve, as do the lumbricals. This is not surprising, because the lumbricals have their proximal attachment on the tendons of the flexor digitorum profundus muscle. Table 13-6 further summarizes hand muscle innervation. This table shows that injury to the lower cervical vertebrae will affect all hand function. Table 13-7 summarizes the segmental innervation. Note that there is some discrepancy among various sources regarding the spinal cord level of innervation.

Hand Function

The human hand performs many functions. The primary function is grasp, or *prehension*. This means that the hand is designed to hold or manipulate objects. There are also many nonprehensile hand functions, such as expressing emotions, scratching, using a fist as a club, and using the open palm, as in pushing down on an armrest to assist in standing. Because no manipulative movement occurs with these types of activities, no further description of nonprehensile function will be made here.

With prehension (grasping or holding an object), the manner in which the hand is used depends on the size, shape, and weight of the object, how that object will be used, and the involvement of the proximal

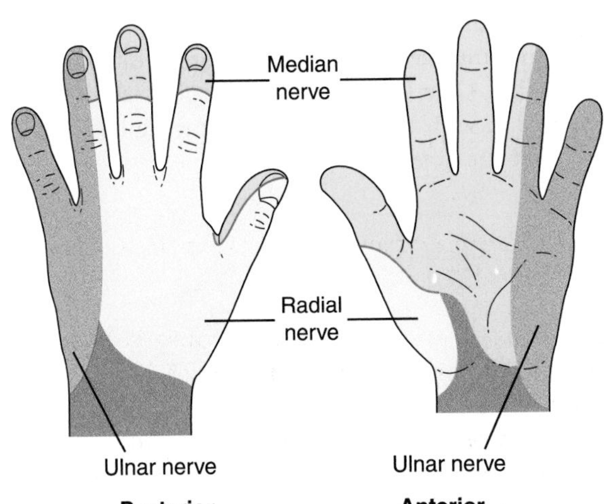

Figure 13-31. Sensory innervation of the hand. Motor innervation follows a similar pattern.

Table 13-6 Innervation of the Muscles of the Hand

Muscle	Nerve	Spinal Segment
Extensor digitorum	Radial	C6, C7, C8
Extensor indicis	Radial	C6, C7, C8
Extensor digiti minimi	Radial	C6, C7, C8
Extensor pollicis longus	Radial	C6, C7, C8
Extensor pollicis brevis	Radial	C6, C7
Abductor pollicis longus	Radial	C6, C7
Flexor digitorum superficialis	Median	C7, C8, T1
Flexor digitorum profundus 1 & 2	Median	C8, T1
4 & 5	Ulnar	C8, T1
Flexor pollicis longus	Median	C8, T1
Flexor pollicis brevis	Median	C6, C7
Abductor pollicis brevis	Median	C6, C7
Opponens pollicis	Median	C6, C7
Lumbricals 1 and 2	Median	C8, T1
Lumbricals 3 and 4	Ulnar	C8, T1
Flexor digiti minimi	Ulnar	C8, T1
Abductor digiti minimi	Ulnar	C8, T1
Opponens digiti minimi	Ulnar	C8, T1
Adductor pollicis	Ulnar	C8, T1
Dorsal and palmar interossei	Ulnar	C8, T1

Table 13-7 Segmental Innervation of the Hand

Spinal Cord Level	C6	C7	C8	T1
Extensor digitorum	X	X	X	
Extensor indicis	X	X	X	
Extensor digiti minimi	X	X	X	
Extensor pollicis longus	X	X	X	
Extensor pollicis brevis	X	X		
Abductor pollicis longus	X	X		
Abductor pollicis brevis	X	X		
Flexor pollicis brevis	X	X		
Opponens pollicis	X	X		
Flexor digitorum superficialis		X	X	X
Flexor digitorum profundus			X	X
Flexor pollicis longus			X	X
Lumbricals			X	X
Flexor digiti minimi			X	X
Abductor digiti minimi			X	X
Opponens digiti minimi			X	X
Adductor pollicis			X	X
Dorsal and palmar interossei			X	X

segments of the upper extremity. Generally speaking, the shoulder girdle and shoulder joint position the hand in space. The elbow allows the hand to move closer or farther away from the body, especially the face. The wrist provides stability while the hand is manipulating objects and is important in the tenodesis action described in Chapter 5. Although much attention tends to focus on the grasping aspect of hand function, release is equally important. Release is the role of the MCP, PIP, and DIP extensors. Without the ability to release, the hand's function is greatly diminished.

Of paramount importance to hand function is sensation. Without intact sensation, an individual must compensate with visual clues to find items, know what is being held, and how hard the object is being grasped. For example, if you were presented with a laundry bag full of clothes and told to find the small box of soap, you could feel around inside the bag until locating the soap. However, if your hand's sensation were not intact, you would have to empty the bag and visually search for the box. A person with an upper extremity amputation who uses a prosthetic device is a good example of having hand function without sensation. That person would need visual feedback to find the soap and to know if the terminal device had grasped it. Hand sensation is provided by the radial, ulnar, and median nerves. Figure 13-31 shows the pattern of sensory distribution. This distribution varies somewhat between individuals and is therefore presented with some variations between authors.

There is an optimal wrist and hand position for the hand to be most effective in terms of strength and precision. This position helps to maintain the optimal length of the extrinsic multijoint muscles and is called the **functional position of the hand.** In this position, the wrist is in a slightly hyperextended (dorsiflexed) position, the MCP and PIP joints of the fingers are slightly flexed, the thumb is in opposition, and the transverse and longitudinal arches are normal. Figure 13-32 illustrates this position. Maintenance of the thenar web is vital to thumb opposition.

Grasps

There are basically two types of prehension: power grips and precision grips. The activity dictates which grip is needed. A **power grip** is used when an object must be held forcefully while being moved about by more proximal joint muscles (holding a hammer or doorknob; Fig. 13-33). Often a power grip involves an isometric contraction with no movement occurring between the hand and the object being held.

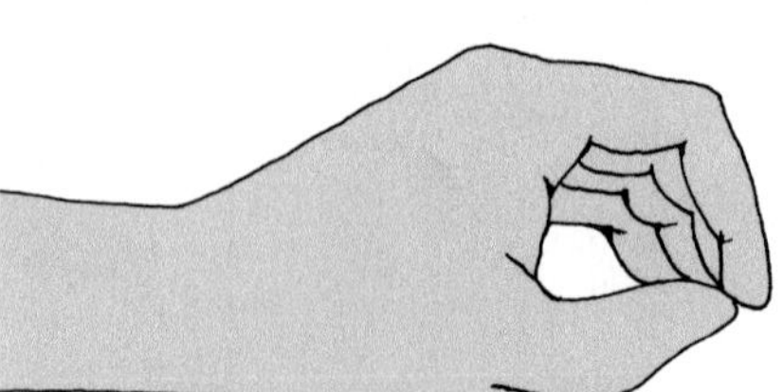

Figure 13-32. Functional position of the wrist and hand. The wrist is in slight hyperextension, the MCP and PIP joints are in some degree of flexion, and the thumb is in opposition.

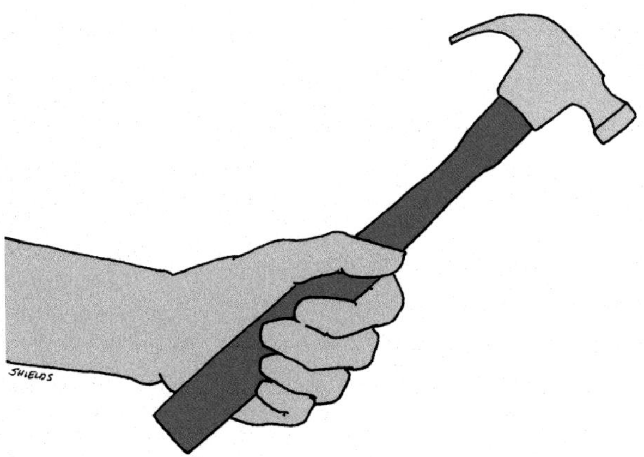

Figure 13-33. Power grip.

A **precision grip,** often referred to as *precision prehension,* is used when an object must be manipulated in a finer type movement, such as holding a pen or threading a needle (Fig. 13-34).

Power Grips

A power grip usually involves a significant amount of force and is considered the most powerful grip. The fingers tend to flex around the object in one direction and the thumb wraps around in the opposite direction, providing a counterforce to keep the object in contact with the palm or fingers. Once the object is firmly set in the hand, it can be moved about in space by more proximal joint musculature. The long finger flexors (extrinsics) grip the object, and the long finger extensors (also extrinsics) assist in holding the wrist in a neutral or slightly extended position. When the thumb is involved, it tends to be in an adducted position.

The three commonly described power grips are cylindrical, spherical, and hook. The **cylindrical grip** (Fig. 13-35) has all the fingers flexed around the object, which usually lies at a right angle to the forearm. The thumb is wrapped around the object in the opposite direction, often overlapping the fingers. Examples of a cylindrical grip would be holding a hammer, a racquet, or a wheelbarrow handle.

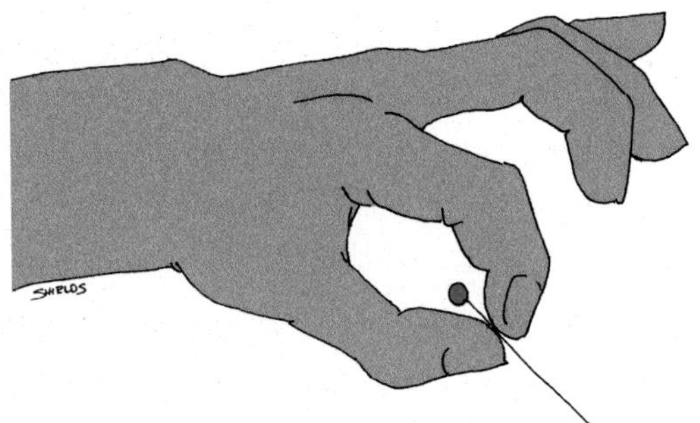

Figure 13-34. Precision grip.

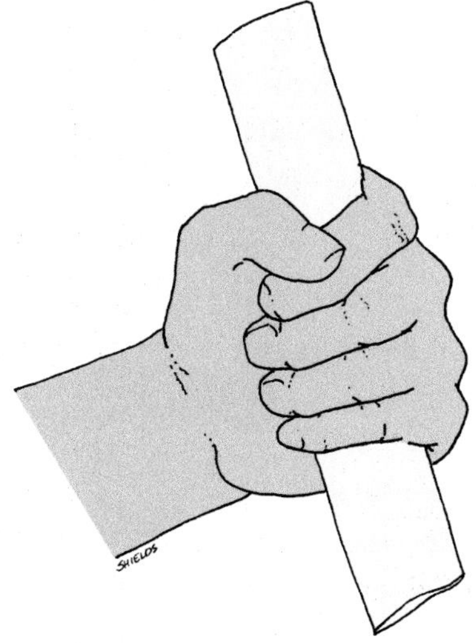

Figure 13-35. Cylindrical grip.

A variation of the cylindrical grip has the fingers flexed around a handle in a graded fashion (Fig. 13-36). The fifth finger joints are flexed the most, and the second finger joints are only partly flexed. The thumb lies parallel and against the handle, and the wrist is in slight ulnar deviation. The advantage of this grip over a cylindrical grip is that it allows a forceful but more controlled use of the tool. Examples of this type of grip would involve holding a golf club or a screwdriver.

A **spherical grip** has all the fingers and thumb abducted around an object, and, unlike the cylindrical grip, the fingers are more spread apart. The palm of the hand is often not involved (Fig. 13-37). Activities involving a spherical grip include holding an apple or a doorknob or picking up a glass by its top.

The **hook grip** involves the second through fifth fingers flexed around an object in a hooklike manner (Fig. 13-38). The MCP joints are extended, and the PIP and DIP joints are in some degree of flexion. The thumb is usually not involved. Therefore, this is the only power grip possible if a person has a median nerve injury and loses the ability to oppose the thumb.

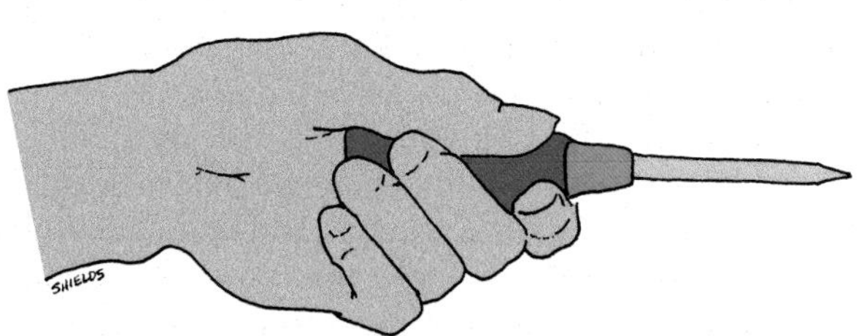

Figure 13-36. Cylindrical grip variation.

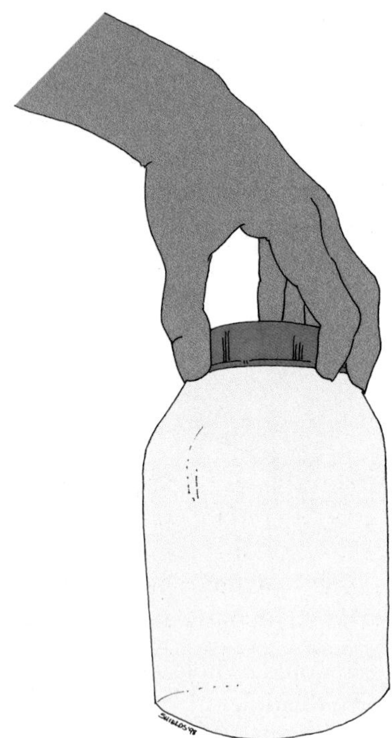

Figure 13-37. Spherical grip.

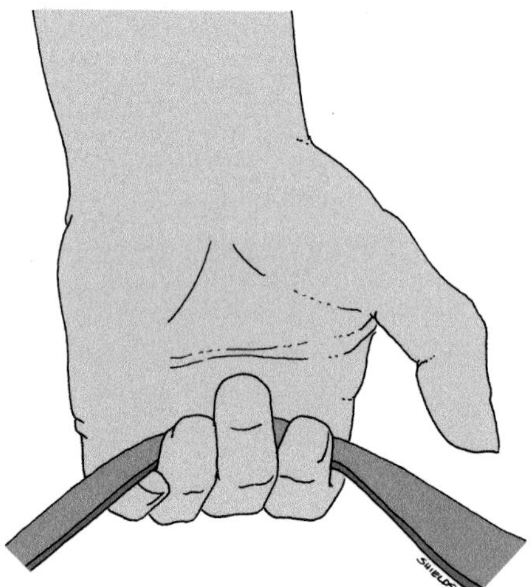

Figure 13-38. Hook grip.

Examples of a hook grip are seen when holding on to a handle, such as on a suitcase, a wagon, or a bucket.

Precision Grips

Precision grips tend to hold the object between the tips of the fingers and the thumb. The intrinsic muscles are involved along with the extrinsics. The thumb tends to be abducted or opposed. These grips provide more fine movement and accuracy. The object is usually small, even fragile. The palm does not tend to be involved, and the proximal joints do not tend to move. There are four commonly recognized types of precision grip.

With the **pad-to-pad grip,** the MCP and PIP joints of the finger(s) are flexed, the thumb is abducted and opposed, and the distal joints of both are extended, bringing the pads of the finger(s) and thumb together. When it involves the thumb and one finger, usually the index finger, it is called a **pinch grip** (Fig. 13-39). It may also involve the thumb and two fingers, usually the index and middle fingers. This is called a tripod grasp, also called a **three-jaw chuck.** If you observe how a power drill holds the drill bit in place, you will see the similarity to this grip (Fig. 13-40). There are three "jaws" pinching in on the drill bit; the entire holding mechanism is called a *chuck.* Holding a pen or pencil would be an example of this grip. This is by far the most common precision grip.

Similar to the pad-to-pad grip, the **tip-to-tip grip** involves bringing the tip of the thumb up against the tip of another digit, usually the index finger, to pick up a small object such as a coin or a pin (see Fig. 13-34). It is also called **pincer grip.** This type of grip becomes difficult, if not impossible, with very long fingernails.

The **pad-to-side grip,** also called *lateral prehension,* has the pad of the extended thumb pressing an object against the radial side of the index finger (Fig. 13-41). This is a strong grip, but it allows less fine movements than the other two types. The terminal device of upper

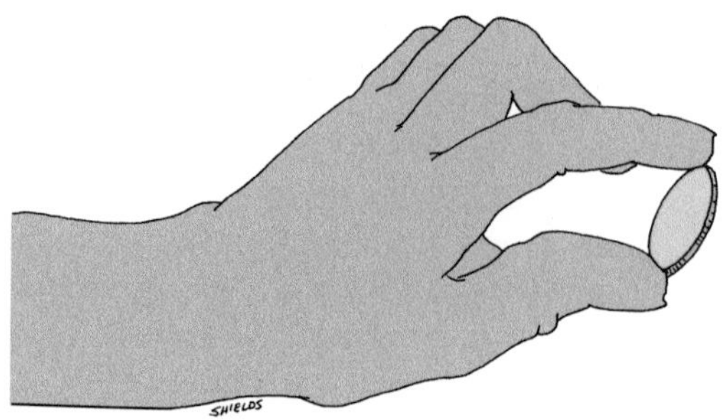

Figure 13-39. Pinch grip.

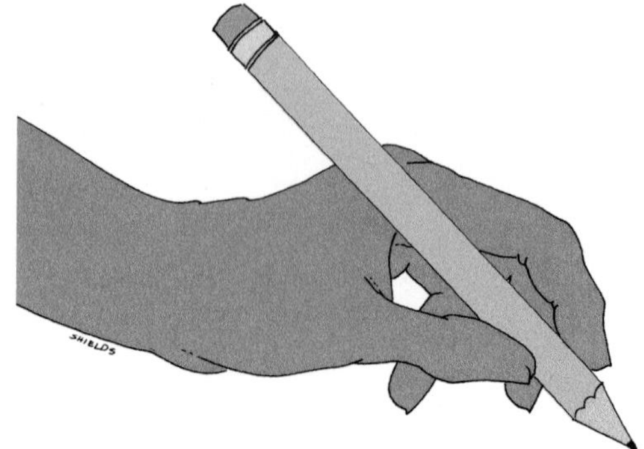

Figure 13-40. Tripod grasp

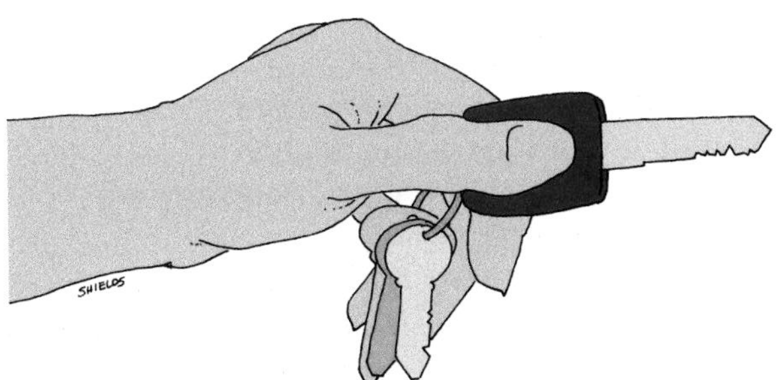

Figure 13-41. Pad-to-side grip.

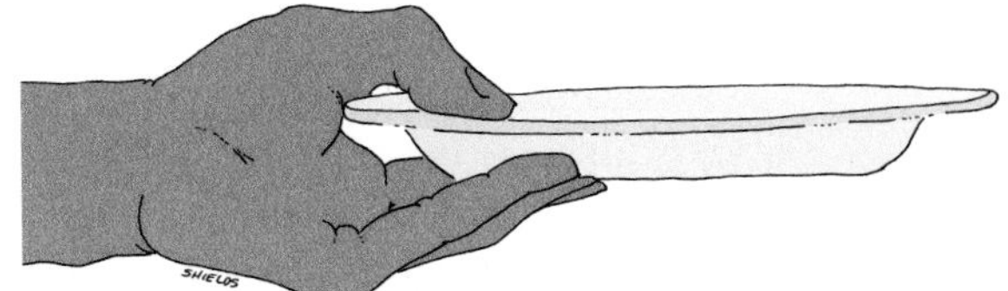

Figure 13-43. Lumbrical grip.

extremity prostheses adapts this type of grip. Also, because this grip does not require an opposed thumb, a person who has lost opposition but has retained thumb adduction can grasp and hold small objects.

The **side-to-side grip,** somewhat similar to pad-to-side grip, requires adduction of the index finger and abduction of the middle finger (Fig. 13-42). It is a weak grip and does not permit much precision. It is perhaps most frequently used to hold a cigarette. It is also used to hold an object, like a pencil, between two fingers while using another pencil or pen. Because the thumb is not involved, this grip could be used in the absence of the thumb.

The **lumbrical grip,** sometimes referred to as the **plate grip,** has the MCP flexed and the PIP and DIP joints extended. The thumb opposes the fingers holding an object horizontal (Fig. 13-43). This grip is usually used when something needs to be kept horizontal, such as a plate or a tray. It is called a lumbrical grip because the action of the lumbrical muscles is to flex the MCP joints while extending the IP joints.

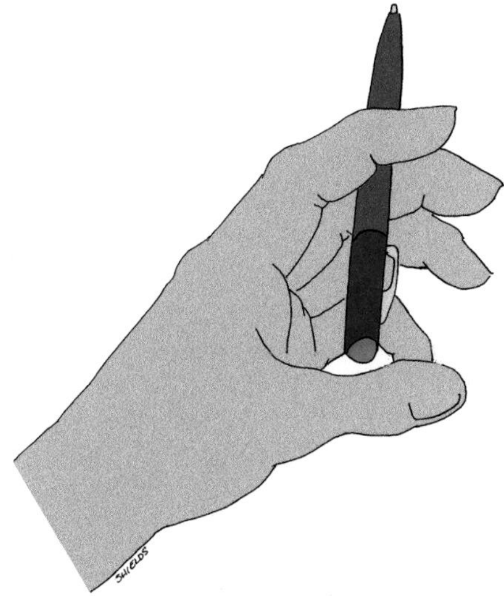

Figure 13-42. Side-to-side grip.

Clinical Application 13-1

Functional Position of the Hand

There is a biomechanical reason why slight wrist hyperextension is part of the functional position for the hand. When the wrist extensors hold the wrist in hyperextension, this allows the long finger flexors to be lengthened over the anterior wrist as they contract (shorten) over the finger joints. This creates an optimal length-tension relationship (contractility potential), and grip strength is maximized.

When wrist immobilization is necessary, a cock-up splint is often used. (See figure below). There are many variations of this type of splint available. What they have in common is that the wrist is maintained in slight hyperextension while the fingers and thumb are able to move. This "functional position" allows for optimal finger function (grip strength), even though the wrist is not moving.

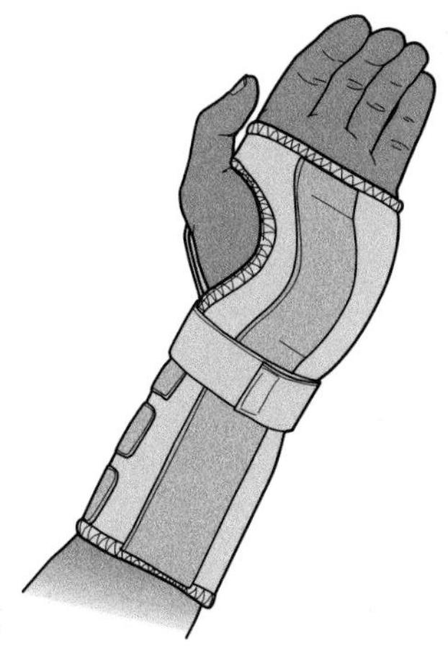

Cock-up wrist splint.

Clinical Application 13-2

Adaptation of Ignition Key with Impaired Lateral Prehension

Certain inflammatory or degenerative conditions, such as rheumatoid or osteoarthritis at the CMC joint, can limit or prevent lateral prehension. Because this motion is required to turn the key in an automobile ignition or door lock, an individual with this impairment may have difficulty with or be unable to complete this task. By placing a fitted block or cylinder over the key to expand its diameter and/or extend its lever arm, an individual can instead use a cylindrical grip, or even a cylindrical grip variation to grasp the block, then use wrist flexion and/or forearm supination to turn the key.

Points to Remember

- Isometric contractions are used to stabilize or hold a body part in position.
- Cylindrical, spherical, and hook grips are used for power hand movements.
- Pad-to-pad, pinch, tripod grasp, tip-to-tip, pad-to-side, side-to-side, and lumbrical grips are used for precision hand movements.
- A convex joint surface glides in the opposite direction of the body segment's movement.
- A concave joint surface glides in the same direction as the body segment's movement.
- In anatomical position, the sagittal plane divides the body into right and left parts. The frontal plane divides the body into front and back parts. The transverse plane divides the body into top and bottom parts.

Review Questions

General Anatomy Questions

1. Which finger and thumb motions occur in:
   a. the frontal plane around the sagittal axis?
   b. the sagittal plane around the frontal axis?
   c. the transverse plane around the vertical axis?
2. Compare the thumb and fingers:
   a. Number of bones
      Thumb ______________
      Finger ______________
   b. Number of joints
      Thumb ______________
      Finger ______________
   c. Names of joints
      Thumb ______________
      Finger ______________
3. Thumb opposition is a combination of what motions?
4. Which of the thumb opposition motions is an accessory motion?
5. What is the purpose of the flexor and extensor retinaculum?
6. a. What structures make up the carpal tunnel?
   b. Which tendons and nerve run through the carpal tunnel?
7. a. What is an extrinsic muscle?
   b. List the extrinsic muscles of the hand.
8. a. What is an intrinsic muscle?
   b. List the intrinsic muscles of the hand.
9. Explain the difference between thenar muscles and hypothenar muscles, and give an example of each.
10. What is the "anatomical snuffbox," and which muscles act as the borders of this area?
11. a. What hand muscle does not have a bony attachment?
    b. To what two tendons does it attach?
    c. What action(s) is/are produced when this muscle contracts?
12. a. What is the shape of the proximal joint surface of the proximal phalanx of the fingers?
    b. What is the shape of the distal joint surface of the finger metacarpals?
    c. Is the joint surface of the proximal phalanx gliding in the same or opposite direction as the finger in MCP flexion/extension?
    d. What direction does the base of the proximal phalanx of the second finger glide during adduction?
13. At what joint does abduction/adduction occur:
    a. in the fingers?
    b. in the thumb?
14. Of the two extrinsic prime movers for finger flexion, which one has the longer moment arm at the MCP joint, and why?

Review Questions—cont'd

15. The joint surface of the base of the first metacarpal has a (an) ____________ shape in the sagittal plane and a (an) ____________ shape in the frontal plane. Therefore, base of the first metacarpal glides in a (an) ____________ direction during CMC abduction and in a (an) ____________ direction during CMC flexion.

Functional Activity Questions

For Questions 1 to 9, identify the type of power or precision grip used in the following activities:

1. Holding the handle of a skillet
2. Pulling a little red wagon
3. Turning pages of a book
4. Fastening a snap or button
5. Carrying a coffee mug by its handle
6. Holding a hand of playing cards
7. Holding an apple
8. Holding on to a barbell
9. Picking up a CD
10. Analyze the following activity in terms of the entire upper extremity action. Hold an infant with your hands on either side of the infant's trunk so that you are looking eye to eye (Fig. 13-44).
    a. A combination of what two types of grasp is used?

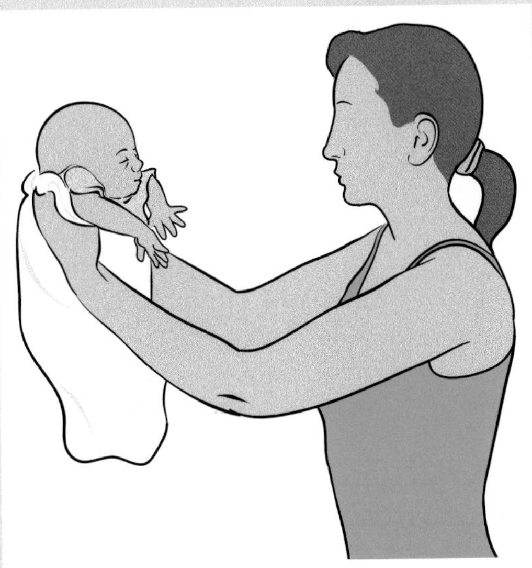

Figure 13-44. Activity analysis: holding a baby.

    b. The wrist is being held in a neutral position by isometric contractions occurring in two different planes. What are the two muscle groups involved?
    c. Name the wrist muscle prime movers of these two muscles groups.
    d. The forearm is in midposition between pronation and supination. What muscle group is holding the elbow in position isometrically?
    e. Name the elbow prime movers of this muscle group.
    f. The shoulder joint is being held in position by isometric contractions occurring in two different planes. What are the two muscle groups involved?
    g. Name the shoulder prime movers of these two muscle groups.
    h. What shoulder girdle positions occur with the shoulder joint positions?
    i. Name the shoulder girdle prime movers.
11. Turning key in lock to lock the door:
    a. What type of grip is used when holding on to the key?
    b. What joint motion is used to turn the key in the lock?

Clinical Exercise Questions

For questions 1 to 5, identify the joint motion (including the joint name) and prime movers involved in the following exercises:

1. Keeping the fingers straight, spread them wide apart; bring them together.
2. With your forearm supinated and the thumb next to the radial side of the index finger, raise the thumb straight up from the palm.
3. Touch the tip of your thumb to the tip of the little finger.
4. Keep the fingers straight and bend at the knuckles.
5. Starting with the thumb next to the radial side of the index finger, move it across the palm toward the little finger.

(continued on next page)

Review Questions—cont'd

6. To facilitate normal arthrokinematics while stretching the third PIP joint into extension, the clinician should place her hands so that the base of the ____________________ glides in a (an) ____________________ direction while the distal end of the bony segment is moved in a (an) ____________________ direction.
7. Describe the position the wrist and fingers must be placed to stretch the extensor digitorum.
8. When tenodesis is used to grasp an object, the long finger ______________ have become ______________ insufficient due to the wrist being placed in a (an) ______________ position.
9. When moving the wrist and fingers into flexion at the same time, the long finger flexors may become ______________ insufficient while the long finger extensors may become ______________ insufficient.

PART III

Clinical Kinesiology and Anatomy of the Trunk

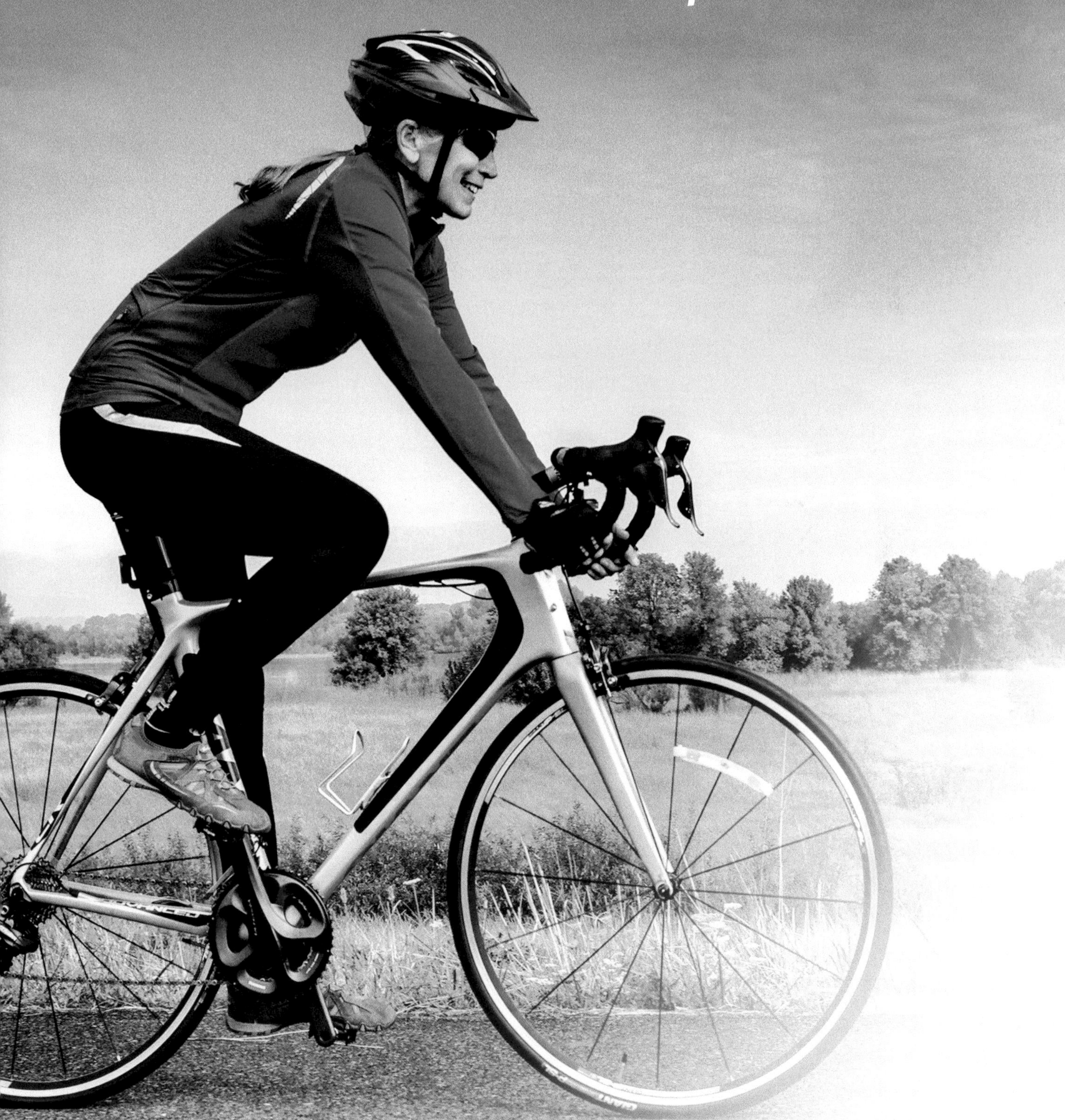

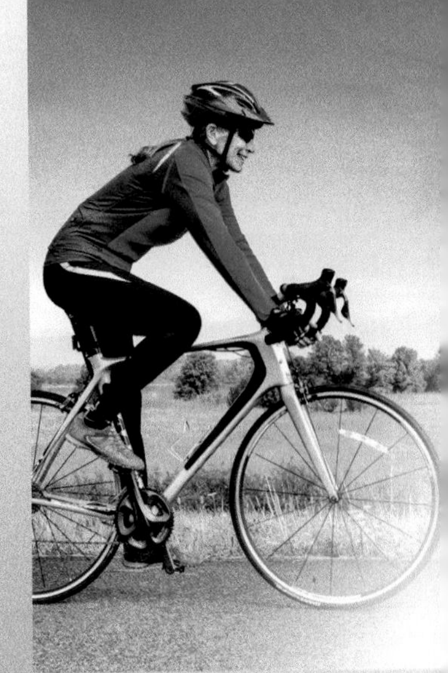

CHAPTER 14
Temporomandibular Joint

Joint Structure and Motions

Bones and Landmarks

Ligaments and Other Structures

Mechanics of Movement

Muscles of the TMJ

Anatomical Relationships

Summary of Muscle Action

Summary of Muscle Innervation

Pathological Conditions

Points to Remember

Review Questions

General Anatomy Questions

Functional Activity Questions

Clinical Exercise Questions

Kinesiology IN ACTION For additional practice activities and videos, please visit www.kinesiologyinaction.com

Joint Structure and Motions

The temporomandibular joint, often referred to as the TMJ, is one of the most frequently used joints in the body. It is used during chewing, swallowing, yawning, talking, and any other activity involving jaw motion. The TMJ is located anterior to the ear and at the posterior superior end of the jaw (Fig. 14-1). It is made up of the mandibular fossa of the temporal bone superiorly, articulating with the condyle of the mandible inferiorly. The TMJ is a synovial joint and is best described as having a modified hinge shape. Because it also allows some gliding motion, it is not a pure hinge joint.

The TMJ consists of two bones, a disk that divides the joint into two joint spaces, a joint capsule, four ligaments, and four main muscles that create five motions. As shown in Figure 14-2, the joint motions are

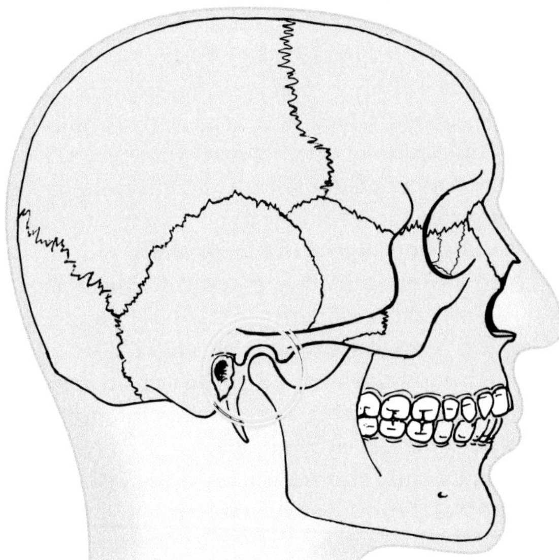

Figure 14-1. The temporomandibular joint (TMJ) is highlighted within the circle (lateral view).

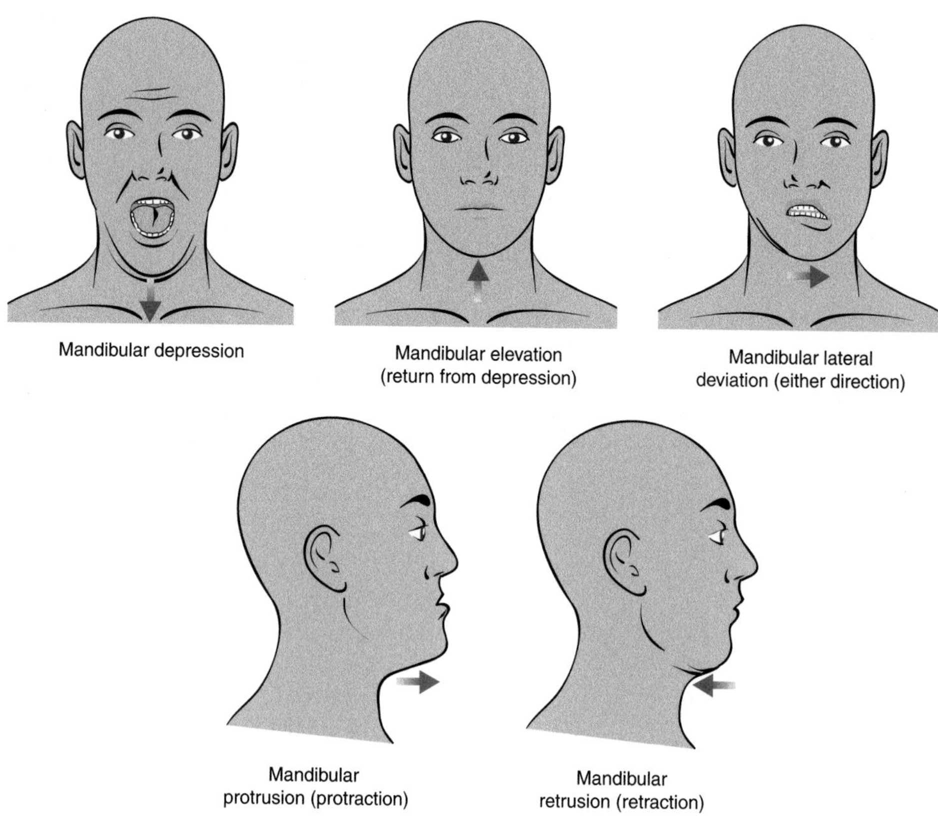

Figure 14-2. TMJ motions.

mandibular depression (opening the mouth); **elevation** (closing the mouth); **lateral deviation** (side-to-side jaw movement); **protrusion,** or *protraction* (moving the jaw forward); and **retrusion,** or *retraction* (moving the jaw posteriorly). Retrusion is basically the return to anatomical position from a protruded position.

When the mandible is at rest, the condyle of the mandible is seated in the mandibular fossa of the temporal bone. The normal resting position of the mandible is lips closed and teeth several millimeters apart. This position is maintained by low levels of activity of the temporalis muscles. The mouth should open far enough for you to be able to put two to three fingers between the front upper and lower teeth.

There is an articular disk that divides the joint space into two separate compartments: a larger **upper joint space** and a smaller **lower joint space**. The superior surface is both concave and convex to accommodate the shape of the fossa. The concave inferior surface of the articular disk accommodates the convex surface of the condyle and allows the joint to remain congruent (compatible) throughout the motion.

Bones and Landmarks

The skull has two parts: the bones of the large cranium cavity, which encase the brain, and the bones of the face (Fig. 14-3). The TMJ is made up of the mandible, a facial bone articulating with the temporal bone, which is a cranial bone. Surrounding bones provide an area for muscle and ligament attachment. The following is a description of the bones and landmarks significant to the TMJ.

The **mandible,** or **mandibular bone** (Figs. 14-4 and 14-5), is shaped somewhat like a horseshoe and articulates with the temporal bone on each side of the cranium. It consists of a body and two upwardly projecting rami (one on each side). Although the mandible is considered one bone, each lateral end articulates with a different temporal bone, forming two identical joints on either side of the cranium. The mandible makes up the inferior part of the face and is often referred to as the *jaw* or *lower jaw*. Its significant landmarks are listed.

Important Landmarks of the Mandible

Angle
Located between the body and the ramus, it is the joining point of the two landmarks. It is often referred to as the *angle of the ramus.*

Body
The horizontal portion of the mandible; the superior surface of the body holds the lower teeth.

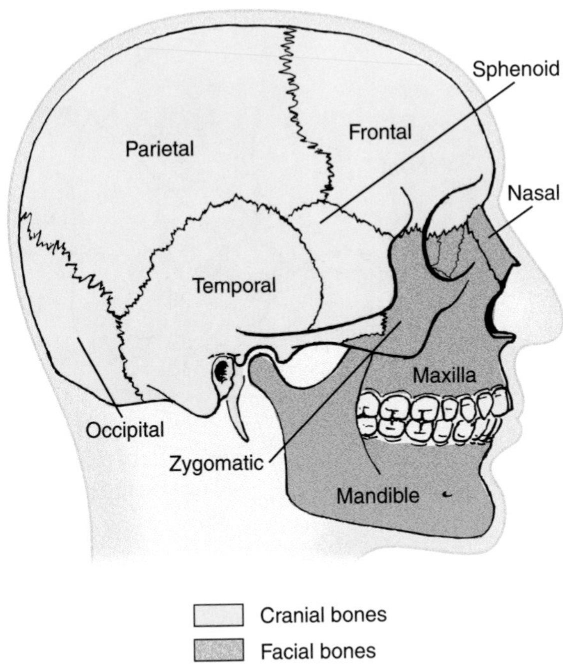

Figure 14-3. Bones of the skull (lateral view).

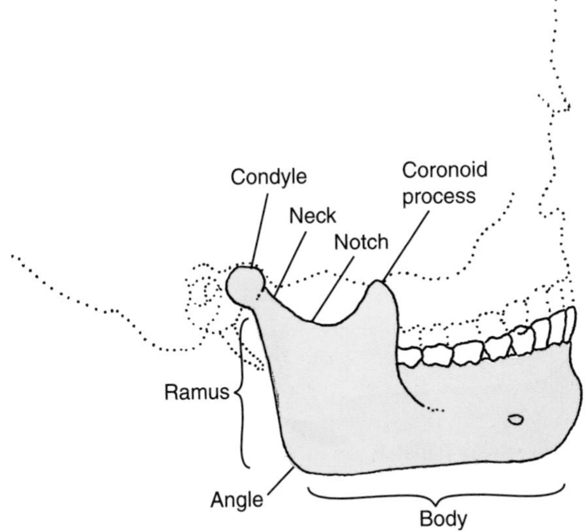

Figure 14-4. Bony landmarks of the mandible (right lateral view).

Condyle
Also called the *condylar process*. It is the posterior projection on the ramus, and it articulates with the temporal bone.

Coronoid Process
Located anterior to the condyle on the ramus. It serves as an attachment for the masseter muscle.

Mental Spine
Located on the interior side (inside) of the mandible near the midline. It serves as an attachment for the geniohyoid muscle.

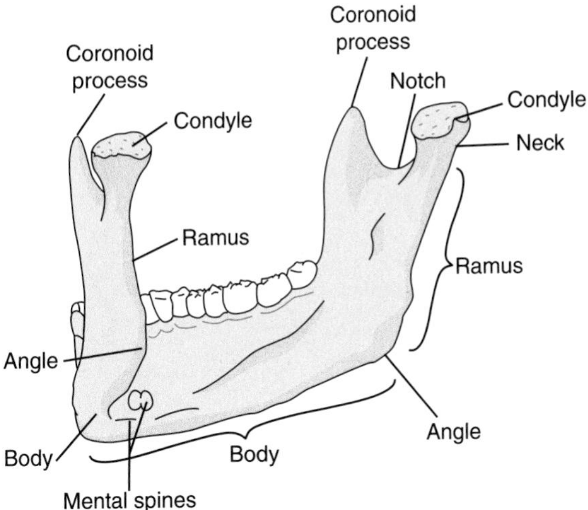

Figure 14-5. Bony landmarks of the mandible (posterior and slightly lateral view).

Neck
Located just inferior to the condyle.

Notch
Located between the condyle and coronoid process on the ramus.

Ramus
The vertical portion of the mandible from the angle to the condyle.

The **temporal bone** is located on the side of the skull posterior to the zygomatic bone, inferior to the parietal bone, posterior to the greater wing of the sphenoid, and anterior to the occipital bone (see Fig. 14-3). The articular portion of the temporal bone consists of the concave articular (mandibular) fossa in the middle, with the convex articular tubercle located anteriorly and the convex postglenoid tubercle located posteriorly (Fig. 14-6). Its main landmarks consist of:

Important Landmarks of the Temporal Bone

Articular Tubercle
Makes up the anterior portion of the articulating surface of the temporal bone. When the mandible is depressed, the condyle of the mandible rests under this landmark.

Mandibular Fossa
Also called the *articular fossa,* it lies anterior to the external auditory meatus and articulates with the condyle of the mandible.

Postglenoid Tubercle
Makes up the posterior wall of the fossa and is located just anterior to the external auditory meatus.

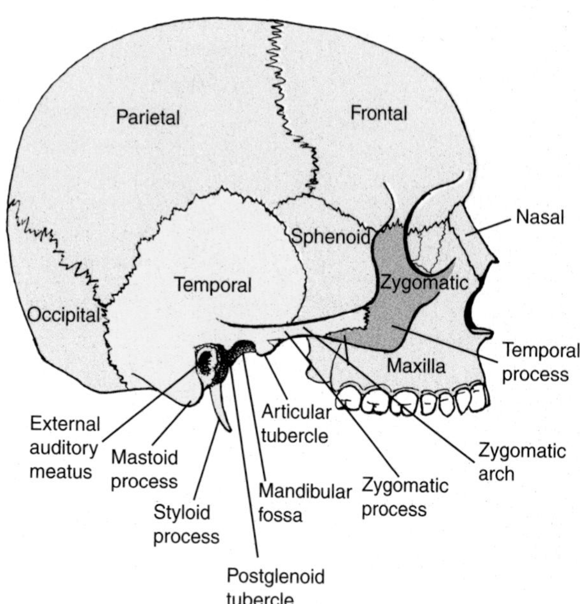

Figure 14-6. Bony landmarks of the temporal and zygomatic bones (right lateral view) with mandible removed.

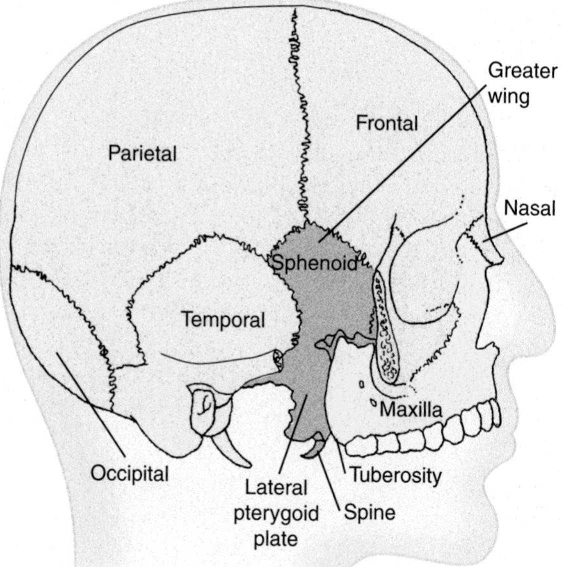

Figure 14-7. Sphenoid and maxillary bones (right lateral view) with zygomatic arch removed.

Styloid Process
A slender projection positioned down and forward from the temporal bone on the inferior, slightly interior surface. It serves as the attachment for various muscles and ligaments.

Mastoid Process
Bony prominence posterior and inferior to the ear, to which the digastric muscle attaches.

External Auditory Meatus
The external opening for the ear, located posterior to the TMJ.

Zygomatic Process
Makes up the posterior portion of the zygomatic arch. It serves as the attachment for the masseter.

The **sphenoid bone** is located at the lateral base of the skull anterior to the temporal bone. It resembles a bat with extended wings (Figs. 14-7 and 14-8). Because of its location, the sphenoid bone connects with six other cranial bones and two facial bones. Only the following external surface features are relevant to TMJ function:

Important Landmarks of the Sphenoid Bone

Greater Wing
A large bony process located deep to the zygomatic arch, posterior to the zygomatic bone, and anterior to the temporal bone. As part of the temporal fossa, it provides attachment for the temporalis and lateral pterygoid muscles.

Lateral Pterygoid Plate
Lies deep to and extends inferiorly under the zygomatic arch. It serves as an attachment for the lateral and medial pterygoid muscles.

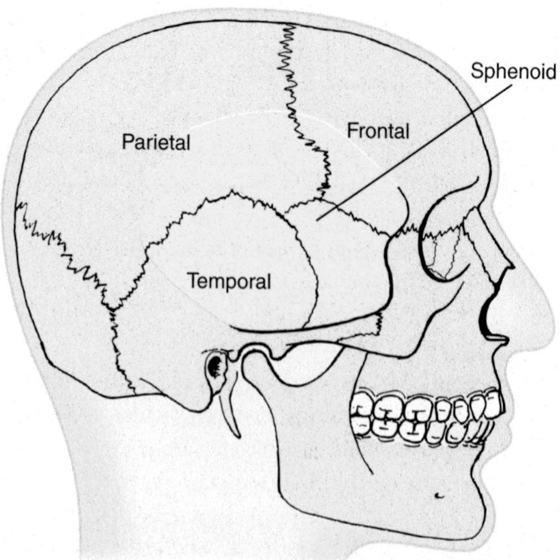

Figure 14-8. Temporal fossa includes portions of the temporal, parietal, frontal, and sphenoid bones (lateral view).

Spine
Lies deep to the mandibular fossa of the temporal bone and provides attachment for the spheno-mandibular ligament.

The **zygomatic bone** forms the prominence of the cheek and contributes the lateral wall and floor of the eye orbit (see Fig. 14-6). The frontal, maxillary, sphenoid, and temporal bones border it. The zygomatic bone along with the zygomatic process of the temporal bone form the zygomatic arch, to which the masseter attaches. Only the following listed features are relevant to TMJ function.

Important Landmarks of the Zygomatic Bone

Temporal Process
Lies posterior and inferior and joins with the zygomatic process of the temporal bone to form the zygomatic arch.

The following are made up of combinations of cranial bones:

Temporal Fossa (Figure 14-8)
Bony floor formed by the zygomatic, frontal, parietal, sphenoid, and temporal bones. It contains the attachment of the temporalis muscle.

Zygomatic Arch (See Fig. 14-6)
Formed by two bones: the zygomatic process of the temporal bone posteriorly and the temporal process of the zygomatic bone anteriorly.

The **maxilla** or **maxillary bone** is commonly called the *upper jaw*. It is located in the middle part of the face and houses the upper teeth (Fig. 14-7). It connects with the nasal bone superiorly and with the zygomatic bone laterally and has one main landmark.

Important Landmark of the Maxilla

Tuberosity
A rounded projection located on the inferior posterior angle. It serves as attachment for the medial pterygoid.

The **hyoid bone** is a horseshoe-shaped bone lying just superior to the thyroid cartilage at about the level of C3. It has no bony articulation but is suspended from the styloid processes of the temporal bones by the stylohyoid ligaments (Fig. 14-9). Its main function is to provide attachment for the tongue muscles. However, it also provides attachment for the suprahyoid and infrahyoid muscles that assist in mandibular depression.

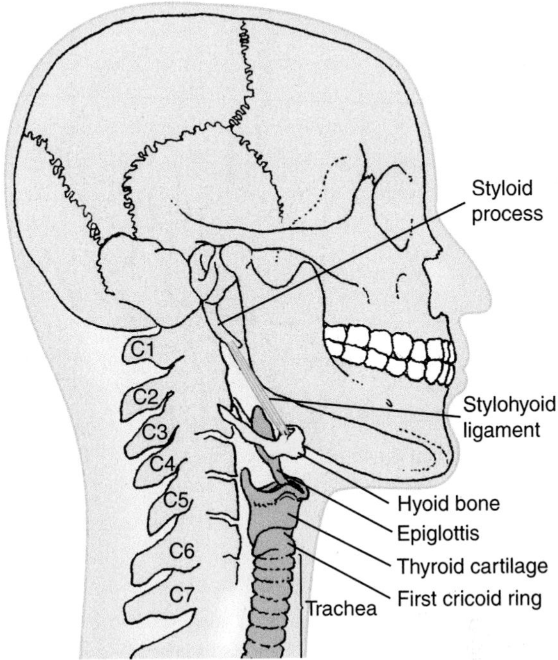

Figure 14-9. The hyoid bone is suspended from the styloid process of the temporal bone by the stylohyoid ligament (right side view).

The **thyroid cartilage** is the largest of the nine cartilages of the larynx. It is commonly called the "Adam's apple" and tends to be more prominent in males. It lies just inferior to the hyoid bone at about the level of C3 to C4 (see Fig. 14-9). It provides attachment for the infrahyoid muscles.

Ligaments and Other Structures

The **lateral ligament** is also known as the **temporomandibular ligament.** Anteriorly, it attaches on the neck of the mandibular condyle and disk, and then runs superiorly to the articular tubercle of the temporal bone (Fig. 14-10). It limits downward, posterior, and lateral motions of the mandible.

The **sphenomandibular ligament** attaches to the spine of the sphenoid bone and runs to the middle of the ramus on the internal surface of the mandible (see Figs. 14-10 and 14-11). It suspends the mandible and limits excessive anterior motion.

The **stylomandibular ligament** runs from the styloid process of the temporal bone to the posterior inferior border of the mandible's ramus (see Figs. 14-10 and 14-11). It lies between the masseter and medial pterygoid muscles and plays a role in limiting excessive anterior motion.

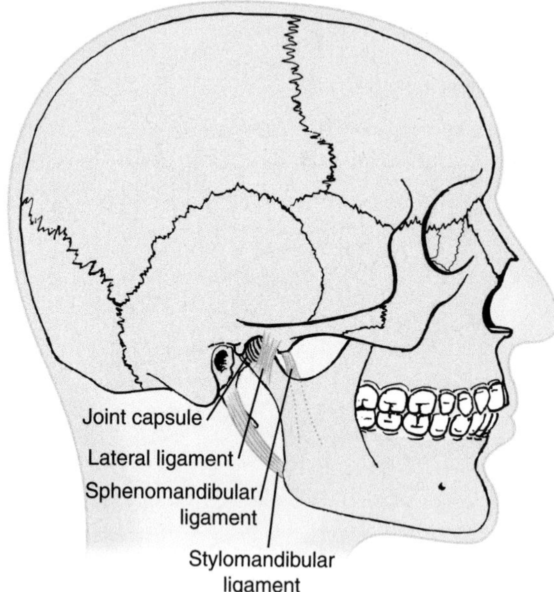

Figure 14-10. The ligaments that suspend and/or limit excessive motion of the mandible (right lateral view). Dotted lines show the sphenomandibular ligament (distal attachment on internal surface).

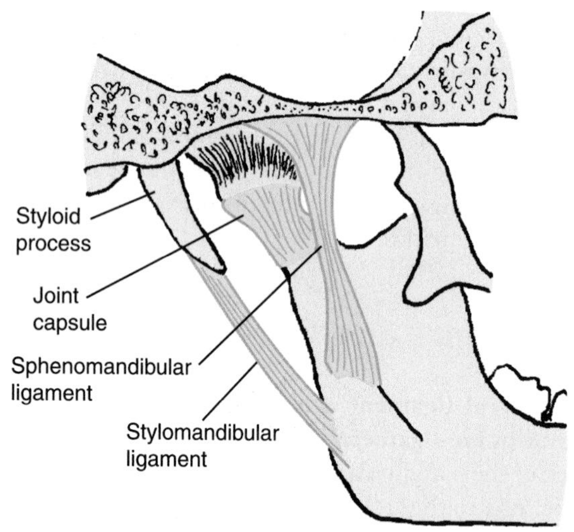

Figure 14-11. Internal surface view of left TMJ shows joint capsule and ligaments. Lateral ligament is not visible from this view.

The **stylohyoid ligament** attaches from the styloid process of the temporal bone to the hyoid bone (see Fig. 14-9). Its function is to hold the hyoid bone in place.

The **joint capsule** envelops the TMJ by attaching superiorly to the articular tubercle and borders of the fossa of the temporal bone. Inferiorly, it attaches to the neck of the condyle of the mandible (see Figs. 14-10 and 14-11).

The **articular disk** of the TMJ is similar to the articular disk of the sternoclavicular joint. It is connected circumferentially to the capsule and tendon of the lateral pterygoid (Fig. 14-12).

Mechanics of Movement

Depression of the mandible (opening the jaw) involves two motions (Fig. 14-13). The first part is accomplished by movement within the lower joint space. This is a convex-on-concave articulation where the mandibular condyle rotates on the disk creating an anterior glide of the condyle while the distal end (ramus/angle) moves posteriorly (see Fig. 14-13A). The second part of the motion occurs in the upper joint space and involves gliding the disk forward and downward under the articular tubercle (see Fig. 14-13B). Because the articular disk is more firmly attached to the mandible than the temporal bone, it allows the disk to move forward with the condyle of the mandible when the mouth opens. It returns posteriorly when the mouth closes. Elevation of the mandible (closing the jaw) is the reverse action. It involves gliding of the disk and condyle posteriorly and superiorly in the upper joint space and rotation of the condyle on the disk creating a posterior glide within the lower joint space. Mandibular elevation and depression occur in the sagittal plane.

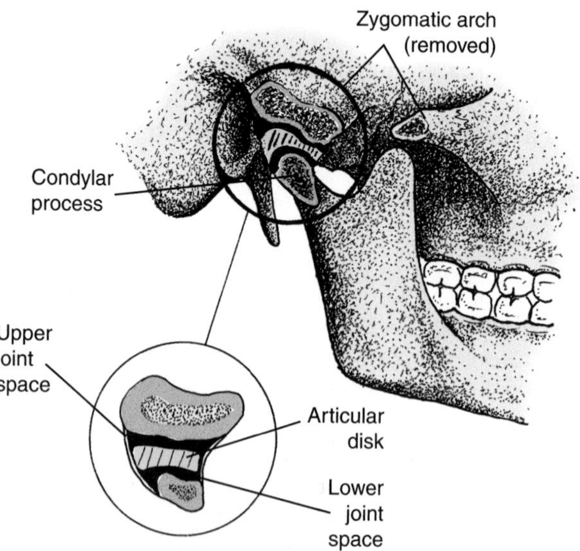

Figure 14-12. Lateral view of the right TMJ with zygomatic arch removed and condylar process cut. This shows the relationship of the mandibular condyle, disk, and mandibular fossa in a closed-jaw position. The articular disk divides the joint space into upper and lower spaces.

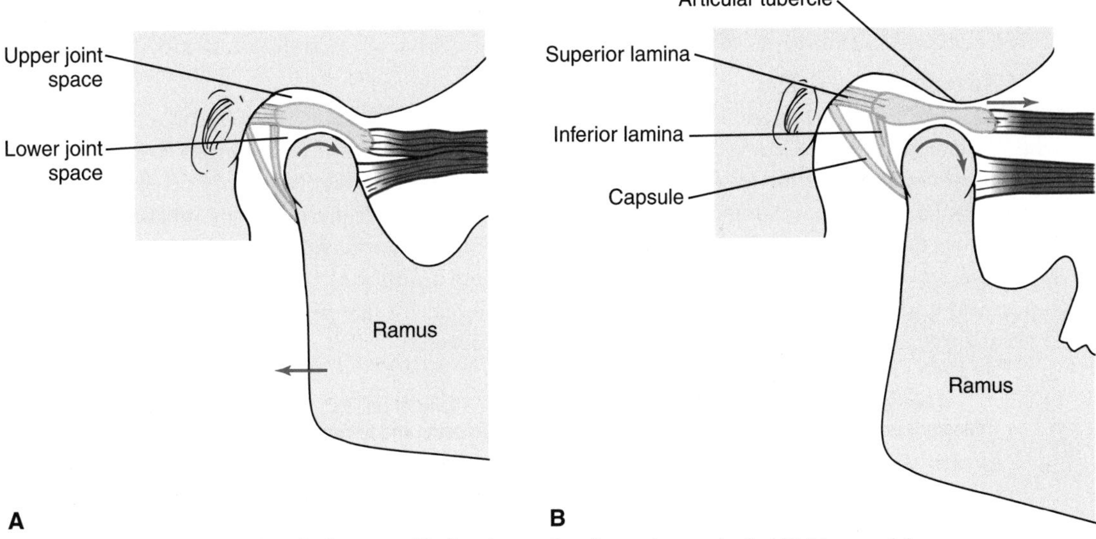

Figure 14-13. Joint motion during mandibular depression (mouth opening). **(A)** The condyle first rotates in the mandibular fossa, and **(B)** the disk then glides downward and forward over the articular tubercle, taking the condyle with it.

Protrusion and retrusion involve anterior-posterior movement within the upper joint space in the horizontal plane. The mandibular condyle and disk move as one unit against the mandibular fossa and articular tubercle of the temporal bone. There is no rotation. Forward and backward motions of all parts of the mandible are equal.

Lateral movement also occurs in the horizontal plane. It involves one condyle rotating in the mandibular fossa while the other condyle glides forward. To move the mandible toward the left, the left condyle will rotate and the right condyle will glide forward (Fig. 14-14). This rotation occurs around a vertical axis.

Muscles of the TMJ

The TMJ is involved in activities such as talking, chewing, biting, swallowing, and yawning. TMJ muscles that have fibers running more vertically will tend to create mandibular elevation or depression, whereas muscles that have fibers running more horizontally will be better aligned to produce protraction and retraction when they contract. Several muscles come into play, often synergistically. The muscles primarily involved are listed below. Unless stated otherwise, the action is considered to be bilateral and occurs at each joint (right and left) simultaneously.

Temporalis	Medial pterygoid
Masseter	Lateral pterygoid

Other muscles involved in TMJ movements are the following:

Suprahyoid muscles	Infrahyoid muscles
Mylohyoid	Sternohyoid
Geniohyoid	Sternothyroid
Stylohyoid	Thyrohyoid
Digastric	Omohyoid

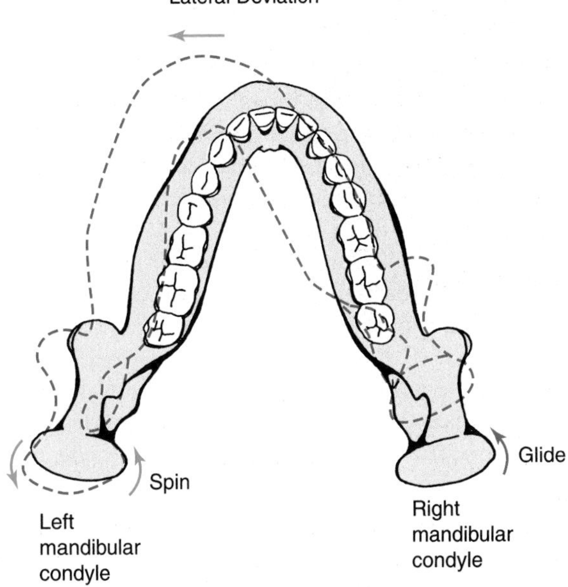

Figure 14-14. Mandibular motion during lateral deviation to the left side (superior view).

Clinical Application 14-1

Mechanical Advantage at the TMJ

The TMJ is designed as a third-class lever system with the force arm (distance from joint axis to muscle attachment) being shorter than the resistance arm (distance from joint axis to contact point of teeth). Contact between the more anterior molars or front teeth creates a long resistance arm and less biting force (Fig. A). When great force is needed in mandibular elevation (i.e., biting down hard), instinct tells us to place the item to be bitten back toward the rear molars (Fig. B).This shortens the resistance arm, which increases the mechanical advantage of the lever system. In other words, the greatest amount of biting force can be generated at the rear molars because the resistance arm is the shortest.

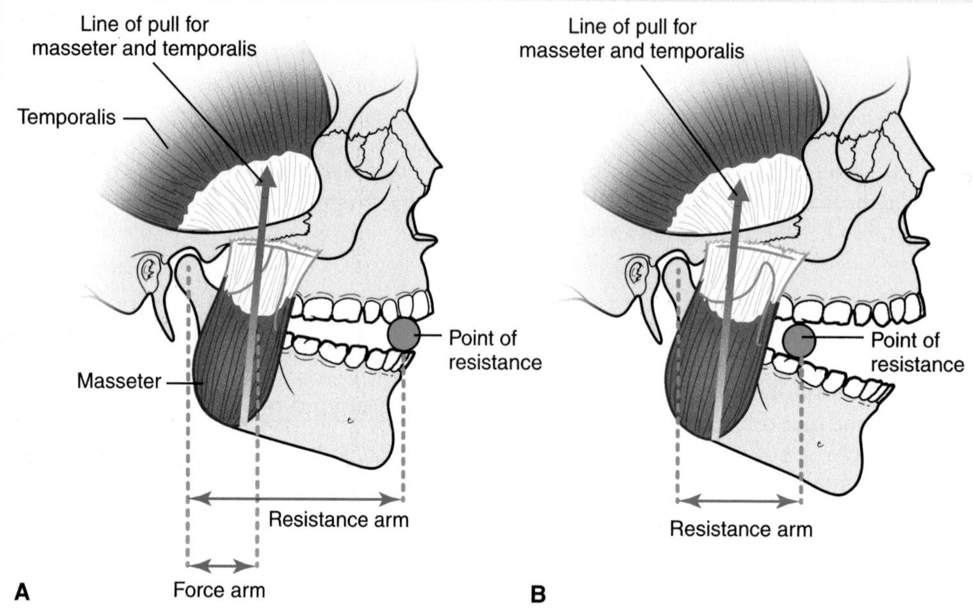

Mechanical advantage at the TMJ. **(A)** Long RA = less biting force; **(B)** Shorter RA = greater biting force.

The **temporalis** is a rather broad and fan-shaped muscle that lies in the temporal fossa (see Figs. 14-8 and 14-15). Because of its fan shape, the more anterior fibers run almost vertically, the middle fibers are at a diagonal, and the posterior fibers are nearly horizontal. From the temporal fossa, the fibers come together to form a tendon that passes deep to the zygomatic arch to insert on the coronoid process and anterior border of the ramus of the mandible. Its primary function is to elevate the mandible. Because of the horizontal direction of the posterior fibers, they also retract the jaw. In side-to-side movements, the temporalis contracts on one side, moving the mandible to the same side (ipsilaterally).

Temporalis Muscle

O	Temporal fossa
I	Coronoid process and ramus of mandible
A	Bilaterally: elevation, retrusion (posterior fibers)
	Unilaterally: ipsilateral lateral deviation
N	Mandibular branch of trigeminal nerve (cranial nerve V)

The powerful **masseter** is a thick, almost quadrilateral-shaped muscle that produces the fullness of the posterior part of the cheek between the mandibular angle and zygomatic arch (Fig. 14-16). It is made up of two parts: the larger, superficial part and the smaller, deep portion. The superficial part arises from the zygomatic process of the maxilla and the inferior border of the zygomatic arch of the temporal bone. The deep part comes from the inferior and medial borders of the zygomatic arch. The two parts run inferiorly and posteriorly, coming together to attach on the angle of the ramus and coronoid process of the mandible. Both parts act as one muscle to elevate

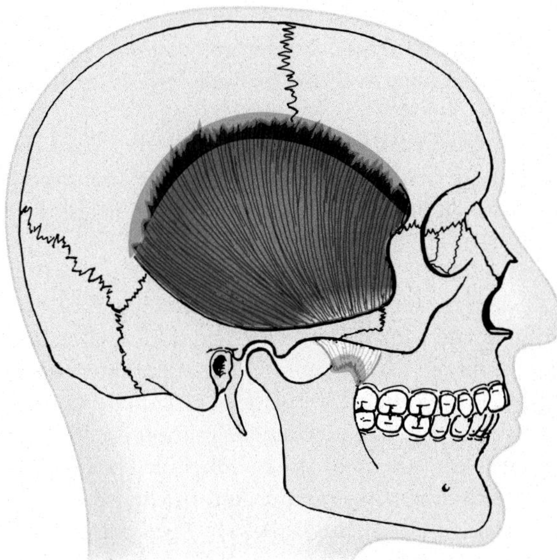

Figure 14-15. Temporalis muscle (lateral view).

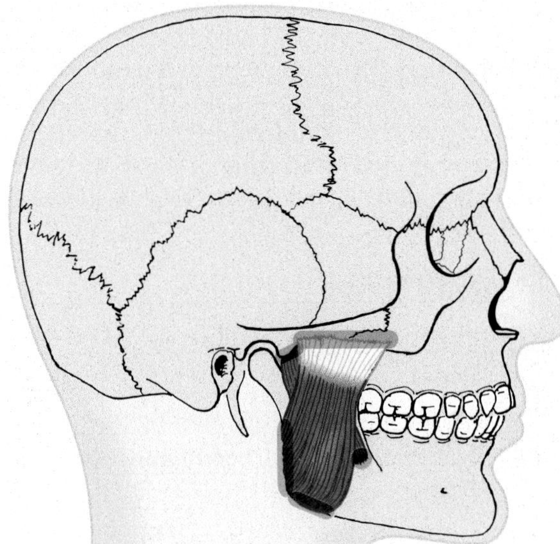

Figure 14-16. Masseter muscle (lateral view).

the mandible (close the jaw). Acting unilaterally, the masseter is an ipsilateral (same side) lateral deviator. The superficial fibers assist in pulling the mandible forward in protrusion.

Masseter Muscle

O	Zygomatic arch of temporal bone and zygomatic process of maxilla
I	Angle of the ramus and coronoid process of mandible
A	Bilaterally: elevation
	Unilaterally: ipsilateral lateral deviation
N	Mandibular branch of trigeminal nerve (cranial nerve V)

Although it is less powerful, the **medial pterygoid** is very similar to the masseter muscle. The medial pterygoid is located on the medial side (inside) of the mandibular ramus (Fig. 14-17), whereas the more superficial masseter is on the lateral side (outside). The medial pterygoid arises from the medial side of the lateral pterygoid plate of the sphenoid bone and the tuberosity of the maxilla. It runs inferiorly, laterally, and posteriorly to attach on the medial side of the ramus and angle of the mandible (Fig. 14-18). Its actions are mandibular elevation (it closes the mouth), protrusion, and contralateral lateral deviation. This deviation occurs when the medial and lateral pterygoid muscles on one side contract together causing the mandible to move to the opposite side.

Medial Pterygoid Muscle

O	Lateral pterygoid plate of the sphenoid bone and tuberosity of the maxilla
I	Ramus and angle of the mandible
A	Bilaterally: elevation, protrusion
	Unilaterally: contralateral lateral deviation
N	Mandibular branch of trigeminal nerve (cranial nerve V)

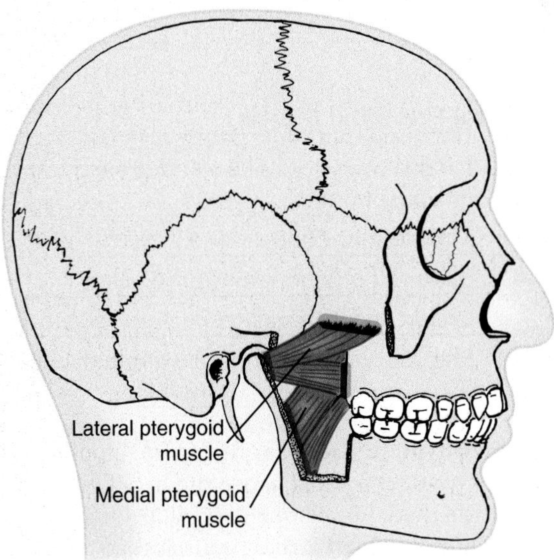

Figure 14-17. Lateral and medial pterygoid muscles (lateral view). The mandible and zygomatic arch are cut to show inside the mandible.

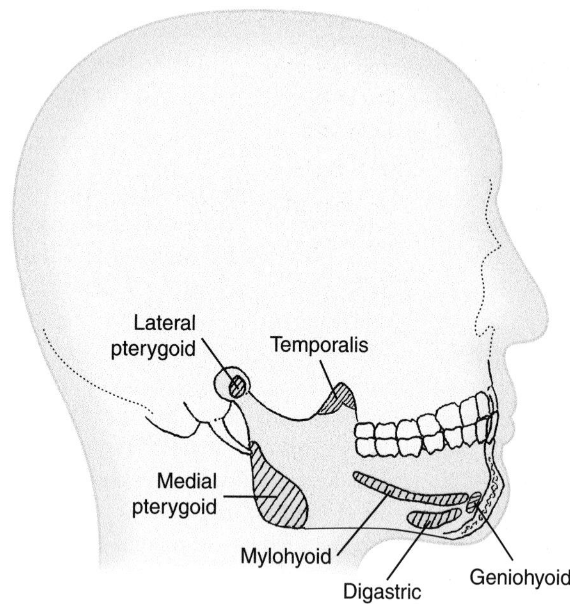

Figure 14-18. Medial (inside) view of mandible showing muscle attachments.

The **lateral pterygoid** muscle is short, thick, and somewhat cone-shaped. It has two heads: superior and inferior. The superior part comes off the lateral surface of the greater wing of the sphenoid bone. The inferior, more horizontal part comes off the lateral surface of the lateral pterygoid plate. Both parts run nearly horizontal in a posterior and lateral direction. They attach on the neck of the mandibular condyle, the articular disk, and the capsule (see Figs. 14-17 and 14-18). This muscle depresses, protrudes, and laterally deviates the mandible to the opposite side (as described for the medial pterygoid).

Lateral Pterygoid Muscle

O	Lateral pterygoid plate and greater wing of the sphenoid
I	Mandibular condyle and articular disk
A	Bilaterally: depression, protrusion
	Unilaterally: contralateral lateral deviation
N	Mandibular branch of trigeminal nerve (cranial nerve V)

The **suprahyoid muscles,** as their name implies, are a group of muscles located above the hyoid bone. They connect the hyoid bone to the skull, primarily to the mandible. Individually, these muscles are known as the mylohyoid, geniohyoid, stylohyoid, and digastric muscles. Although their primary function is to elevate the hyoid during swallowing, they can assist in mandibular depression when they reverse their muscle action, which requires the infrahyoid muscles to stabilize the hyoid bone. Therefore, these muscles will be described here in terms of their importance to the TMJ only.

The **mylohyoid** is a broad muscle that runs from the interior (inside) medial part of the mandible to the superior border of the hyoid bone (Figs. 14-18 through 14-20). The **geniohyoid** is a narrow muscle located superior to the mylohyoid (see Fig. 14-19). It attaches to the mental spine on the inside midline of the mandible and runs down to the hyoid. In Figure 14-20, the geniohyoid can be seen on the right side with the mylohyoid and digastric muscles reflected out of the way. In this view from under the mandible, the geniohyoid muscle is deep to the mylohyoid. The **digastric** muscle has two bellies connected in the middle by a tendon (Figs. 14-20 and 14-21). The anterior belly goes from the internal inferior surface of the mandible near the midline posteriorly and inferiorly, where it attaches to the tendinous inscription at the hyoid bone. The tendon is held in place by a fibrous sling attached to the hyoid bone. From this point, the posterior belly runs posterior and superior to attach to the mastoid process of the temporal bone. This pulleylike tendon is an example of how a muscle changes its line of pull. The **stylohyoid** is almost parallel to the digastric muscle. It attaches to the styloid process of the temporal bone and goes to the hyoid bone (see Fig. 14-20).

Mylohyoid Muscle

O	Interior medial mandible
I	Hyoid
A	Assists in depressing mandible
N	Branch of trigeminal nerve (cranial nerve V)

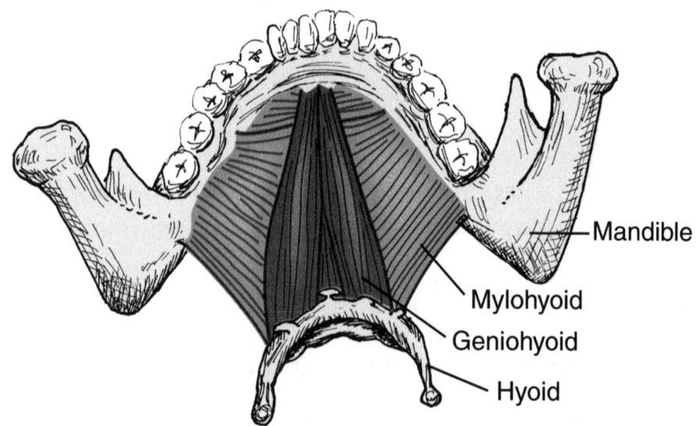

Figure 14-19. Muscles of the floor of the mouth. Posterior superior view (looking down toward the front inside of the mandible).

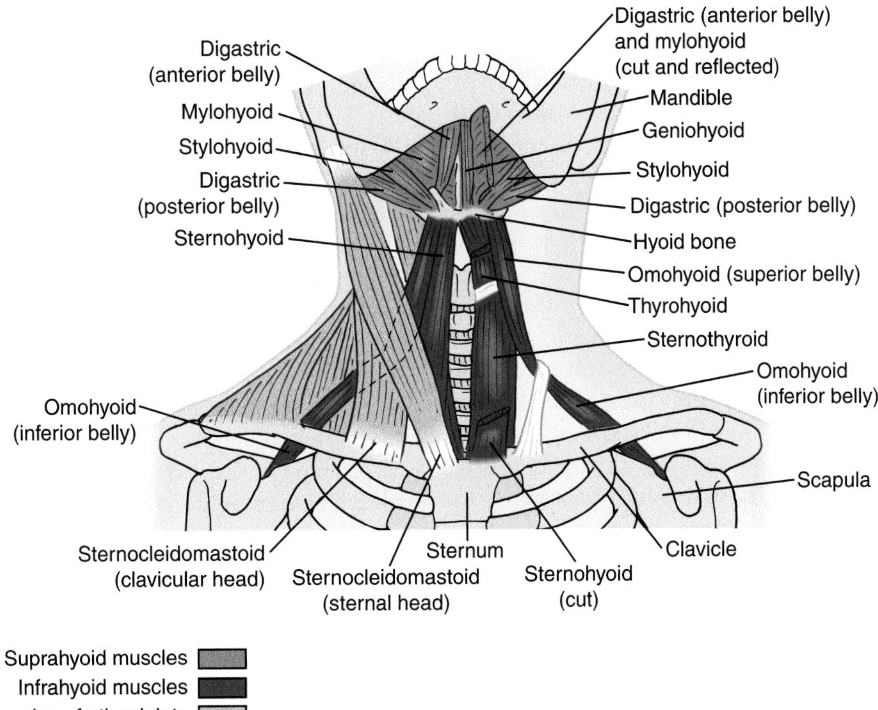

Figure 14-20. Suprahyoid and infrahyoid muscles.

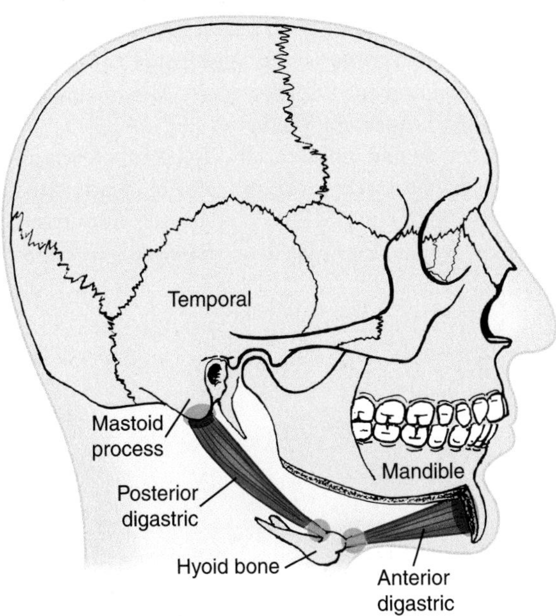

Figure 14-21. Digastric muscle (right lateral view) with the mandible cut away to show anterior attachment.

Geniohyoid Muscle

O	Mental spine of mandible
I	Hyoid
A	Assists in depressing mandible
N	C1 via hypoglossal nerve (cranial nerve XII)

Stylohyoid Muscle

O	Styloid process of temporal bone
I	Hyoid
A	Assists in depressing mandible
N	Branch of facial nerve (cranial nerve VII)

Digastric Muscle

O	Anterior: internal inferior mandible
	Posterior: mastoid process
I	Via pulleylike tendon to hyoid
A	Assists in depressing mandible
N	Mandibular branch of trigeminal nerve (cranial nerve V) and branch of facial nerve (cranial nerve VII)

As their name implies, the **infrahyoid muscles** are located below the hyoid bone and serve to depress it (see Fig. 14-20). Individually, these muscles are known as the sternohyoid, sternothyroid, thyrohyoid, and omohyoid muscles. They stabilize the hyoid bone, allowing the suprahyoid muscles to depress the mandible. These muscles will be described here in terms of their importance to the TMJ only.

The **sternohyoid** is a thin, narrow muscle that runs vertically next to the midline from the posterior aspect of the medial end of the clavicle, sternoclavicular ligament, and sternal manubrium. It is covered distally by the sternocleidomastoid muscle. Like all the infrahyoid muscles, the sternohyoid attaches to the inferior border of the hyoid bone. The **sternothyroid muscle** is shorter, wider, and lies deep to the sternohyoid, running vertically from the sternal manubrium and cartilage of the first rib to the thyroid cartilage. It indirectly pulls down on the hyoid bone by pulling down on the thyroid cartilage, which, in turn, is connected to the hyoid bone via the thyrohyoid muscle. The **thyrohyoid** is a short, rectangular muscle that acts much like a continuation of the sternothyroid muscle. It runs vertically from the thyroid cartilage to the inferior border of the hyoid bone. The thyrohyoid serves to close the laryngeal opening, thus preventing food from entering the larynx during swallowing. In terms of the TMJ, it pulls down on the hyoid bone, stabilizing it so that the suprahyoid muscles can assist in depressing the jaw.

The **omohyoid** has two bellies connected by a tendon in between, much like the digastric muscle. The inferior belly comes off the superior border of the scapula and runs mostly horizontally. At the tendinous insertion, the muscle changes direction, and the superior belly runs mostly vertically to the inferior border of the hyoid bone. The tendon is held in place by a fibrous sling attached to the clavicle that allows the muscle to make an almost right-angle turn. This is another example of an internal fixed pulley changing a muscle's line of pull. This muscle also stabilizes the hyoid bone by pulling down on it.

Sternohyoid Muscle

O	Medial end of clavicle, sternoclavicular ligament, and manubrium of sternum
I	Inferior border of hyoid bone
A	Stabilize hyoid bone
N	C1 to C3 via hypoglossal nerve (cranial nerve XII)

Sternothyroid Muscle

O	Manubrium of sternum and cartilage of the first rib
I	Thyroid cartilage
A	Stabilize hyoid bone
N	C1 to C3 via hypoglossal nerve (cranial nerve XII)

Thyrohyoid Muscle

O	Thyroid cartilage
I	Inferior border of hyoid bone
A	Stabilize hyoid bone
N	C1 to C3 via hypoglossal nerve (cranial nerve XII)

Omohyoid Muscle

O	Superior border of the scapula
I	Inferior border of hyoid bone
A	Stabilize hyoid bone
N	C1 to C3 via hypoglossal nerve (cranial nerve XII)

Note that the geniohyoid, sternohyoid, sternothyroid, and omohyoid are innervated by either C1 or C1 to C3 via the hypoglossal nerve. Clinically, that means that with a lesion involving C1 to C3, these muscles would be paralyzed, but with a lesion of the hypoglossal nerve inside the skull, these muscles would be unaffected.

Anatomical Relationships

There are four prime movers of the temporomandibular joint and many assistive movers. The temporalis and masseter are most superficial. The muscle belly of the temporalis lies above the zygomatic arch, and the belly of the masseter lies below (Fig. 14-22). Deep to these muscles at the level of the zygomatic arch and inside the mandible are the lateral and medial pterygoids. The medial pterygoid is deep to the lateral pterygoid (Fig. 14-23).

Also deep to the masseter and lying in a horizontal direction is the buccinator muscle. It is not considered a muscle of the TMJ because it does not cross the joint. However, it does play an assistive role in chewing

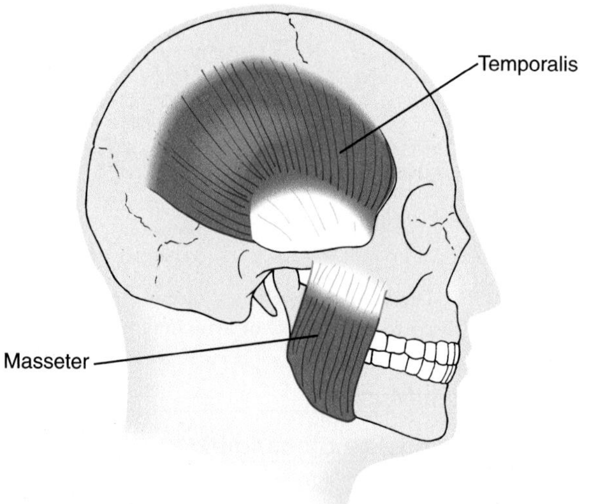

Figure 14-22. Temporalis and masseter muscles.

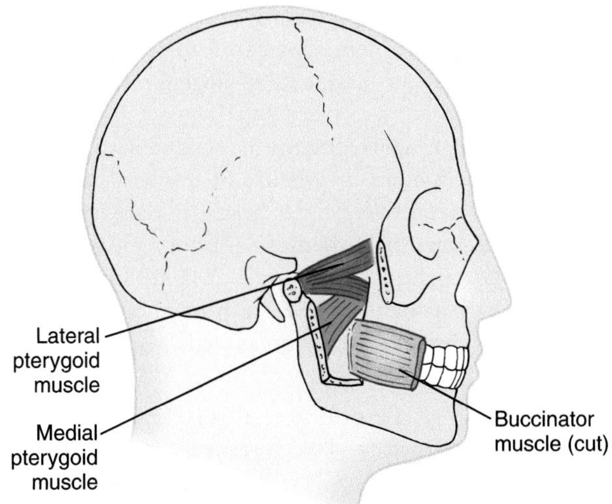

Figure 14-23. Pterygoid and buccinator muscles.

by pressing the cheeks against the teeth. It forms the lateral wall of the mouth and is better known as the "whistling" muscle, because it compresses the cheeks. The buccinator basically runs from the lips posteriorly to just below and above the molars on the mandible and maxilla, respectively (see Fig. 14-23).

There are two groups of assistive muscles: the suprahyoid and infrahyoid (see Fig. 14-20). These are deep muscles that work as a team to assist in mandibular depression. The infrahyoid group stabilizes the hyoid muscle. With the suprahyoid group's distal attachment stabilized, they can assist in mandibular depression.

Summary of Muscle Action

Table 14-1 summarizes the actions of the prime movers of the temporomandibular joint.

Summary of Muscle Innervation

Innervation of the TMJ muscles comes from cranial nerve V, the trigeminal nerve. If the assisting muscles of the suprahyoid and infrahyoid group are included, innervation additionally comes from cranial nerves VII and XII (the facial and hypoglossal nerves, respectively). The hypoglossal nerve communicates with the first three cervical nerves as well. Table 14-2 summarizes the innervation of all TMJ muscles.

Table 14-1 Prime Movers of the TMJ Joint

Mandibular Action	Muscle
Elevation	Temporalis, masseter, medial pterygoid
Depression	Lateral pterygoid
Protrusion	Lateral pterygoid, medial pterygoid
Retrusion	Temporalis (posterior)
Ipsilateral lateral deviation	Temporalis, masseter
Contralateral lateral deviation	Medial pterygoid, lateral pterygoid

Table 14-2 Innervation of TMJ Muscles

Muscle	Nerve	Cranial Nerve Number
Temporalis	Trigeminal (mandibular branch)	CN V
Masseter	Trigeminal (mandibular branch)	CN V
Lateral pterygoid	Trigeminal (mandibular branch)	CN V
Medial pterygoid	Trigeminal (mandibular branch)	CN V
Suprahyoid group		
Mylohyoid	Trigeminal	CN V
Geniohyoid	C1 via hypoglossal	CN XII
Stylohyoid	Facial	CN VII
Digastric	Trigeminal, facial	CN V, VII
Infrahyoid group		
Sternohyoid	C1 to C3 via hypoglossal	CN XII
Sternothyroid	C1 to C3 via hypoglossal	CN XII
Thyrohyoid	C1 via hypoglossal	CN XII
Omohyoid	C1 to C3 via hypoglossal	CN XII

Pathological Conditions

TMJ Dysfunction

When an individual has pain or dysfunction in the temporomandibular joint, it is not uncommon to hear it described by a layperson as "having TMJ." This, of course, is inaccurate, as the term TMJ refers to the joint itself and not the dysfunction.

There are many potential sources of temporomandibular dysfunction (TMD). "Clicking" in the jaw can occur when the articular disk is not positioned correctly. Clenching or grinding of the teeth is a common nighttime problem that can lead to TMD. This repetitive stress can also lead to degeneration of the joint surfaces.

TMJ problems are frequently associated with cervical dysfunction. Changes in posture of the cervical spine change the orientation of the head in space, and this in turn can alter the TMJ muscle line of pull, length-tension relationships, and overall TMJ mechanics. For this reason, treatment of TMD almost always involves treatment of the cervical region as well.

Clinical Application 14-2

Postural Influences

Forward-head, rounded-shoulder posture creates an increased convex curve on the anterior aspect of the cervical region. This places the suprahyoid and infrahyoid muscles on stretch, which can pull the mandible into a position of retrusion and subsequent malalignment during occlusion (bite) (See figure.)

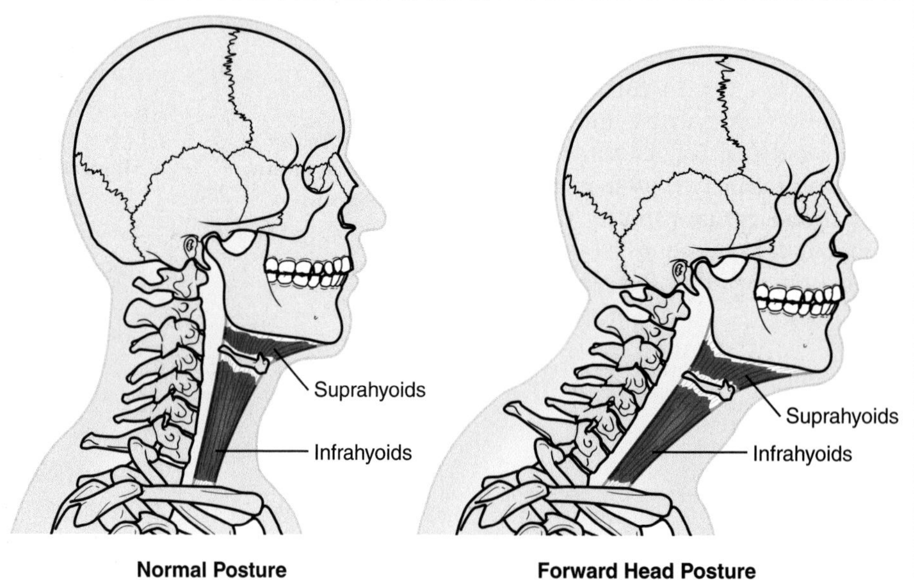

Postural influences.

Points to Remember

- The trigeminal nerve is the fifth cranial nerve, which has both sensory and motor components.
- The sensory component of the trigeminal nerve involves the facial area, whereas the motor component involves the chewing muscles.
- The facial nerve is the seventh cranial nerve, which also has sensory and motor components.
- The sensory component of the facial nerve involves the tongue area, whereas the motor component involves the muscles of the face.

Review Questions

General Anatomy Questions

1. The zygomatic arch is made up of which two bones?
2. What are synonymous terms for the following TMJ motions?
   a. Opening the jaw
   b. Closing the jaw
   c. Moving the jaw posteriorly
   d. Moving the jaw anteriorly
   e. Moving the jaw toward the side
3. Name the two bones and their articular surfaces that make up the temporomandibular joint.
4. What muscle can be palpated superior and anterior to the ear?
5. What muscle makes up the fullness of the posterior portion of the cheek?
6. What muscles work like a pulley?
7. Which would impair function of the TMJ more: damage to the mandibular division of CN V or damage to CN VII?
8. Two motions occur during mandibular depression: (1) the disk and condyle glide forward and inferiorly, and (2) the mandible rotates anteriorly on the disk. Which occurs first?
9. Lateral deviation of the mandible to the left involves both spinning and gliding motions. Describe how that happens.
10. What is another term for "Adam's apple"?

Functional Activity Questions

1. Forming the letter *O* with your lips requires what motion of the TMJ and contraction of what muscle that flattens the cheek?
2. Biting off a tough piece of bread is usually done by placing it in one side of the mouth.
   a. The biting action requires what motion of the TMJ?
   b. Which side of the jaw experiences some distraction?
   c. Which side of the jaw experiences some compression?
   d. Identify the force (*F*) and resistance (*R*) in this example.
   e. What class lever system is the TMJ functioning as with respect to this motion?
   f. What would happen to the force and resistance arms if the bread was moved to the front teeth instead?
   g. How does this change the amount of force the muscles need to generate in order to bite through the bread?
3. Grinding your teeth could involve motions in the sagittal plane and frontal plane. What are these motions?
4. Clenching your teeth requires what TMJ motion and involves what muscles?
5. What portion of the temporalis is the most effective line of pull when biting down hard, and why?
6. As you stand in anatomical position, what TMJ muscles are working to resist the force of gravity? How are they contracting?

Clinical Exercise Questions

1. Sit in a good posture position with your hands on each side of your jaw. Move your jaw from side to side against slight resistance.
   a. What is the joint motion?
   b. What type of contraction (isometric, concentric, or eccentric) is occurring?
   c. Name the muscles responsible for moving the jaw to the right.
2. Sit in a good posture position with your index and middle fingers on the anterior surface of your lower jaw in the midline. Without allowing your fingers to move, push against them with your lower jaw.
   a. What is the joint motion?
   b. What type of muscle contraction (isometric, concentric, or eccentric) is occurring?
   c. Name the muscles responsible for moving the jaw to the forward.

(continued on next page)

Review Questions—cont'd

3. Sit in a good posture position with your thumb beneath your chin. Open your mouth against slight pressure (Fig. 14-24).
   a. What is the joint motion?
   b. What type of muscle contraction (isometric, concentric, or eccentric) is occurring?
   c. Name the primary muscle responsible for moving the mouth.
   d. Name the muscle group that assists with this action
   e. The TMJ muscles in what group are acting as stabilizers during this activity? Describe what structure they are stabilizing and what motion they are preventing.

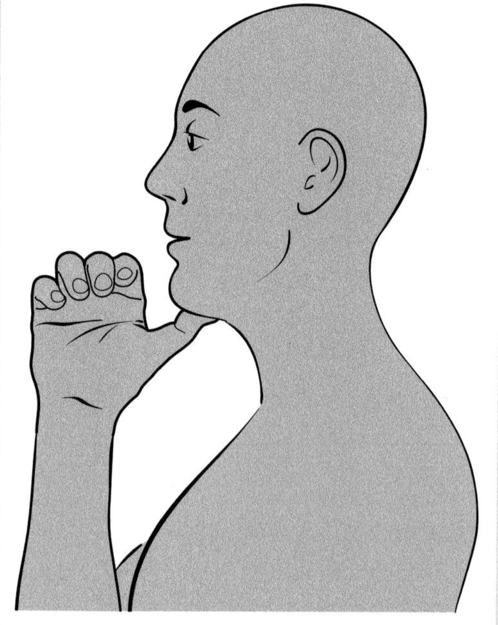

Figure 14-24. Opening mouth against slight pressure.

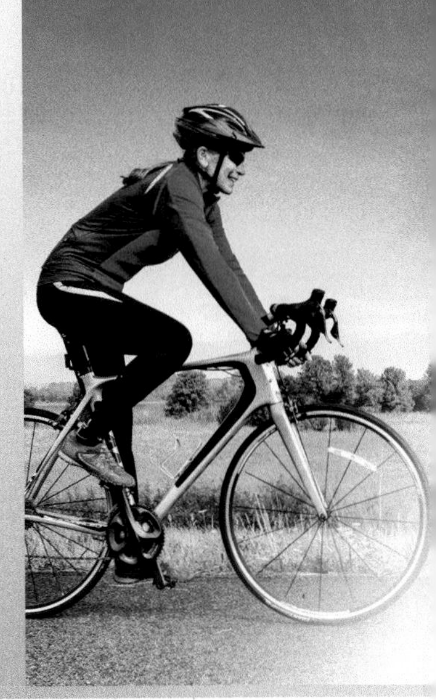

CHAPTER 15
Neck and Trunk

Vertebral Curves
Clarification of Terms
Joint Motions
Bones and Landmarks
Joints and Ligaments
Other Soft Tissue Structures
Muscles of the Neck and Trunk
Muscles of the Cervical Spine
Muscles of the Trunk
Anatomical Relationships
Summary of Muscle Actions
Summary of Muscle Innervation
Common Vertebral Column Pathologies
Points to Remember
Review Questions
General Anatomy Questions
Functional Activity Questions
Clinical Exercise Questions

The vertebral column establishes and maintains the longitudinal axis of the body. Because it is a multijointed rod, the motions of the column occur due to the combined motions of individual vertebrae.

The spinal column provides a pivot point for motion and support of the head at the cervical region. The weight of the head, shoulder girdle, upper extremities, and trunk are transmitted through the vertebral column. The vertebral column encases the spinal cord and is therefore able to protect it. Not only does this multijointed rod provide movement, but also the arrangement of these segments provides effective shock absorption and transmission.

The skeleton of the head is the skull, which sits atop the vertebral column. The skull is made up of two parts: the cranium and the facial skeleton. The skull forms a protective cavity (cranium) for the brain and supports the facial bones. Because the sensory organs for sight, hearing, taste, and smell are located within the head, it is important that the head be able to move freely. This occurs through movements at various levels of the cervical spine.

Vertebral Curves

The vertebrae are arranged in a manner that forms anterior-posterior (concave/convex) curves in the vertebral column, which can be seen from the side (Fig. 15-1). In the cervical and lumbar regions, the curves are concave posteriorly; in the thoracic and sacral regions, they are convex posteriorly. These curves provide the vertebral column with much more strength and resilience, approximately 10 times more than if it were a straight rod. Table 15-1 summarizes the curves of the vertebral column.

Clarification of Terms

The term *spine* can be used in more than one way. The spinal cord is made of nervous tissue. The *spinal column*

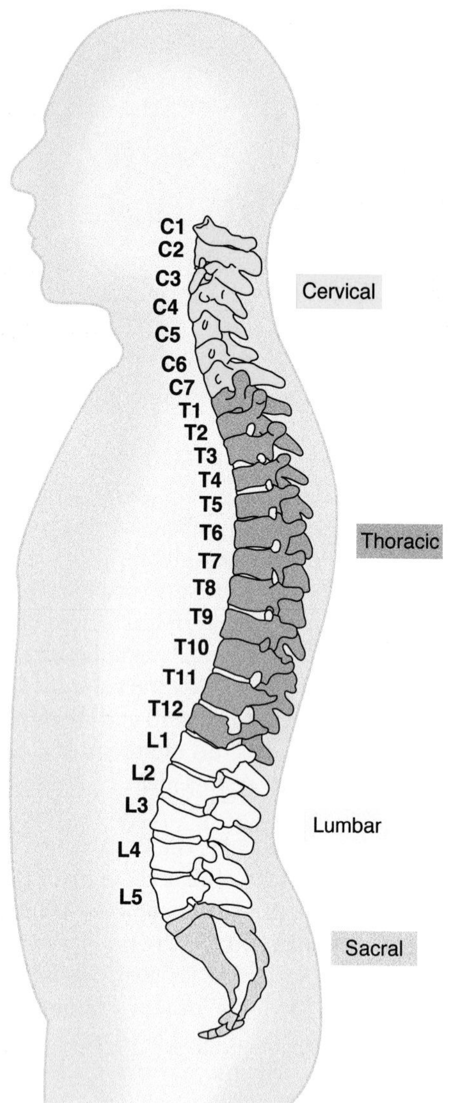

Figure 15-1. Anterior-posterior curves of the vertebral column (lateral view).

and *vertebral column* are synonymous terms referring to the bony components housing the spinal cord.

Another term that needs clarification is *facet.* A **facet** is a small, smooth, flat surface on a bone. Facets, as will be discussed, are found on thoracic vertebrae at the point of contact with a rib (see Fig. 15-9). A **facet joint,** often called an apophyseal joint, is the articulation between the superior articular process of the vertebra below with the inferior articular process of the vertebra above (see Fig. 15-5).

Table 15-1 Vertebral Segments

Segment	Number	Anterior Curve
Cervical	7	Convex
Thoracic	12	Concave
Lumbar	5	Convex
Sacral	5 (fused)	Concave

Joint Motions

Given that the typical intervertebral articulations are composed of cartilaginous joints (intervertebral joints) and plane-shaped joints (facet joints), one would not expect to see more than a small amount of gliding/bending from any individual segment. Because there are so many intervertebral articulations stacked up in a series, however, the total sum of spinal motion is actually quite substantial. Depending on what part of the vertebral column is moving, motion can be occurring in either the cervical, thoracic, or lumbar regions or in all three simultaneously.

The vertebral column as a whole is considered to be triaxial. Therefore, it has movement in all three planes (Fig. 15-2). **Flexion, extension,** and **hyperextension** occur in the sagittal plane around a frontal axis. **Lateral bending,** also sometimes called *side bending* or *lateral flexion,* occurs in the frontal plane around a sagittal axis. This motion *always* occurs to the same side on which the muscle is located. For example, the right quadratus lumborum laterally bends the trunk to the right. With right lateral bending of the trunk, the head moves to the right and the right shoulder lowers. **Rotation** occurs in the transverse plane around a vertical axis. Alignment of the facet joints will greatly determine the amount of rotation and other motions possible.

The cervical spine allows movement and positioning of the head. The articulation between the head and C1 (atlas) is called the **atlantooccipital (AO) joint.** The main motion here is **flexion** and **extension,** as when nodding your head "yes." There is also some lateral bending. Most **rotation** of the head on the neck, as in shaking your head "no," occurs at the **atlantoaxial (AA) joint** (C1 and C2). The muscles having the most control over moving the head on the neck are the prevertebral muscles anteriorly and the suboccipital muscles posteriorly. Obviously, to have the ability to move the head on the neck, a muscle must have an attachment on the head and on the cervical region.

The AO joint motions of flexion, extension, and lateral bending, as well as AA joint rotation, are almost always combined with movement of the C3 to C7 cervical segments. For example, AO flexion usually occurs with cervical flexion, AO lateral bending usually occurs with cervical lateral bending, and AA rotation with cervical rotation.

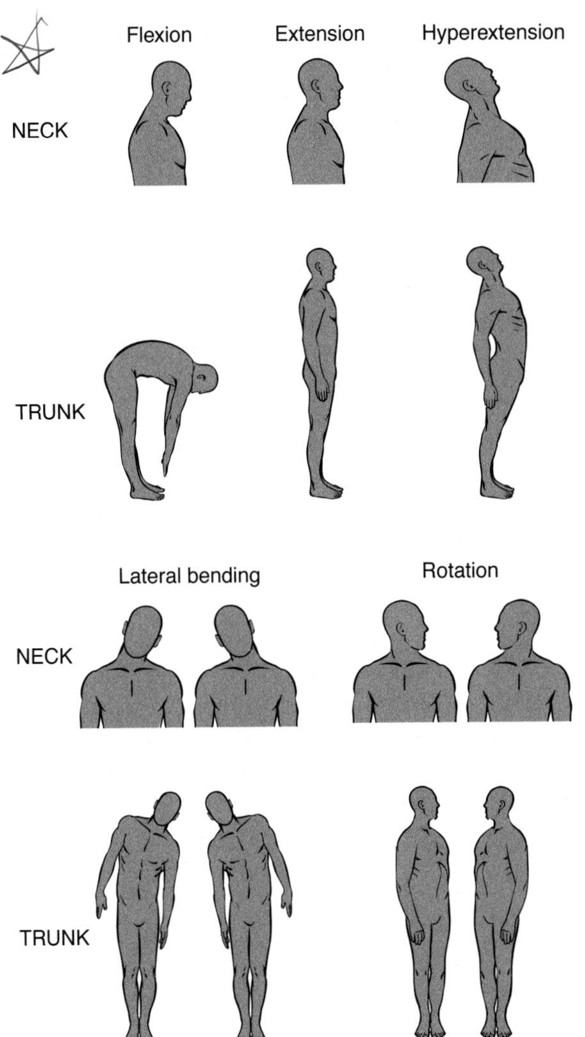

Figure 15-2. Motions of the neck and trunk.

While all of the spinal motions presented so far are angular motions, there are two linear motions that need to be examined. Tucking your chin in involves the head flexing on C1 (AO joint), as well as the neck (C2 to C7) extending. This combined motion is sometimes referred to as **axial extension** or *cervical retraction.* Conversely, extending the head on C1 and flexing the neck (C2 to C7) is called *cervical protraction.* This moves the head anteriorly through space. A relaxed forward head posture or looking at a computer screen through bifocals tends to accentuate cervical protraction. "Standing up straight" emphasizes axial extension.

Bones and Landmarks

The skull is made up of 22 separate bones and is considered to be the skeleton of the head (Fig. 15-3A, B). We

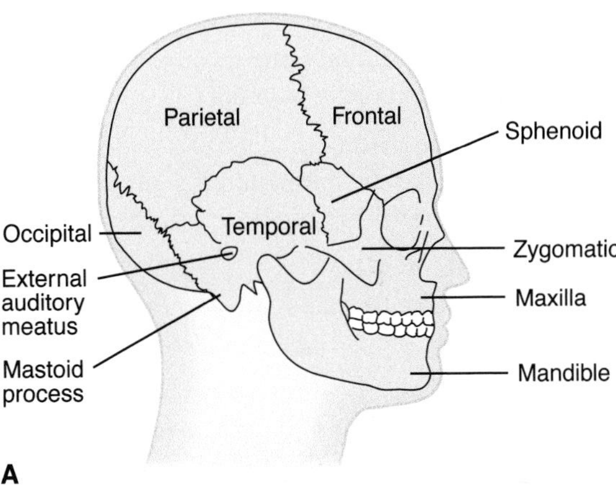

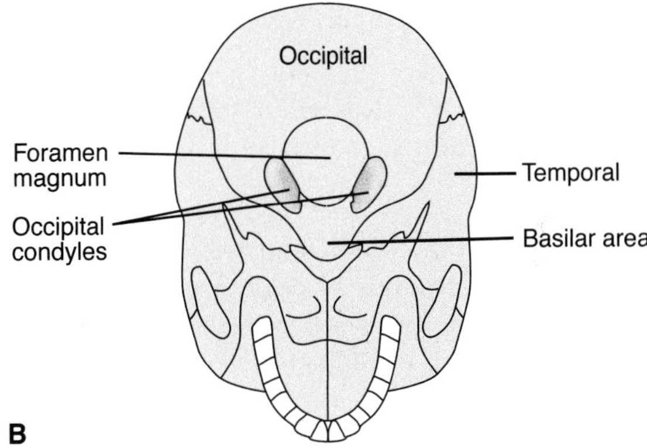

Figure 15-3. Bones of the skull as viewed from **(A)** the lateral view and **(B)** below the base of the skull.

will discuss only those bones associated with movement of the vertebral column.

Important Bony Landmarks of the Skull

Occipital Bone
Also called the occiput, it forms the posterior inferior part of the cranium.

Occipital Protuberance
The small prominence in the center of the occiput (not pictured)

Nuchal Line
The ridge running horizontally along the back of the head from the occipital protuberance toward the mastoid processes (not pictured)

Basilar Area
Refers to the base, or inferior portion of the occiput

Foramen Magnum
Opening in the occipital bone through which the spinal cord enters the cranium

Occipital Condyles
Located lateral to the foramen magnum on the occiput; provides articulation with the atlas (C1)

Temporal Bone
Forms part of the base and lateral inferior sides of the cranium

Mastoid Process
Bony prominence behind the ear to which the sternocleidomastoid muscle attaches

Vertebrae (plural of *vertebra*) differ in size and shape but generally have the same layout (Fig. 15-4). The typical parts of a vertebra are listed below.

Important Bony Landmarks of the Vertebrae

Body
Being primarily a cylindrical mass of cancellous bone, it is the anterior portion of the vertebra and the major weight-bearing structure. It is not present in the atlas (C1) (see Fig. 15-7). Between C3 and S1, bodies become progressively larger, bearing progressively more weight (see Fig. 15-10).

Neural Arch
Also called the *vertebral arch,* it is the posterior portion of the vertebra, with many different parts.

Vertebral Foramen
Opening formed by the joining of the body and neural arch through which the spinal cord passes.

Pedicle
Portion of the neural arch just posterior to the body and anterior to the lamina

Lamina
Posterior portion of the neural arch that unites from each side in the midline

Transverse Process
Formed at the union of the lamina and pedicle, the lateral projections of the arch to which muscles and ligaments attach

Vertebral Notches
Depressions located on the superior and inferior surfaces of the pedicle, and are so named (see Fig. 15-10).

Intervertebral Foramen (Fig. 15-5)
Opening formed by the superior vertebral notch of the vertebra below and the inferior vertebral notch of the vertebra above.

Articular Process
Projecting superiorly and inferiorly off the posterior surface of each lamina, and so named. Superior articular processes face posteriorly or medially, whereas inferior processes face anteriorly or laterally (see Fig. 15-10).

Spinous Process
The most posterior projection on the neural arch; located at the junction of the two laminae. It serves as a point of attachment for many muscles and ligaments and can be palpated throughout the length of the vertebral column.

Between adjacent vertebrae is an **intervertebral disk** that articulates with the bodies of the vertebrae (see Fig. 15-5).

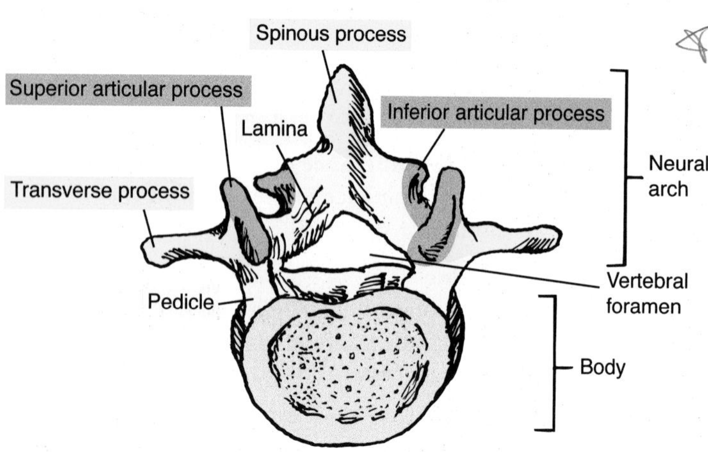

Figure 15-4. Body landmarks of the anterior and posterior portions of a typical vertebra.

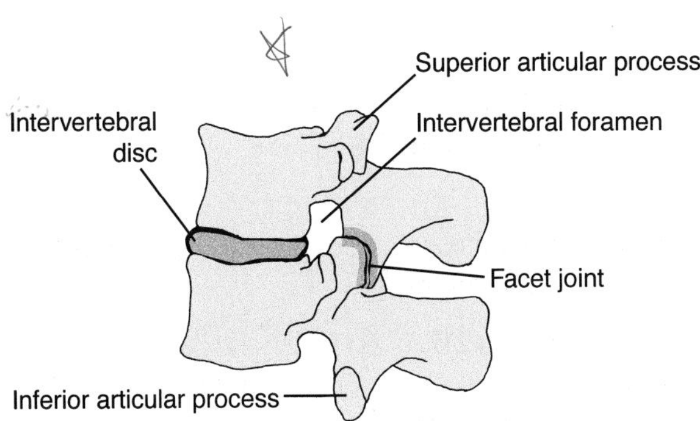

Figure 15-5. Lateral view of two vertebrae showing the intervertebral foramen and the facet joint. Both are formed by parts from each vertebra. The vertebrae are separated anteriorly by the intervertebral disk.

There are 23 disks beginning between C2 and C3. Their main function is to absorb and transmit shock and maintain flexibility of the vertebral column. The disks make up approximately 25% of the total length of the vertebral column.

Annulus Fibrosus

The outer portion of the disk consisting of several concentrically arranged fibrocartilaginous rings that serve to contain the nucleus pulposus (see Fig. 15-6).

Nucleus Pulposus

Pulpy, gelatinous substance with a high water content in the center of the disk (see Fig. 15-6). At birth, it is approximately 80% water, decreasing to less than 70% at 60 years of age. In part, this explains why an individual loses height with advanced age.

There are a few vertebrae with distinguishing characteristics that must be identified. They are listed below.

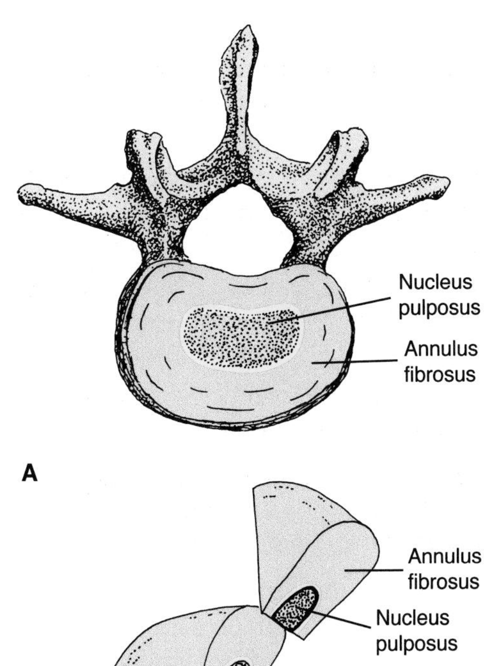

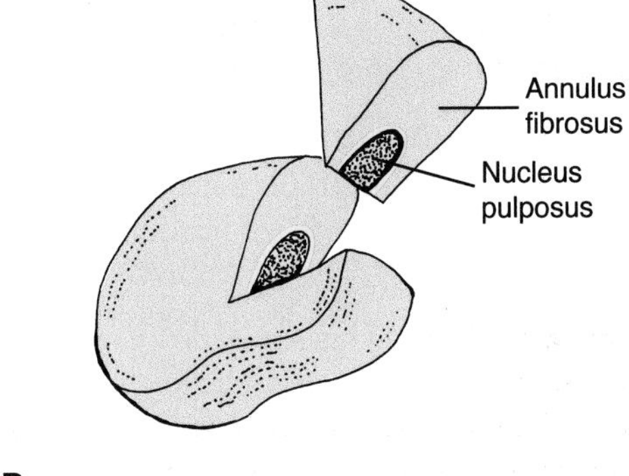

Figure 15-6. Two parts of the intervertebral disk. **(A)** Viewed from above, the nucleus pulposus cannot be seen, as it is surrounded by the annulus fibrosus. Its approximate location is shown within the yellow line. **(B)** The longitudinal section view shows the relationship between the annulus fibrosus and the nucleus pulposus.

Vertebrae with Unique Bony Landmarks

Atlas (C1)

The first cervical vertebra upon which the cranium rests (Fig. 15-7). Because it supports the globe of the head, it is named after the Titan in Greek mythology who held up the earth. The atlas is ring-shaped and has no body or spinous process.

Anterior Arch

The anterior portion of C1.

Axis (C2)

The second cervical vertebra (Fig. 15-8) is so named because it forms the pivot that allows rotation of the atlas (C1), which supports the head. It also has no body.

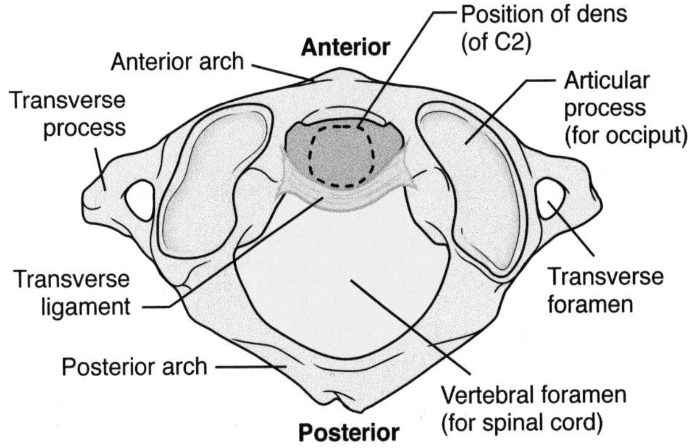

Figure 15-7. Parts of the first cervical vertebra (C1), also called the *atlas* (superior view).

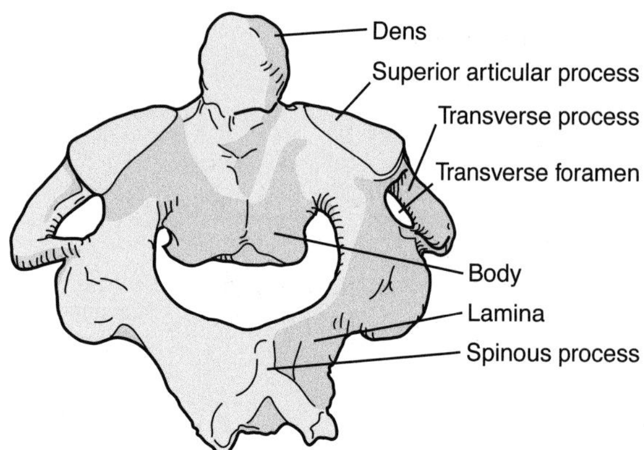

Figure 15-8. Parts of the second cervical vertebra (C2), also called the *axis* (posterior view).

Dens
Also called the *odontoid process;* large vertical projection located anteriorly on the axis. Cervical rotation occurs through its articulation with the atlas. It takes the place of the vertebral body that exists at the other levels below C2.

C7
Also known as *vertebra prominens* because of its long and prominent spinous process. It resembles a thoracic vertebra and can be easily palpated with the neck in flexion.

Transverse Foramen
Holes or openings in the transverse process of each of the cervical vertebra through which the vertebral artery passes (see Figs. 15-7 and 15-8)

Costal Facet
Located on the sides of the bodies and transverse processes of thoracic vertebrae only (Fig. 15-9). It is here that the ribs articulate with the vertebrae.

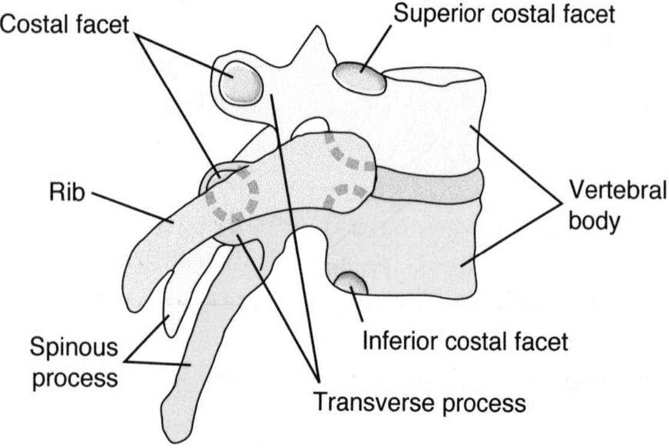

Figure 15-9. Costal facets of the thoracic vertebrae (lateral view). Dotted line indicates costal facet is deep to the rib.

Although the cervical, thoracic, and lumbar vertebrae have many of the same parts, there are differences among them (Fig. 15-10; Table 15-2).

Joints and Ligaments

Atypical Vertebral Articulations

Head and C1

The cervical spine begins with two very different articulations. The **atlantooccipital joints** (also known as the *AO joints*) are formed by the right and left occipital condyles articulating with the superior articular facets of the atlas (C1). This union is strong and supports the weight of the head. Each of the AO joints formed at the union of the occipital condyles and the superior articular processes of the atlas are synovial joints, with a synovial membrane enclosed in a joint capsule. The anterior atlantooccipital membrane is an extension of the anterior longitudinal ligament, which is somewhat thin superiorly. The tectorial membrane is a continuation of the posterior longitudinal ligament. Attached to the occipital bone on the inside of the foramen magnum, the tectorial membrane serves as a sling to support the spinal cord as it enters the vertebral column. The posterior atlantooccipital membrane serves to secure the weight of the head on the neck.

C1 and C2

The articulations between the atlas and the axis are the **atlantoaxial joints** (also known as AA joints), of which there are three. The **median atlantoaxial joint** (Fig. 15-11) consists of a synovial articulation between the odontoid process (dens) of the axis and the anterior arch of the atlas anteriorly and the transverse ligament posteriorly. The two **lateral atlantoaxial joints** are between the articular processes of C1 and C2 vertebrae (see Fig. 15-11).

The **transverse ligament** runs from one side of the atlas to the other and divides the atlas into an anterior and posterior compartment (see Fig. 15-7). The dens (odontoid process) projects upward into the anterior compartment of the atlas, whereas the spinal cord passes through the posterior compartment. The transverse ligament is crucial for keeping the dens from displacing posteriorly in the vertebral foramen and damaging the spinal cord. (see Fig. 15-7). Degeneration of the ligaments sometimes occurs in people with severe arthritis, which then allows posterior slippage of the dens.

Typical Vertebral Articulations

The articulations between adjacent vertebrae from C2 through S1 are all basically the same (Fig. 15-5). The

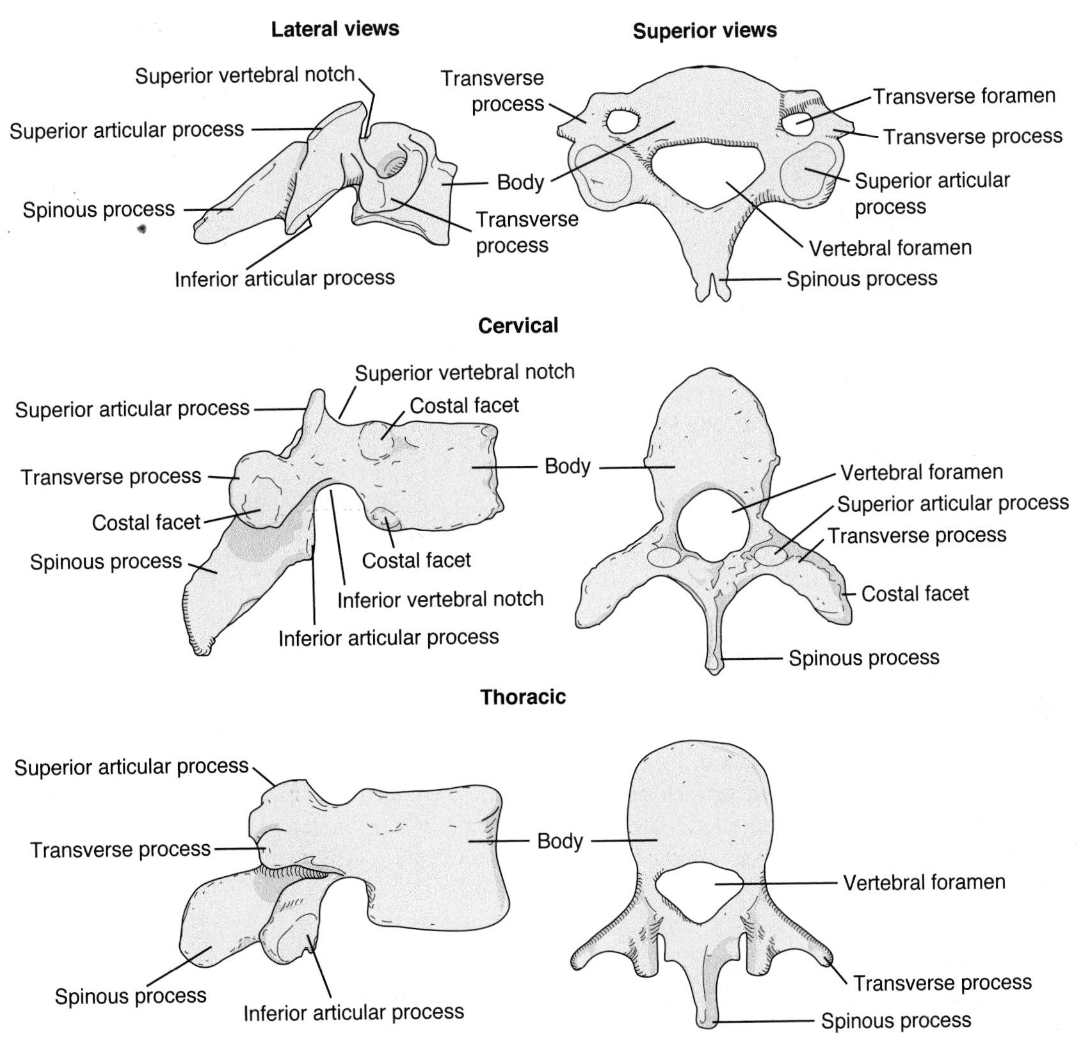

Figure 15-10. Comparison of cervical, thoracic, and lumbar vertebrae.

Table 15-2 Parts of the Vertebrae

	Cervical	Thoracic	Lumbar
Size	Smallest	Intermediate	Largest
Body shape	Small oval	Heart-shaped, with facets that connect with ribs	Large oval
Vertebral foramen	Large, triangular	Smallest	Intermediate
Transverse process	Foramen for vertebral artery; laterally	Facets that connect with ribs; long, thick, point posteriorly and laterally	No foramen or articulation
Spinous process	Short, stout, bifid	Long, slender, points inferiorly	Thick, points posteriorly
Superior articular process	Faces upward, medially, and posteriorly	Faces posteriorly and laterally	Faces posteriorly
Inferior articular process	Faces laterally	Faces anteriorly and medially	Faces anteriorly
Vertebral notches	Equal depth	Deeper inferior notches	Deeper inferior notches

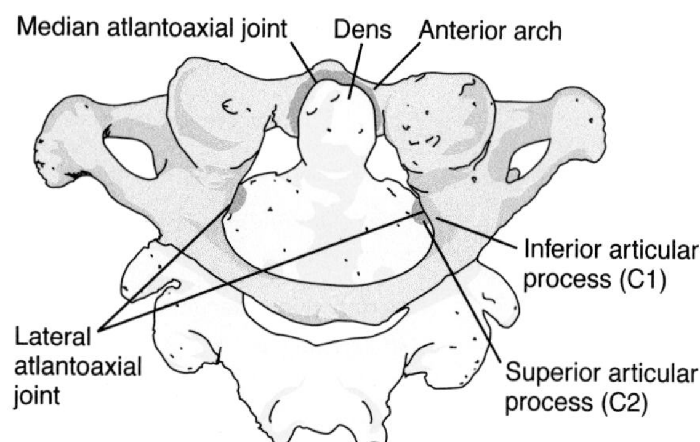

Figure 15-11. The relationship of C1 sitting on top of C2, showing the three atlantoaxial joints (posterior view).

strong, weight-bearing **intervertebral joint** occurs anteriorly on the vertebra between vertebral bodies. These are cartilaginous joints that allow only a slight degree of motion.

The posterior portion of the vertebra has two articulations (one on each side) called **facet joints** (also known as *apophyseal* or *zygapophyseal joints;* see Fig. 15-5). Each facet joint is formed by the articulation between a superior articular process of the vertebra below and an inferior articular process of the vertebra above. At each vertebral level, there are two facet joints (right and left). Each facet joint is a plane-shaped synovial joint enclosed in a joint capsular ligament.

By the direction they face, these facet joints largely determine the type and amount of motion possible (Fig. 15-12) at that part of the vertebral column. The articular processes in the lumbar area are positioned in the sagittal plane, favoring flexion and extension. Articular processes in the thoracic area are positioned in the frontal plane, favoring rotation and lateral bending. The attachment of ribs to the vertebra and the long downward sloping spinous process contributes to the limited flexion and extension. The cervical spine moves freely because the articular processes are located diagonally between the sagittal and frontal planes. The cervical region supports the head and allows a great deal of motion of the head on the neck, allows for the spinal cord to enter the vertebral canal from the brain, and allows for entrance and exit of the major blood vessels in the skull.

Many ligaments hold these vertebrae together (Fig. 15-13). The **anterior longitudinal ligament** runs down the vertebral column on the anterior surface of the bodies and tends to prevent excessive hyperextension. It is thin superiorly and thick inferiorly, where it fuses to the sacrum. It is found in the thoracic and lumbar regions just deep to the aorta. The **posterior longitudinal ligament (PLL)** runs along the vertebral bodies posteriorly, inside and along the anterior border

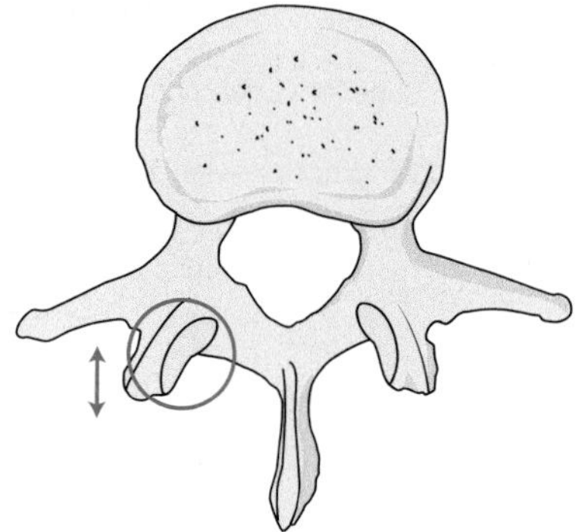

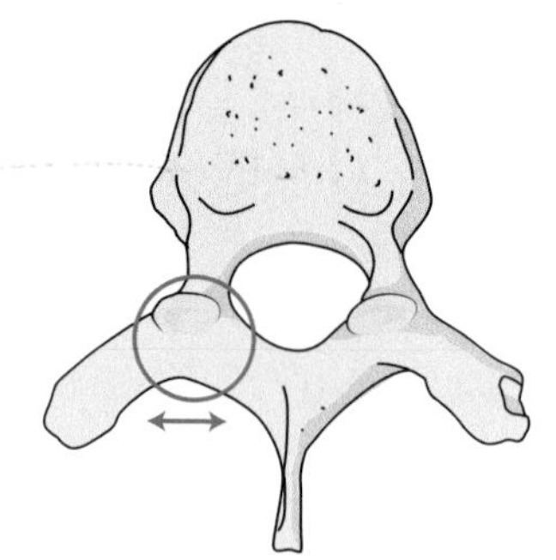

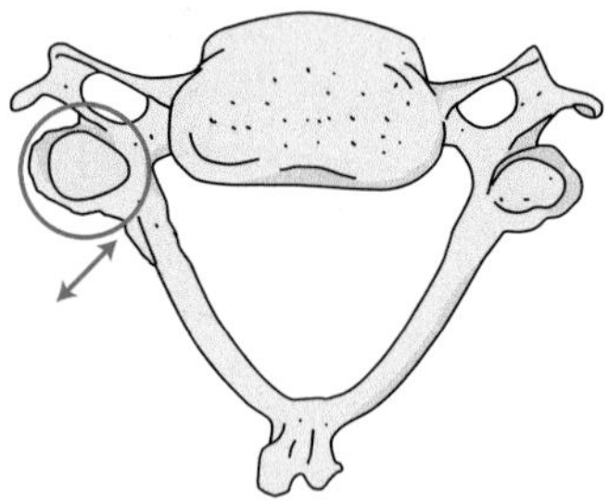

Figure 15-12. The direction in which facet joints are aligned will determine the type of motions allowed (superior view). Note that only the superior articular processes are shown in this view.

of the vertebral foramina. Its purpose is to prevent excessive flexion and to act as a barrier between the intervertebral disk and the spinal cord. It is thick superiorly, where it helps support the skull. It is thinner and more narrow inferiorly, which contributes to instability and increased disk injury in the lumbar region. The **ligamentum flavum** creates the posterior border of the vertebral canal by connecting adjacent laminae anteriorly. It is highly elastic so it can effectively lengthen during movement of the nearby facet joints but can also assist the PLL in preventing excessive flexion. The **supraspinal ligament** extends from the seventh cervical vertebra distally to the sacrum attaching posteriorly along the tips of the spinous processes. The **interspinal**

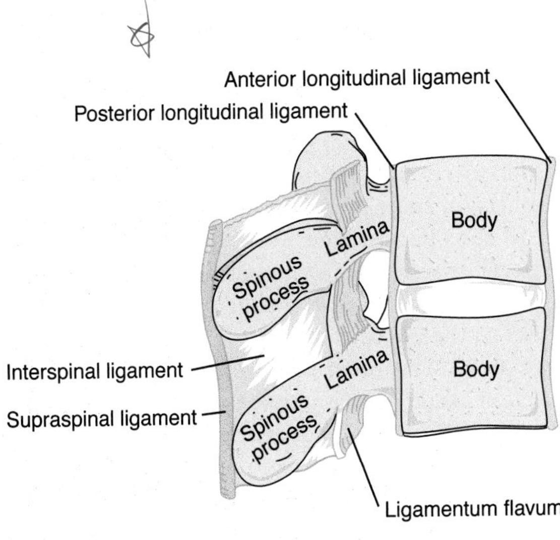

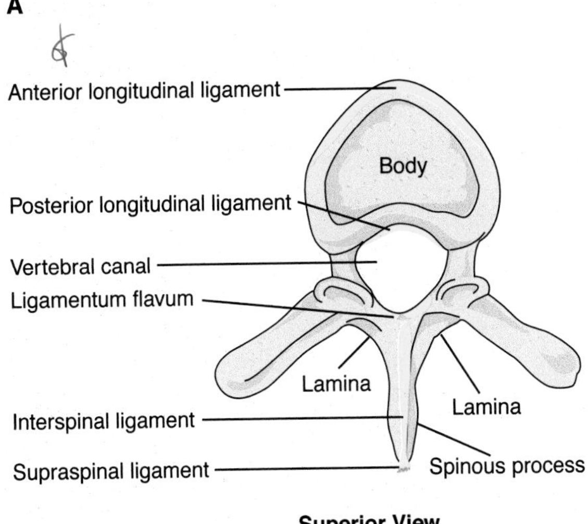

Figure 15-13. Vertebral ligaments. **(A)** Sagittal section view showing the ligaments inside and outside the vertebral canal. **(B)** Superior view showing the attachments of the ligaments on the vertebra.

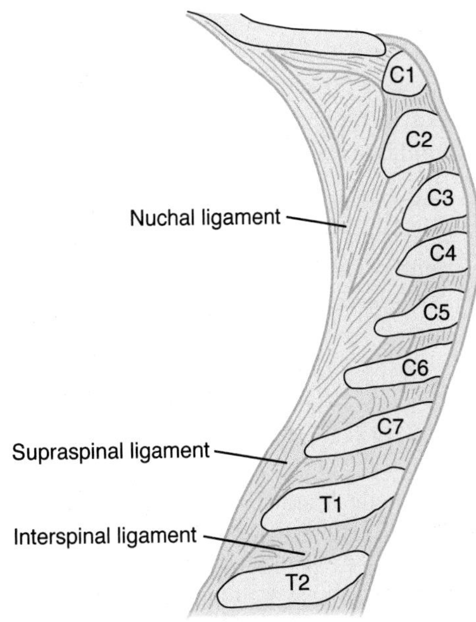

Figure 15-14. The nuchal ligament (ligamentum nuchae) becomes the supraspinal ligament in the cervical region (lateral view).

ligament runs between successive spinous processes. The very thick **ligamentum nuchae** (nuchal ligament) takes the place of the supraspinal and interspinal ligaments in the cervical region (Fig. 15-14).

In anatomical position, the majority of the weight-bearing load goes through the anterior portion of the vertebral column (vertebral bodies and intervertebral disks), and only a small portion goes through the posterior portion (facet joints). During flexion, (1) the load shifts anteriorly placing greater compressive forces at the intervertebral disk, (2) the anterior portion of the annulus fibrosus is compressed, causing the nucleus pulposus to move posteriorly, and (3) the size of the vertebral foramen and the intervertebral foramen increases, affording greater space for the spinal cord and nerve roots in these regions.

During extension, the opposite occurs: (1) a greater portion of the weight-bearing load is transferred to the facet joints, (2) the posterior portion of the annulus is compressed causing the nucleus pulposus to move anteriorly, and (3) the size of the vertebral and intervertebral foramen decreases, thereby reducing the space of the neural structures in these regions.

Why is this important? Knowledge of these mechanics allows a therapist to instruct an individual in how to move in such a way that removes pressure from pain-sensitive structures. For example, someone with a herniated disk will benefit from extension exercises because there is less load on the disks and because the nucleus pulposus moves anteriorly away from the spinal cord, whereas a person with spinal stenosis will respond better to the flexed position which creates more space for the spinal cord and spinal nerves.

Other Soft Tissue Structures

Abdominal Aponeurosis

A sheet-like tendon connecting the oblique and transverse abdominis muscles to their attachments to the linea alba

Linea Alba

A fibrous band running vertically in the midline from the xiphoid process to the pubic symphysis. It provides attachment for the transverse abdominis and two oblique muscles.

Thoracolumbar Fascia

Similar to the abdominal aponeurosis, it provides a broad area of fascial attachment posteriorly for the erector spinae and latissimus dorsi muscles.

Muscles of the Neck and Trunk

Muscles of the neck and trunk are numerous and can be divided generally into anterior and posterior muscles (Table 15-3). (The quadratus lumborum muscle is the one exception; it is located in the midline of the frontal plane and is neither an anterior nor a posterior muscle.) The clinical significance of the anterior or posterior location is function. As with most other joints, anterior muscles flex and posterior muscles extend. Only those muscles that are clinically important from an exercise standpoint will be discussed here. Other muscles will be summarized in charts and illustrations.

Muscles of the Cervical Spine

Generally speaking, muscles located anterior to the cervical vertebral column are neck flexors. The largest flexor, the **sternocleidomastoid muscle,** is a long, superficial, straplike muscle that originates as two heads from the medial aspect of the clavicle and the superior end of the sternum (Fig. 15-15). It runs superiorly and posteriorly to insert on the mastoid process of the temporal bone. When both contract bilaterally, it flexes the neck; when it contracts unilaterally, it laterally bends and rotates the face to the opposite side. For example, when the right sternocleidomastoid muscle contracts, your neck rotates so that you are looking over your left shoulder. Hence, it rotates to the opposite side. Note that when describing rotation, "face" is often used in place of "head." This is done for clarity. The motion is the same. Because it attaches on the head, it can affect head motion. Looking at the muscle's line of pull from the side, you can see that it passes anterior to the frontal axis in the lower cervical segments, which allows it to flex the neck (cervical flexion), and posterior to the frontal axis in the upper cervical region, allowing the sternocleidomastoid to hyperextend the head. This accentuates the "forward-head" position common in faulty posture. To neutralize this action, one should always "tuck the chin" before doing such activities as sit-ups.

Sternocleidomastoid Muscle

O	Sternum and clavicle
I	Mastoid process
A	Bilaterally: flexes neck, hyperextends head Unilaterally: laterally bends the neck; rotates face to the opposite side
N	Accessory nerve (cranial nerve XI); second and third cervical nerves

Table 15-3 Vertebral Muscles

	Neck	Trunk
Anterior	Sternocleidomastoid Scalenes (3) Prevertebral group (4)	Rectus abdominis External oblique Internal oblique Transverse abdominis
Posterior	Erector spinae group (3) Splenius capitis Splenius cervicis Suboccipital group (4)	Erector spinae group (3) Transversospinalis group (3) Interspinales Intertransversarii
Lateral		Quadratus lumborum

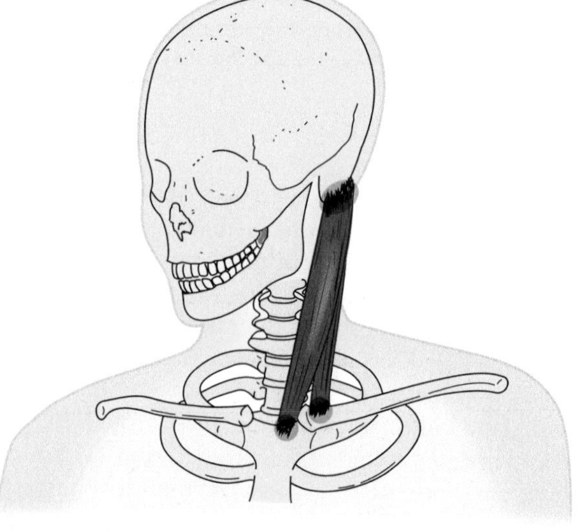

Figure 15-15. Sternocleidomastoid muscle (anterior view).

Deep to the sternocleidomastoid muscle lie the three **scalene muscles** (Fig. 15-16). The **anterior scalene muscle** originates on the transverse processes of C3 through C6 and inserts into the superior surface of the first rib. The **middle scalene muscle** originates on the transverse processes of C2 through C7; it, too, inserts into the superior surface of the first rib. The **posterior scalene muscle,** the smallest and deepest muscle, originates from C5 through C7 and inserts into the second rib. Because they all perform the same action and are located close to each other, functionally it is not necessary to differentiate between them. Located laterally at the neck, they are very effective in laterally bending the cervical spine. Because they are close to the frontal axis, they are only assistive in flexion.

Scalene Muscles

O	Transverse processes of the cervical vertebrae
I	First and second ribs
A	Bilaterally: assists in neck flexion
	Unilaterally: neck lateral bending
N	Lower cervical nerves (C3 to C8)

There is an anterior group of muscles often referred to as the **prevertebral muscles.** They are located deep and run along the anterior portion of the cervical vertebrae (Fig. 15-17). These muscles have a role in flexing either the neck or the head. Because of their small size in relation to other neck flexors, perhaps their greatest role is maintaining postural control and "tucking" the chin. Table 15-4 summarizes their locations and actions.

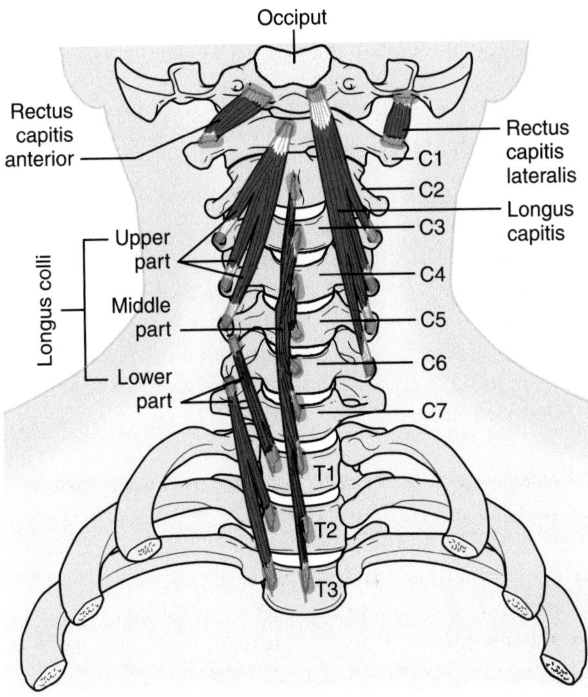

Figure 15-17. Prevertebral muscles (anterior view). Note that the anterior skull has been cut away to view the attachments on the occiput.

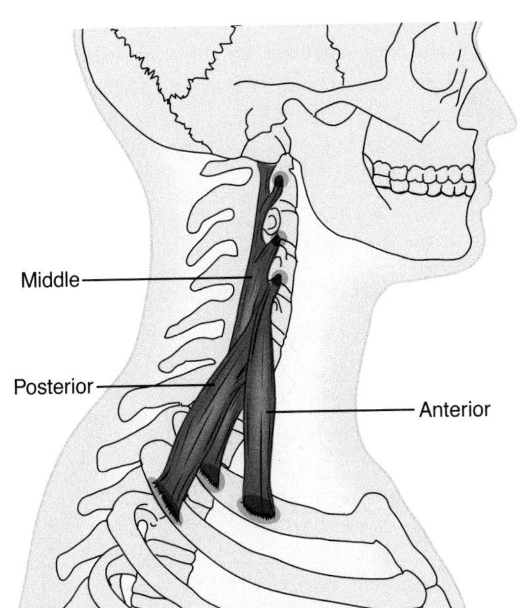

Figure 15-16. Three parts of the scalene muscles (lateral view).

Several small muscles in the neck serve as anchors for the hyoid bone and the tongue. Except for the platysma, these muscles are illustrated in Figures 15-17 and 15-30. The hyoid bone is unique in that it has no bony articulation. It functions as a primary support for the tongue and its numerous muscles. The influence of these muscles on motions of the cervical spine is assistive at best. These muscles approach the base of the skull from all directions. Table 15-5 summarizes the actions of these muscles.

The **suboccipital muscles** are clustered together below the base of the skull posteriorly and move only the head (Fig. 15-18). The muscles work together to extend the head, with a rocking motion of the occipital condyles on the atlas (AO joint), or to rotate it to the same side by pivoting the skull and atlas around the odontoid process of the axis (AA joint). These muscles also have a stabilizing role during head movement. Primarily, the rectus capitis posterior major and minor and the oblique capitis superior stabilize the AO joint, and the oblique capitis inferior stabilizes the AA joint. Table 15-6 summarizes these muscles.

Table 15-4 Prevertebral Muscles (Anterior)

Muscle	Origin	Insertion	Action
Longus colli	Upper part: transverse processes of C3 through C5 Middle part: bodies of C5 through T3 Lower part: bodies of T1 through T3	Upper: Anterior tubercle of C1 Middle: Bodies of C2 through C6 Lower: Transverse processes of C5 to C6	Flexes neck, assists in lateral bending
Longus capitis	Transverse processes of C3 through C6	Occipital bone	Flexes head and upper neck
Rectus capitis anterior	Atlas (C1)	Occipital bone	Flexes head, stabilizes AO joint
Rectus capitis lateralis	Transverse process of atlas	Occipital bone	Laterally bends head, stabilizes AO joint

Table 15-5 Muscles of the Mouth and Hyoid Bone

Group	Muscle	Action
Superficial cervical	Platysma	Draws lower lip down and out, tensing skin over neck
Suprahyoid	Digastric Stylohyoid Mylohyoid Geniohyoid	Raises hyoid bone and/or tongue
Infrahyoid	Sternohyoid Sternothyroid Thyrohyoid Omohyoid	Lowers hyoid bone

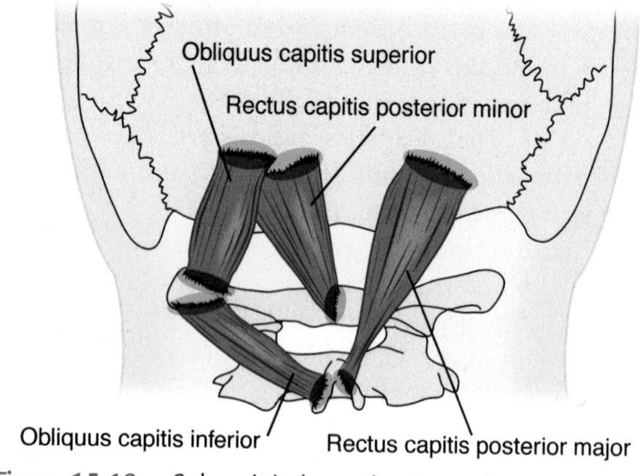

Figure 15-18. Suboccipital muscles (posterior view).

The muscles located superficially along the posterior vertebral column are known as the **erector spinae group,** which will be discussed later in more detail with the trunk muscles. These muscles provide postural control over the gravitational pull of the head into flexion; they act as extensors to bring the head back from the flexed position. The deepest back muscles (transversospinalis, interspinales, and intertransversarii) will also be described in the trunk section, as that is where the majority of these muscles are located.

Deep to the erector spinae are the **splenius capitis** and **splenius cervicis muscles.** As their names imply, they attach to the head and to the cervical spine. The splenius capitis muscle is the more superficial of the two. They both attach from the spinous processes of the lower cervical and upper thoracic vertebrae, and they run superiorly and laterally to the lateral occiput (capitis) and transverse processes of the upper cervical vertebrae (cervicis), respectively (see Fig. 15-19). When the muscles on only one side contract, they rotate and laterally bend the face and neck to the same side. However, when both sides contract, they extend the neck, and the splenius capitis extends the head on the neck.

Splenius Capitis Muscles

O	Lower half of nuchal ligament; spinous processes of C7 through T3
I	Lateral occipital bone; mastoid process
A	Bilaterally: extend head and neck Unilaterally: laterally bend and rotate the face to same side
N	Middle and lower cervical nerves

Splenius Cervicis Muscles

O	Spinous processes of T3 through T6
I	Transverse processes of C1 through C3
A	Bilaterally: extend neck Unilaterally: laterally bend and rotate the face to same side
N	Middle and lower cervical nerves

Table 15-6 Suboccipital Muscles (Posterior)

Muscle	Location	Head Motion
Obliquus capitis superior	Posterior	Extension and stabilization of AO joint
Obliquus capitis inferior	Posterior	Extension, lateral bending, rotation to the same side, and stabilization of AA joint
Rectus capitis posterior minor	Posterior	Extension and stabilization of AO joint
Rectus capitis posterior major	Posterior	Extension, lateral bending, rotation to the same side, and stabilization of AO joint

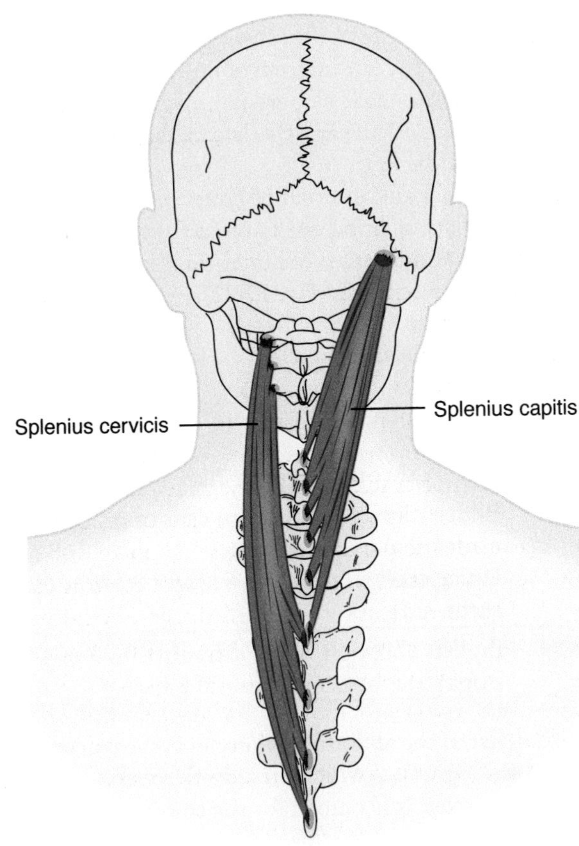

Figure 15-19. Splenius capitis and cervicis muscles (posterior view).

It should be noted that the upper trapezius and levator scapula can assist the splenius capitis and cervicis under certain conditions. If the scapula is fixed, they can function in reverse muscle action. Instead of moving the scapula on the head and neck as in shoulder girdle motion, the head and neck can move on the scapula. The upper trapezius can rotate the face to the opposite side and laterally bend to the same side, whereas the levator scapula both rotates and laterally bends to the same side.

Muscles of the Trunk

Spanning the anterior trunk in the midline is the **rectus abdominis** muscle. The two sides are separated from each other by the linea alba. The rectus abdominis muscle arises from the crest of the pubis and inserts into the costal cartilages of the fifth, sixth, and seventh ribs. Three tendinous intersections divide the muscle horizontally into smaller units (Fig. 15-20). Located in the anterior midline, the rectus abdominis muscle is a strong trunk flexor that, along with the other anterior trunk muscles, compresses the abdominal contents.

Rectus Abdominis Muscles

O	Pubic crest
I	Xiphoid process and costal cartilages of fifth to seventh ribs
A	Trunk flexion; compression of abdomen
N	Seventh through 12th intercostal nerves

The **external oblique muscle** is a large, broad, flat muscle (Fig. 15-21A) that lies superficially on the

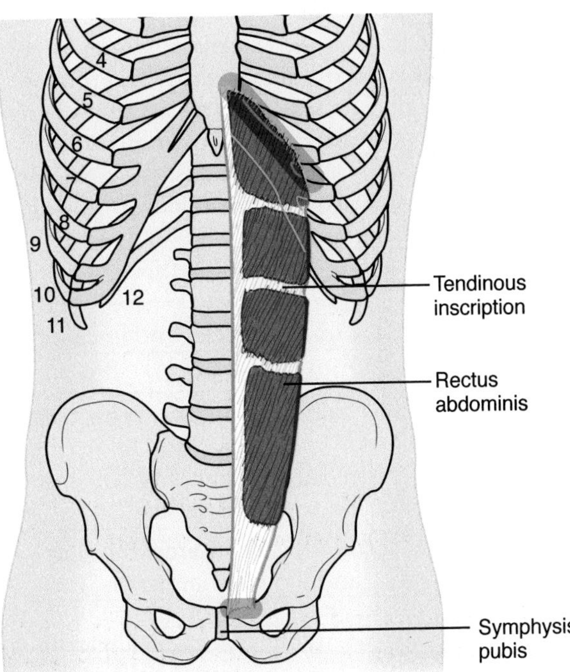

Figure 15-20. Rectus abdominis muscle (anterior view). Note that the muscle is shown only on the left side.

Clinical Application 15-1

Doing a Proper Sit-up

When doing a sit-up, the trunk flexors (abdominals) will move the trunk toward the femur (trunk flexion) if the legs are not stabilized, but when doing a sit-up with the legs stabilized, the hip flexors will be engaged in a reverse muscle action, moving the trunk toward the femur (trunk flexion). If the objective is to strengthen the abdominals and not the hip flexors, the legs should not be stabilized when doing a sit-up.

To further work the abdominals, in addition to not stabilizing the feet, the hips and knees should be flexed. This will put the hip flexors on a slack, making them less able to contribute to trunk flexion.

anterolateral abdomen. Its originates from the anterior half of the iliac crest, pubic tubercle, and, via the abdominal aponeurosis, into the linea alba at the midline, and runs superiorly and laterally to insert on the fifth through twelfth ribs laterally. The fiber direction of each external oblique muscle can be depicted by the direction in which your fingers run when placing your hands *into* your front pockets at about a 45-degree angle. Viewed together, the fibers of the left and right external oblique muscles form the shape of a *V.* When both sides contract, they flex the trunk and compress the abdominal contents. When one side contracts, that external oblique laterally bends the trunk toward the same side, but rotates the trunk to the opposite side. This means that the right external oblique muscle rotates the right side of the trunk toward the midline. Visualize the right shoulder moving forward toward the midline, causing the face to move to the left.

External Oblique Muscle

O	Iliac crest, pubic tubercle, and linea alba
I	Lower eight ribs laterally
A	Bilaterally: trunk flexion; compression of abdomen Unilaterally: lateral bending to same side; rotation to opposite side
N	Eighth through 12th intercostal, iliohypogastric, and ilioinguinal nerves

Located deep to and running at right angles to the external oblique muscle is the **internal oblique muscle.** It originates from the lateral half of the inguinal ligament, the anterior two-thirds of the iliac crest, and thoracolumbar fascia. It then runs superiorly and medially to insert into the inferior borders of the last five ribs and, via the abdominal aponeurosis, into the linea alba (Fig. 15-21B). Viewed together, the fibers of the left and right internal oblique muscles form the shape of an inverted *V.* When both sides contract, they flex the trunk and compress the abdominal contents. When one side contracts, that internal oblique laterally bends the trunk (to the same side). It also rotates the trunk to the same side. Visualize the right shoulder rotating back and toward the right, causing the face to move to the right. With the left internal oblique muscle rotating the trunk to the same side, visualize the left shoulder rotating back and toward the left causing the face to move toward the left.

The external and internal obliques on the same side of the body act as antagonists to each other. However, the external and internal obliques on opposite sides of the body act as agonists (Fig. 15-22).

Internal Oblique Muscle

O	Inguinal ligament, iliac crest, thoracolumbar fascia
I	Eighth through twelfth ribs, linea alba
A	Bilaterally: trunk flexion; compression of abdomen Unilaterally: lateral bending; rotation to same side
N	Eighth through 12th intercostal, iliohypogastric, and ilioinguinal nerves

The deepest of the abdominal muscles is the **transverse abdominis** muscle, which lies deep to the internal oblique muscles. It is named for the transverse, or horizontal, direction of its fibers. It originates from the lateral third of the inguinal ligament, the inner lip of the iliac crest, the thoracolumbar fascia posteriorly, and the inner surfaces of the costal cartilage of the lower seven ribs. The inguinal ligament runs from the anterior superior iliac spine of the ilium to the pubic tubercle (see Fig. 18-13). The transverse abdominis spans the abdomen horizontally to insert into the abdominal aponeurosis, linea alba, and the pubic crest. (see Fig. 15-21C). Because of its horizontal line of pull, it plays no effective part in moving the trunk. However, it does work with the other abdominal muscles to compress and support the abdominal contents. This is important in activities such as coughing, sneezing, laughing, forced expiration, and "bearing down" during childbirth or while having a bowel movement.

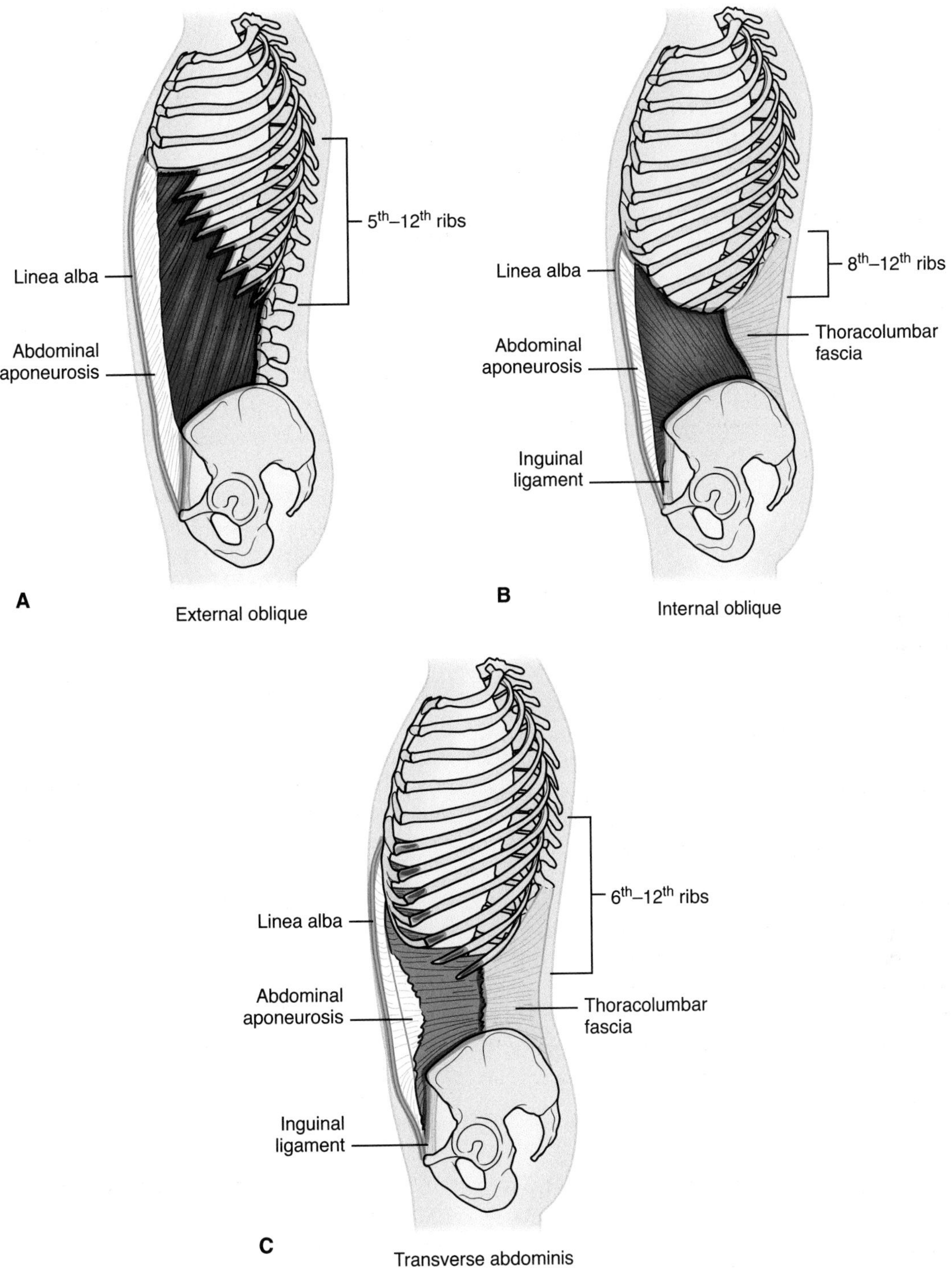

Figure 15-21. Three layers of abdominal muscles (anterior view). The external oblique is superficial, the internal oblique lies underneath it, and the transverse abdominis is the deepest layer.

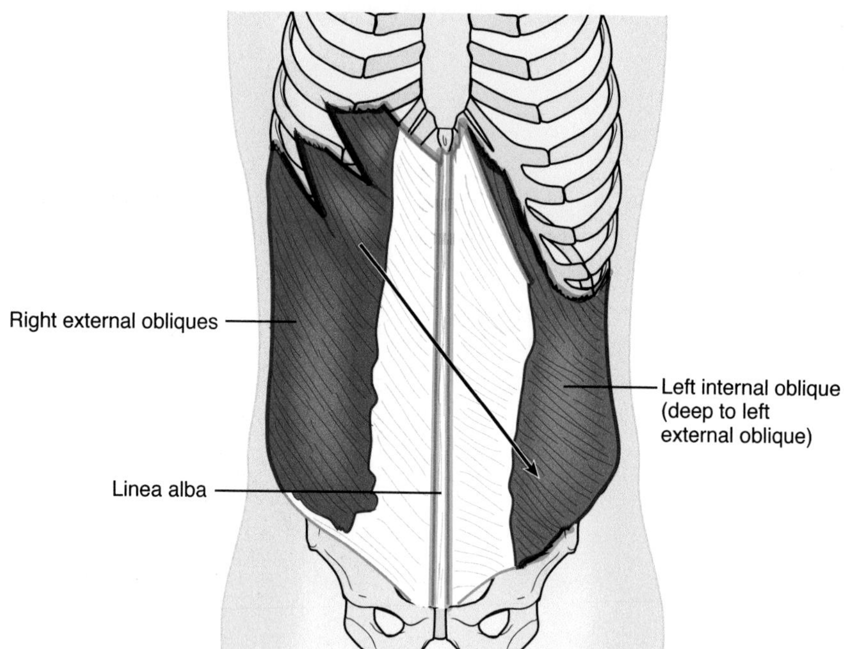

Figure 15-22. External and internal obliques working as agonists and antagonists in trunk rotation.

Transverse Abdominis Muscle

O	Inguinal ligament, iliac crest, thoracolumbar fascia, and costal cartilages of the last seven ribs
I	Pubic crest, abdominal aponeurosis, and linea alba
A	Compression of abdomen
N	Seventh through 12th intercostal, iliohypogastric, and ilioinguinal nerves

There are many groups of posterior muscles, which are summarized in Table 15-7. Some general statements can be made regarding their attachments and actions (Fig. 15-23). Generally speaking, regardless of the number of vertebrae spanned, muscles attaching from spinous process to spinous process have a vertical line of pull; thus, they extend (Fig. 15-23A). Because they are located in the midline, there is only one set of them. Muscles that run from transverse process to transverse process have a vertical line of pull lateral to the midline. When acting unilaterally, they laterally bend; when acting bilaterally, they extend (Fig. 15-23B). Muscles attaching from rib to rib have the same line of pull as those attaching between transverse processes. Being more lateral, muscles attaching to ribs are even more

Table 15-7 Posterior Trunk Muscles

Attachments	Action	Muscles
Spinous process to spinous process	Extension	Spinalis (ES) Interspinales
Transverse process to transverse process	Extension, lateral bending	Longissimus (ES) Intertransversarii
Spinous process to transverse process	Extension, rotation to same side	Splenius cervicis
Transverse process to spinous process	Extension, rotation to opposite side	Semispinalis (T) Multifidus (T) Rotatores (T)
Transverse process to rib, or rib to rib	Extension, lateral bending	Iliocostalis (ES)

ES, erector spinae group; T, transversospinalis group.

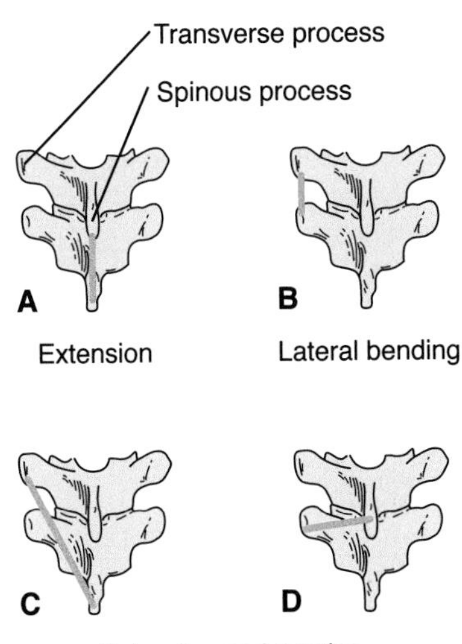

Figure 15-23. Line of pull determines muscle action as summarized for posterior trunk muscles.

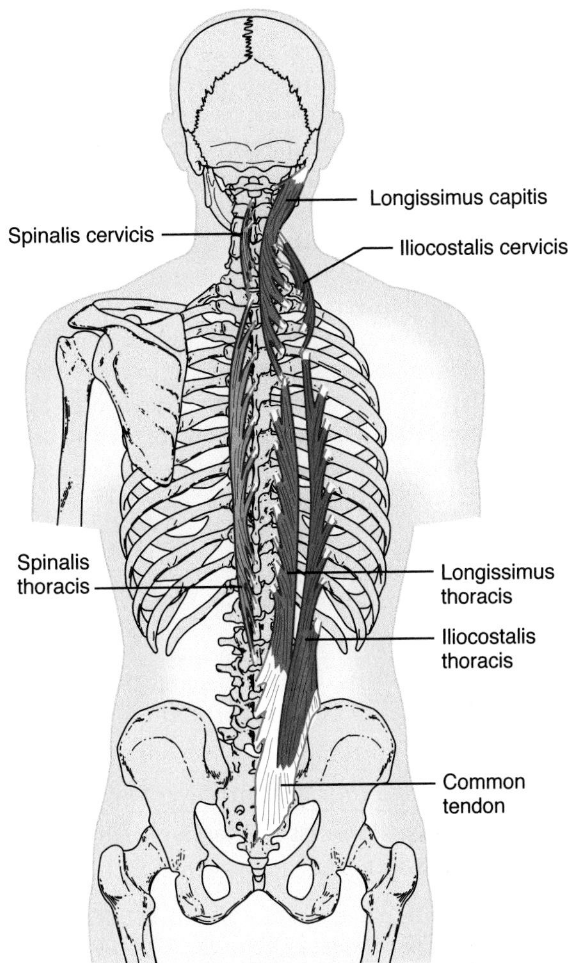

Figure 15-24. Three parts of the erector spinae muscle group (posterior view). Note that the spinalis group is more medial, the iliocostalis group is more lateral, and the longissimus group runs in the middle.

effective at lateral bending because they have a greater distance between the lateral bending axis of rotation at the spine and the line of pull of the muscle, creating a larger moment arm. Muscles attaching from spinous process to transverse process or from transverse process to spinous process have an oblique line and therefore extend bilaterally and rotate unilaterally (Fig. 15-23C, D). In Figure 15-23C, with the lower attachment fixed, these muscles will rotate the trunk above to the same side. In Figure 15-23D, with the lower attachment fixed, these muscles will rotate the trunk above to the opposite side. Of these posterior muscles, shorter muscles are more effective at rotation, and longer muscles are more effective at extension.

The superficial layer of back extensors is a group of muscles called the **erector spinae muscles,** sometimes called the *sacrospinalis muscle group.* It is a massive and complex muscle group occupying the groove on each side of the vertebral column. It lies deep to the thoracolumbar fascia, serratus posterior superior and inferior, posterior shoulder girdle muscles in the cervical area, and the splenius capitis and cervicis muscles. It lies superficial to the transversospinalis muscles.

The erector spinae can be subdivided into three groups that run mostly vertical along the vertebral column and connect spinous processes, transverse processes, and ribs (Fig. 15-24). It originates as a broad, thick tendon attached to the posterior sacrum, posterior iliac crest, lumbar spinous processes, and supraspinal ligaments. It then splits into three vertically running parts: iliocostalis, longissimus, and spinalis.

As a whole, the erector spinae ascends the length of the back, but its three columns are composed of shorter bundles of muscles; one bundle originating as another is inserting. Each muscle bundle spans from 6 to 10 segments between bony attachments. All three portions act as one in extending the vertebral column and laterally bending it to the same side. Because the upper portion of the longissimus inserts on the mastoid process, it can also rotate the head to the same side.

The most medial group is the **spinalis muscle group,** which primarily attaches to the nuchal ligament and spinous processes of the cervical and thoracic vertebrae. The portion of this group that attaches to the occiput also attaches to the transverse processes of the cervical vertebrae. Located near the midline, these muscles are prime movers in trunk extension.

The intermediate muscles, the **longissimus muscle group,** are located lateral to the spinalis muscle group, attaching to the transverse processes from the occiput to the sacrum. Because these muscles are lateral to the midline and have a vertical line of pull, they produce lateral bending to the same side when contracting unilaterally and produce extension when contracting bilaterally. The upper fibers of the longissimus group attach to the occiput and therefore can contribute to extension and lateral bending of the head on the neck.

The **iliocostalis muscles** are the most lateral group, attaching primarily to the ribs posteriorly. Superiorly, they attach to transverse processes, and inferiorly they attach to the sacrum and ilium. Because of their lateral position, these muscles are excellent at lateral bending. Acting bilaterally, they are effective extensors. These three groups of muscles generally are referred to as the *erector spinae muscle group,* and therefore will be summarized as a group.

Erector Spinae Muscles

Iliocostalis portion	
O	iliac crest, lower ribs
I	angles of ribs, upper ribs, and transverse processes of cervical vertebrae
Longissimus portion	
O	transverse processes at lower levels
I	transverse processes at upper levels, mastoid process
Spinalis portion	
O	spinous processes below
I	spinous processes above
A	Bilaterally: extend neck and trunk Unilaterally: Rotate head and laterally bend neck and trunk to the same side
N	Spinal nerves

The deepest of the back extensor muscles is a group of three muscles called the **transversospinalis (transverse spinal) muscle group** (Fig. 15-25). They get their name from their attachments. They have an oblique line of pull, essentially attaching from a transverse process to the spinous process of a vertebra above; therefore, they are very effective at rotation to the opposite side (see Fig. 15-23D). The *semispinalis* muscles tend to span five or more vertebrae; the *multifidus* muscles tend to span two to four vertebrae; and the *rotatores* muscles, the shortest and deepest of this group, span only one vertebra. Unilaterally, these muscles rotate to the opposite side and bilaterally extend the spine. The semispinalis is the most superficial muscle of the transversospinalis group and runs from the lower thoracic region to the base of the skull. Therefore, it has an additional role in extension and rotation of the head. The multifidus lies underneath the semispinalis and runs from the sacrum to the lower four or five cervical vertebrae. The rotators are the deepest of the transversospinalis muscles and are primarily in the thoracic region. All of the transversospinalis muscles lie in the groove between the transverse and spinous processes of the vertebrae. Perhaps of more functional importance is the role that these muscles, especially the multifidus and rotatores, play as stabilizers of the vertebral column.

Transversospinalis Muscles

O	Transverse processes
I	Spinous processes of vertebrae above
A	Bilaterally: extend neck and trunk Unilaterally: rotate head, neck, and trunk to opposite side
N	Spinal nerves

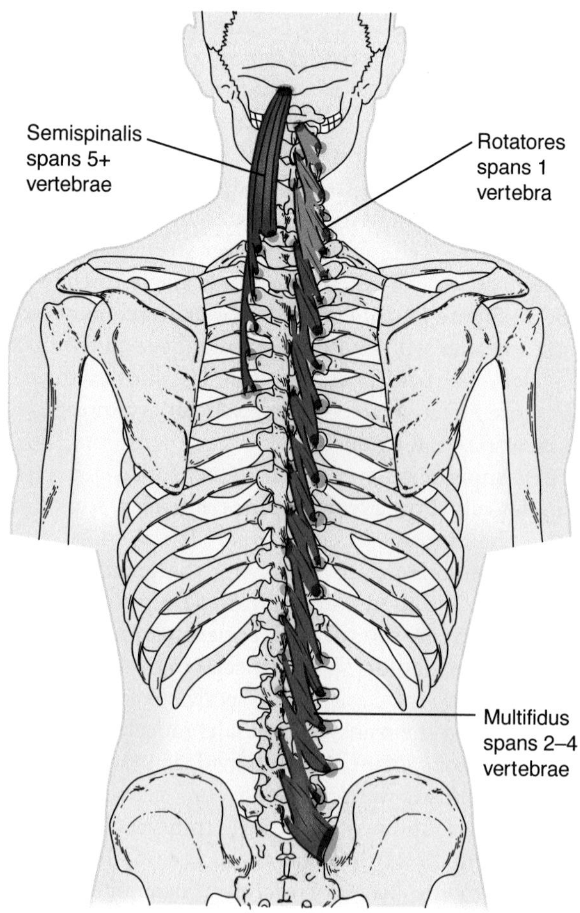

Figure 15-25. Transversospinalis muscle group (posterior view). For illustration purposes, muscles are shown in different parts of the vertebral column. In fact, all run greater lengths than shown of the vertebral column in layers.

Like the transversospinalis muscle group, these next two muscles are located deep, but they have a vertical, not oblique, line of pull. Therefore, they must be considered separately. The names of the interspinales and intertransversarii muscles indicate where they attach. The **interspinales muscles** attach from the spinous process below to the spinous process above throughout most of the vertebral column (Fig. 15-26). With this vertical line of pull in the midline, they are effective extensors. The **intertransversarii muscles** attach from the transverse process below to the transverse process above, and they appear throughout most of the vertebral column (Fig. 15-27). They are effective at lateral bending. Both play a role in stabilizing the vertebral column during movement of the trunk.

Interspinales Muscles

O	Spinous process below
I	Spinous process above
A	Neck and trunk extension
N	Spinal nerves

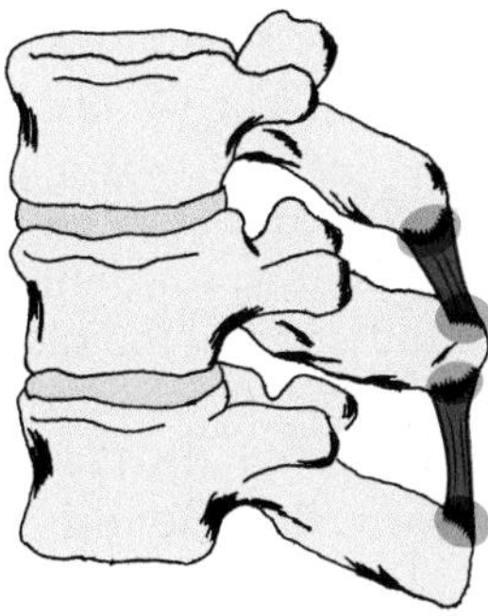

Figure 15-26. Interspinales muscles (lateral view).

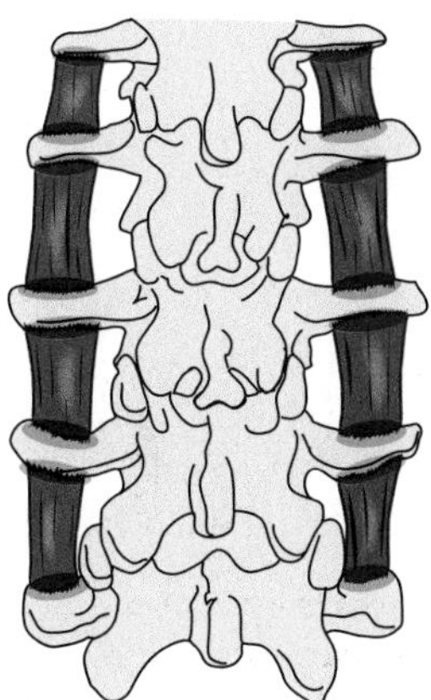

Figure 15-27. Intertransversarii muscles (posterior view).

Intertransversarii Muscles

O	Transverse process below
I	Transverse process above
A	Neck and trunk lateral bending to the same side
N	Spinal nerves

The **quadratus lumborum muscle** is a deep muscle that originates from the iliac crest. It runs superiorly to insert into the last rib and transverse processes of all lumbar vertebrae (Fig. 15-28). Because it is located in the anterior-posterior midline, it does not have a function of flexion or extension; being vertical, it has no role in rotation. However, being lateral to the midline makes it effective at lateral bending. It has another function that occurs when its origin is pulled toward its insertion (reverse muscle action). The action is called *hip hiking,* or *elevation,* of one side of the pelvis. This is an important function to anyone with a long leg cast or fused knee because it allows the foot to clear the floor without bending the knee. A small degree of hip hiking occurs normally as the foot reaches up to the next step during stair climbing.

Clinical Application 15-2

Role of Compressive Forces in Spinal Stability

When the spinal flexors and extensors perform a cocontraction, this creates a downward pull that compresses the vertebrae together. This compression makes the vertebrae less prone to unwanted shearing movements and helps to keep the spine stable. Further stability can be achieved by increasing the intraabdominal pressure, which forms a natural "corset" around the spine. To increase intraabdominal pressure, the abdominals compress the trunk anteriorly while the muscles that attach to the thoracolumbar fascia (internal oblique, transverse abdominis, latissimus dorsi) compress the trunk posteriorly. For this reason, patients with lower back pain may be instructed to "brace" before lifting by performing an isometric contraction of their core muscles. Simply stated, core muscles are muscles that stabilize and move the trunk of the body, especially the abdominals and muscles of the back.

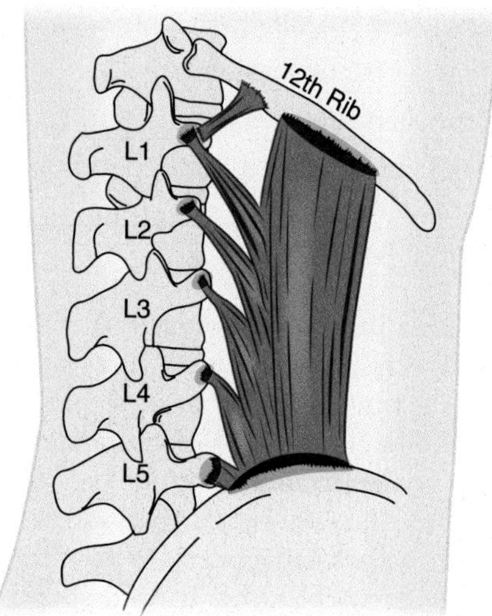

Figure 15-28. Quadratus lumborum muscle (lateral view).

Quadratus Lumborum Muscle

O	Iliac crest
I	Twelfth rib, transverse processes of all five lumbar vertebrae
A	Trunk lateral bending
N	Twelfth thoracic and first lumbar nerves

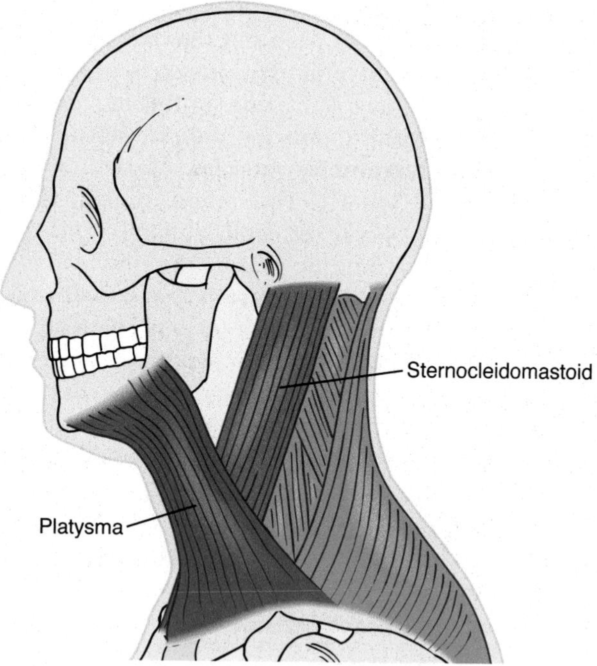

Figure 15-29. Platysma muscle (side view).

Anatomical Relationships

Looking at the anterior neck, the most superficial muscle is the very broad, thin platysma muscle (Fig. 15-29). This muscle covers a large portion of the anterior and lateral neck. It participates in facial expression and has no function at the neck. Beneath the platysma and running diagonally from the medial clavicle out and up to the mastoid process behind the ear is the sternocleidomastoid muscle (Fig. 15-30). Deep to the sternocleidomastoid are the infrahyoid muscles, which align more vertically in the anterior neck region. Looking under the chin, you would see the suprahyoid muscles. The prevertebral muscles are the deepest muscle group, lying next to the vertebral column (not visible in Fig. 15-30, see Fig. 15-17).

From a lateral view, the platysma covers all but the upper half of the sternocleidomastoid (see Fig. 15-29).

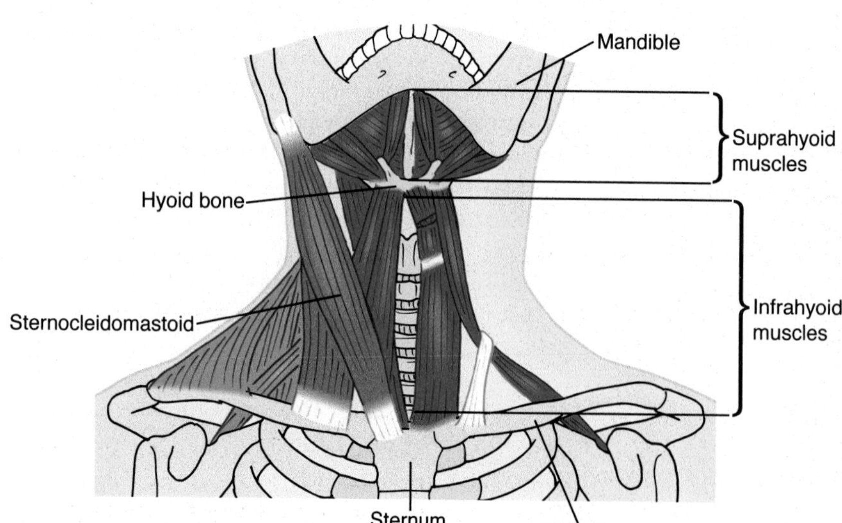

Figure 15-30. Muscles of the neck (anterior view).

Because the sternocleidomastoid runs diagonally from posterior-superior to anterior-inferior, it covers portions of the infrahyoid muscles anteriorly and the three scalene muscles near the midline laterally (Fig. 15-31). The posterior scalene is not visible. Posteriorly, the sternocleidomastoid covers portions of the levator scapulae and splenius capitis near their superior attachments. The upper trapezius is the most superficial muscle posteriorly.

There are several layers of muscles in the posterior neck (Fig. 15-32). As mentioned earlier, the most superficial muscle is the upper trapezius (see Fig. 9-13). This muscle has been removed in Figure 15-32 to show the splenius capitis partially covering the splenius cervicis. Beneath these muscles is the semispinalis portion of the transversospinalis group. This group covers the erector spinae (not visible in Fig. 15-32). The deepest layer in the neck includes the shortest muscles: the suboccipital muscles (near the head) and the interspinales and intertransversarii muscles. These last two muscles are also not visable in Fig. 15-32.

The trunk muscles are divided into anterior and posterior muscles. There are four layers of muscles on the abdominal, or anterior, trunk wall (Fig. 15-33). The rectus abdominis lies the most superficial and is in the midline. The external oblique muscle is superficial on the sides of the abdominal wall and is just underneath the rectus femoris anteriorly. Directly under the external oblique muscle lies the internal oblique. The transverse abdominis is the deepest of the abdominal muscles; its fibers run in a horizontal direction.

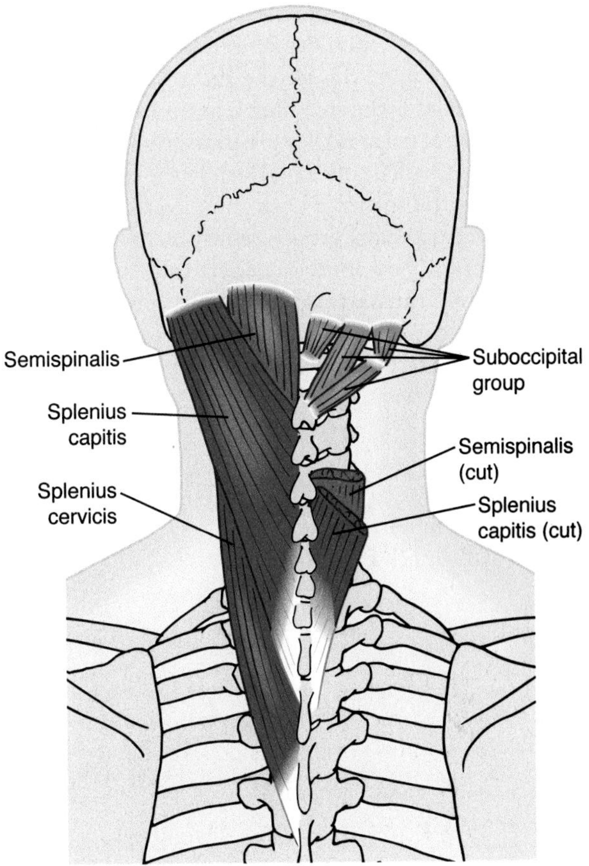

Figure 15-32. Muscles of the neck (posterior view).

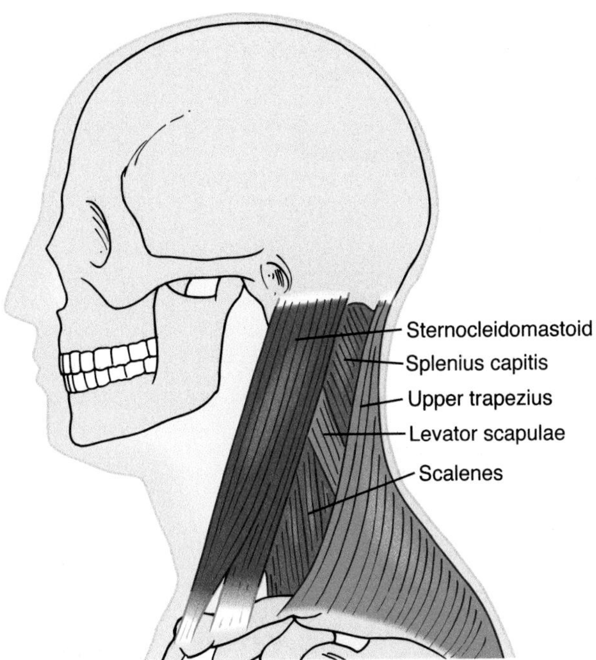

Figure 15-31. Muscles of the neck (lateral view).

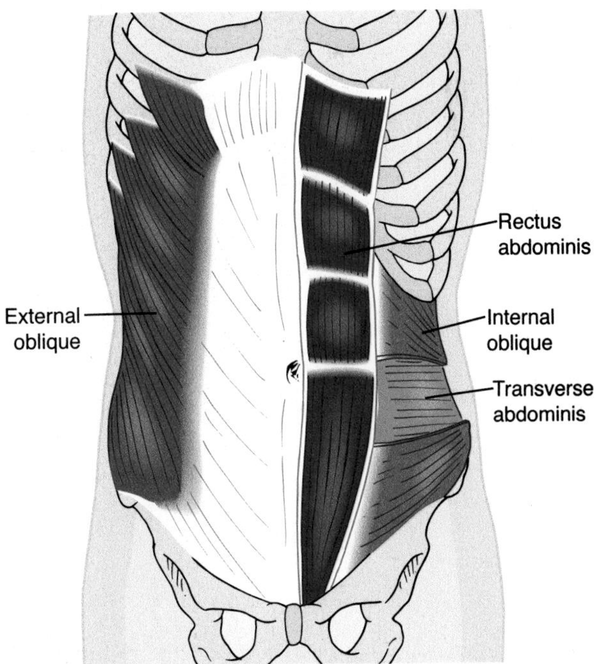

Figure 15-33. Muscles of the trunk (anterior view). Note that the muscles are shown only on one side, and a portion of the internal oblique has been cut away to show the transverse abdominis deep to it.

The posterior trunk muscles are located deep to the shoulder girdle and shoulder joint muscles (see Fig. 9-22). As shown in Figure 15-34, the most superficial layer of back muscles is the erector spinae muscle group: iliocostalis (lateral column), longissimus (middle column), and spinalis (medial column). Deep to the erector spinae muscles are the intrinsic back muscles that belong to the transversospinalis group (semispinalis, multifidus, and rotators). These muscles lie vertically in the groove between the transverse and spinous processes. The deepest muscles of the trunk are the one-joint interspinal and intertransversarii muscles. The interspinal muscles are not visible in Figure 15-34.

Summary of Muscle Actions

Table 15-8 summarizes the muscle actions of the prime movers of the neck and trunk.

Summary of Muscle Innervation

Most muscles of the neck and trunk do not receive innervation from branches or terminal nerves of a plexus. Because they tend to be groups that span several vertebral levels, their innervation typically reflects that. Generally speaking, they receive innervation from spinal nerves at various levels. For example, a spinal cord injury at T12 will not cause paralysis of all erector spinae muscles but will cause only paralysis of those located below that level.

Common Vertebral Column Pathologies

Thoracic outlet syndrome is a general term referring to compression of the neurovascular structures (brachial plexus and subclavian artery and vein) that run from the

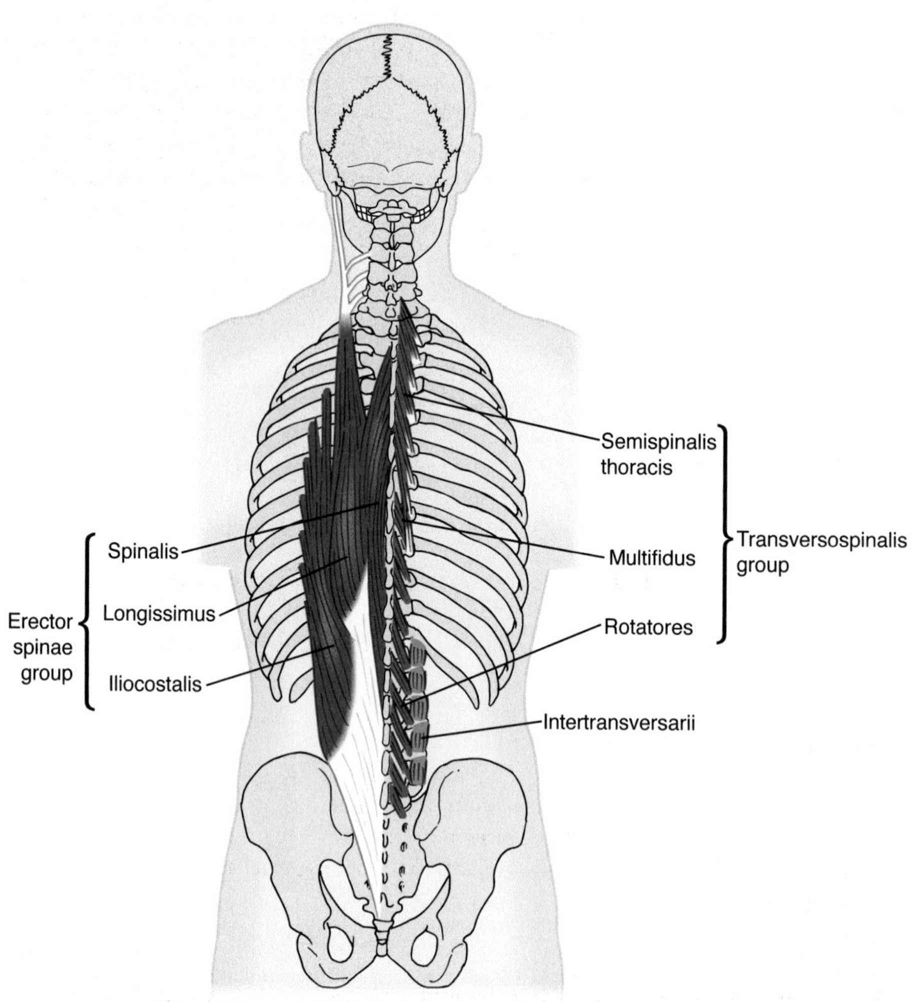

Figure 15-34. Muscles of the trunk (posterior view).

Clinical Application 15-3

Mechanics of Lifting: "Lift with Your Legs, Not with Your Back"

"Lifting with the legs," commonly referred to as a *squat lift,* is achieved with hips and knees flexed, and the trunk in a relatively upright position. "Lifting with the back" is a *forward bent lift,* in which the hips and spine are flexed and the knees are extended. A squat lift increases compressive forces on the intervertebral disks, and a forward bent lift increases anterior shearing forces on the spine. Because the spine is able to resist compressive forces better than shearing forces, a squat lift reduces the risk of spinal injury.

The length of the resistance arm must also be considered. The weight of any object lifted in front of the body will cause a flexion force at the spine. This force must be offset by contraction of the spinal extensors. Using a squat-type lift and holding the object close to the trunk both decreases the length of the resistance arm and reduces the amount of spinal extensor contraction force needed.

neck through the axilla. The thoracic outlet is located between the first rib, the clavicle, and the scalene muscles. The brachial plexus and subclavian artery pass between the anterior and middle scalene muscles, the first rib, and the clavicle. A variety of signs and symptoms can occur, depending on the structures involved. **Torticollis** (from the Latin *tortus,* meaning "twisted," and *collum,* meaning "neck") is a deformity of the neck in which the person's head is laterally bent to one side and rotated toward the other side. It is also known as *wryneck.* **Sciatica** is pain that tends to run down the posterior thigh and leg. It is caused by pressure on the sciatic nerve roots and usually is symptomatic of an underlying pathology such as a herniated lumbar disc.

The vertebral column has a normal anterior-posterior curvature. **Lordosis** is an abnormally increased curve of the lumbar spine. The layman's term is *swayback.* **Flat back** is an abnormally decreased lumbar curve. **Kyphosis** is an abnormally increased thoracic curve. Any amount of lateral curve is a pathological condition known as **scoliosis.**

Spondylosis (spinal osteoarthritis) is a degenerative disorder of vertebral structure and function. It may result from bony spurs, thickening of ligaments, and decreased disk height that results from reduced water content of the nucleus pulposus, a normal part of the aging process. All of these problems may lead to nerve

Table 15-8 Prime Movers of the Neck and Trunk

Action	Muscle
Head (Occiput on C1)	
Flexion	Prevertebral group
Extension	Suboccipital group
Neck	
Flexion	Sternocleidomastoid
Extension	Splenius capitis, splenius cervicis, erector spinae, transversospinalis, interspinales
Lateral bending	Sternocleidomastoid, splenius capitis, splenius cervicis, scalenes, erector spinae, intertransversarii
Rotation (same side)	Splenius capitis, splenius cervicis
Rotation (opposite side)	Sternocleidomastoid, transversospinalis
Trunk	
Flexion	Rectus abdominis, external oblique, internal oblique
Extension	Erector spinae, transversospinalis, interspinales
Lateral bending	Quadratus lumborum, erector spinae, internal oblique, external oblique, intertransversarii
Rotation same side	Internal oblique
Rotation opposite side	External oblique, transversospinalis
Compression of abdomen	Rectus abdominis, external oblique, internal oblique, transverse abdominis

root and spinal cord compression. **Spinal stenosis** is a narrowing of the vertebral canal that houses the spinal cord. It is also possible to have stenosis of the intervertebral foramen through which the nerve roots pass. **Herniated disks** occur when there is a weakness or degeneration of the annulus fibrosus (outer layer). This allows a portion of the nucleus pulposus to bulge, or herniate, through the annulus. It becomes symptomatic when the herniation puts pressure on the spinal cord or, more commonly, on the nerve root. L4 and L5 are the most common sites for disk lesions, and the fourth and fifth lumbar nerve roots are the most commonly affected. **Ankylosing spondylitis,** a chronic inflammation of the vertebral column and sacroiliac joints, leads to fusion. It is a progressive rheumatic disease; over time, it can lead to a total loss of spinal mobility.

The lumbar spine is the most injured region of the human body. It bears the majority of our body weight plus the weight of anything we carry. The body's center of gravity is located anterior to the second sacral vertebra. Most movement of the lumbar spine occurs between L4 and L5 and between L5 and S1. Not surprisingly, most disk herniations occur at these two levels. The thinness of the posterior longitudinal ligament in the lumbar spine contributes to the increased disk herniation in this region. **Spondylolysis** is a vertebral defect in the pars interarticularis (the part of the lamina between the superior and inferior articular processes). This defect is most commonly seen in L5 and less commonly in L4. **Spondylolisthesis** usually results from a fracture, or giving way, of a defective pars interarticularis. One vertebra slips forward in relation to an adjacent vertebra, usually L5 slipping anterior on S1.

Compression fractures typically result in the collapse of the anterior (body) portion of the vertebrae. They are usually caused by trauma in the lumbar region or by osteoporosis in the thoracic region. This type of fracture does not commonly cause spinal cord damage and paralysis, because the fracture is usually stable. A stable fracture does not have progressive displacement or dislocation. Unstable fractures, or **fractures with dislocation,** usually result in spinal cord injury and paralysis. A fracture involving C2, commonly called a **hangman's fracture,** typically occurs when there is a forceful, sudden hyperextension of the head. Striking the head against the windshield in a motor vehicle accident is often the cause. This is usually a stable fracture, but without proper care and handling, it could become unstable. Spinal cord paralysis at this level usually results in death because respiration stops.

Whiplash is the layman's term used to describe a type of cervical sprain in which the head and neck suddenly and forcefully hyperextends then flexes, like the cracking of a whip. This commonly occurs during a rear-end car accident. When the head and neck hyperextend, soft tissue structures (muscles, ligaments, joint capsules) on the anterior side of the neck are stretched. This is followed quickly by a forceful cervical flexion. This results in the overstretching of soft tissue structures on the posterior side. The severity of the injury will dictate the amount of muscle, capsular, and ligamentous pain, and possible joint instability.

Points to Remember

- When a muscle contracts, it knows no direction; it simply shortens.
- When a muscle contracts, it usually moves its insertion (more movable end) toward its origin (more stable end).
- A muscle insertion is usually the distal end and the more movable end.
- A muscle origin is usually the proximal end and the more stable end.
- Reversal of muscle action occurs when the origin becomes more movable and moves toward the insertion, which has become more stable.
- Concentric contractions occur when the body part is moving against gravity.
- Eccentric contractions occur when the body part is moving in the same direction as the pull of gravity.
- Isometric contractions occur when a muscle contracts but no significant joint motion occurs.
- The muscle group contracting isometrically is the same group as if the joint were contracting concentrically.

Review Questions

General Anatomy Questions

1. Describe neck and trunk motions in:
   a. the frontal plane around the sagittal axis
   b. the transverse plane around the vertical axis
   c. the sagittal plane around the frontal axis
2. You are handed a cervical, thoracic, and lumbar vertebra. What identifying features help you distinguish among them?
3. What structural features allow the thoracic vertebrae to rotate but not flex?
4. What structural features allow the lumbar vertebrae to flex but not rotate?
5. Name the ligament that extends over the spinous processes from the occiput to C7 and from C7 to the sacrum.
6. What is the name of the series of ligaments that connect the lamina above to the lamina below along the length of the vertebral column?
7. With respect to the ligaments that support the spine:
   a. Name the ligaments that attach to the bodies of the vertebrae and run the length of the vertebral column.
   b. Name the primary motion that each of these ligaments limits.
8. Why does the quadratus lumborum muscle not play a role in trunk flexion, extension, or rotation?
9. Which posterior muscle groups are the most superficial?
10. A muscle on the right side of the trunk will always produce lateral bending to which side?
11. Name all of the joints that move when atlantoaxial rotation occurs. Identify the type/classification of each of these joints.
12. What is/are the most common level(s) for a herniated disk, and why?
13. During AO joint extension, name the bony segment that is gliding and the direction of the glide.
14. With respect to spinal flexion and extension, describe what happens to:
    a. the lumbar curve
    b. the intervertebral foramen size
    c. the annular portion of the disk
    d. the nucleus portion of the disk?
    e. the load on the intervertebral disk?
    f. the load on the facet joints?
15. Describe the role of the transverse ligament.

Functional Activity Questions

Identify the main **cervical** positions in the following activities:

1. Sleeping on your stomach
2. Cradling the telephone between your ear and shoulder
3. Looking at the top of a tall building from the street below
4. Lying supine on a sofa with your head propped up on a pillow or the sofa's arm
5. Painting the ceiling

For questions 6 to 10, identify the main **trunk** action in the following activities:

6. Preparing to hit a tennis ball with a backhand swing with the racket in your right hand (Fig. 15-35)

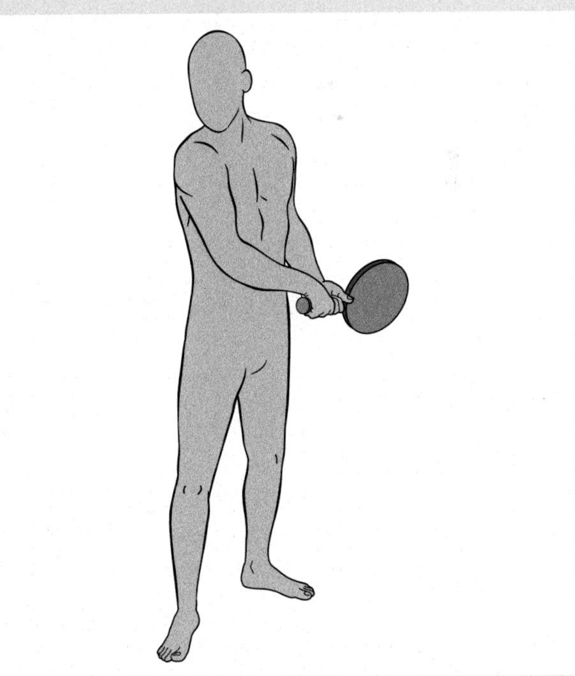

Figure 15-35. Preparing to hit with tennis backswing.

(continued on next page)

Review Questions—cont'd

7. Hitting the tennis ball with the backhand swing (Fig. 15-36)

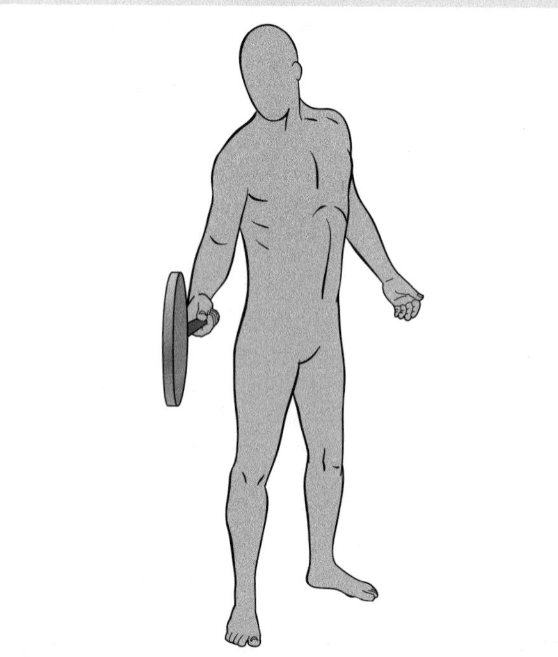

Figure 15-36. Hitting with backswing.

8. Reaching down to pick up a suitcase beside you (Fig. 15-37)

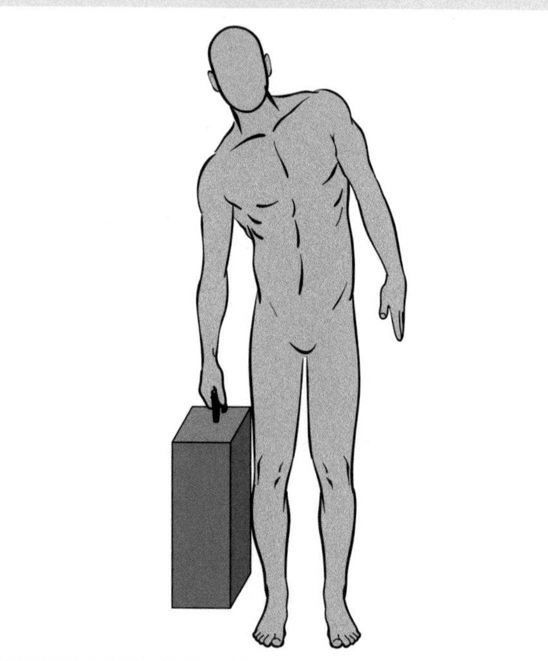

Figure 15-37. Picking up suitcase.

9. The follow-through of punting a football
10. Doing a backward handstand
11. As the pelvis rises up on one side while ascending a step, what muscle is contracting, and what type of action is it performing?
12. While bending forward to pick up a light object from the floor:
    a. What force is causing the forward bending?
    b. What spinal muscles are contracting, and what type of contraction are they performing?
13. While lifting a suitcase up off the floor (Fig. 15-37), what muscle is contracting and what type of contraction is it performing? (Be sure to identify if the muscle is on the right or the left side.)

Clinical Exercise Questions

Head and Neck

1. Lie prone with your head and shoulders over the edge of the table and head down. Tuck your chin in and raise your head to anatomical position.
    a. What joint motion is occurring in the neck as you tuck in your chin?
    b. What joint motion is occurring in the neck as you raise your head?
    c. What type of contraction (isometric, concentric, eccentric) occurs as you raise your head?
    d. What type of contraction (isometric, concentric, eccentric) occurs as you hold your head in anatomical position while in this prone position?
    e. What are the prime movers that are working to raise your head?
2. Sitting or standing with your head and neck in anatomical position, press your right hand against the right side of your head. Try to move your head but resist any motion with your hand.
    a. What joint motion is occurring (or attempting to occur)? (Be sure to state if the direction of motion is toward the right or left.)
    b. What type of contraction (isometric, concentric, or eccentric) is occurring?
    c. What are the prime movers of this joint motion? (Be sure to identify if these muscles are on the right or the left.)

Review Questions—cont'd

3. While lying supine, lean your head toward your right shoulder without moving the shoulder. Both stretching and strengthening are occurring here. In answering the questions below, be sure to indicate whether you are referring to the right or left side.
   a. What joint motion is occurring (or attempting to occur)?
   b. What muscle group is being stretched?
   c. What are the prime movers of this joint motion?
   d. What muscle group is being strengthened?
   e. What are the prime movers of this joint motion?
4. Which cervical muscle would be stretched if you leaned your head toward the right shoulder and rotated your head to the left? Be sure to identify if this muscle is on the right or the left side.
5. From a supine position, tuck your chin and raise your head off the mat, hold for the count of five, then return to the starting position.
   a. Is the head flexing or extending on C1 as you tuck in your chin?
   b. What type of contraction (isometric, concentric, or eccentric) is occurring as you tuck the chin?
   c. What is the muscle group involved in tucking your chin?
   d. Is your neck flexing or extending as you raise your head?
   e. What type of contraction is occurring as you raise your head?
   f. What muscles are prime movers in this joint motion?
   g. What type of contraction is occurring as you hold your head for the count?
   h. What muscles are prime movers in this action?
   i. Is neck flexion or extension occurring as you return to the starting position?
   j. What type of contraction is occurring with this motion?
   k. What muscles are involved with this action?

Trunk

1. Sit in a chair with your legs abducted. Drop your head and shoulders forward, bending at hips and trunk until your shoulders are between your knees.
   a. Is trunk flexion or extension occurring in this activity?
   b. Are the trunk flexors or extensors being stretched?
   c. What muscles are being stretched?
2. Lie supine with your knees extended and your arms at your sides. First, press your lower back to the mat, and then curl your trunk. Lift your head and shoulders up (keeping your chin down) until your scapulae leave the floor.
   a. Is trunk flexion or extension occurring in this activity?
   b. What type of contraction (isometric, concentric, or eccentric) is occurring?
   c. What muscles are prime movers in this trunk motion?
3. Repeat the action of the exercise in question 2, except this time have someone hold down your feet. In this exercise, the hip flexors are contracting.
   a. Is the trunk motion still the same as in question 1?
   b. Are the hips flexing or extending?
   c. Is the hip muscle moving its origin toward its insertion or its insertion toward its origin?
   d. What is the kinesiology term for a muscle that contracts in this direction?
   e. Describe how holding the feet down allows certain hip muscles to contract.
4. Lie supine with your knees bent and feet flat. Put your right hand behind your head. Lift your right shoulder and scapula off the mat toward your left knee.
   a. What two trunk motions are occurring (flexion, extension, right rotation, left rotation, right lateral bending, or left lateral bending)?
   b. What type of contraction (isometric, concentric, or eccentric) is occurring?
   c. What muscles are causing these trunk motions? Be sure to indicate on which side the muscle is contracting.
5. While maintaining the plank position (position at the end of a full push-up with hands on the floor, elbows extended, and bearing weight on the toes):
   a. What motion does gravity want to impose on the lumbar spine?
   b. What muscle group needs to contract to resist the motion that gravity wants to impose?
   c. How are these muscles contracting?

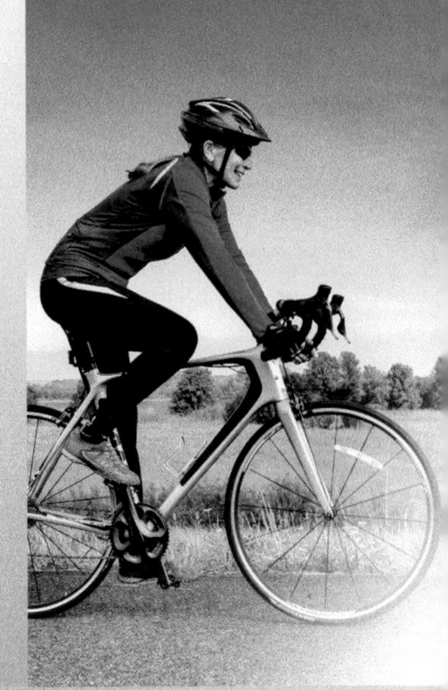

CHAPTER 16
Respiratory System

The Thoracic Cage
Bones and Landmarks
Joints of the Thorax
Movements of the Thorax
Structures of Respiration
Mechanics of Respiration
Phases of Respiration
Muscles of Respiration
Diaphragm Muscle
Intercostal Muscles
Accessory Inspiratory Muscles
Accessory Expiratory Muscles
Anatomical Relationships
Diaphragmatic Versus Chest Breathing
Summary of Innervation of the Muscles of Respiration
Common Respiratory Conditions or Pathologies
Review Questions
General Anatomy Questions
Functional Activity Questions
Clinical Exercise Questions

Kinesiology IN ACTION For additional practice activities and videos, please visit www.kinesiologyinaction.com

Simply stated, the main function of the respiratory system is to supply oxygen to and eliminate carbon dioxide from the lungs. The respiratory organs are the conduits through which air enters and exits the lungs. The thorax provides bony protection to the lungs and assists in the air exchange. Although a brief description of the passage of air through the respiratory organs will be given, the main focus of this chapter will be the bony and muscular mechanisms that make air exchange possible.

The Thoracic Cage

The thorax consists of the sternum, the ribs and costal cartilages, and the thoracic vertebrae (Fig. 16-1). It is bounded anteriorly by the sternum, posteriorly by the bodies of the 12 thoracic vertebrae, superiorly by the clavicle, and inferiorly by the diaphragm. The thorax is wider from side to side than it is from front to back. The thoracic, or chest, cavity lies inside the thorax. It is within this cavity that the lungs, heart, and other vital structures are located.

Bones and Landmarks

The **rib cage** serves to attach the vertebral column posteriorly to the sternum anteriorly. Due to these attachments, movement within the thoracic spine is very limited. The chest organs (heart, lungs, aorta, thymus gland, portion of the trachea, esophagus, lymph nodes, and important nerves) are housed within and protected by the rib cage. Each side has 12 ribs, for a total of 24.

The upper seven ribs (also called **true ribs**) attach directly to the sternum anteriorly. Ribs 8 through 10 are called **false ribs,** because they attach indirectly to the sternum via the costal cartilage of the seventh rib. The 11th and 12th ribs are called **floating ribs,** because they have no anterior attachment.

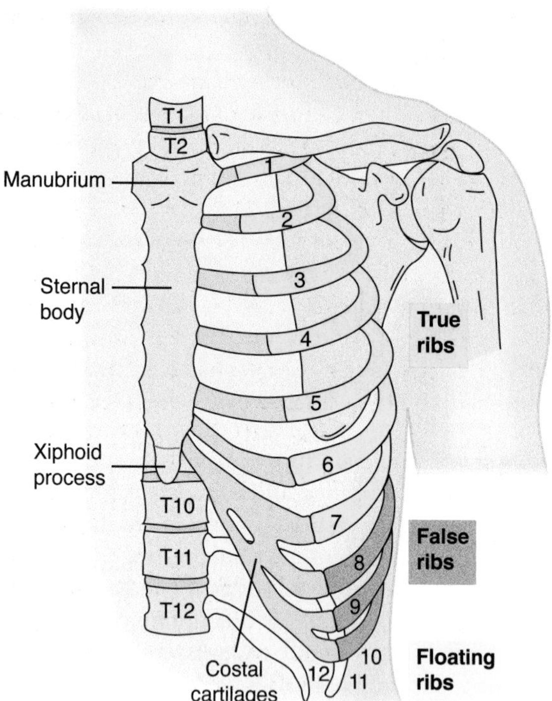

Figure 16-1. Thoracic cage (anterior view).

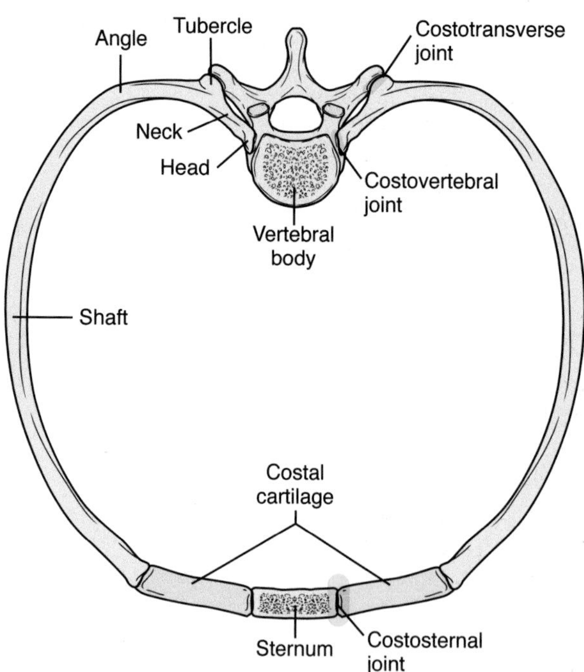

Figure 16-2. Costovertebral and costotransverse joints with rib landmarks (superior view).

Bony Landmarks of the Ribs

A typical **rib** has the following significant landmarks (Fig. 16-2):

Head
Located at the vertebral end, it articulates with vertebral body

Neck
Narrowed portion of the rib between the head and tubercle

Tubercle
Prominence at the junction of the neck and the shaft. It has a facet for articulation with the transverse process of the vertebra

Facet
A term sometimes used to describe a smooth, flat surface where one bone articulates with another

Angle
That part of the rib where it has the greatest curvature

Shaft
Is thin, flat and very curved

Sternal End
End of the rib connecting to the costal cartilages

Intercostal Space
Area between ribs where the muscles are located

Costal Cartilage
Bars of hyaline cartilage that connect the ribs to the sternum. They provide the elasticity allowing the rib cage mobility needed during the phases of respiration.

Bony Landmarks of the Sternum

The **sternum** is the long, flat bone in the midline of the anterior chest wall. Its shape resembles a dagger, and it consists of three parts: manubrium, body, and xiphoid process (see Fig. 16-1).

The *manubrium* (Latin for "handle") is the superior part, the *body* is the middle and longest part, and the *xiphoid process* (Greek for "sword") is the inferior tip portion. The ribs, sternum, and vertebral bodies form the thorax.

Bony Landmarks of the Thoracic Vertebra

Specific to **thoracic vertebra** are the following landmarks:

Costal Facet
Located superiorly and inferiorly on the sides of the vertebral bodies and on the transverse processes

of thoracic vertebrae (see Fig. 15-9). It is here that the ribs articulate with the vertebrae. Sometimes the facets are referred to as **demifacets** (In Latin, *demi* means "half") when the costal facet is located partially on two adjacent vertebral bodies. That term will not be used in this text.

Joints of the Thorax

The ribs mainly articulate with the vertebrae in two areas: (1) the bodies of the vertebrae and (2) the transverse processes. These joints are called costovertebral and costotransverse joints, respectively (Fig. 16-2). At the **costovertebral joint,** the **costal facet** of the vertebral body articulates with the head of the rib. It is located laterally and posteriorly on the body, near the beginning of the neural arch. Some ribs articulate partially with two adjacent bodies. These articulations are with the superior part of the vertebral body below and the inferior part of the vertebral body above. With the **costotransverse joint,** the costal facet is located on the anterior tip of the transverse process of the vertebra. It articulates with the tubercle of the rib. Figure 16-3 shows the costal facets.

The costal cartilages articulate with the sternum at the **chondrosternal joints.** Like the costovertebral articulations, the chondrosternal joints are plane-shaped synovial joints.

Movements of the Thorax

Because most of the ribs attach anteriorly and posteriorly, there is little movement. However, **elevation** and **depression** of the rib cage do occur as a result of gliding at the costovertebral and costotransverse joints posteriorly and at the chondrosternal joints anteriorly. These movements are associated with inspiration and expiration, respectively.

As you inhale, the rib cage moves up and out, increasing the medial-lateral diameter of the chest. Accordingly, as you exhale, the rib cage returns to its starting position by moving down and in, decreasing the medial-lateral chest diameter. This type of movement has been compared to the up and down movement of a bucket handle (Fig. 16-4A). When the handle is resting against the side of the bucket, it is comparable to the lowered position of the rib cage during expiration. As the handle (the lateral aspect of the ribs) moves up and away from the bucket (the vertebral column and sternum), it is comparable to the increased mediolateral diameter of the rib cage during inspiration.

In addition to a change in medial-lateral diameter, there is a change in the anterior-posterior diameter of the chest. This is called the *pump-handle effect* (Fig. 16-4B). As you inhale, the sternum and ribs move upward and outward (forward), increasing the anterior-posterior diameter of the chest. This is comparable to the pump

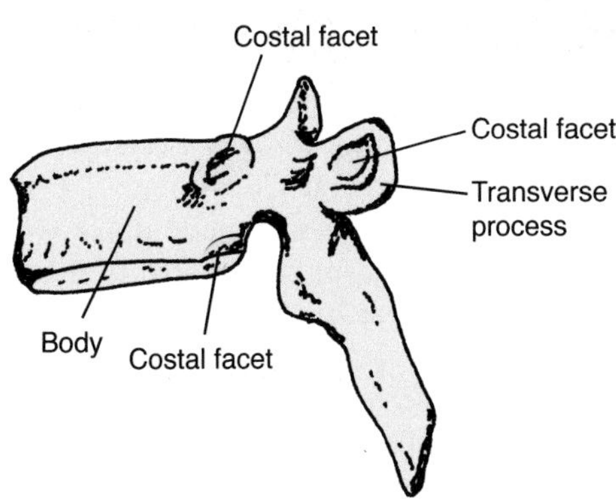

Figure 16-3. Costal facets on the thoracic vertebra (lateral view).

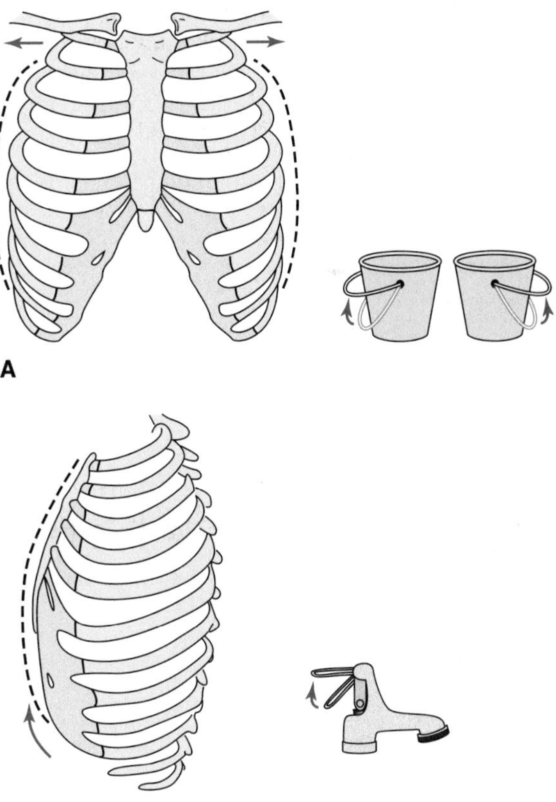

Figure 16-4. Comparison of thorax movements during breathing with movements of bucket and pump handles. **(A)** Medial-lateral chest diameter and **(B)** anterior-posterior chest diameter.

handle moving up. Conversely, as the ribs and sternum are lowered, the diameter of the anterior-posterior thorax decreases, resulting in expiration. This movement is comparable to the pump handle moving back down.

Structures of Respiration

Respiratory structures can be divided into upper and lower airway tracts (Fig. 16-5). The **upper respiratory tract** consists of the nasal cavity, oral cavity, pharynx, and larynx. The **lower respiratory tract** is made up of the trachea and bronchial tree. To allow the airways to remain open, all structures, down to the smallest bronchi, are made up of cartilaginous material. The **nose** is mostly made up of relatively soft cartilage and consists of the two nostrils, also called the *nares.* Only the upper part of the nose, or bridge, is bony. The two nostrils lead into the **nasal cavity.** The nasal septum, formed by the vomer and part of the ethmoid bones, separates the nasal cavity into two fairly equal chambers. The ethmoid, sphenoid, and a small part of the frontal bone form the roof of the nasal cavity, whereas the palatine and part of the maxillae bones form the floor. These floor bones also make up the hard palate of the mouth. The functions of the nasal cavity are to warm, filter, and moisten the air you breathe in.

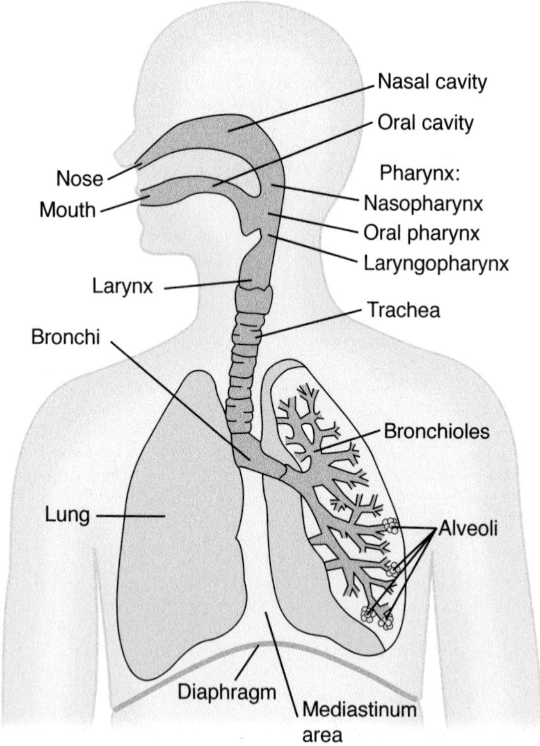

Figure 16-5. The respiratory structures are divided into the upper and lower airway tracts (anterior view). Note that the left lung is cut in cross section to show terminal airway structures.

If you breathe through your mouth, air enters the **oral cavity,** moving over the lips and tongue and into the pharynx. The roof of the mouth consists of the bony hard palate and the fibrous soft palate. The uvula is the soft tissue structure that hangs down in the middle at the back of the mouth; it is part of the soft palate. The function of the soft palate is to close off the opening between the nasal and oral pharynx during such activities as swallowing, blowing, and certain speech sounds. The soft palate forces food and liquids down into the throat during swallowing and forces air out through the mouth when blowing and speaking.

Once air passes through the nasal cavity, it enters the pharynx through the nasopharynx. The **pharynx,** or throat, has three parts: the nasal pharynx, which has primarily a respiratory function; the oral pharynx, which receives food from the mouth; and the laryngopharynx. This last part, the larynogopharynx, is located between the base of the tongue and the entrance to the esophagus. Next, air passes into the **larynx,** or voice box. The larynx is located between the pharynx and the trachea, anterior to vertebrae C4 through C6. Anteriorly, it is fairly easy to locate by the laryngeal prominence, or *Adam's apple,* which tends to be more prominent in men than in women. The larynx consists of cartilage, ligaments, muscles, and the vocal cords. Its function is to (1) act as a passageway for air between the pharynx and trachea, (2) prevent food or liquid from passing into the trachea, and (3) generate speech sounds. When you swallow, the epiglottis, which is one of the cartilaginous structures of the larynx, closes over the vocal cords, allowing food or liquids to pass into the esophagus but not into the trachea, thus preventing aspiration of food or drink into the lungs. The glottis is the opening between the vocal cords and the area where sound is produced. It is also an important part of the cough mechanism, which is important for keeping the airways clear.

Passing out of the larynx, air then enters the **trachea,** commonly called the *windpipe.* It is located anterior to the esophagus and vertebrae C6 through T4. To keep the airway open, the trachea is made up of C-shaped cartilage on all sides, except posteriorly. It divides into right and left **main stem bronchi.** The right bronchus is shorter and wider and subdivides into three **lobar bronchi** (upper, middle, and lower), with one going to each lobe of the lung. The longer, narrower left bronchus subdivides into two lobar bronchi (upper and lower). As the bronchi continue to divide, they become progressively smaller, narrower, and more numerous. The trachea, bronchi, and their subdivisions are sometimes referred to as the *bronchial tree.* The smallest bronchi, which are less than 1 mm in diameter, are called **bronchioles.** It is at this point that the airway becomes noncartilaginous. The **alveolus** (plural, *alveoli*) is at the very end of the bronchial tree subdivision. These saclike alveoli cluster around the terminal bronchioles much like grapes on their stem. The alveoli exchange oxygen for carbon dioxide and vice versa.

When the trachea divides into the right and left bronchi, they each enter a lung. The **lungs** are somewhat triangular, being wider and concave at the bottom. This concave shape fits with the convex dome shape of the diaphragm located below. The right lung has an upper, middle, and lower lobe, whereas the left lung has an upper and lower lobe. A double-walled sac, called the **pleura,** encases each lung. The outer wall of the pleura lines the chest wall and covers the diaphragm, and the inner wall adheres to the lung. The pleural cavity lies between the two walls, and the **mediastinum** lies between the lungs. The mediastinum contains several structures, including the heart, esophagus, and several vital blood vessels and nerves.

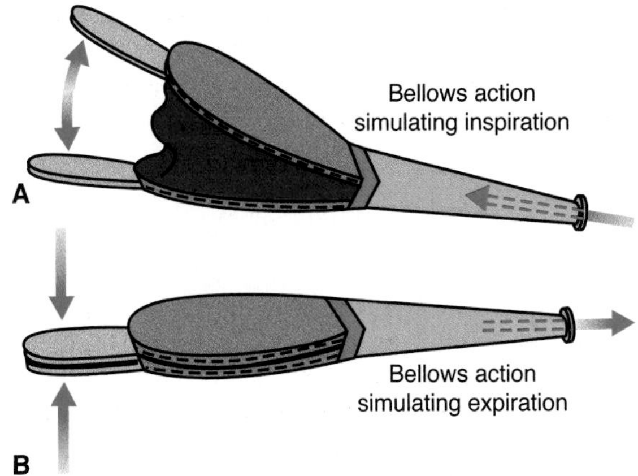

Figure 16-6. **(A)** Simulation of inspiration. As the handles of the bellows are pulled apart, air is brought into the bellows. As the ribs elevate and the diaphragm moves down, the thoracic cavity gets larger and air is pulled into the lungs. **(B)** Simulation of expiration. As the handles of the bellows are pushed together, air is pushed out of the bellows. Similarly, as the ribs move downward and the diaphragm moves upward, the thoracic cavity gets smaller and air is pushed out of the lungs.

Mechanics of Respiration

The lungs are passive during the process of breathing. Although the pleural cavities around the lungs are closed, the insides of the lungs are in communication with the outside atmosphere and are subject to its pressure. It is important to remember that air flows from higher pressure to lower pressure until pressure is equalized. During inspiration, the size of the thoracic cavity increases, causing the pressure within the thorax to decrease and forcing air into the lungs. You can simulate this inspiration action by pulling apart the handles of a bellows (Fig. 16-6A). When the handles are pulled apart, the bellows become larger as air rushes into them. The reverse happens during expiration. Similarly, the thoracic cavity returns to its smaller size, pressure in the thorax increases, and air is forced out of the lungs. You can simulate expiration by pushing the handles of the bellows together, making them smaller and forcing air out of them (Fig. 16-6B).

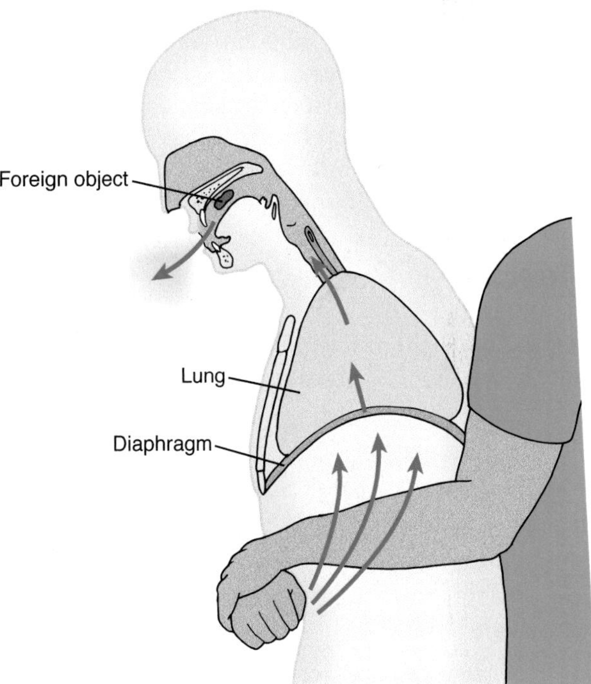

Figure 16-7. Heimlich maneuver.

Using the Heimlich maneuver to dislodge a foreign object from the pharynx or larynx of someone who is choking demonstrates the mechanics of expiration. To perform the Heimlich, stand behind the choking victim and put both arms around the victim's waist. With one hand curled into a fist, place it between the umbilicus and the rib cage. Cover your fist with the other hand, and perform a quick, forceful, upward thrust (Fig. 16-7). This forces the diaphragm upward and compresses the lungs, forcing air and the foreign object out of the victim's trachea. This action can be compared with a forceful artificial cough.

Phases of Respiration

Inspiration is commonly divided into three phases of increasing effort: quiet, deep, and forced. **Quiet inspiration** occurs when an individual is resting or sitting quietly. The diaphragm is responsible for approximately 70% of quiet inspiration and external intercostal muscles are the prime movers. The actions of quiet inspiration increase during **deep inspiration.** A person needs more oxygen and therefore breathes harder. Muscles that can pull the ribs up are being called into action. **Forced inspiration** occurs when an individual is working very hard, needs a great deal of oxygen, and is in a state of "air hunger." The muscles of quiet and deep inspiration are working, as are muscles that stabilize or elevate the shoulder girdle; this directly or indirectly elevates the ribs.

Expiration is divided into two phases: quiet and forced. **Quiet expiration** is mostly a passive action. It occurs through relaxation of the diaphragm and the external intercostal muscles, elastic recoil of the thoracic wall and tissue of the lungs and bronchi, and gravity pulling the rib cage down from its elevated position. There is some debate as to whether the internal intercostals play a significant or any role in quiet expiration. Some sources claim that they have a role, whereas others claim that they do not become effective until forced expiration.

Forced expiration uses muscles that can pull down on the rib as well as muscles that can compress the abdomen, forcing the diaphragm upward.

Muscles of Respiration

Respiration is the result of changes in thoracic volume, hence thoracic pressure. There are two ways of changing thoracic volume: (1) moving the ribs and (2) lowering the diaphragm. Either action requires muscles. The primary muscles during respiration are the diaphragm and the intercostal muscles. The role of accessory muscles, which come into play during forced respiration, can be determined by noting whether a muscle's action pulls the ribs up (inspiration) or pulls them down (expiration). There has been a great deal of controversy over which muscles are active during which phases of respiration. In recent years, more refined electromyographic (EMG) instruments and techniques may have helped to clarify the roles of various muscles. Because there have been numerous studies conducted, many of which disagree, the waters are still cloudy.

Diaphragm Muscle

The thoracic cavity is separated from the abdominal cavity by the diaphragm muscle, a large, sheetlike, dome-shaped muscle (Fig. 16-8). It has a somewhat circular origin on the xiphoid process anteriorly, on the lower six ribs laterally, and on the upper lumbar vertebrae posteriorly. Its insertion is rather unique. Because the muscle is somewhat circular, it inserts into itself at the broad central tendon. Three openings in the diaphragm muscle allow passage of the esophagus, the aorta, and the inferior vena cava. Because the insertion (central tendon) is higher than the origin, the diaphragm muscle descends when it contracts (Fig. 16-9). This makes the thoracic cavity larger and the abdominal cavity smaller, causing inspiration. Very forced inspiration may lower the dome as much as 4 inches.

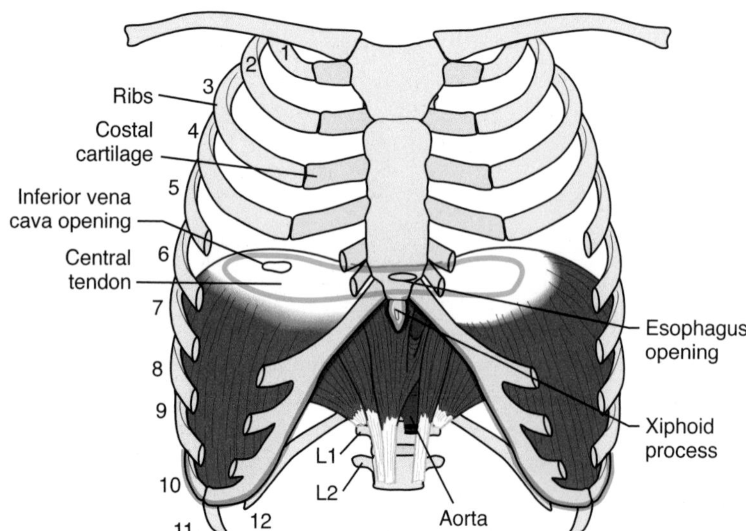

Figure 16-8. Diaphragm muscle (anterior view).

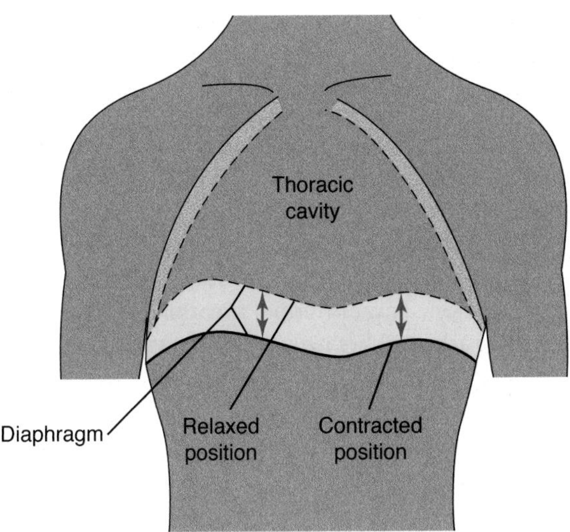

Figure 16-9. Movement of the diaphragm (anterior view). When the diaphragm contracts, it descends, making the thoracic cavity larger. As in the bellows example, this allows air to be pulled into the lungs. When it relaxes, it moves upward, decreasing the size of the thoracic cavity and forcing air out of the lungs.

Diaphragm Muscle

O	Xiphoid process, ribs, lumbar vertebrae
I	Central tendon
A	Inspiration
N	Phrenic nerve (C3, C4, C5)

Intercostal Muscles

The intercostal muscles occupy each of the eleven intercostal spaces and run at right angles to each other (Fig. 16-10). The most superficial muscles are the **external intercostal muscles,** which run in a diagonal direction inferiorly and medially from the lower border of the rib above to the superior border of the rib below (Fig. 16-11). They extend from the from the rib tubercle posteriorly to the costal cartilage anteriorly. They elevate the ribs below by pulling up on them from their attachment on the rib above.

Anteriorly, the external intercostal muscles run in the same direction as the external oblique muscles of the abdomen. Together the fibers of the left and right external intercostals form a *V.* Similarly, the internal intercostal muscles, which run in the opposite direction, form the shape of an inverted *V.*

If you view these two sets of muscles posteriorly, the direction of their fibers is just the opposite from their direction anteriorly. Posteriorly, the external intercostals on the right and left sides when viewed together are in the shape of an inverted *V,* whereas the internal intercostals on both sides, if they could be viewed, would be seen in the shape of a *V.* This seems contrary to what was described in the previous paragraph. To clearly understand how this change occurs, take a pencil and place it diagonally next to the sternum of a skeleton (or your partner). Next, move the pencil around the rib cage posteriorly toward the vertebral column without changing the *direction* of the pencil. Notice that the pencil (muscle fibers) direction posteriorly is opposite to what it was in front. Although the fibers have not changed direction, the ribs have curved 180 degrees, causing this apparent change in direction.

External Intercostal Muscles

O	Rib above
I	Rib below
A	Elevate ribs during inspiration
N	Intercostal nerve (T2 through T6)

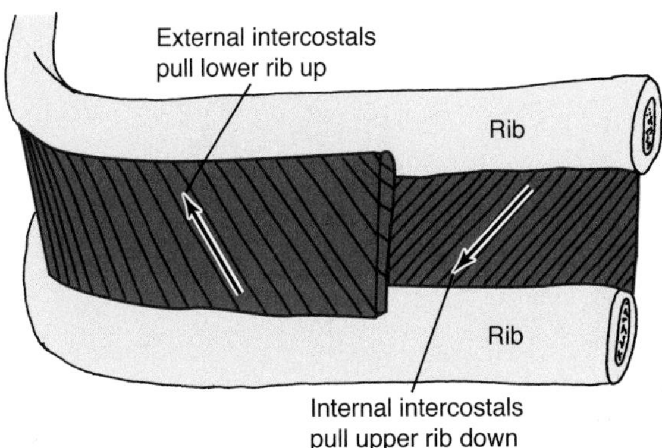

Figure 16-10. Direction of the fibers of the external and internal intercostal muscles (anterior view).

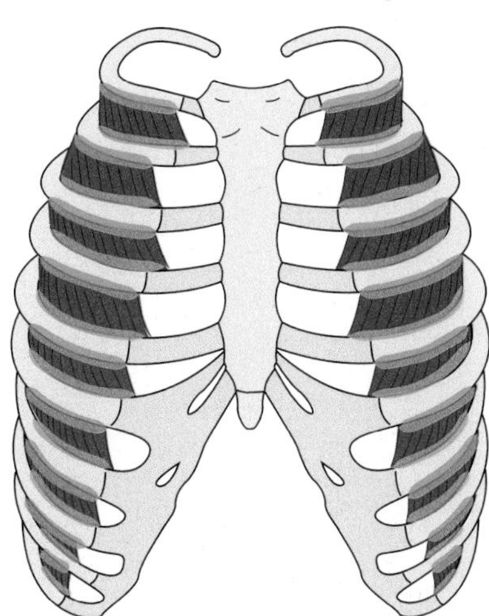

Figure 16-11. External intercostal muscles (anterior view).

The fibers of the **internal intercostal muscles** run at a 90-degree angle to the external intercostal muscles and therefore perform the opposite action. They run in a diagonal direction superiorly and medially from the rib below to the rib above (Fig. 16-12) and extend from the side of the sternum to the angle of the rib. They lie deep to the external intercostals throughout most of their attachment, except they extend farther anteriorly than the external intercostals, so are superficial at this point. They depress the ribs by pulling down on the rib above.

Internal Intercostal Muscles

O	Rib below
I	Rib above
A	Depress ribs during expiration
N	Intercostal nerve (T2 through T6)

Accessory Inspiratory Muscles

Accessory muscles of inspiration assist the diaphragm and external intercostals in pulling up on the rib cage. Some of these muscles demonstrate reverse muscle action by pulling from origin toward insertion, not from insertion toward origin. For example, the **sternocleidomastoid** usually pulls from its insertion on the skull toward the sternum, causing the head to move. During inspiration, the head and neck extensors neutralize this flexion action, thereby stabilizing the head and neck. The sternocleidomastoid now pulls the sternum up toward the head (Fig. 16-13). Pulling in this direction will elevate the rib cage.

Like the sternocleidomastoid, the **scalenes** usually move the head and neck. However, when the head and

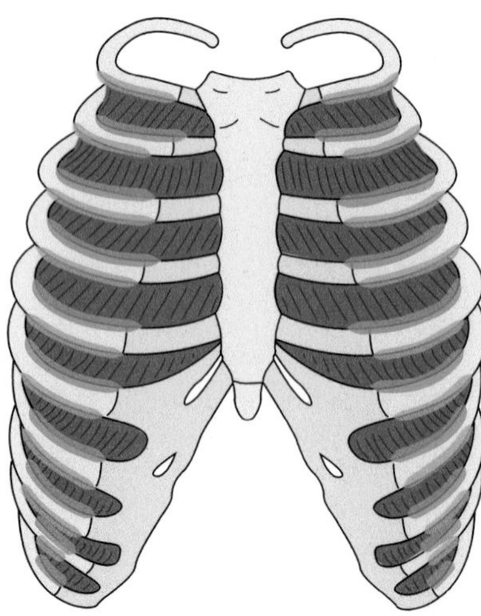

Figure 16-12. Internal intercostal muscles (anterior view).

Clinical Application 16-1

Paradoxical Breathing

An important role that both intercostal muscles play is that of stabilizing or stiffening the intercostal spaces during inspiration and expiration. Without them, this space would be "sucked in" during inspiration and "ballooned out" during expiration. This abnormal breathing is known as paradoxical breathing. It decreases an individual's vital capacity—the amount of air that can be forcibly exhaled from the lungs after inhaling as deeply as possible. This is evident immediately after a person sustains a high spinal injury, when there is flaccid paralysis of the trunk muscles and the diaphragm is the only respiratory muscle working. As the person moves out of the period of spinal shock and the paralysis becomes more spastic, the chest wall stiffens and vital capacity improves.

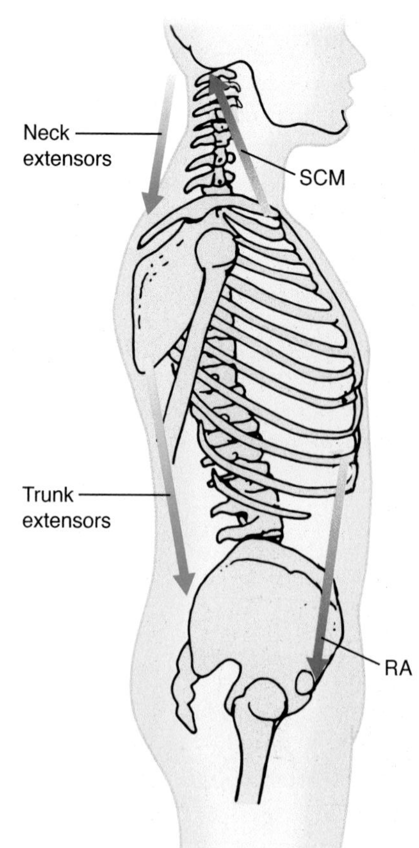

Figure 16-13. Sternocleidomastoid (SCM) muscle pulling up (assisting in inspiration) and rectus abdominis (RA) pulling down (assisting in expiration) (lateral view).

neck are stabilized as was described with the sternocleidomastoid, they can elevate the first and second ribs, assisting in inspiration. There is conflicting evidence about whether the scalenes are active in quiet inspiration as well as in deep inspiration.

Athletes who have just completed a sprint commonly put their hands on their hips while trying to "catch their breath." This position braces the arms, making it a closed-chain action. It also elevates the shoulder girdle, which changes the line of pull of the **pectoralis major** to a more vertical direction. These two changes now allow the muscle to pull the sternum toward the humerus in a reverse action, pulling up on the rib cage, and thus increasing the diameter of the rib cage. In this posture, the **pectoralis minor** is in a position to elevate the third through fifth ribs through reverse action because the thoracic spine is extended and the scapulae are stabilized. Individuals with chronic obstructive pulmonary disease commonly brace their arms against the arms of a chair to accomplish the same thing (Fig. 16-14).

Posteriorly, the shoulder girdle muscles that attach on the vertebral column and the scapula, such as the levator scapula, upper trapezius, and rhomboids, all perform scapular elevation. As such, they contribute toward inspiration in that scapular elevation can exert an upward pull on the rib cage via the scapula's connection to the clavicle.

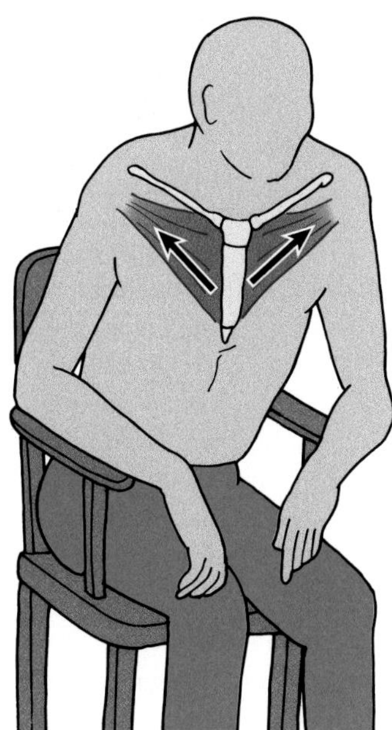

Figure 16-14. The pectoralis major muscle assisting with inspiration in a reversal of muscle action by pulling the sternum toward the humerus, which is stabilized by resting the forearms on the arms of the chair (closed-chain action).

Accessory Expiratory Muscles

Accessory expiratory muscles operate in similar ways, except that they pull down on the rib cage. For example, the **rectus abdominis** usually flexes the trunk by pulling the sternum toward the pubis. However, when the trunk extensors neutralize the trunk flexion action, the spine becomes stabilized. The rectus abdominis is now able to assist with expiration by pulling the rib cage down (see Fig. 16-13). This stabilizing action of the trunk extensors can explain why a person with a back injury feels pain when coughing or sneezing. The stabilizing action causes the erector spinae muscles to contract. The **quadratus lumborum** pulls the lower ribs toward the iliac crest in the same fashion. This provides a stable origin for the diaphragm and allows the central tendon to be effectively pulled downward during inspiration.

Many of the accessory breathing muscles have already been discussed with the vertebral column (see Chapter 15) or the shoulder girdle (see Chapter 9). Those that have not been discussed here or in previous chapters are illustrated in Figures 16-15 and 16-16 and listed in Table 16-1, alongside a summary of the phases of respiration.

Anatomical Relationships

Many muscles attach to the rib cage, including those of the neck and trunk, the shoulder girdle, the shoulder, and the respiratory muscles. The main respiratory muscles are the deepest, whereas the accessory muscles lie

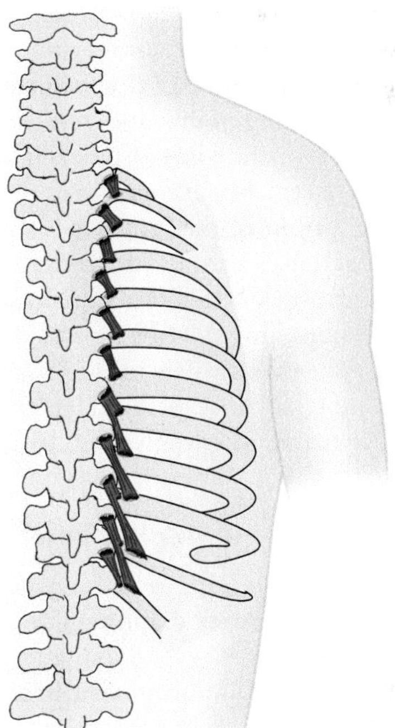

Figure 16-15. Levator costarum muscles (posterior view).

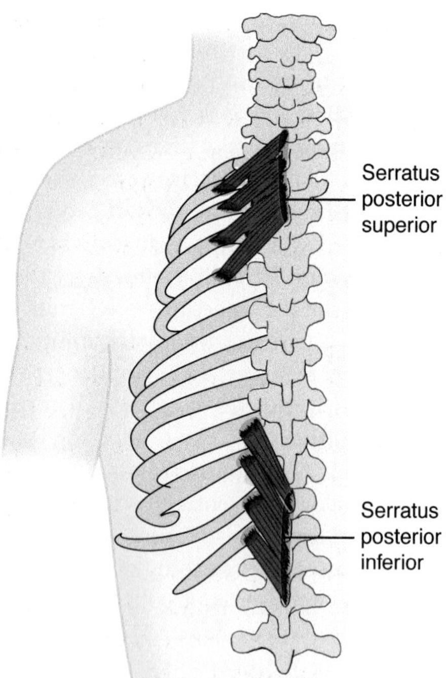

Figure 16-16. Serratus posterior superior and inferior muscles (posterior view).

Table 16-1 Phases of Respiration

Inspiration

Elevation (raising) of ribs and increase in size of the thoracic cavity via descent of the diaphragm muscle and expansion of the thoracic cavity

Phase	Muscles
Quiet inspiration	Diaphragm (primary muscle) External intercostals
Deep inspiration	Muscles of quiet inspiration plus accessory muscles: Sternocleidomastoid Scalenes Pectoralis major Levator costarum Serratus posterior superior
Forced inspiration	Muscles of quiet and deep inspiration plus accessory muscles: Levator scapula Upper trapezius Rhomboids Pectoralis minor

Expiration

Depression (lowering) of ribs and decrease in size of the thoracic cavity

Phase	Muscles
Quiet expiration	Relaxation of diaphragm and external intercostals (primary muscles) Elastic recoil of thoracic wall, lungs, and bronchi Gravity Internal intercostals in assistive role
Forced expiration	Internal intercostals plus accessory muscles External oblique Internal oblique Transverse abdominis Rectus abdominis Quadratus lumborum Serratus posterior inferior

more superficial. As described earlier, any muscle that attaches to the rib cage, even indirectly (as is the case with the levator scapula), and exerts an upward pull can perform as an accessory inspiratory muscle. Figure 16-17 shows most of the muscles listed in Table 16-1.

Anteriorly, the rectus abdominis, external and internal obliques, and quadratus lumborum have attachments on the ribs and can pull down in a similar fashion. The transverse abdominis does not exert a pull on the ribs, but its horizontal line of pull is inward against the abdominal viscera, which compresses the abdominal cavity, forcing air out of the lungs. It is most effective in expulsion actions such as coughing, vomiting, or defecating. The serratus posterior superior and inferior muscles assist in pulling the ribs up and down, respectively. They are the intermediate muscle layer in the back between the more superficial shoulder girdle muscles and the deeper trunk muscles (see Fig. 16-16).

Diaphragmatic Versus Chest Breathing

There are two methods of breathing that we may employ at various times: diaphragmatic and chest breathing. Some people may tend to use one more commonly than the other. **Diaphragmatic breathing** is the most efficient method of breathing and requires the least amount of energy. The diaphragm lowers when it contracts, causing the abdomen to move out, the lungs to expand, and air to flow into the lungs. When the diaphragm relaxes, it returns to its elevated position, the abdomen moves in, the lungs recoil, and air flows out of the lungs. When sitting or standing, the gravitational pull on the abdominal viscera also tends to lower

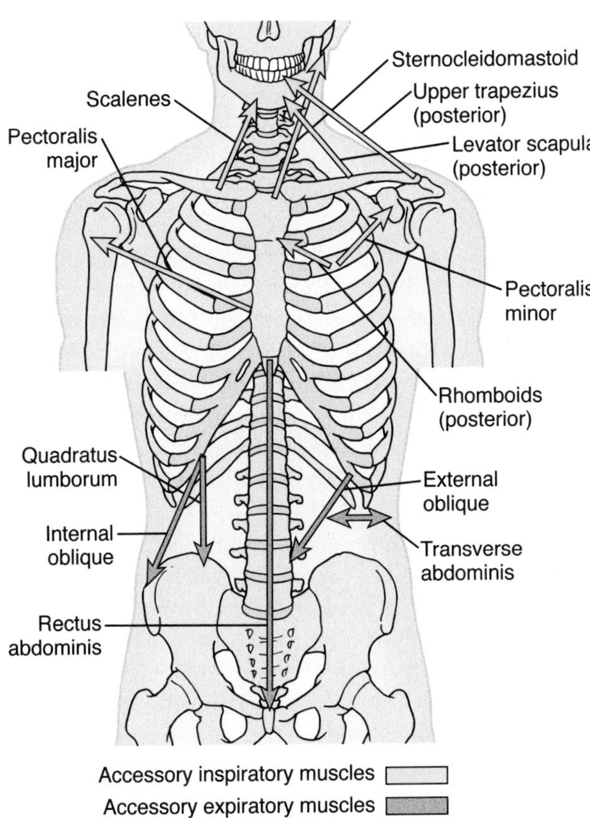

Figure 16-17. Muscles of respiration (anterior view).

the diaphragm. However, when lying down, gravity's effect on the abdominal viscera tends to push the diaphragm up into the thoracic cavity, making the diaphragm work harder. This gravitational effect provides the rationale for elevating the head of the bed of an individual with respiratory difficulty. The elevated position allows easier breathing.

Certain habits, conditions, or pathologies will not allow the diaphragm to work effectively. In those cases, the upper chest and rib cage must play a major role in lifting the ribs up and out during inspiration, without the usual support from the diaphragm. **Chest breathing** requires greater effort and is much less efficient than diaphragmatic breathing. As described earlier, during inspiration, the rib cage moves up and out (both in a medial-lateral direction and in an anterior-posterior direction), the lungs expand, and air flows into the lungs. During expiration, the rib cage relaxes, the lungs recoil, and air flows out of the lungs. Chest breathing draws a much smaller volume of air into the lungs. With shorter breaths, the individual must breathe more rapidly. A person who chest breathes is more prone to hyperventilate and faint.

To increase your awareness of the two methods of breathing, lie supine in a comfortable position with pillows under your knees and head. Place one hand on your upper chest and the other hand on your stomach, just below your ribs. Breathe in slowly through your nose with your mouth closed. With diaphragmatic breathing, you will notice that the hand on your stomach moves up and down as you breathe in and out. There should be little or no movement of the hand on your chest. With chest breathing, the opposite occurs. You will notice movement of the hand on your chest instead of the one on your stomach.

A century ago, it was considered fashionable for women to wear dresses with tightly laced corsets. Aesthetically, this made for a small waist, but functionally it forced the internal organs up against the diaphragm, greatly restricting its effectiveness and forcing women to become chest breathers. No wonder the literature is full of accounts of women "swooning" or fainting. Today, we have the "designer jeans syndrome." Tight-fitting clothing, belts, and waistbands restrict diaphragmatic breathing and force a person to chest breathe. Extremely obese people and women in the later stages of pregnancy cannot effectively contract the diaphragm; therefore, they also tend to chest breathe.

Summary of Innervation of the Muscles of Respiration

Muscles of respiration, like other trunk muscles, receive innervation from spinal nerves at various levels, primarily in the thoracic region. The notable exception is the diaphragm muscle, which is innervated by the phrenic nerve. The phrenic nerve arises from the third, fourth, and fifth cervical nerves. This is functionally significant because an individual with a spinal cord injury at C3 or above cannot breathe unassisted and will be dependent on a ventilator. Inspiration in individuals with a cervical spinal cord injury below C3 will have impaired respiration. They can breathe unassisted, although activities such as coughing, yelling, or taking deep breaths will be limited. Not only are the intercostal muscles active, but other accessory breathing muscles are necessary as well. Activities requiring forced inspiration or expiration are affected to the degree that the accessory breathing muscles are weakened or paralyzed.

Valsalva's Maneuver

Valsalva's maneuver occurs when people hold their breath and attempt to exhale. Several things can happen. Forcibly exhaling while keeping the mouth closed and nose pinched shut forces air into the eustachian tubes and increases pressure inside the eardrum. This is sometimes helpful in "clearing your ears," which may have become blocked from diving or quickly descending from a high elevation.

Prolonged breath-holding and straining forces exhalation against the closed glottis. This increases intrathoracic pressure, which traps blood in veins and prevents it from entering the heart. When the breath is released, intrathoracic pressure drops, and the trapped blood is quickly propelled through the heart, increasing the heart rate (tachycardia) and blood pressure. Immediately, reflex bradycardia (slowed heart rate) follows. This event can have no consequences, or it can lead to cardiac arrest.

Young children having a temper tantrum sometimes take several deep, fast breaths, then stick their thumb in their mouth and blow hard without releasing any air. This can cause them to get dizzy and pass out. During exertion, adults may take a deep breath and blow hard or "bear down" without exhaling. Because this maneuver helps to create intraabdominal pressure and strong contraction of the abdominal muscles that help to stabilize the spine and keep the trunk tight during a heavy lift, it may be done purposefully during exercise. It is also commonly done during childbirth, moving up in bed, straining when urinating, defecating, vomiting, coughing, or sneezing.

A healthy heart can usually withstand these sudden and changing demands. However, for a weakened heart, it can lead to cardiac arrest. Therefore, when exercising, it is a good general rule to breathe out slowly and avoid holding your breath.

Common Respiratory Conditions or Pathologies

An **upper respiratory infection (URI)** is any infection confined to the nose, throat, and larynx. The larynx marks the transition between the upper and lower airways. The common cold is perhaps the most frequent URI. Other URIs include influenza (flu), laryngitis, and rhinitis (inflammation of the nasal mucosa).

Lower respiratory infections (LRIs) involve structures from the trachea to the alveoli. **Pneumonia** is perhaps the most common LRI. It is an inflammation of the alveoli caused by a bacterial or viral infection. Pneumonia can affect an entire lobe (lobar pneumonia) or can be scattered throughout the entire lung (bronchopneumonia). Bronchopneumonia is more common in the very young and very old. "Walking pneumonia" is so named because, in most cases, the disease is not severe enough to confine the individual to bed or to be hospitalized. Bronchitis, emphysema, and asthma are other common LRIs. **Bronchitis** involves the bronchi and their many subdivisions. In **emphysema,** the walls of the alveoli become distended and lose their elasticity due to chronic bronchial obstruction. **Asthma** symptoms are usually due to a spasm of the bronchial walls, which makes exhalation very difficult.

Hyperventilation occurs commonly during rapid breathing when more carbon dioxide is removed from the system than is being produced metabolically. A common treatment for hyperventilation involves breathing into a paper bag to "rebreathe" carbon dioxide. A **stitch** is a temporary condition common in runners. It is a localized, sharp pain, usually felt just below the rib cage and commonly caused by a cramp in the diaphragm. **Hiccups** are involuntary spasms of the diaphragm accompanied by rapid closure of the glottis which produces short, sharp, inspiratory sounds.

Pleurisy is a quiet, painful condition caused by inflammation of the pleura. A **pneumothorax,** or *collapsed lung,* occurs by introducing air into or otherwise destroying the vacuum of the pleural cavity, thereby reducing ventilation capacity.

Rib separation refers to a dislocation between the rib and its costal cartilage. A **rib dislocation** is the displacement of the costal cartilage from the sternum. **Flail chest** occurs when four or more ribs are fractured in two places (comminuted). This causes that part of the chest wall to collapse rather than expand during inspiration. Conversely, the chest wall will also expand during expiration.

Clinical Application 16-2

Biomechanical Impediments to Respiration

With advancing age, **arthritis and joint degeneration** are common sources of motion limitation in the thoracic spine, costovertebral, costotransverse, and/or chondrosternal joints. Reduced motion at any of these joints will impair rib elevation/depression and the thorax's ability to increase and decrease in size.

Forward-head, rounded-shoulder posture in an individual of any age pulls the thoracic spine into flexion, limiting the expansion between the ribs during inspiration, thus reducing the volume of air taken into the lungs. This may not impair function at rest, but can lead to inadequate air exchange during increased respiratory demand.

Scoliosis in the thoracic spine can be another cause for reduced respiratory function. The scoliotic curve places the spine in a position of lateral bending where the ribs separate on the convex side of the curve and are closer together on the concave side of the curve. Rib depression will be limited on the side of the convexity, and rib elevation will be limited on the concave side of the curve. Therefore, respiratory ability can be adequate at rest but become inadequate when increased physical activity is required.

Review Questions

General Anatomy Questions

1. What bony structures make up the thorax?
2. The costovertebral and costotransverse joints involve what bony structures?
3. The chondrosternal joints involve what structures?
4. What type of movement is allowed at the joints named in questions 2 and 3?
5. How do (a) movements of the thorax and (b) movements of the diaphragm affect inspiration and expiration?
6. What is the muscle origin of all accessory inspiratory muscles in relation to the rib cage?
7. The line of pull of the right and left external intercostal muscles forms a *V* shape in front similar to the right and left external obliques. However, in the back, they have the opposite line of pull. Why?
8. The diaphragm has only one bony attachment. How is the other end attached? How does the muscle work?
9. When you talk, are you doing so during inspiration, expiration, or both?
10. How do the accessory muscles assist with breathing?
11. Answer the following questions about mechanical analogies for the thorax and lungs.
    a. Medial and lateral expansion of the thorax can be compared to __________ handle motion.
    b. Anterior-posterior expansion of the thorax can be compared to __________ handle motion.
    c. Inflation and deflation of the lungs can be compared to an object known as a(an) __________.
12. What is the functional significance with regard to respiration between a person with a C3 spinal cord injury and a person with an injury at C5?

Functional Activity Questions

Identify the phase(s) of respiration occurring during the activities in questions 1 to 5:

1. Blowing up a balloon
2. Holding your breath for the count of 15
3. Sneezing
4. Whistling a tune
5. Sitting quietly

(continued on next page)

Review Questions—cont'd

6. At the end of a 100-yard dash, please describe:
   a. What stabilizing muscles are contracting to allow the abdominals to assist with expiration? Why are they needed?
   b. How is the pectoralis minor contracting, and what action is produced?
   c. How are the levator scapula, upper trapezius, and rhomboids contracting, and what motion they are working together to produce?
   d. How does the action produced by the muscles in (c) help the pectoralis minor assist with inspiration?

Clinical Exercise Questions

1. Lie supine in a comfortable position with a pillow under your knees and head. Place your right hand on your upper chest and your left hand on your stomach, just below your ribs. Breathe in slowly through your nose with your mouth closed.
   a. What type of breathing is occurring if your *right* hand is moving up and down?
   b. What type of breathing is occurring if your *left* hand is moving?
2. Lying in the same position, place one hand on your stomach and the other hand over your mouth. Cough. What muscles do you feel contract?
3. Place one hand on your chest and the other on the anterior lateral side of your neck. Sniff strongly (as if you had a runny nose).
   a. What movement occurs at your chest?
   b. Did you feel any muscle contraction at your neck?
   c. What phase of respiration occurs when sniffing, and what neck muscles reversed their muscle action to produce the sniffing?
4. Sit in a chair with your elbows supported on the armrests. Place your right hand on the left side of your chest with your fingers pointing up toward the left shoulder. Take a deep breath.
   a. What rib movement occurred, and in what phase of respiration did it occur?
   b. What accessory breathing muscle is working?
   c. What type of chain activity is occurring?

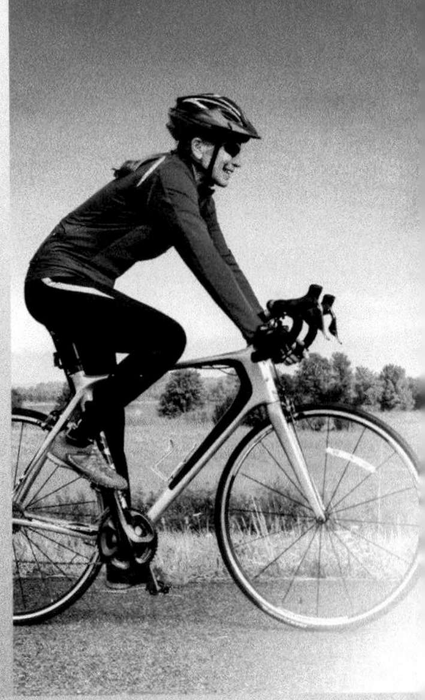

CHAPTER 17
Pelvic Girdle

Structure and Function

False and True Pelvis

Sacroiliac Joint

Pubic Symphysis

Lumbosacral Joint

Pelvic Girdle Motions

Muscle Control

Review Questions

General Anatomy Questions

Functional Activity Questions

Clinical Exercise Questions

Kinesiology IN ACTION For additional practice activities and videos, please visit www.kinesiologyinaction.com

Structure and Function

Four bones make up the **pelvic girdle:** the sacrum, the coccyx, and the two innominate bones. Innominate bones are also known as the hip bones or os coxae. To avoid confusion with the hip joint, the hip bone will be referred to as the innominate bone. Each irregularly shaped innominate bone is composed of the ilium, the ischium, and the pubis, which are fused together into one bone. The joints or articulations in the pelvic girdle include the right and left **sacroiliac joints** posterolaterally, the **symphysis pubis** anteriorly, and the **lumbosacral joint** superiorly (Fig. 17-1).

The pelvic girdle, also referred to as the **pelvis,** performs several functions. Perhaps most important to movement and posture is that it supports the weight of the body through the vertebral column and passes that force on to the innominate bones via the sacrum. Conversely, it receives the ground forces generated when the foot contacts the ground and transmits them upward toward the vertebral column. During walking, the pelvic girdle moves as a unit in all three planes, allowing relatively smooth motion. In addition, the

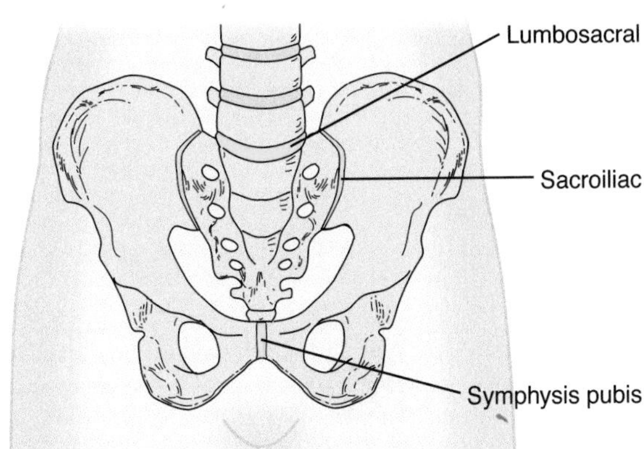

Figure 17-1. Joints of the pelvic girdle (anterior view).

pelvic girdle supports and protects the pelvic viscera, provides attachment for muscles, and makes up the bony portion of the birth canal in females.

False and True Pelvis

Several terms are commonly used when referring to the birth canal within the pelvis. Therefore, it is appropriate to briefly describe a few of these terms and identify some of the differences between the male and female bony pelvis.

The **false pelvis,** also called the *greater* or *major pelvis,* is the bony area between the iliac crests and superior to the pelvic inlet. The **pelvic inlet** can be seen by drawing a line between the sacral promontory posteriorly and the superior border of the symphysis pubis anteriorly (Fig. 17-2). There are no pelvic organs within the false pelvis.

The **true pelvis,** also called the *lesser* or *minor pelvis,* lies between the pelvic inlet and the pelvic outlet. The **pelvic outlet** can be seen by drawing a line from the tip of the coccyx to the inferior surface of the pubic symphysis (see Fig. 17-2). The true pelvis area makes up the **pelvic cavity.** It contains portions of the gastrointestinal (GI) tract, the urinary tract, and some reproductive organs. In females, it forms the *birth canal.*

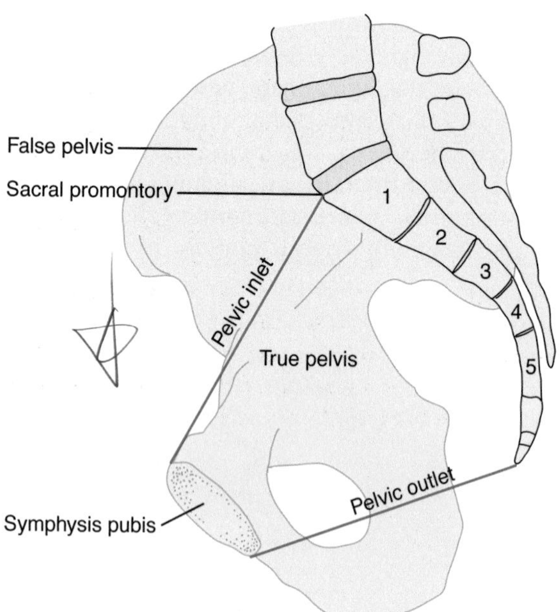

Figure 17-2. Pelvic inlet and outlet, sagittal section. The bony area between them is called the *true pelvis,* which makes up the pelvic cavity. The bony area above the pelvic inlet is called the *false pelvis.*

There are several differences between the male and female pelvis (Fig. 17-3). The superior opening into the pelvic cavity is more oval in females and more heart-shaped in males. The pelvic cavity is also shorter and less funnel-shaped in females, and the sacrum is shorter and less curved. The iliac walls are not as vertical, and the acetabula (plural of acetabulum) and ischial tuberosities are farther apart in females. These features make the area within the female pelvic cavity greater than the longer, funnel-shaped cavity of the male pelvis. In addition, the pelvic arch is wider and more rounded in females. The differences in these arches can be represented visually with your hand: form an arch by extending the thumb and index finger on one hand (in females) or by extending the index and middle finger (in males).

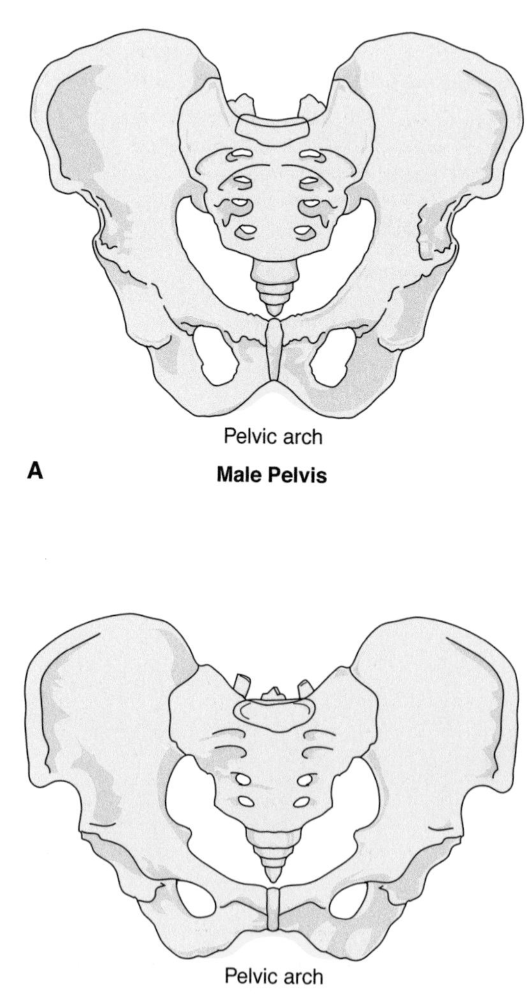

Figure 17-3. Comparison of the male and female pelvis (anterior view). **(A)** Male pelvis. **(B)** Female pelvis.

Sacroiliac Joint

Joint Structure and Motions

The **sacroiliac joint,** commonly referred to as the **SI joint,** is a synovial, nonaxial joint between the sacrum and the ilium. It is described as a plane joint, but its articular surfaces are very irregular. It is this irregularity that helps to lock the two surfaces together.

The function of the sacroiliac joint is to transmit weight from the upper body through the vertebral column to the innominate bones. It is designed for great stability and has very little mobility. Like other synovial joints, its articular surface is lined with hyaline cartilage. Synovial membrane lines the nonarticular portions of the joint. It has a fibrous capsule reinforced by ligaments.

SI Joint Motion

The actual type and amount of movement occurring at the SI joint is the subject of considerable controversy. However, it is generally accepted that the motions that do occur at the SI joint are nutation and counternutation (Fig. 17-4).

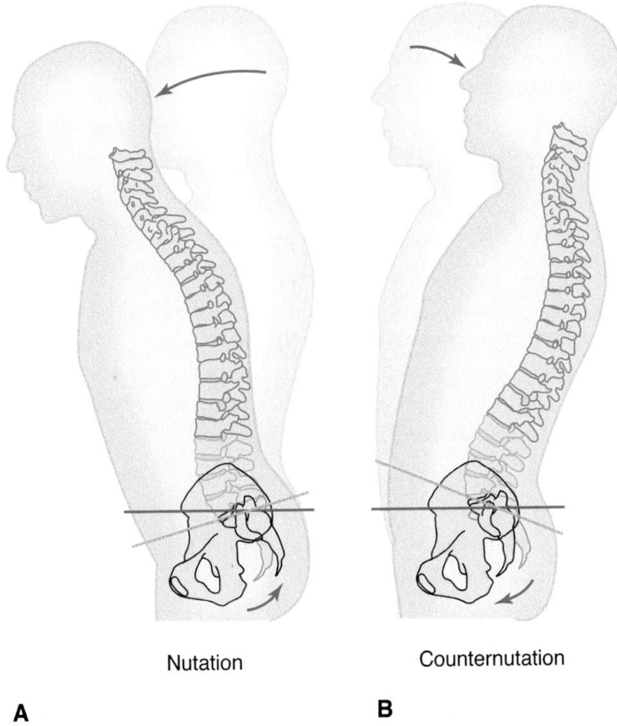

Nutation

Counternutation

A

B

Figure 17-4. Sacroiliac joint motions. **(A)** Nutation occurs when the sacral promontory moves anteriorly and inferiorly while the tip of the coccyx moves in the opposite direction. **(B)** Counternutation occurs when the sacral promontory moves posteriorly and superiorly while the tip of the coccyx moves in the opposite direction.

Nutation, sometimes referred to as *sacral flexion,* occurs when the base of the sacrum (on the superior end) moves anteriorly and inferiorly. This causes the inferior portion of the sacrum and the coccyx to move posteriorly. The pelvic outlet becomes larger and can be visualized by drawing a line from the tip of the coccyx to the bottom surface of the pubic symphysis (see Fig. 17-2).

Counternutation, sometimes called *sacral extension,* refers to the opposite motion. The base of the sacrum moves posteriorly and superiorly, causing the tip of the coccyx to move anteriorly. The pelvic inlet becomes larger. The pelvic inlet can be visualized by drawing a line from the base of the sacrum across to the top of the symphysis pubis.

The amount of motion that occurs in nutation and counternutation is minimal, and it can occur only in conjunction with other joint motions. Nutation occurs with trunk flexion or hip extension. Conversely, counternutation occurs with trunk extension or hip flexion. These motions are also important during childbirth. When the baby moves through the pelvic inlet during the early stages of labor, the anterior-posterior (A-P) diameter needs to be larger. Therefore, the SI joints are in counternutation. In the later stages of labor, when the baby passes through the pelvic outlet, it is important that this A-P diameter has increased. Putting the SI joints in nutation increases the A-P diameter.

Bones and Landmarks

The two bones of the SI joint are the sacrum and the ilium, the latter of which is the superior portion of the innominate bone. The **sacrum** is wedge-shaped and consists of five fused sacral vertebrae. It is located between the two innominate bones and makes up the posterior border of the bony pelvis. Its anterior surface, often called the *pelvic surface,* is concave (Fig. 17-5). Because it is tilted, the sacrum articulates with the fifth lumbar vertebra at an angle referred to as the *lumbosacral angle.* The significant landmarks of the **sacrum** are listed below (Figs. 17-5 and 17-6).

Important Bony Landmarks of the Sacrum

Base
Superior surface of S1

Promontory
Ridge projecting along the anterior edge of the body of S1

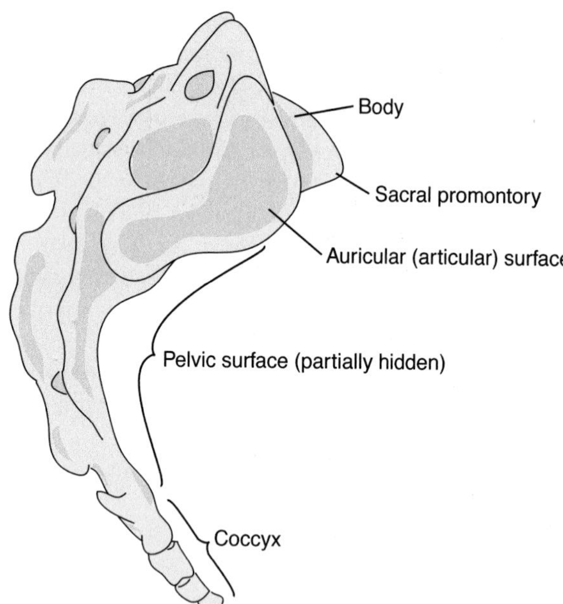

Figure 17-5. Sacrum (lateral view).

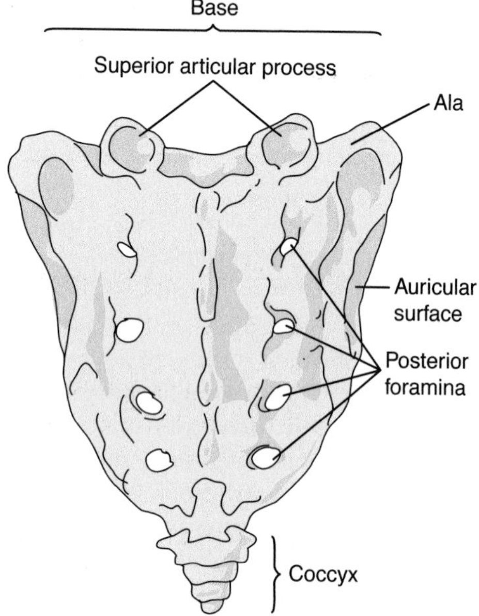

Figure 17-6. Sacrum (posterior view).

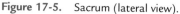

Superior Articular Process
Located posteriorly on the base, it articulates with the inferior articular process of L5.

Ala
Lateral flared wings that are actually fused transverse processes

Foramina
Located on the anterior (pelvic) and dorsal surfaces are four pairs of foramina. They serve as the exit for the anterior and posterior divisions of the sacral nerves. The anterior foramina are larger.

Auricular Surface
Named because its shape is similar to the external ear (*auricular* is Latin for "earlike"). It is located on the lateral surface of the sacrum and articulates with the ilium. The irregular surface assists in locking the two surfaces together, providing greater stability.

Pelvic Surface
Concave anterior surface

The **ilium** will be described in more detail in Chapter 18. The ilium makes up the superior part of the innominate bone. Landmarks relevant to the sacroiliac joint are listed below (Fig. 17-7).

Important Bony Landmarks of the Ilium

Iliac Tuberosity
Large, roughened area between the posterior portion of the iliac crest and the auricular surface. It serves as an attachment for the interosseous ligament.

Auricular Surface
Named for its earlike shape, it is the articular surface of the ilium with the sacrum. It is located inferior and anterior to the iliac tuberosity.

Iliac Crest
Superior ridge of the ilium, the bony area felt when you place your hands on your hips

Posterior Superior Iliac Spine
Often abbreviated PSIS, it is the posterior projection of the iliac crest and serves as an attachment for the posterior sacroiliac ligaments.

Posterior Inferior Iliac Spine
Often abbreviated PIIS, it lies inferior to the PSIS and serves as an attachment for the sacrotuberous ligaments

Greater Sciatic Notch
Formed by the ilium superiorly and the ilium and ischium inferiorly

Greater Sciatic Foramen
Formed from the greater sciatic notch by ligamentous attachments. The sacrotuberous ligament forms the posterior medial border of the foramen, and the sacrospinous ligament forms the inferior border (Figs. 17-8 and 17-9). The sciatic nerve passes through this opening.

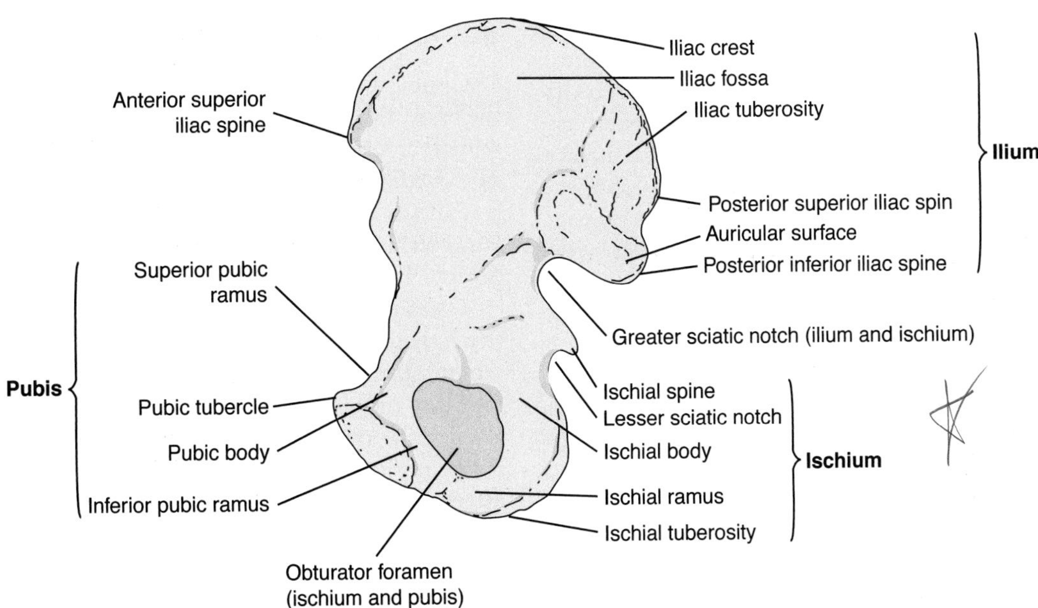

Figure 17-7. Right innominate bone (medial view).

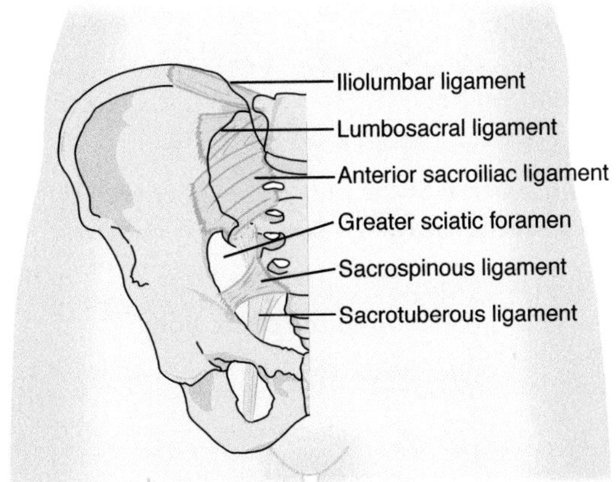

Figure 17-8. Ligaments of the pelvis (anterior view).

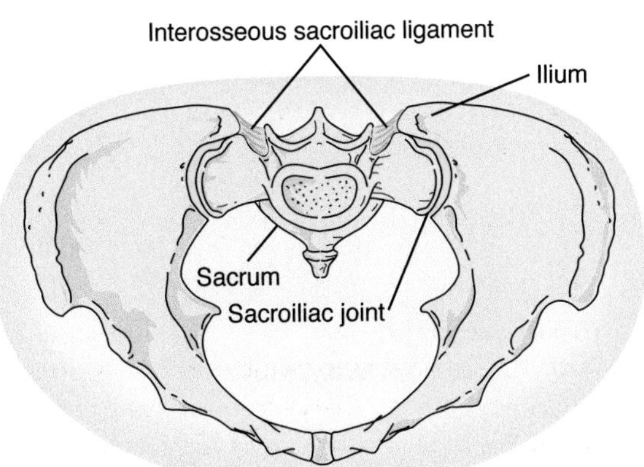

Figure 17-9. Cross section of the sacroiliac joints (superior view).

The **ischium** will also be described in more detail in Chapter 18. The portions of the ischium pertaining to the sacroiliac joint are as follows (see Fig. 17-7):

Important Bony Landmarks of the Ischium

Ischial Body
Makes up all of the ischium superior to the tuberosity

Lesser Sciatic Notch
Smaller concavity located on the posterior body between the greater sciatic notch and the ischial tuberosity

Ischial Spine
Located on the posterior body and between the greater sciatic and lesser sciatic notches. It provides attachment for the sacrospinous ligament.

Ischial Tuberosity
The blunt, rough projection on the inferior part of the body. It is a weight-bearing surface when you are sitting.

Ligaments

Because the sacroiliac joint is meant to absorb a great deal of stress while providing great stability, it is heavily endowed with ligaments. The **anterior sacroiliac ligament** is a broad, flat ligament on the anterior (pelvic) surface connecting the ala and pelvic surface of the sacrum to the auricular surface of the ilium (see Fig. 17-8). It holds together the anterior portion of the joint. The **interosseous sacroiliac ligament** is the deepest, shortest, and strongest of the sacroiliac ligaments (see Fig. 17-9). It fills the roughened area immediately above and behind the auricular surfaces and the anterior sacroiliac ligament. It also connects the tuberosities of the ilium to the sacrum.

The posterior sacroiliac ligament comprises two parts (Fig. 17-10). The **short posterior sacroiliac ligament** runs more obliquely between the ilium and the upper portion of the sacrum on the dorsal surface. It prevents forward movement of the sacrum. The **long posterior sacroiliac ligament** runs more vertically between the posterior superior iliac spine and the lower portion of the sacrum. It prevents downward movement of the sacrum.

Three accessory ligaments further reinforce the sacroiliac joint and are seen in Figures 17-8 and 17-10. The **sacrotuberous ligament** is a very strong, triangular ligament running from between the PSIS and PIIS of the ilium, from the posterior and lateral side of the sacrum inferior to the auricular surface, and from the coccyx. These fibers come together to attach on the ischial tuberosity. It serves as an attachment for the gluteus maximus and prevents forward rotation of the sacrum. The **sacrospinous ligament** is also triangular and lies deep to the sacrotuberous ligament. It has a broad attachment from the lower lateral sacrum and coccyx on the posterior side. It then narrows to attach to the spine of the ischium. These two ligaments convert the greater sciatic notch into a foramen through which the sciatic nerve passes. The **iliolumbar ligament** connects the transverse process of L5 with the iliac crest. It is described in more detail in the "Lumbosacral Joint" section.

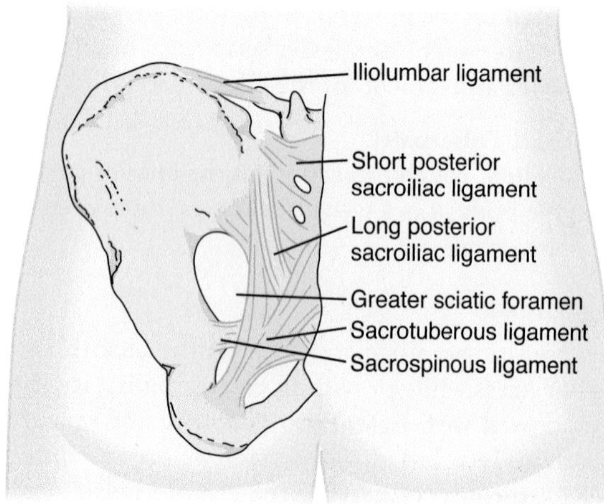

Figure 17-10. Ligaments of the pelvis (posterior view).

Pubic Symphysis

The pubic symphysis joint is located in the midline of the body (Fig. 17-11). The right and left pubic bones are joined anteriorly and form the pubic symphysis. A fibrocartilage disk lies between the two bones. Because it is an amphiarthrodial joint, there is little movement. However, it becomes much more moveable in women during childbirth.

The pubic symphysis is held together primarily by two ligaments (see Fig. 17-11). The **superior pubic ligament** attaches to the pubic tubercles on each side of the body and strengthens the superior and anterior portions of the joint. The **inferior pubic ligament** attaches between the two inferior pubic rami. It strengthens the inferior portion of the joint.

Landmarks

The **pubis** will be described in greater detail in Chapter 18. The landmarks relevant to the pubic symphysis are listed below (see Fig. 17-7).

Important Bony Landmarks of the Pubis

Body
Main portion of the pubic bone, between the two projections (rami)—superior and inferior

Superior Ramus
Superior projection of the pubic body

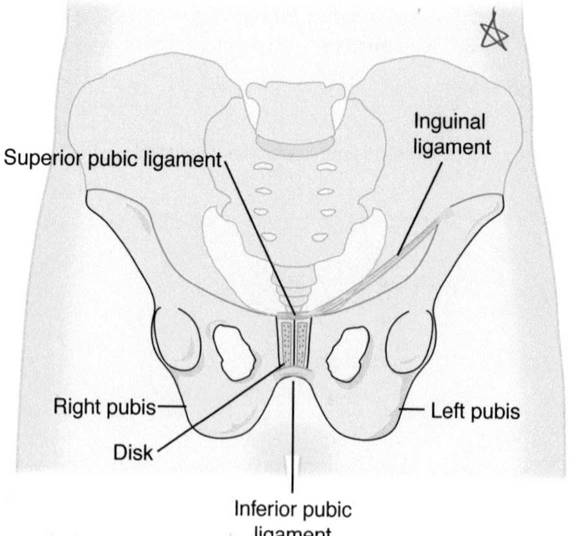

Figure 17-11. Pubic symphysis, frontal view with pubic bone cut away.

Inferior Ramus
Inferior projection of the pubic body that provides attachment for the inferior pubic ligament

Tubercle
Projects anteriorly on the superior ramus near the midline and provides attachment for the superior pubic ligament

Lumbosacral Joint

Joint Structure and Ligaments

The lumbosacral joint is made up of the fifth lumbar vertebra and the first sacral vertebra. The articulation between these vertebrae is the same as that for all other vertebrae. The bodies of these two bones are separated by an intervertebral disk and are held together at the bodies by the anterior and posterior longitudinal ligaments. The vertebrae articulate at the articular processes (inferior articular process of L5 and superior articular process of S1). The ligaments holding together this portion of the joint are the supraspinal and interspinal ligaments and the ligamentum flava. All of these ligaments are described in Chapter 15.

Two additional ligaments specifically hold the lumbosacral joint together (see Fig. 17-8). The **iliolumbar ligament** attaches on the transverse process of L5 and runs inferiorly and laterally to the posterior portion of the inner lip of the iliac crest. This ligament limits the rotation of L5 on S1, and it assists the articular processes in preventing L5 from moving anteriorly on S1. The **lumbosacral ligament** also attaches on the transverse process of L5. It runs inferiorly and laterally to attach on the ala of the sacrum, where its fibers intermingle with the fibers of the anterior sacroiliac ligament.

Lumbosacral Angle

The lumbosacral angle is responsible for creating the lumbar lordosis, and indirectly for creating the rest of the spinal curves. Having an optimal lumbosacral angle generates the optimal degree of curvature throughout the rest of the spine, as can be seen in Figure 17-12. The lumbosacral angle is determined by drawing one line parallel to the ground and another line along the base of the sacrum. This angle will increase as the pelvis tilts anteriorly and will decrease as the pelvis tilts posteriorly. The optimal lumbosacral angle is approximately 30 degrees. As the lumbar lordosis increases, the angle increases. This causes the shearing stresses of L5 on S1 to increase. Forward movement of L5 on S1 is prevented by ligamentous restraint, and the shape and fit of the inferior articular process of L5 is seated inside and behind the

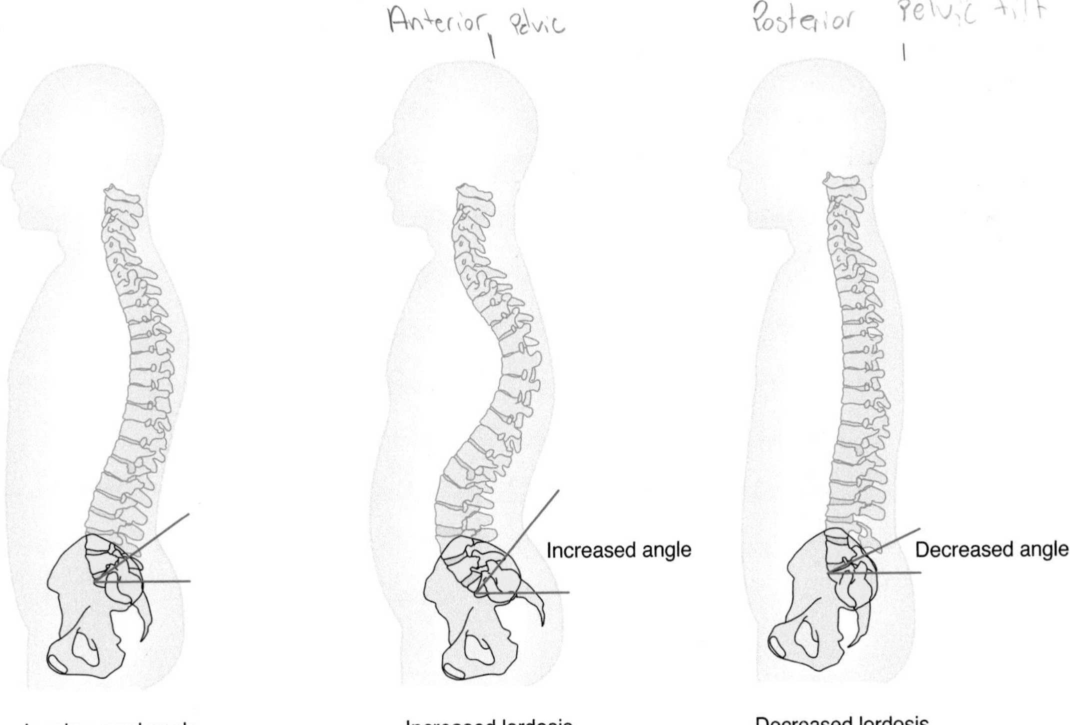

Figure 17-12. The lumbosacral angle is determined by drawing one line parallel to the ground and another line along the base of the sacrum. The angle increases or decreases as lumbar lordosis increases or decreases, respectively.

superior articular process of S1. Conversely, as the lumbar lordosis decreases, lumbosacral angle decreases.

Pelvic Girdle Motions

The joints directly involved in pelvic girdle movement include the two hip joints and the lumbar joints, particularly the lumbosacral articulation between L5 and S1. Pelvic motions occur in all three planes. When you stand in an upright position, the pelvis should be level; in the sagittal plane, the anterior superior iliac spine (ASIS, see Fig. 17-7) and the pubic symphysis should be in the same vertical plane (Fig. 17-13). **Anterior tilt** occurs when the pelvis tilts forward, moving the ASIS anterior to the pubic symphysis. **Posterior tilt** occurs when the pelvis tilts backward, moving the ASIS posterior to the pubic symphysis. These motions are shown in Figure 17-13.

Keeping the body upright when the pelvis tilts forward requires the joints above and below the pelvis to move in the opposite direction. Therefore, when the pelvis tilts anteriorly, the lumbar portion of the vertebral column goes into hyperextension and the hip joints flex. Thus, when a person with a hip flexion contracture stands in the upright position, the pelvis tilts anteriorly and the lumbar region hyperextends. Conversely, a person with tight hamstrings may stand with the pelvis tilted posteriorly and the lumbar curve flattened.

In the frontal plane, the iliac crests should be level (Fig. 17-14). You can assess this by placing your thumbs on the ASISs and determining whether your thumbs are at the same level. **Lateral tilt** occurs when the two iliac crests are not level. Because the pelvis moves as a unit, one side moves up as the other side moves down (Fig. 17-15). Therefore, a point of reference must be used. *The side that is unsupported (or non–weight-bearing) will be the point of reference.* When you walk, the pelvis is level when both legs are in contact with the ground. However, when one leg leaves the ground (swing phase), it becomes unsupported and the pelvis on that side drops slightly. It is impossible to drop the pelvis on the weight-bearing side. Therefore, the point of reference for lateral tilt is the unsupported, or less supported, side. Figure 17-16 illustrates a left lateral tilt. The person bears weight on the right leg while lifting the left leg from the ground. The left side of the pelvis becomes unsupported and drops, or laterally tilts to the left.

To keep the body balanced, joints directly above and below will shift in the opposite direction. Notice in

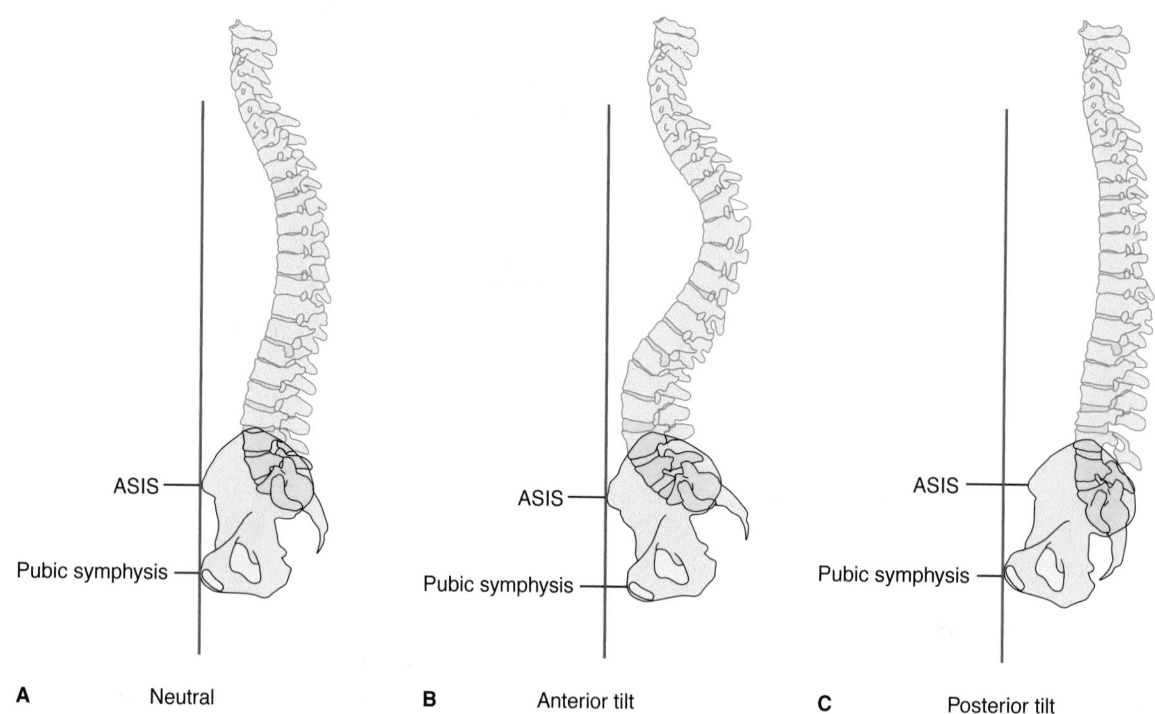

Figure 17-13. Pelvic movement in the sagittal plane. **(A)** The anterior superior iliac spine (ASIS) and the pubic symphysis should be in the same vertical plane. **(B)** Anterior tilt occurs when the pelvis tilts forward, moving the ASIS anterior to the pubic symphysis. **(C)** Posterior tilt occurs when the pelvis tilts backward, moving the ASIS posterior to the pubic symphysis.

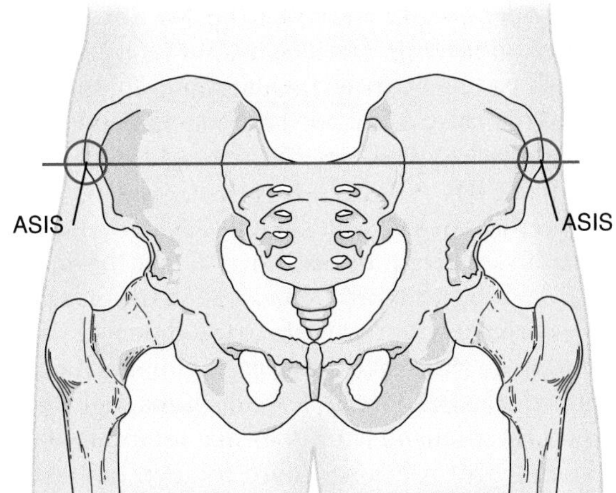

Figure 17-14. Pelvic movement in the frontal plane. When standing upright on both feet, the iliac crests and the ASISs should be level.

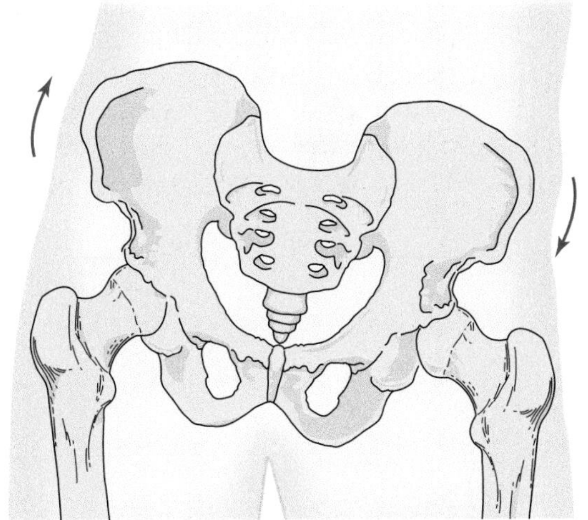

Figure 17-15. Left lateral tilt (anterior view). One side of the pelvis moves up while the other side moves down.

Figure 17-17 that as the pelvis tilts (drops) to the right, the vertebral column laterally bends to the left. While the weight-bearing hip joint (left) adducts, the unsupported hip joint (right) becomes more abducted.

Although this discussion has centered on one side of the pelvis dropping below the level of the other side, it is possible to raise the pelvis on the unsupported side. This is commonly called *hip hiking*, which is actually a misnomer. More accurately, it should be called *pelvic hiking*. When a person walks with a long leg cast or a brace, hip hiking helps the foot clear the floor during the swing phase. Shifting from one ischial tuberosity to the other while sitting also involves raising the pelvis on one side. This motion is useful in allowing some pressure relief.

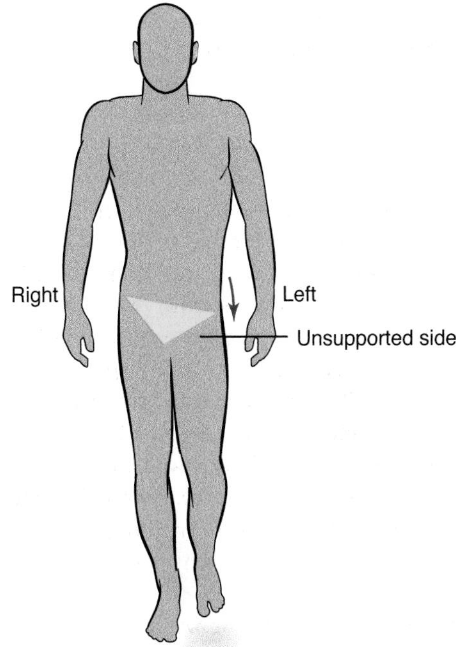

Figure 17-16. Left lateral tilt (anterior view). When one leg leaves the ground, the pelvis on that side becomes unsupported. This causes the pelvis on that side to drop slightly. Therefore, lateral tilt is named by the unsupported side.

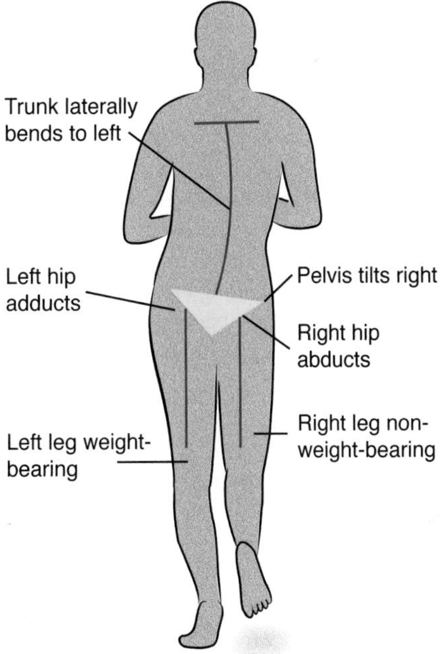

Figure 17-17. Other joint motions affected by pelvic tilting. As the pelvis tilts to the right, the vertebral column laterally bends to the left. The left hip joint (the weight-bearing side) adducts and the right hip joint (the non-weight-bearing side) abducts.

Pelvic rotation occurs in the transverse plane around a vertical axis when one side of the pelvis moves forward or backward in relation to the other side. Looking down on the pelvis, the significant landmarks again are the left and right ASISs. In the anatomical (neutral) position (Fig. 17-18A), the left and right ASISs should be in the same plane. In Figure 17-18B and C, the red dot represents the femoral head and the red circle around it is the acetabulum. *The non–weight-bearing side of the pelvis is the point of reference* for describing the direction of pelvic rotation. In Figure 17-18B, the left leg is weight-bearing and the right leg is swinging forward. In this example, the right side of the pelvis rotates forward, moving the right ASIS in front of the left ASIS. Right forward pelvic rotation is the result of the left acetabulum rotating *medially* on the stationary left femoral head in a closed-chain motion. This is actually left hip rotation in a reverse muscle action. If the right leg swings backward (Fig. 17-18C), the left acetabulum rotates *laterally* on the stationary left femoral head in a closed-chain motion. This results in right backward pelvic rotation (left hip rotation in a reverse muscle action) so that the right ASIS is now behind the left ASIS. If you orient the page of the book so that the pelvis in (B) and (C) are in the same plane as in (A), it may be easier to visualize the hip rotation by noting the direction the foot is pointing. In other words, in (B), rotate the page about 45 degrees clockwise; in (C), rotate the page about 45 degrees counterclockwise. Figure 17-18B shows right pelvic forward rotation and left hip medial rotation, whereas (C) shows right pelvic backward rotation and left hip lateral rotation. The combinations of joint motions that occur during walking are described in greater detail in Chapter 22. However, a summary of some of the associated joint motions are listed in Table 17-1.

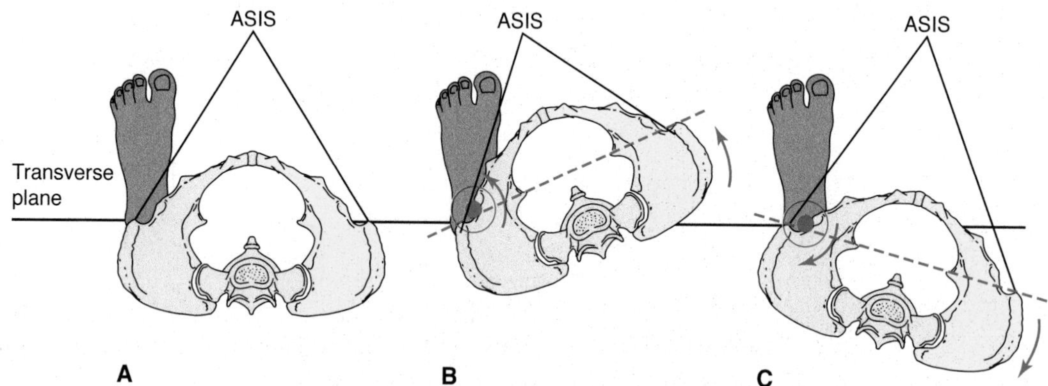

Figure 17-18. Pelvic rotation in the transverse plane (superior view). **(A)** In the anatomical (neutral) position, both ASISs are in the same plane (shown as black line). **(B)** With forward rotation, the right side of the pelvis moves forward. This causes the left side of the pelvis to rotate around the femoral head, resulting in left hip medial rotation. **(C)** With backward rotation, the right side of the pelvis moves backward. This causes the left side of the pelvis to rotate on the femoral head, resulting in left hip lateral rotation.

Table 17-1 Associated Motions of the Pelvic Girdle, Vertebral Column, and Hip Joints

Pelvic Girdle	Vertebral Column	Hip
Anterior tilt	Hyperextension	Flexion
Posterior tilt	Flexion	Extension
Lateral tilt (unsupported side)	Lateral bending (to supported side)	Adduction: weight-bearing side Abduction: non-weight-bearing side
Rotation (forward)	Rotation: to opposite side	Medial rotation: weight-bearing side
Rotation (backward)	Rotation: to opposite side	Lateral rotation: weight-bearing side

Muscle Control

The pelvis is moved and controlled by groups of muscles acting as force couples. As the pelvis tilts in the anterior-posterior direction, the opposing muscle groups provide movement and control (Fig. 17-19). To tilt the pelvis anteriorly, the lumbar trunk extensors, primarily the erector spinae, pull up posteriorly while the hip flexors pull down anteriorly. Conversely, to tilt the pelvis posteriorly, the trunk flexors (primarily the abdominals) pull up anteriorly while the hip extensors (gluteus maximus and hamstrings) pull down posteriorly (Fig. 17-20). In both cases, these muscle groups are acting as a force couple by pulling in opposite directions and causing the pelvis to tilt.

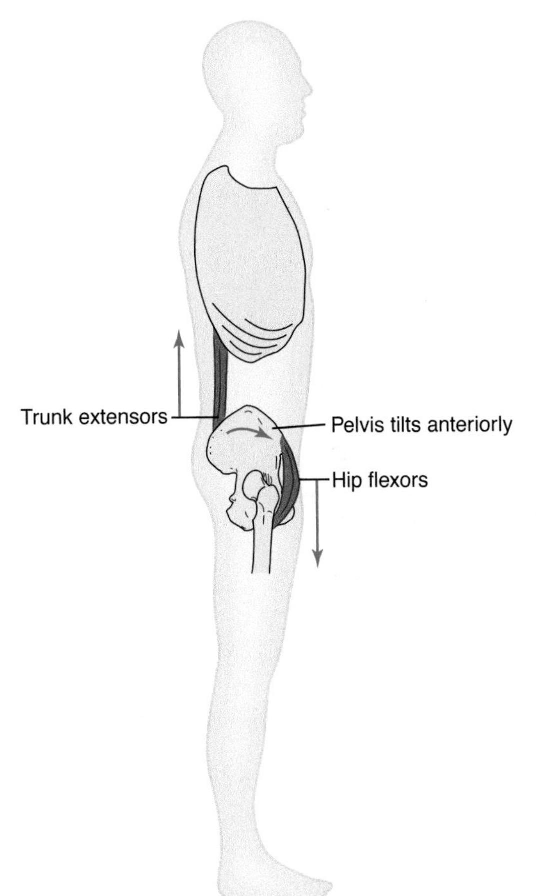

Figure 17-19. Force couple causing anterior pelvic tilt (lateral view). The trunk extensors pulling up (posteriorly) and the hip flexors pulling down (anteriorly) cause the pelvis to tilt anteriorly.

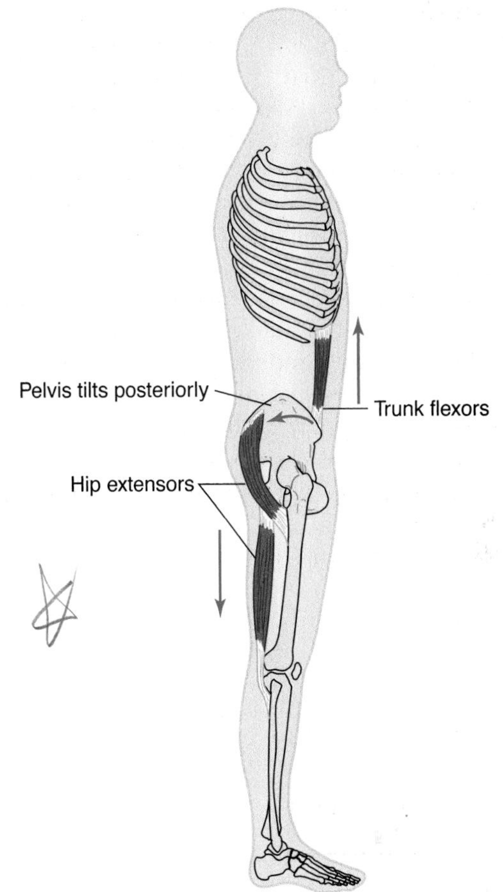

Figure 17-20. Force couple causing posterior pelvic tilt (lateral view). The trunk flexors pulling up (anteriorly) and the hip extensors pulling down (posteriorly) cause the pelvis to tilt posteriorly.

Without any muscle action, the force of gravity can tilt the pelvis laterally when that leg becomes unsupported. However, to control or limit the amount of lateral tilting, muscle groups on opposite sides of the body also work as a force couple. Using the example shown in Figure 17-21, in a reversal of muscle action, the left trunk lateral benders (primarily the erector spinae and quadratus lumborum) pull up on the left side of the pelvis while the right hip abductors (gluteus medius and minimus) pull down on the right side to keep the pelvis fairly level.

By preventing pelvic motion, all of these same muscle groups can work together to provide stability. Pelvic and trunk control are necessary to provide the stable foundation upon which the head and extremities can move.

Clinical Application 17-1

Muscular Implications of Chronic Poor Posture

An individual who stands with a **habitual anterior tilt** puts the lumbar vertebral column in hyperextension and the hips in flexion. Over time, the trunk extensor and hip flexor muscles adaptively shorten and become tight (Fig. A).

The opposite happens to the trunk flexors and hip extensors. The trunk flexors are lengthened over the abdomen and the hip extensors are lengthened over the gluteal region. As a result, they become overstretched and weakened.

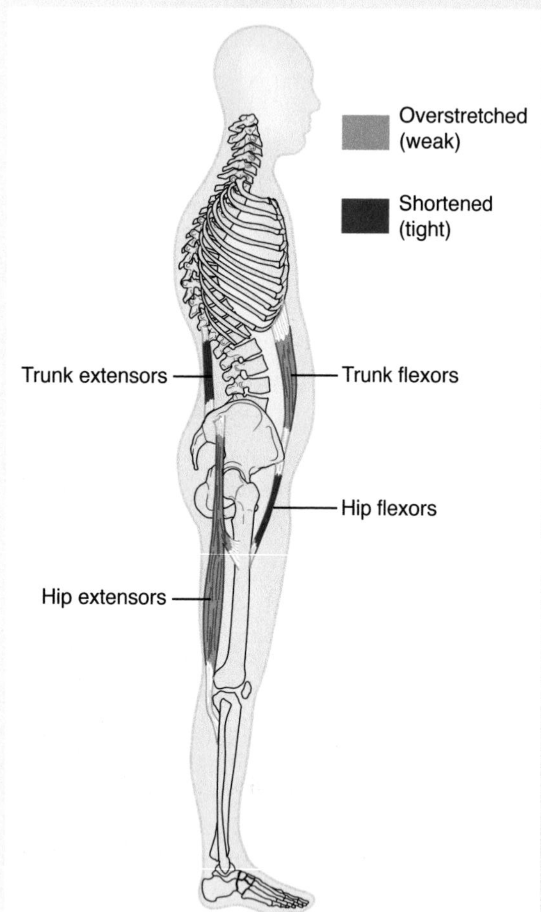

A. Habitual Anterior Tilt Posture

With a **habitual posterior tilt,** the normal lumbar curve is reduced and the hips become slightly hyperextended. In this position, the hip extensors are shortened while the trunk extensors are lengthened (Fig. B). An individual with a habitual posterior tilt posture will have hip extensor and trunk flexor tightness. The trunk extensors and hip flexors will be overstretched and weakened.

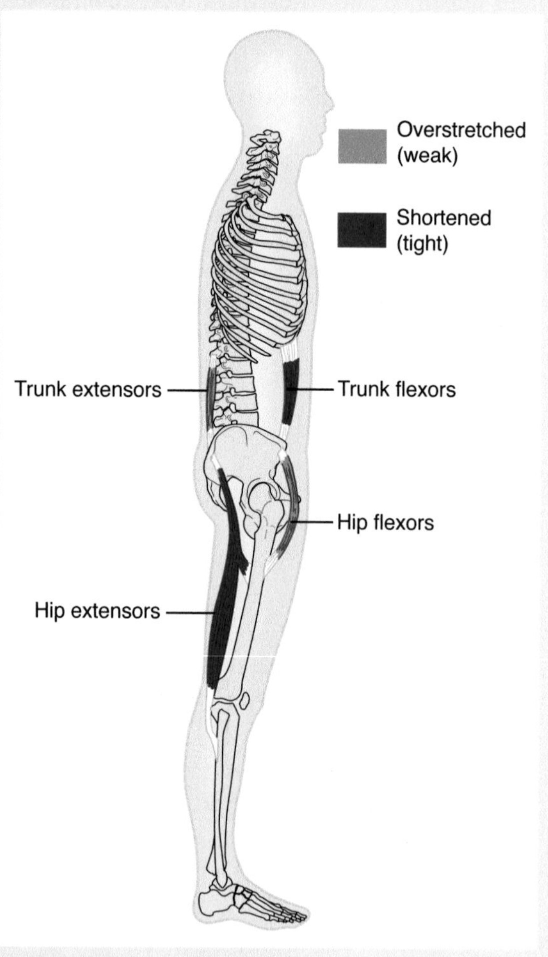

B. Habitual Posterior Tilt Posture

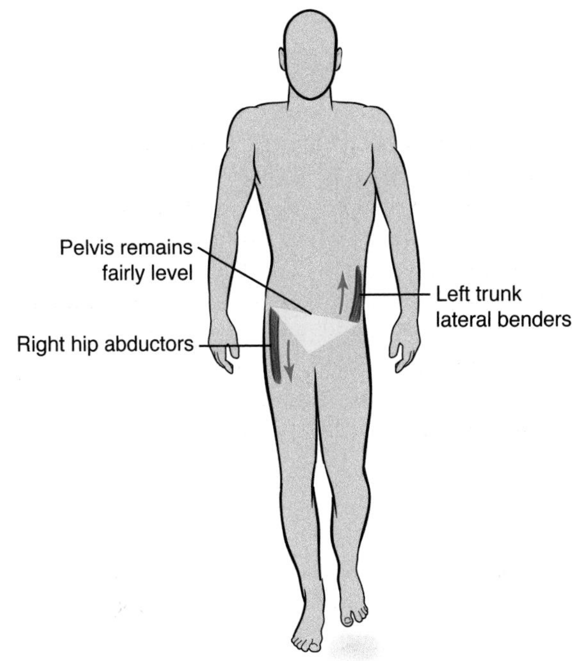

Figure 17-21. Force couple keeps the pelvis level in the frontal plane. In a reversal of muscle action, the left trunk lateral benders pull up while the right hip abductors pull down. This keeps the pelvis fairly level as opposed to letting the pelvis drop on the unsupported side.

Review Questions

General Anatomy Questions

1. What pelvic girdle motions occur in the following?
   a. The sagittal plane around the frontal axis
   b. The frontal plane around the sagittal axis
   c. The transverse plane around the vertical axis
2. a. Concentric contraction of the right quadratus lumborum would cause the pelvis to laterally tilt to which side?
   b. Another term for this motion is ____________________.
3. Motion occurs at the lumbosacral joint when the pelvis tilts anteriorly and posteriorly and at what other distal joint?
4. What associated hip joint motion occurs when the pelvis tilts:
   a. anteriorly?
   b. posteriorly?
   c. laterally?
5. What associated hip joint motions occur when the left side of the pelvis rotates:
   a. forward?
   b. backward?
6. What associated lumbar motion occurs when the pelvis tilts:
   a. anteriorly?
   b. posteriorly?
   c. laterally?
7. If a person maintained a posture in which the pelvis was tilted excessively in an anterior position:
   a. What muscle groups would tend to be tight?
   b. What muscle groups would tend to be weak?
8. If an individual has a scoliotic curve that is convex to the left, and assuming the scoliosis was caused by a true leg length discrepancy, which would be the short leg?
9. A decreased lumbosacral angle causes the anterior shearing force of L5 on S1 to increase/decrease __________.
10. Name two ligaments that help prevent anterior shearing of L5 on S1.

(continued on next page)

Review Questions—cont'd

Functional Activity Questions

Identify the position of the pelvis in the following activities:

1. Lying supine, bring your right leg up to your chest.
2. Kneeling on your hands and knees, let your trunk sag downward.
3. Kneeling on your hands and knees, arch your back.
4. Stand with your left foot on a telephone book and your right foot on the floor with weight on both feet. Identify the position of right and left hip joints in terms of abducted or adducted positions (Fig. 17-22).

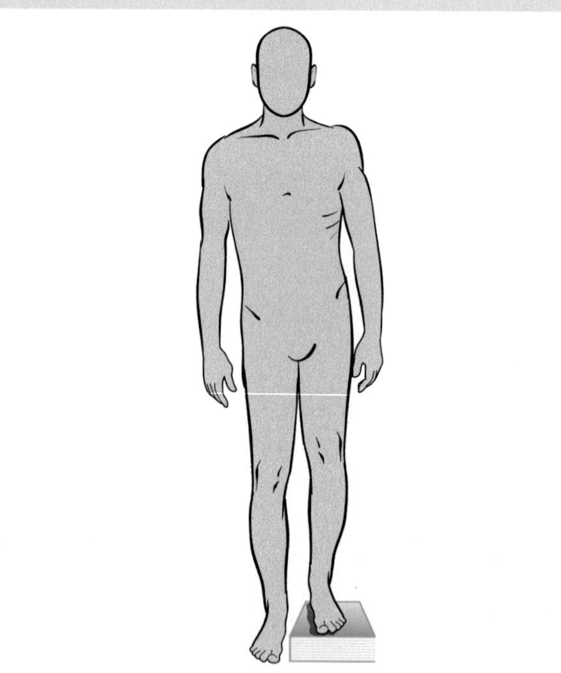

Figure 17-22. Standing with one foot on a telephone book and the other foot on the floor.

5. During an anterior pelvic tilt:
   a. What hip muscle group helps to generate this motion?
   b. What hip muscle needs to contract as a stabilizer while the muscle group in (a) is contracting?
   c. What trunk muscle group helps to generate this motion?
   d. What trunk muscle group needs to contract as a stabilizer while the muscle group in (c) is contracting?

Clinical Exercise Questions

1. Lie supine with your knees flexed and the soles of your feet flat on the mat. Place your hand in the small of your back (lumbar curve). Push your back against your hand. Identify the main trunk, pelvic, and hip joint motions. Which muscles contribute to this force couple action?
   Motions:
   Muscles:
2. Standing in anatomical position, lift your left foot off the ground while keeping your hip and knee joints extended. Identify the main pelvic and hip joint motions. Which muscles contribute to this force couple action?
   Motions:
   Muscles:

PART IV

Clinical Kinesiology and Anatomy of the Lower Extremities

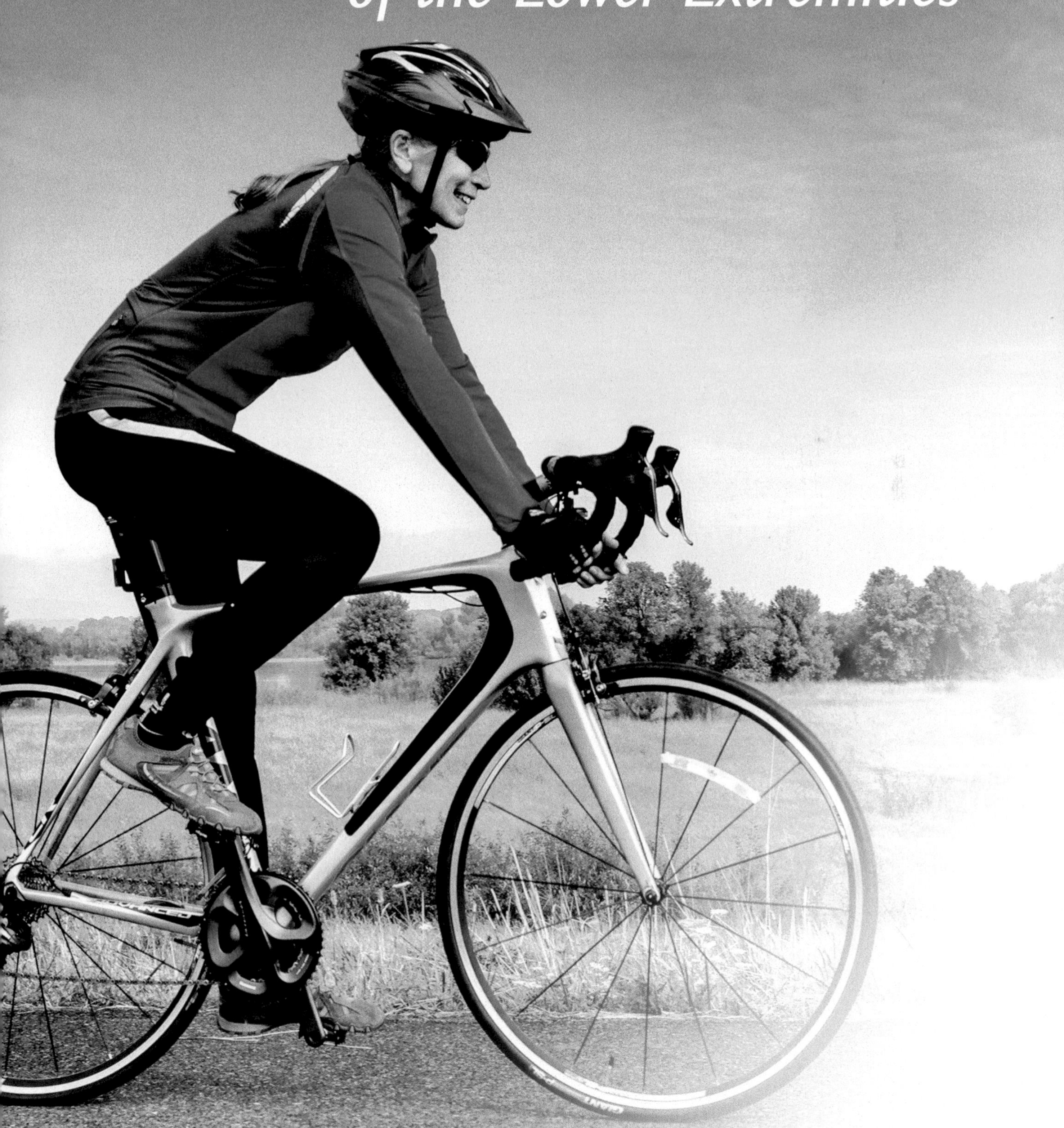

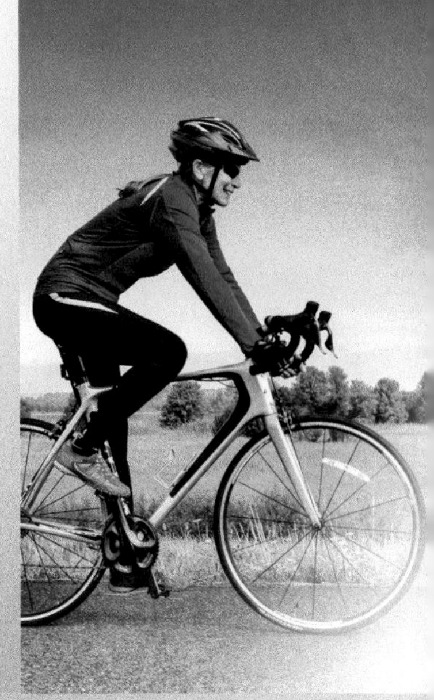

CHAPTER 18 Hip Joint

Joint Structure and Motions
Bones and Landmarks
Ligaments and Other Structures
Muscles of the Hip
Anatomical Relationships
Common Hip Pathologies
Summary of Muscle Action
Summary of Muscle Innervation
Points to Remember
Review Questions
General Anatomy Questions
Functional Activity Questions
Clinical Exercise Questions

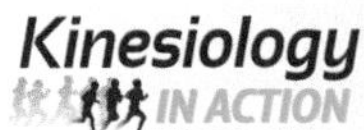

For additional practice activities and videos, please visit www.kinesiologyinaction.com

The lower extremity includes the pelvis, thigh, leg, and foot (Fig. 18-1). Bones of the pelvis are the two innominate bones (hip bones), the sacrum, and the coccyx. To avoid confusion with the hip joint, the hip bone will be referred to as the innominate bone. The innominate bone consists of three bones (ilium, ischium, and pubis) fused together. The thigh contains the femur and the patella. The leg includes the tibia and fibula, and the foot includes seven tarsal bones, five metatarsals, and 14 phalanges. Table 18-1 summarizes the bones of the lower extremity.

Joint Structure and Motions

The **hip** joint is the most proximal of the lower extremity joints. It is very important in weight-bearing and walking activities. Like the shoulder, it is a ball-and-socket joint. The rounded, or convex-shaped, femoral head fits into and articulates with the concave-shaped acetabulum (Fig. 18-2). The convex femoral head slides in the direction opposite the movement of the thigh. Unlike the shoulder, the hip is a very stable joint and therefore sacrifices some range of motion. Conversely, the shoulder, which allows a great deal of motion, is not as stable.

Being a triaxial joint, the hip has motion in all three planes (Fig. 18-3). **Flexion, extension, and hyperextension** occur in the sagittal plane, with approximately 120 degrees of flexion and 15 degrees of hyperextension. Extension is the return from flexion. **Abduction and adduction** occur in the frontal plane, with about 45 degrees of abduction. Adduction is usually thought of as the return to anatomical position, although there is approximately an additional 25 degrees of motion possible beyond the anatomical position. In the transverse plane, **medial and lateral rotations** are sometimes referred to as *internal* and *external rotation,* respectively. There are approximately 45 degrees of rotation possible in each direction from the anatomical position.

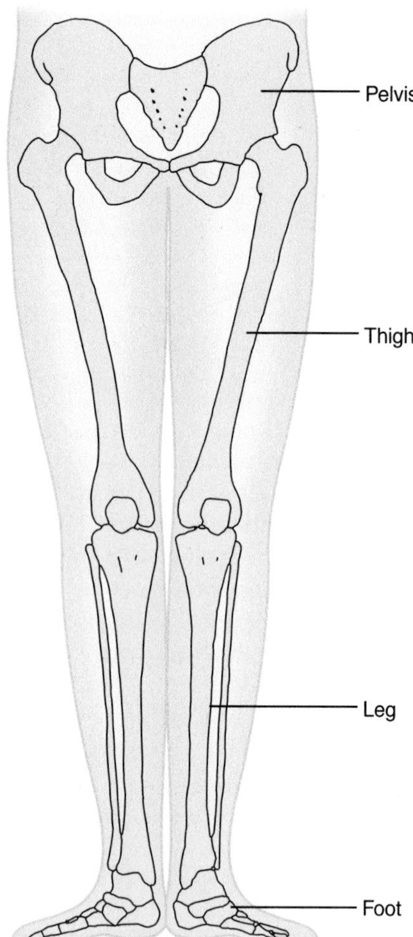

Figure 18-1. Bones of the lower extremities (anterior view).

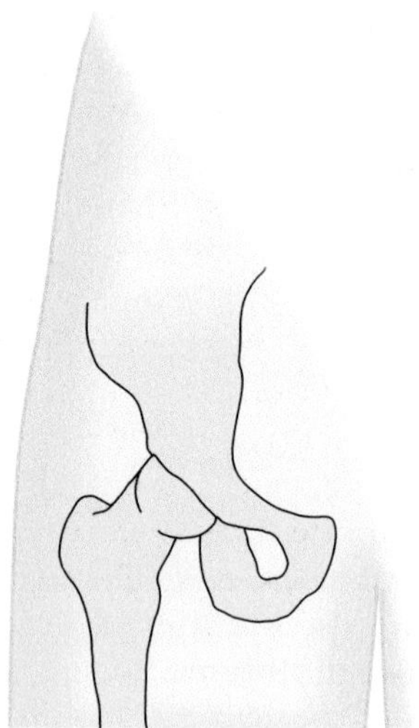

Figure 18-2. Hip joint (anterior view).

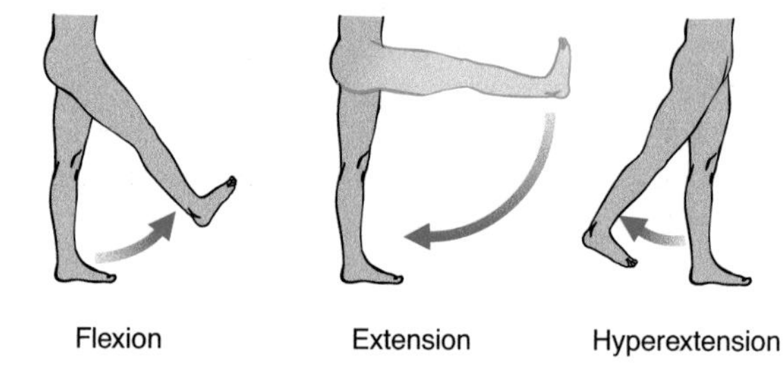

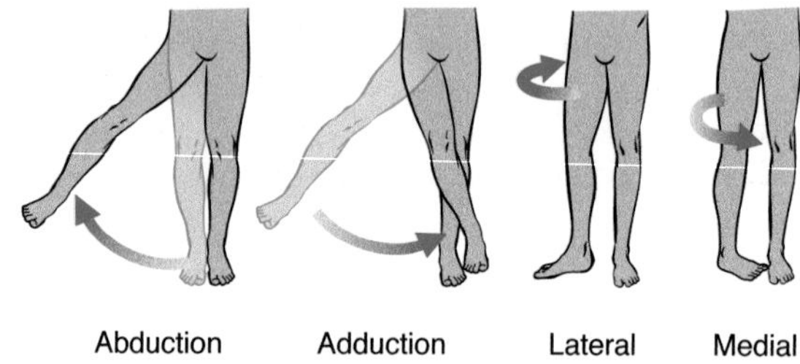

Figure 18-3. Motions of the hip.

Table 18-1 Bones of the Lower Extremity

Region	Bones	Individual Bones
Pelvis	Innominate	Ilium, ischium, pubis
	Sacrum	
	Coccyx	
Thigh	Femur	
	Patella	
Leg	Tibia	
	Fibula	
Foot	Tarsals (7)	Calcaneus, talus, cuboid, navicular, cuneiform (3)
	Metatarsals (5)	First through fifth
	Phalanges (14)	Proximal (5), middle (4), distal (5)

The end feel of all hip joint motions, except flexion, is **firm** because of tension in the capsule, ligaments, and muscles. For hip flexion, the end feel is **soft** because of contact between the anterior thigh and the abdomen.

Arthrokinematics

The hip is in the open-packed position when it is in 30 degrees of flexion, 30 degrees of abduction, and a small degree of lateral rotation. This is the position where maximal joint surface movement is possible. The hip joint is a convex-on-concave articulation where the head of the femur glides in the opposite direction from the distal end of the bone. For example, when the femur moves laterally in hip abduction, the femoral head glides medially. In other words, they move in opposite directions. During hip adduction, the femur moves medially while the femoral head glides laterally (Fig. 18-4). The same movement pattern occurs for hip flexion/extension, and medial-lateral rotation, respectively. In each movement, the femoral head (articular surface) glides one way and the femur (distal end of bone) moves in the opposite direction.

When these accessory motions of the femoral head are limited, a mobilizing force that moves the head of the femur into the direction of restriction can help restore motion. For example, a posterior glide of the head of the femur will promote stretching of the posterior capsule and increased flexion and medial rotation, whereas an anterior glide will stretch the anterior capsule and increase extension and lateral rotation.

The two innominate bones are connected to each other anteriorly and to the sacrum posteriorly. The sacrum is also connected distally to the coccyx. These four bones (the two innominate bones, the sacrum, and the coccyx) are collectively known as the **pelvis,** or **pelvic girdle** (Fig. 18-5). Note that the pelvis does not include the femur.

Bones and Landmarks

As mentioned earlier, the hip joint is made up of the innominate bone and the femur. The innominate bone is irregularly shaped and actually consists of three bones—the ilium, the ischium, and the pubis (Fig. 18-6). By adulthood, these bones fuse together.

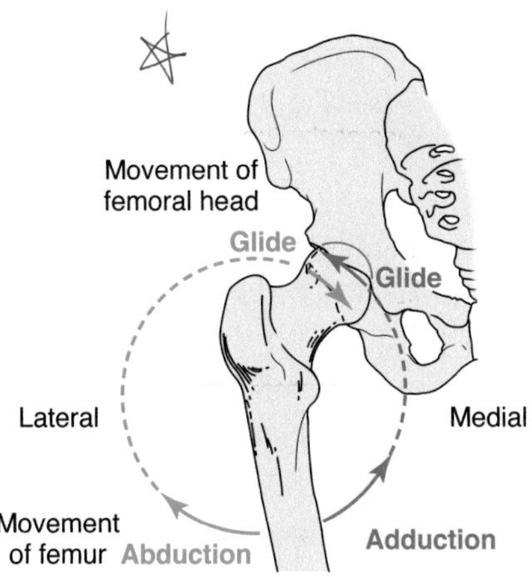

Figure 18-4. Arthrokinematic motion at hip joint. Convex joint surface moves in opposite direction of the femur during hip abduction/adduction.

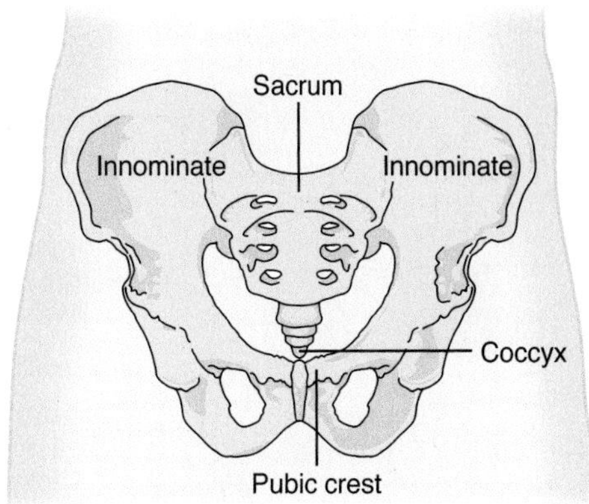

Figure 18-5. Bones of the pelvis (anterior view).

The fan-shaped **ilium** makes up the superior portion of the innominate bone. Its significant landmarks are listed below (Figs. 18-6 and 18-7).

Important Bony Landmarks of the Ilium

Iliac Fossa

Large, smooth, concave area on the internal surface to which the iliac portion of the iliopsoas muscle attaches

Iliac Crest

Bony part that your hands rest on when you put your hands on your hips. Its borders are the

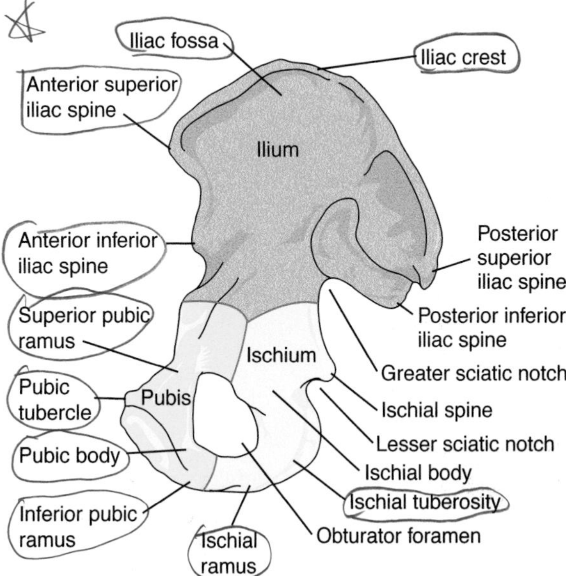

Figure 18-6. Right innominate bone (medial view) consists of the ilium, ischium, and pubis. The greater sciatic notch, acetabulum, and obturator foramen are formed by different combinations of these bones.

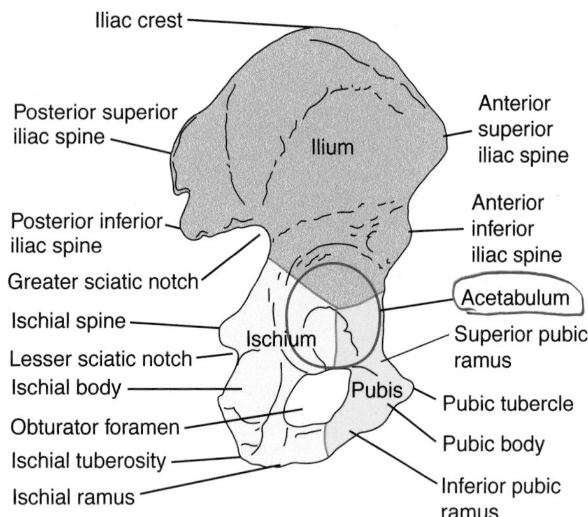

Figure 18-7. Right innominate bone (lateral view).

anterior superior iliac spine and the posterior superior iliac spine.

Anterior Superior Iliac Spine (ASIS)
The projection on the anterior end of the iliac crest. The tensor fascia lata and sartorius muscles and the inguinal ligament attach here.

Anterior Inferior Iliac Spine (AIIS)
The projection to which the rectus femoris attaches is on the AIIS.

Posterior Superior Iliac Spine (PSIS)
It is the posterior projection on the iliac crest.

Posterior Inferior Iliac Spine (PIIS)
Located just below the PSIS.

The **ischium** is the posterior inferior portion of the innominate bone. Its significant landmarks are listed below (see Figs. 18-6 and 18-7).

Important Bony Landmarks of the Ischium

Ischial Body
Makes up about two-fifths of the acetabulum

Ischial Ramus
Extends medially from the body to connect with the inferior ramus of the pubis. The adductor magnus, obturator externus, and obturator internus muscles attach here.

Ischial Tuberosity
Rough, blunt projection of the inferior part of the body, which is weight-bearing when you are sitting. It provides attachment for the hamstring and adductor magnus muscles.

Ischial Spine
Located on the posterior portion of the body between the greater and lesser sciatic notches. It provides attachment for the sacrospinous ligament.

The **pubis** forms the anterior inferior portion of the innominate bone. It can be divided into three parts—the body and its two rami (see Figs. 18-6 and 18-7).

Important Bony Landmarks of the Pubis

Pubic Body
Externally forms about one-fifth of the acetabulum and internally provides attachment for the obturator internus muscle

Superior Ramus
Lies superiorly between the acetabulum and the body and provides attachment for the pectineus muscle

Inferior Ramus
Lies posterior, inferior, and lateral to the body. Provides attachment for the adductor magnus and brevis and gracilis muscles.

Symphysis Pubis
A cartilaginous joint connecting the bodies of the two pubic bones at the anterior midline

Pubic Tubercle
Projects anteriorly on the superior ramus near the symphysis pubis and provides attachment for the inguinal ligament

The following are made up of combinations of the innominate bones (see Fig. 18-7):

Acetabulum
A deep, cup-shaped cavity that articulates with the femur. It is made up of nearly equal portions of the ilium, ischium, and pubis.

Obturator Foramen
A large opening surrounded by the bodies and rami of the ischium and pubis and through which pass blood vessels and nerves

Greater Sciatic Notch
Large notch just below the PIIS that is actually made into a foramen by the sacrospinous and sacrotuberous ligaments (see Fig. 17-8). The sciatic nerve, piriformis muscle, and other structures pass through this opening.

The **femur** is the longest, strongest, and heaviest bone in the body. A person's height can roughly be estimated to be four times the length of the femur (Moore, 1985). It articulates with the innominate bone to form the hip joint and has significant landmarks (Fig. 18-8).

Important Bony Landmarks of the Femur

Head
The rounded portion covered with articular cartilage articulating with the acetabulum

Neck
The narrower portion located between the head and the trochanters

Greater Trochanter
Large projection located laterally between the neck and the body of the femur, providing attachment for the gluteus medius and minimus and for most deep rotator muscles

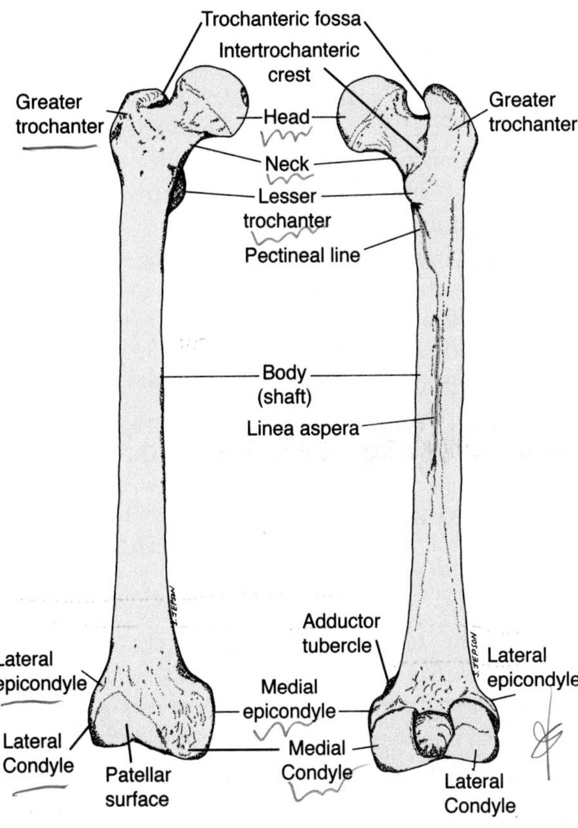

Figure 18-8. Right femur.

Lesser Trochanter
A smaller projection located medially and posteriorly just distal to the greater trochanter, providing attachment for the iliopsoas muscle

Trochanteric Fossa
Medial surface of the greater trochanter

Intertrochanteric Crest
The smooth ridge between greater and lesser trochanters. Serves as attachment for quadratus femoris.

Body
The long, cylindrical portion between the bone ends; also called the *shaft.* It is bowed slightly anteriorly.

Medial Condyle
Distal medial end

Lateral Condyle
Distal lateral end

Lateral Epicondyle
Projection proximal to the lateral condyle

Medial Epicondyle
Projection proximal to the medial condyle

Adductor Tubercle
Small projection proximal to the medial epicondyle to which a portion of the adductor magnus muscle attaches

Linea Aspera
Prominent longitudinal ridge or crest running down the middle third of the posterior shaft of the femur to which many muscles attach

Pectineal Line
Runs from below the lesser trochanter diagonally toward the linea aspera. It provides attachment for the adductor brevis.

Patellar Surface
Located between the medial and lateral condyle anteriorly. It articulates with the posterior surface of the patella.

The **tibia** will be discussed in more detail in Chapter 19, but it is important to identify one landmark now (Fig. 18-9).

Important Bony Landmark of the Tibia

Tibial Tuberosity
Large projection at the proximal end, in the midline. It provides attachment for the patellar tendon.

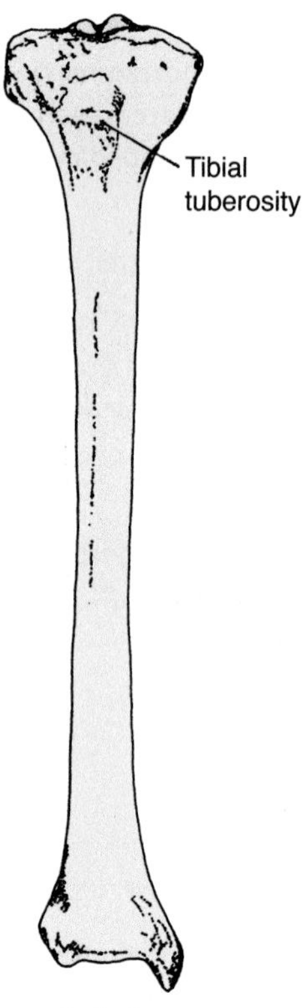

Figure 18-9. Right tibia (anterior view).

Ligaments and Other Structures

Like all synovial joints, the hip has a fibrous **joint capsule.** It is strong and thick, and it covers the hip joint in a cylindrical fashion. It attaches proximally around the lip of the acetabulum and distally to the neck of the femur (Fig. 18-10). It forms a cylindrical sleeve that encloses the joint and most of the femoral neck.

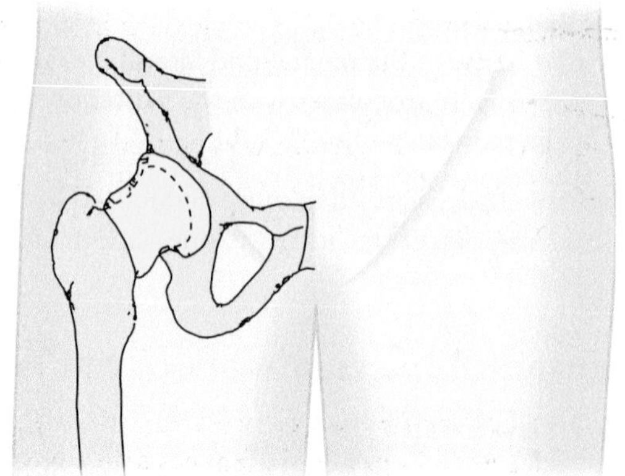
Figure 18-10. Hip joint capsule (anterior view).

Three ligaments reinforce the capsule: the iliofemoral, the pubofemoral, and the ischiofemoral ligaments (Fig. 18-11). The most important of these ligaments is the **iliofemoral ligament.** It reinforces the capsule anteriorly by attaching proximally to the AIIS and crossing the joint anteriorly. It splits into two parts distally to attach to the intertrochanteric line of the femur. Because it resembles an inverted *Y,* it is often referred to as the *Y ligament.* It is also known as the *ligament of Bigelow.* Its main function is to limit hyperextension.

The **pubofemoral ligament** spans the hip joint medially and inferiorly. It attaches from the medial part of the acetabular rim and superior ramus of the pubis and runs down and back to attach on the neck of the femur. Like the iliofemoral ligament, it limits hyperextension. In addition, it limits abduction.

The **ischiofemoral ligament** covers the capsule posteriorly. It attaches on the ischial portion of the acetabulum, crosses the joint in a lateral and superior direction, and attaches on the femoral neck. Its fibers limit hyperextension and medial rotation.

All three of these ligaments attach along the rim of the acetabulum and cross the hip joint in a spiral fashion to attach on the femoral neck. The combined effect of this spiral attachment is to limit motion in one direction (hyperextension) while allowing full motion (flexion) in the other direction. Therefore, these ligaments are slack in flexion and become taut as the hip joint moves into hyperextension. If you thrust your hips forward so that they are in front of the shoulders and knees, you cause the line of gravity (LOG) to pass posterior to the axis of rotation for the hip joint. This allows you to stand in the upright position without using any muscles by essentially resting or hanging on the iliofemoral ligament. This is the basis for the standing posture of an individual with paralysis following spinal cord injury (Fig. 18-12).

The depth of the acetabulum is increased by the fibrocartilaginous **acetabular labrum,** which is located around the rim. The free end of the labrum surrounds the femoral head and helps to hold the head in the acetabulum.

Although the **inguinal ligament** has no function at the hip joint, it should be identified because of its presence. It runs from the ASIS to the pubic tubercle and is the landmark that separates the anterior abdominal wall from the thigh (Fig. 18-13). When the external iliac artery and vein pass under the inguinal ligament, their names change to the *femoral artery* and *vein.*

The **iliotibial band** or **tract** is the very long, tendinous portion of the tensor fascia lata muscle (see Fig. 18-26). It attaches to the anterior portion of the iliac crest and runs superficially down the lateral side of the thigh to attach to the tibia. Both the gluteus maximus and

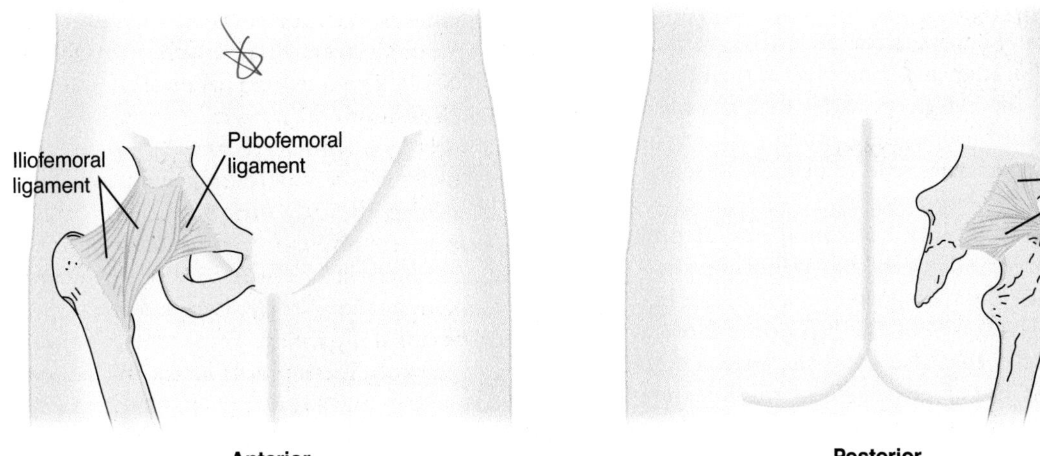

Figure 18-11. Hip joint capsule is reinforced by three ligaments: the iliofemoral, the pubofemoral, and the ischiofemoral ligaments.

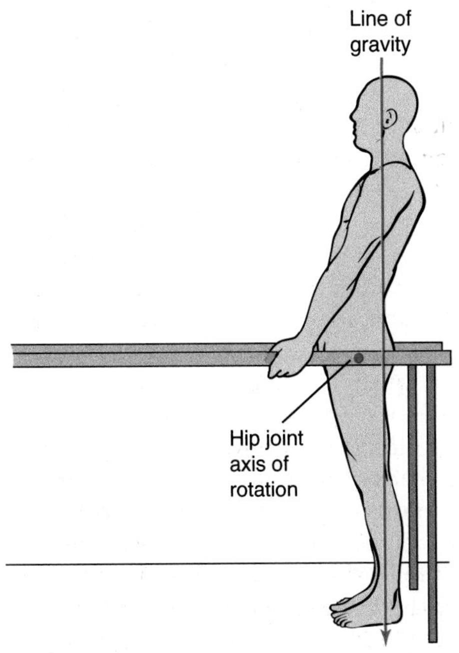

Figure 18-12. The spiral attachment of the hip ligaments tends to limit hyperextension. Positioning the hips forward of the shoulders and knees causes the line of gravity to run posterior to the axis of rotation for the hip joint, creating a natural extension force at the hip. This is referred to as "hanging on the Y ligament."

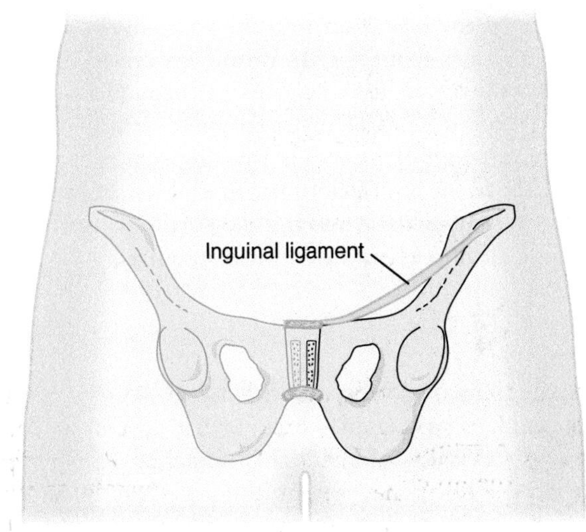

Figure 18-13. Inguinal ligament (anterior view).

tensor fascia lata muscles have fibers attaching to the iliotibial band.

The end feel of all hip joint motions, except flexion, is **firm** because of tension in the capsule, ligaments, and muscles. For hip flexion, the end feel is **soft** because of contact between the anterior thigh and the abdomen.

Adductor Hiatus

The adductor hiatus is the gap or opening in the distal attachment of the adductor magnus between the linea aspera and the adductor tubercle. It is significant because the femoral artery and vein pass through this opening to reach the posterior surface of the knee, where their name changes to *popliteal artery* and *vein* (see Fig. 18-18C).

Muscles of the Hip

There are many similarities between the shoulder and hip joints. Like the shoulder, the hip has a group of one-joint muscles that provide most of the control, and it has a group of longer, two-joint muscles that provide the range of motion. These muscles can also be grouped according to their location and somewhat by their function. For example, the anterior muscles with a vertical line of pull tend to be flexors, lateral muscles tend to be abductors, posterior muscles tend to be extensors, and medial muscles tend to be adductors.

Muscles that have a more horizontal line of pull and cross the anterior side of the hip are medial rotators, and those that cross the posterior side of the hip are lateral rotators. Several of the hip prime movers are two-joint muscles that also cross the knee. Those muscles that cross the anterior side of the knee are knee extensors, whereas the posterior muscles are knee flexors. Table 18-2 classifies the hip muscles by location and function.

The **iliopsoas muscle** is actually two muscles with separate proximal attachments and a common distal attachment (Fig. 18-14). The iliacus muscle portion arises from the iliac fossa, and the psoas major muscle portion comes from the transverse processes, bodies, and intervertebral disks of the T12 through L5 vertebrae. These muscles blend together to attach on the lesser trochanter of the femur. The iliopsoas muscle is a prime mover in hip flexion. Because of its attachment on the vertebrae, the psoas muscle portion contributes to trunk flexion when the femur is stabilized.

Table 18-2 Muscles of the Hip

Muscle Group	One-Joint Muscles	Two-Joint Muscles
Anterior	Iliopsoas	Rectus femoris Sartorius
Medial	Pectineus Adductor magnus Adductor longus Adductor brevis	Gracilis
Posterior	Gluteus maximus	Semimembranosus
	Deep rotators (6)	Semitendinosus
		Biceps femoris (long head)
Lateral	Gluteus medius, gluteus minimus	Tensor fascia lata

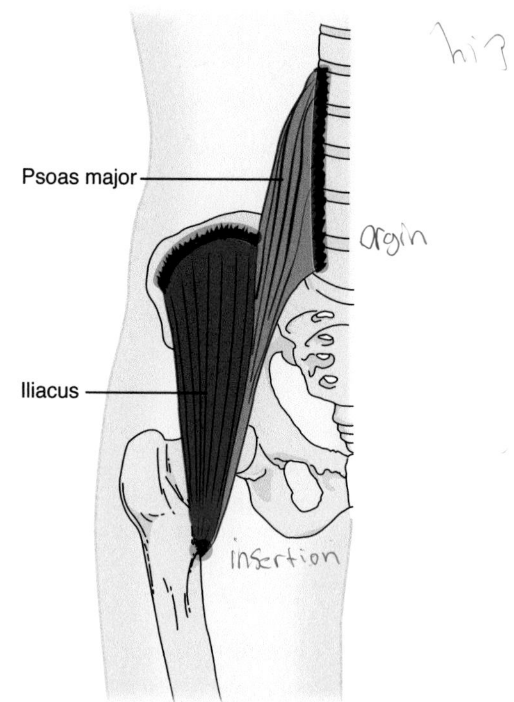

Figure 18-14. The iliopsoas muscle is made up of the psoas major and the iliacus (anterior view).

Iliopsoas Muscle

O	Iliac fossa, anterior and lateral surfaces of T12 through L5
I	Lesser trochanter
A	Hip flexion
N	Iliacus portion: femoral nerve (L2, L3) Psoas major portion: L2 and L3

The **rectus femoris muscle** is part of the quadriceps muscle group and is the only one of that group to cross the hip joint (Fig. 18-15). Its proximal attachment is on the AIIS. It runs almost straight down the thigh, where it is joined by the three vasti muscles to blend into the quadriceps tendon (also called the *patellar tendon*). This tendon encases the patella, crosses the knee joint, and attaches to the tibial tuberosity. The rectus femoris muscle is a prime mover in hip flexion and knee extension.

Rectus Femoris Muscle

O	AIIS
I	Tibial tuberosity
A	Hip flexion, knee extension
N	Femoral nerve (L2, L3, L4)

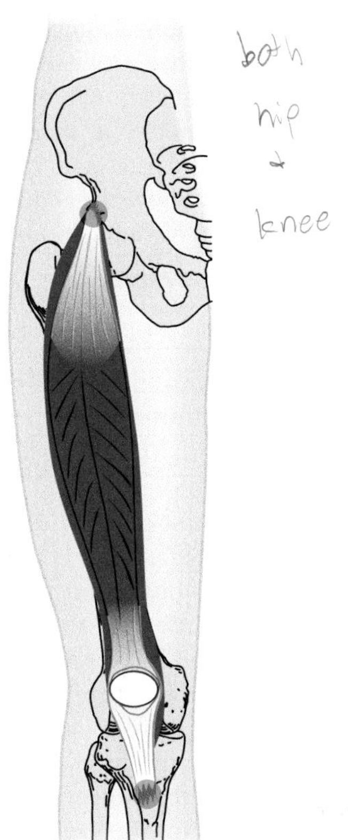

Figure 18-15. Rectus femoris muscle (anterior view).

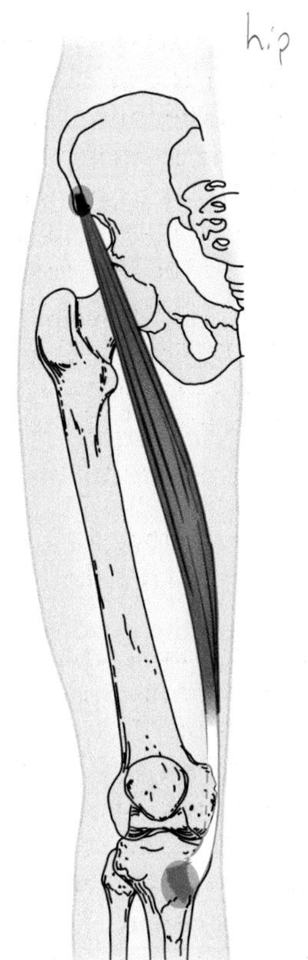

Figure 18-16. Sartorius muscle (anterior view).

The **sartorius muscle** is the longest muscle in the body (Fig. 18-16). This straplike muscle arises from the ASIS. It runs diagonally across the thigh from lateral to medial and proximal to distal to cross the medial knee joint posteriorly. Because of its line of pull, it is capable of flexing, abducting, and laterally rotating the hip and flexing the knee. However, it is not considered a prime mover in any one of these motions. It is most efficient when doing all four motions at the same time. An example of this motion is when you cross your legs by putting one foot on the opposite knee.

Sartorius Muscle

O	ASIS
I	Proximal medial aspect of tibia
A	Combination of hip flexion, abduction, lateral rotation, and knee flexion
N	Femoral nerve (L2, L3)

Located medial to the iliopsoas muscle and lateral to the adductor longus muscle is the **pectineus muscle.** Its origin is on the superior ramus of the pubis, and its insertion is on the pectineal line of the femur (Fig. 18-17). Because it spans the hip joint anteriorly and medially, it provides hip flexion and adduction.

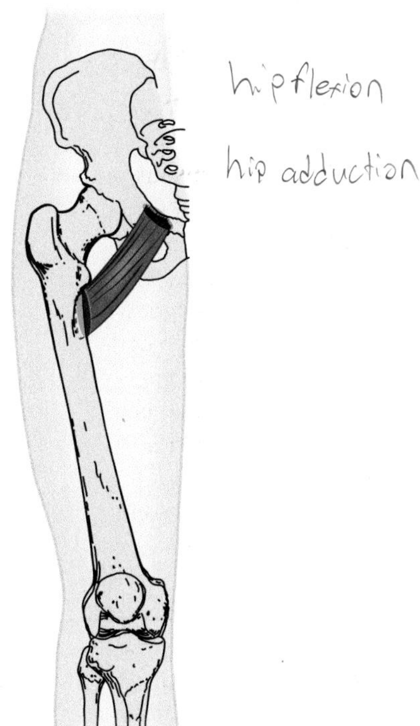

Figure 18-17. Pectineus muscle (anterior view). Note that the distal attachment is on the posterior femur.

Pectineus Muscle

O	Superior ramus of pubis
I	Pectineal line of femur
A	Hip flexion and adduction
N	Femoral nerve (L2, L3)

There are three other one-joint hip adductors, all with the same first name (Fig. 18-18). The **adductor longus muscle,** the most superficial of the three, originates from the anterior surface of the pubis near the tubercle and inserts on the middle third of the linea aspera of the femur. Because it is superficial, its tendon can easily be felt in the anteromedial groin. Being able to palpate this tendon is important when checking for correct fit of the quadrilateral socket of an above-knee prosthesis. It is a prime mover in hip adduction.

Adductor Longus Muscle

O	Pubis
I	Middle third of the linea aspera
A	Hip adduction
N	Obturator nerve (L2, L3, L4)

The **adductor brevis muscle** implies by its name that it is shorter than the other adductor muscles. It lies deep to the adductor longus muscle but superficial to the adductor magnus muscle. It arises from the inferior ramus of the pubis and inserts on the pectineal line and proximal linea aspera above the adductor longus muscle. It is a prime mover in hip adduction.

Adductor Brevis Muscle

O	Pubis
I	Pectineal line and proximal linea aspera
A	Hip adduction
N	Obturator nerve (L2, L3)

The largest and deepest of the adductors is the **adductor magnus muscle.** It arises from the ischial tuberosity and ramus of the ischium and inferior ramus of the pubis. It makes up most of the bulk on the medial thigh. Its fibers fan out in a downward and lateral direction to insert along the entire linea aspera and on the adductor tubercle. There is an interruption called the adductor hiatus, in the distal attachment between the linea aspera and adductor tubercle. The femoral artery and vein pass through this opening. After these structures have passed through to the posterior surface, their

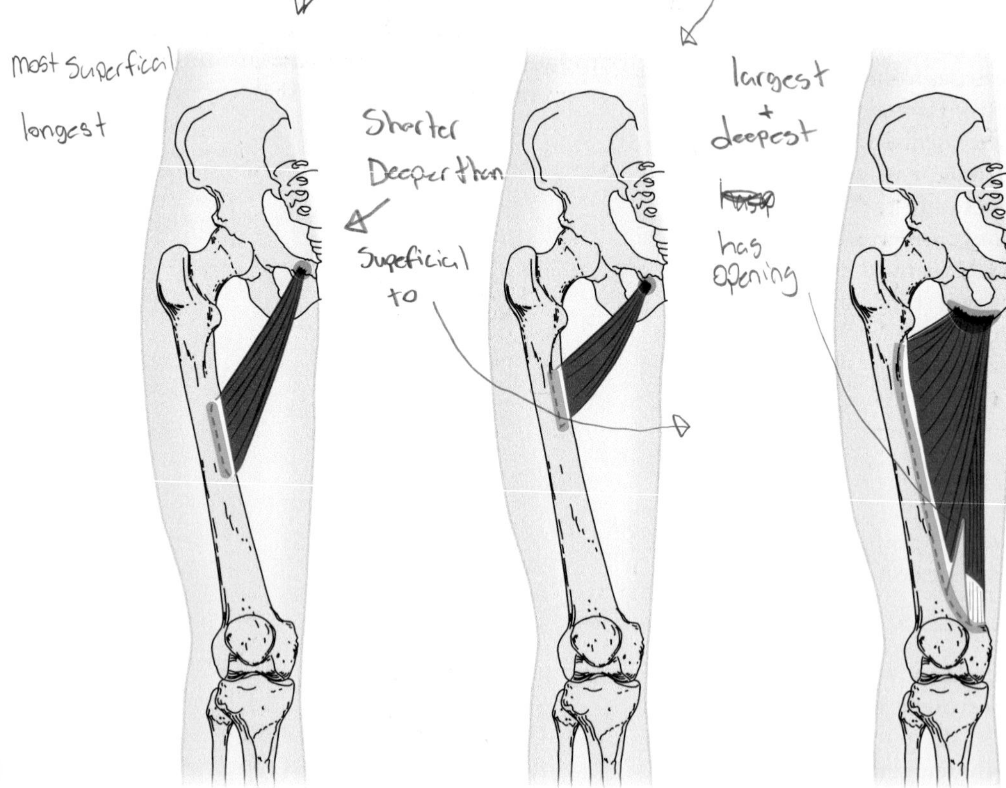

Figure 18-18. Three adductor muscles (anterior view). Note that the distal attachments are on the posterior femur.

names become the *popliteal artery* and *vein,* respectively. Because of its size, the adductor magnus muscle is a very strong hip adductor. Because the lower fibers have a near vertical line of pull, it can assist in hip extension.

Adductor Magnus Muscle

O	Ischium and pubis
I	Entire linea aspera and adductor tubercle
A	Hip adduction
N	Obturator and sciatic nerve (L2, L3, L4)

The only hip adductor that is a two-joint muscle is the **gracilis muscle** (Fig. 18-19). It arises from the symphysis and inferior ramus of the pubis and descends the thigh medially and superficially. It crosses the knee joint posteriorly and curves around the medial condyle to attach distally on the anteromedial surface of the proximal tibia. It assists with knee flexion.

Gracilis Muscle

O	Pubis
I	Anteromedial surface of proximal end of tibia
A	Hip adduction
N	Obturator nerve (L2, L3)

The **gluteus maximus muscle** can be described as a large, thick, one-joint, quadrilateral muscle located superficially on the posterior buttock (Fig. 18-20). It arises from the general area of the posterior sacrum, coccyx, and ilium, and it runs in a diagonal direction distally and laterally to the posterior femur, inferior to the greater trochanter. Some fibers also attach to the iliotibial band. Because it spans the hip joint posteriorly in this diagonal direction, it is very strong in hip extension, hyperextension, and lateral rotation.

Gluteus Maximus Muscle

O	Posterior sacrum and ilium
I	Posterior femur distal to greater trochanter and to iliotibial band
A	Hip extension, hyperextension, lateral rotation
N	Inferior gluteal nerve (L5, S1, S2)

There are six small, deep, mostly posterior muscles that span the hip joint in a horizontal direction, and they all laterally rotate the hip. Because they all work together to produce the same motion, their individual attachments are not functionally important; therefore, they can be grouped together as the **deep rotator muscles** (Fig. 18-21). However, the piriformis is the best known of

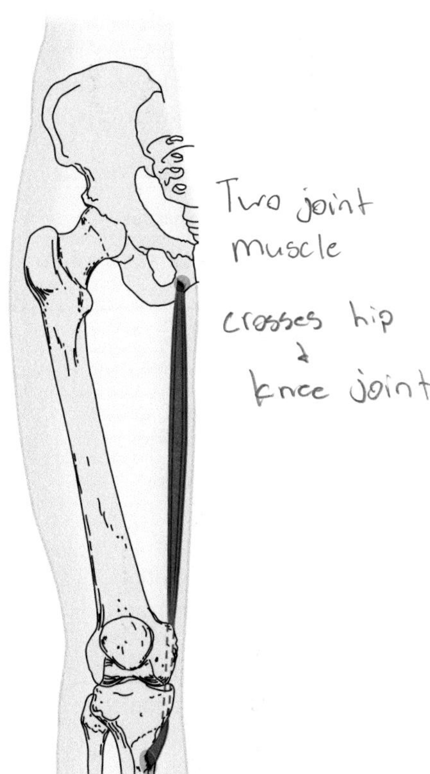

Figure 18-19. Gracilis muscle (anterior view). Note that it passes behind the knee but attaches anteriorly.

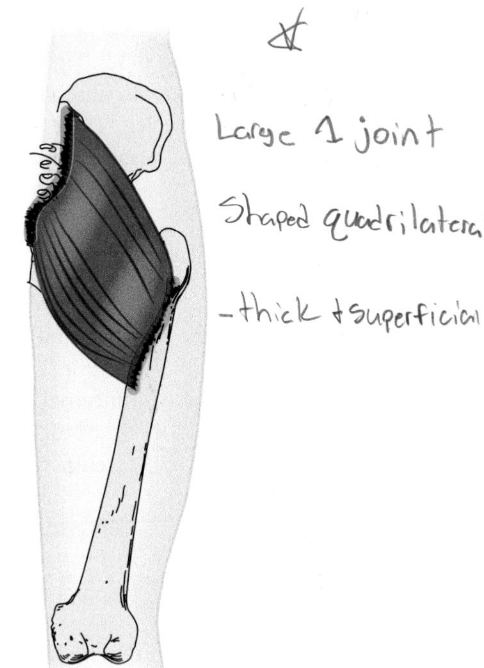

Figure 18-20. Gluteus maximus muscle (posterior view).

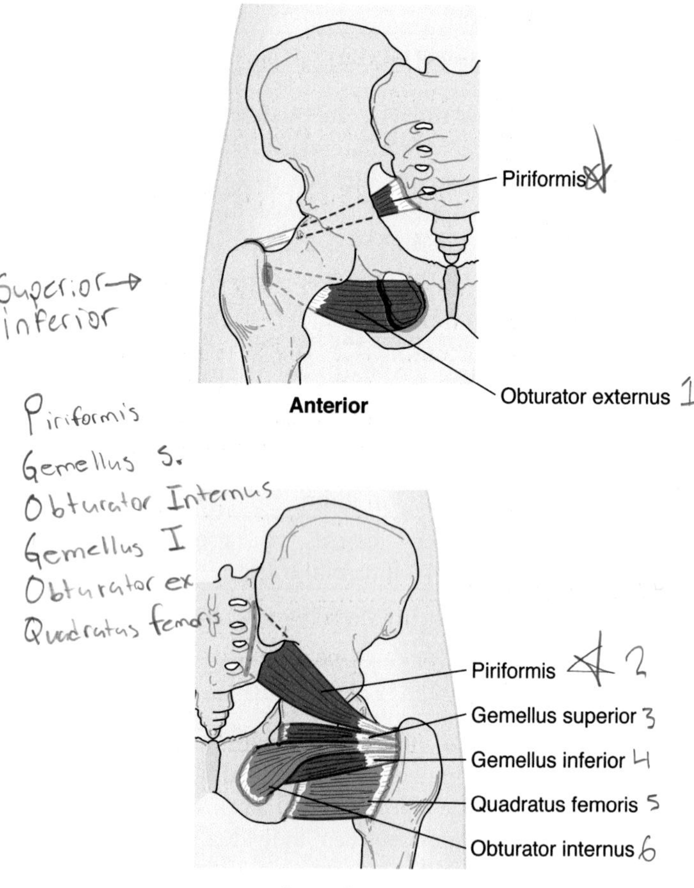

Figure 18-21. Deep rotator muscles.

this group, perhaps because of its close relationship to the sciatic nerve (see Fig. 6-32). Tightness of the piriformis can compress the sciatic nerve resulting in radiating pain down the back of the leg. Table 18-3 summarizes the attachments and innervation of the deep rotator muscles.

Deep Rotator Muscles

O	Anterior sacrum, ischium, pubis
I	Greater trochanter area
A	Hip lateral rotation
N	Numerous (see Table 18-3)

Three muscles that are known collectively as the **hamstring muscles** cover the posterior thigh. They consist of the semimembranosus, the semitendinosus, and the biceps femoris muscles (Fig. 18-22). They have a common site of origin on the ischial tuberosity.

The **semimembranosus muscle** runs down the medial side of the thigh, deep to the semitendinosus muscle, and inserts on the posterior surface of the medial condyle of the tibia. The **semitendinosus muscle** has a much longer and narrower distal tendon that spans the knee joint posteriorly and then moves anteriorly to attach to the anteromedial surface of the tibia with the gracilis and sartorius muscles. The **biceps femoris muscle** has two heads and runs down the thigh laterally on the posterior side. The long head arises with the other two hamstring muscles on the ischial tuberosity, but the short head arises from the lateral lip of the linea aspera of the femur. Both heads join together, spanning the knee posteriorly to attach laterally on the head of the fibula and, by a small slip, to the lateral condyle of the tibia. Because they span the knee posteriorly, they flex the knee. The long head, because it spans the hip joint posteriorly, extends the hip.

Semimembranosus Muscle

O	Ischial tuberosity
I	Posterior surface of medial condyle of tibia

Table 18-3 Deep Rotator Muscles

Muscle	Proximal Attachment	Distal Attachment	Innervation
Obturator externus	External surface of inferior two-thirds of obturator foramen	Trochanteric fossa	Obturator nerve
Obturator internus	Internal surface of most of obturator foramen	Medial surface of greater trochanter	Nerve to obturator internus
Quadratus femoris	Ischial tuberosity	Intertrochanteric crest	Nerve to quadratus femoris
Piriformis	Anterior sacrum	Medial surface of greater trochanter	L5, S1, S2
Gemellus superior	Ischial spine	Medial surface of greater trochanter	Nerve to obturator internus
Gemellus inferior	Ischial tuberosity	Medial surface of greater trochanter	Nerve to quadratus femoris

Clinical Application 18-1

Piriformis Stretch Position

The piriformis is a prime mover in hip lateral rotation. However, when the hip is flexed to 90 degrees or more, its line of pull shifts anterior of the hip axis for rotation, causing it to contribute toward medial rotation instead. It is for this reason that the piriformis can be stretched by placing the hip in *lateral rotation* (while also flexed). The piriformis is the only deep lateral rotator that functions this way.

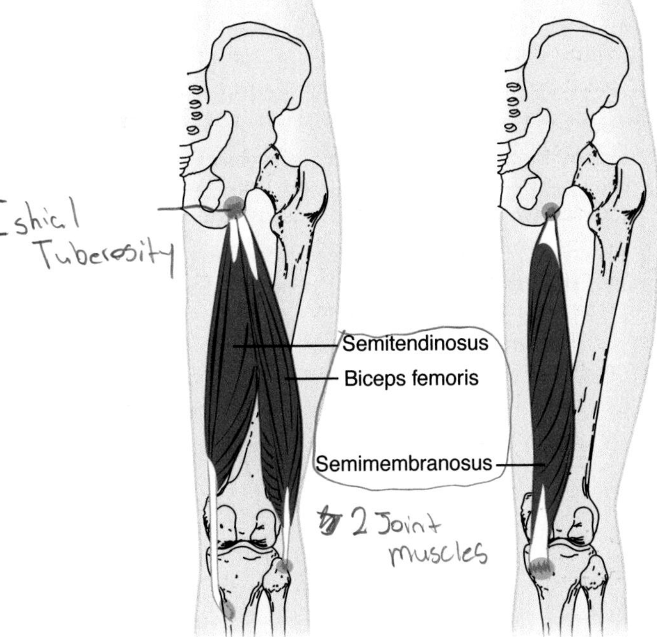

Figure 18-22. Hamstring muscles (posterior view).

A	Hip extension and knee flexion
N	Sciatic nerve – tibial division (L5, S1, S2)

Semitendinosus Muscle

O	Ischial tuberosity
I	Anteromedial surface of proximal tibia
A	Hip extension and knee flexion
N	Sciatic nerve – tibial division (L5, S1, S2)

Biceps Femoris Muscle

O	Long head: ischial tuberosity Short head: lateral lip of linea aspera
I	Fibular head
A	Long head: hip extension and knee flexion Short head: knee flexion
N	Long head: sciatic nerve – tibial division (L5, S1, S2) Short head: common fibular (peroneal) nerve (L5, S1, S2)

The other two gluteal muscles are more laterally located. The **gluteus medius muscle** is triangular, much like the deltoid muscle of the shoulder (Fig. 18-23). It attaches proximally to the outer surface of the ilium and distally to the lateral surface of the greater trochanter. Because it spans the hip joint laterally, the gluteus medius muscle can abduct the hip. Its anterior fibers are able to assist the gluteus minimus muscle in medially rotating the hip.

Gluteus Medius Muscle

O	Outer surface of the ilium
I	Lateral surface of the greater trochanter
A	Hip abduction
N	Superior gluteal nerve (L4, L5, S1)

Clinical Application 18-2

Positioning for a Straight Leg Raise

During a straight leg raise in the supine position, the hip flexors move the leg against gravity. For this to occur, the hip flexor origin (pelvis) must be stabilized to prevent a reverse muscle action that would create an anterior pelvic tilt (see Figure 1). This stabilization is achieved primarily by: (1) abdominal muscle contraction and (2) bending the opposite hip and knee. Both of these actions help lock the pelvis in a posterior direction, which helps resist the anterior tilting force exerted by the hip flexor muscles.

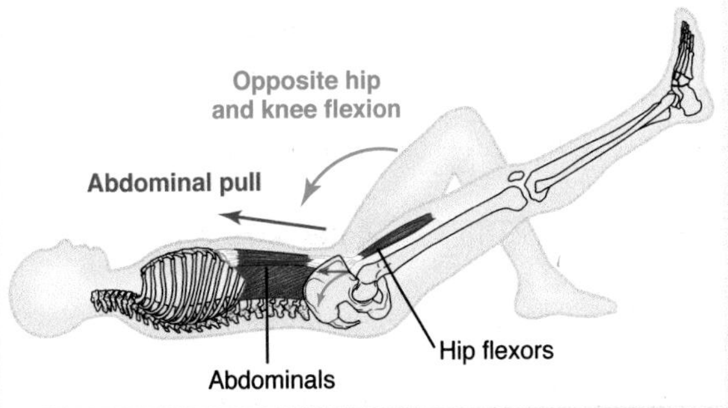

Figure 1 Straight leg raise (SLR).

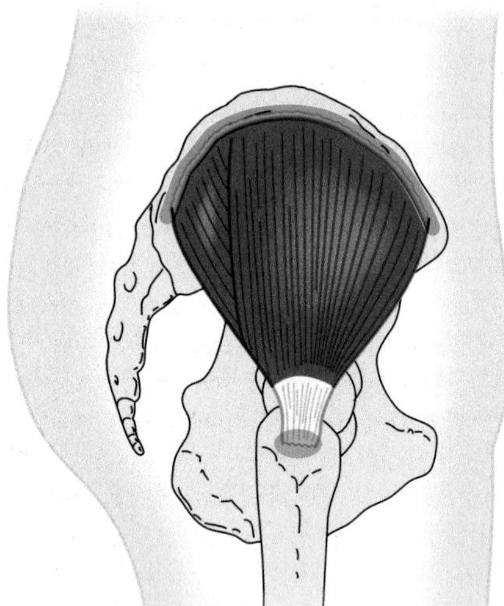

Figure 18-23. Gluteus medius muscle (lateral view).

The smallest and deepest of the three gluteal muscles, the **gluteus minimus muscle** lies deep and inferior to the gluteus medius muscle on the lateral ilium (Fig. 18-24). Its broad proximal attachment extends from near the greater sciatic notch to almost as far forward as the anterior border, near the ASIS. The distal attachment is on the anterior aspect of the greater trochanter. This gives the gluteus minimus muscle a somewhat diagonal line of pull, making it able to medially rotate the hip. Because it spans the hip joint laterally, it also abducts the hip.

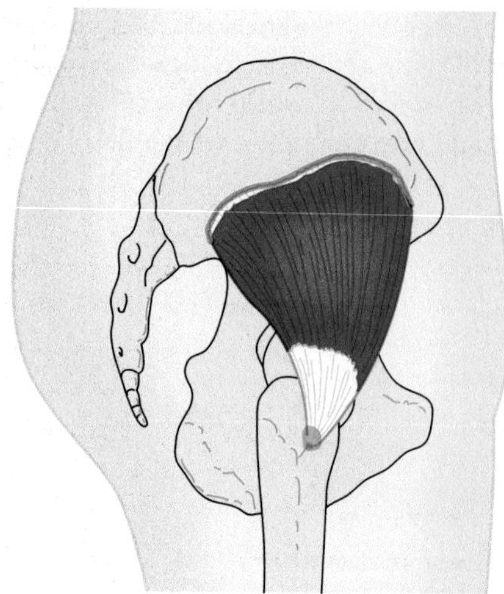

Figure 18-24. Gluteus minimus muscle (lateral view).

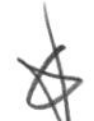

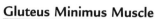

Gluteus Minimus Muscle

O	Lateral surface of the ilium
I	Anterior surface of the greater trochanter
A	Hip abduction, medial rotation
N	Superior gluteal nerve (L4, L5, S1)

Attaching to the ilium and the femur and spanning the hip joint laterally, these two gluteal muscles have another very important function. When you stand on one leg, the gluteus medius and minimus muscles contract to keep the pelvis fairly level and to prevent the opposite side of the pelvis from dropping too much (lateral tilt) when you stand on one leg (Fig. 18-25). This occurs every time you pick up one leg, as when walking. Weakness or loss of these muscles results in a "Trendelenburg gait." For example, because the pelvis moves as a whole, if your right hip abductors are weak, the left side of your pelvis will drop significantly when you stand on your right leg and lift your left leg off the ground.

The **tensor fascia lata muscle** is a very short muscle with a very long tendinous attachment (Fig. 18-26). It arises from the ASIS, crosses the hip joint laterally and slightly anteriorly, and then attaches to the long fascial band called the *iliotibial band,* which proceeds down the

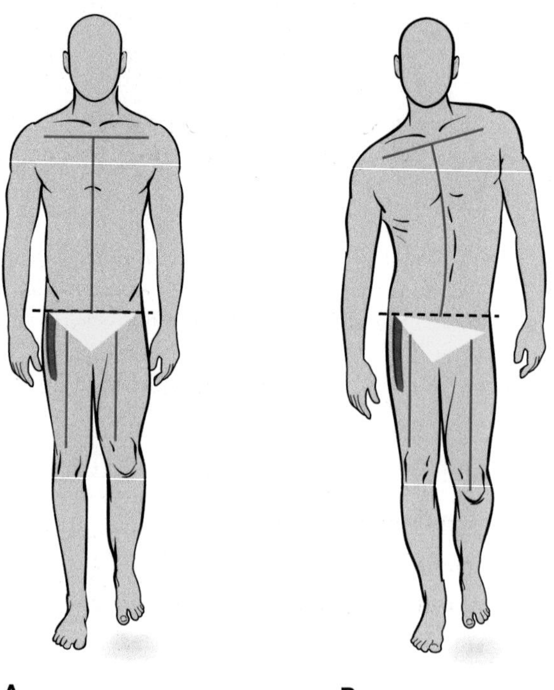

Figure 18-25. Anterior view. **(A)** In reverse muscle action, the right hip abductors contract to keep the pelvis steady when the left leg is lifted. **(B)** When right hip abductors are weak, the left side of the pelvis drops.

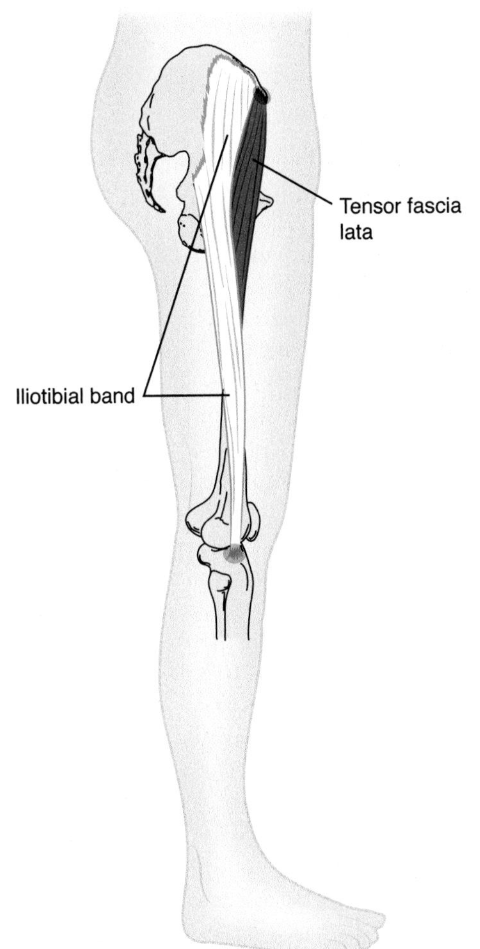

Figure 18-26. Tensor fascia lata muscle (lateral view). The very long, tendinous portion of this muscle is known as the *iliotibial band.*

lateral thigh and attaches to the lateral condyle of the tibia. It is a hip abductor, but due to its slight anterior position, it is perhaps strongest when performing a combination of flexion and abduction. Stated another way, it is most efficient when abducting in a slightly anterior direction.

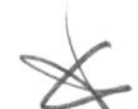

Tensor Fascia Lata Muscle

O	ASIS
I	Lateral condyle of tibia
A	Combined hip flexion and abduction
N	Superior gluteal nerve (L4, L5, S1)

Anatomical Relationships

Table 18-2 organizes the hip muscles into four groups based on location. Using this grouping, the anatomical relationships of the hip muscles can be easily discussed by adding one other factor: superficial muscles versus deep muscles.

Starting anteriorly, there are two superficial muscles: the tensor fascia lata and the sartorius, which have their origins on the ASIS (Fig. 18-27). They make an inverted *V* from their common attachment. The tensor fascia lata runs down toward the knee and slightly laterally, whereas the sartorius runs down in a medial direction. Between these two muscles lies the rectus femoris, which runs straight down toward the knee. Moving medially from the sartorius are the iliopsoas, pectineus, adductor longus, and gracilis muscles. Deep to the adductor longus, near the hip joint, is the adductor brevis. Because the adductor magnus fans out along the entire linea aspera, it is deep to both the adductor longus and brevis and gracilis (Fig. 18-28).

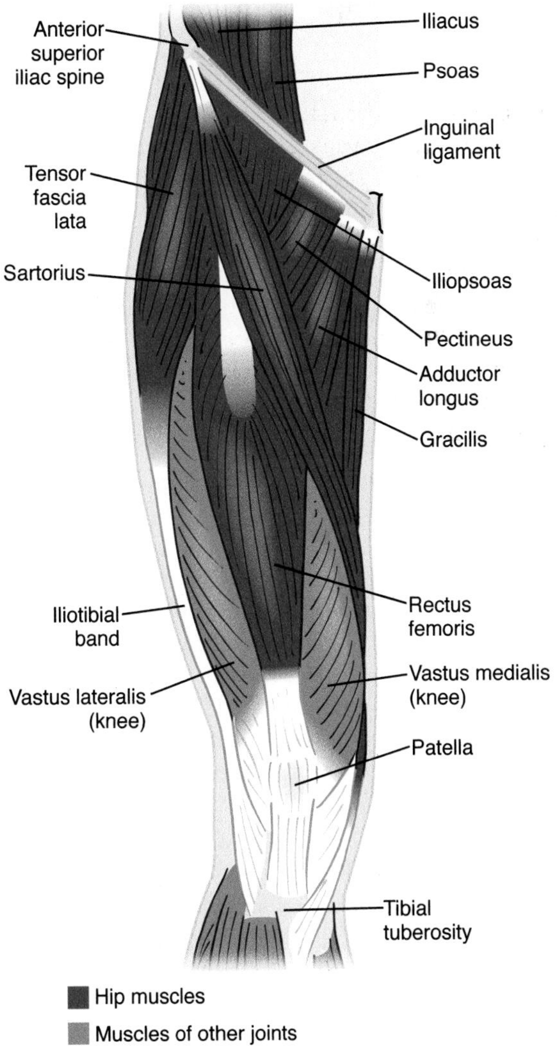

Figure 18-27. Anterior superficial muscles (right leg).

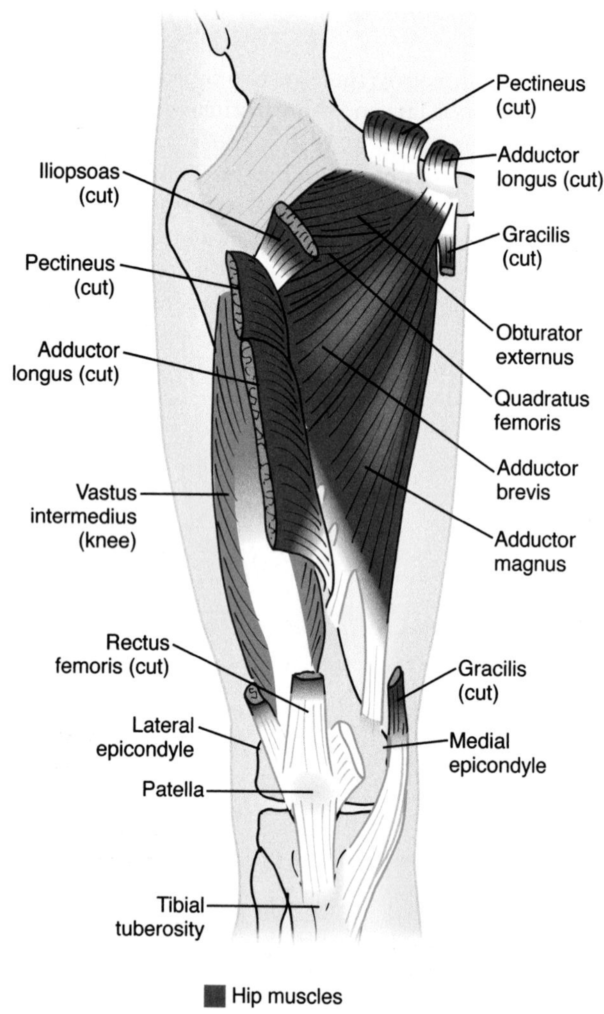

Figure 18-28. Anterior deep muscles (right leg).

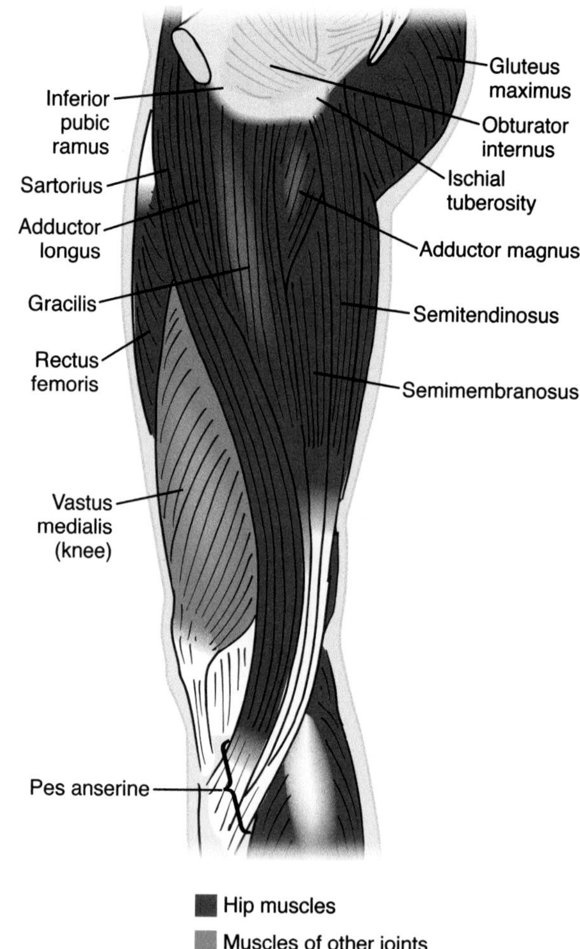

Figure 18-29. Medial muscles (right leg).

Viewing the hip joint region from the medial side superficially, the sartorius, the upper portion of the adductor longus, the gracilis, and the upper half of the adductor magnus can be seen from front to back, followed by the medial hamstrings (Fig. 18-29). From this medial view, you can see that most of the adductor longus and much of the adductor brevis and adductor magnus lie deep.

On the posterior side, the gluteus maximus covers the proximal posterior hip region (Fig. 18-30). Distal to the gluteus maximus, and taking up most of the posterior thigh, are the hamstring muscles. Deep to the gluteus maximus and slightly more lateral is the gluteus medius, and deeper still is the gluteus minimus (Fig. 18-31). The deep rotators are the deepest muscles; you can see five of the six deep rotators in the figure. The hamstring muscles are deep to the gluteus maximus at their proximal attachment on the ischial tuberosity.

Viewing the proximal hip from the lateral side in Figure 18-32, you can see the gluteus maximus posteriorly, the iliotibial band laterally, and the tensor fascia lata anteriorly. The gluteus medius lies deep to these structures, and the gluteus minimus lies deep to the gluteus medius.

Common Hip Pathologies

The hip joint is the site of many orthopedic conditions that occur throughout life and can affect lower extremity alignment. **Congenital hip dislocation,** or **dysplasia,** occurs when an unusually shallow acetabulum causes the femoral head to slide upward. The joint capsule remains intact, though stretched. **Legg-Calvé-Perthes disease,** or **coxa plana,** is a condition in which the femoral head undergoes necrosis. It is usually seen in children between the ages of 5 and 10 years.

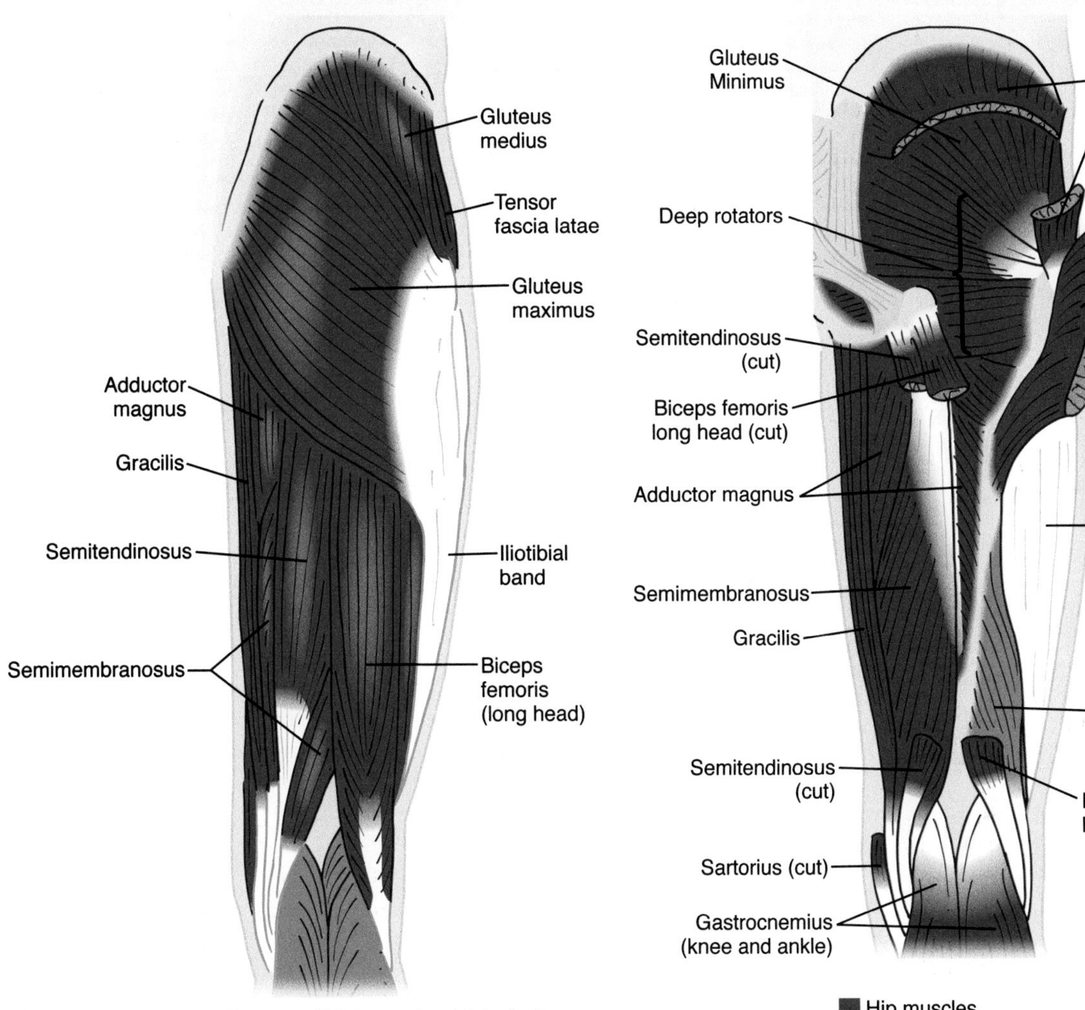

Figure 18-30. Posterior superficial muscles (right leg).

Figure 18-31. Posterior deep muscles (right leg).

During the course of the disease, it may take about 2 to 4 years for the head to die, revascularize, and then remodel. **Slipped capital femoral epiphysis** is seen in children during the growth-spurt years. The proximal epiphysis slips from its normal position on the femoral head.

The angle between the shaft and the neck of the femur in the *frontal plane* is referred to as the **angle of inclination,** which normally is 125 degrees. This angle varies from birth to adulthood. At birth, the angle may be as great as 170 degrees, but by adulthood the angle decreases significantly. However, factors such as congenital deformity, trauma, or disease may affect the angle. **Coxa valga** is characterized by a neck-shaft angle greater than 125 degrees (Fig. 18-33). Because this angle is "straighter," it tends to make the limb longer, thus placing the hip in an adducted position during weight-bearing. **Coxa vara** is a deformity in which the neck-shaft angle is less than the normal 125 degrees. Because it is "more bent," it tends to make the involved limb shorter, dropping the pelvis on that side during weight-bearing.

The angle between the shaft and the neck of the femur in the *transverse plane* is called the **angle of torsion,** which normally has the head and neck rotated outward from the shaft approximately 15 to 25 degrees. Looking down on the femur (Fig. 18-34A), you can see the femoral head and neck superimposed on the shaft. The shaft is best shown here by a line through the femoral condyles, which attach to the shaft distally. As the shaft rotates, so do the condyles. An increase in this angle is called **anteversion,** which forces the hip joint into a more medially rotated position (Fig. 18-34B). This causes a person to walk more "toed in."

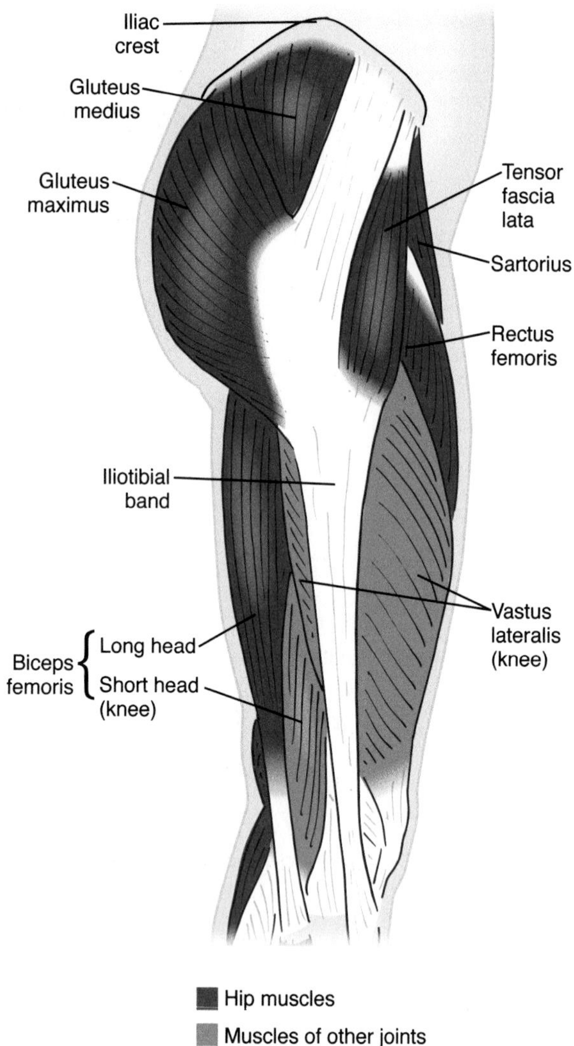

Figure 18-32. Lateral muscles (right leg).

A decrease in the angle of torsion is called **retroversion.** This forces the hip joint into a more laterally rotated position, causing the person to walk more "toed out" (Fig. 18-34C).

Osteoarthritis is a degeneration of the articular cartilage of the joint. It may result from trauma or wear and tear and is typically seen later in life. It is commonly treated with a total joint replacement. **Hip fractures** tend to be of two types: intertrochanteric and femoral neck. These are very common among elderly people, usually resulting from falls. High-impact trauma such as motor vehicle accidents may cause hip fractures in younger individuals.

Iliotibial band syndrome is an overuse injury causing lateral knee pain. It is commonly seen in runners

Clinical Application 18-3

Assistive Device Use on Opposite Side

An assistive device, such as a cane, is often used to relieve hip pain and/or compensate for weakness in the hip abductors. While it may seem logical to use the cane on the same side as the painful hip, it should be placed in the opposite hand (see Fig. 2). A wider base of support is created between the cane and the involved leg. This allows the cane to share in the weight-bearing demand, directly reducing the weight that the involved hip needs to bear.

The upward force from the cane prevents lateral tilt of the pelvis on the non-weight-bearing side, thus reducing the contraction force needed from the hip abductors on the weak/painful side. As a result, the hip abductors do not have to contract as hard and therefore do not produce as much compressive force on the involved hip. Holding the cane in the opposite hand also promotes a normal arm swing during gait.

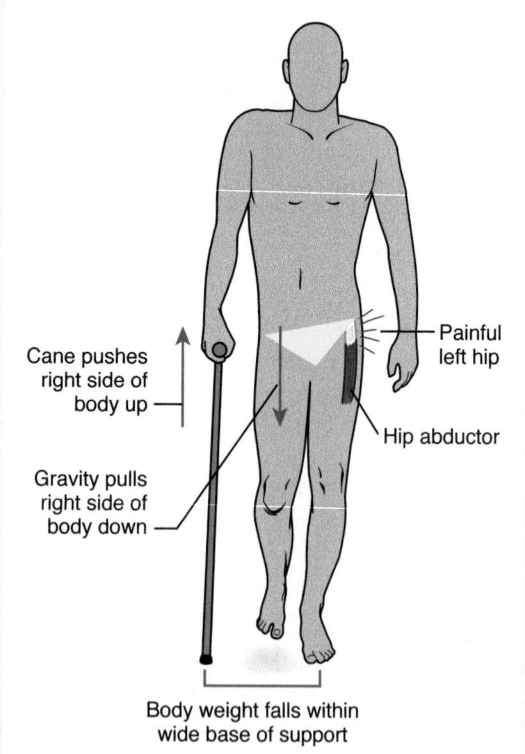

Figure 2 Assistive devise use on opposite side.

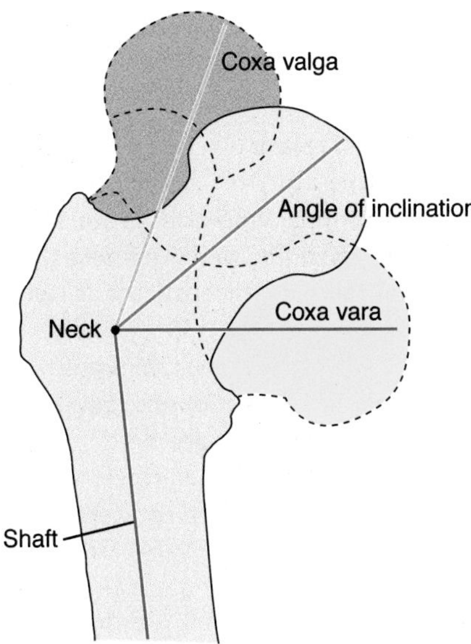

Figure 18-33. Angle of inclination is normally about 125 degrees. Coxa valga is an angle greater than 125 degrees, and coxa vara is an angle less than 125 degrees.

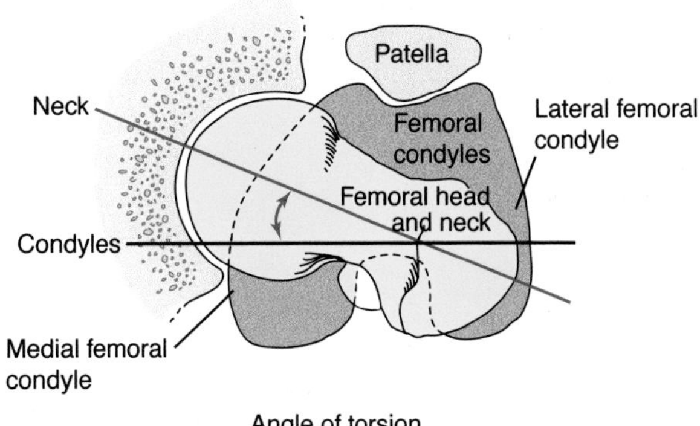

A

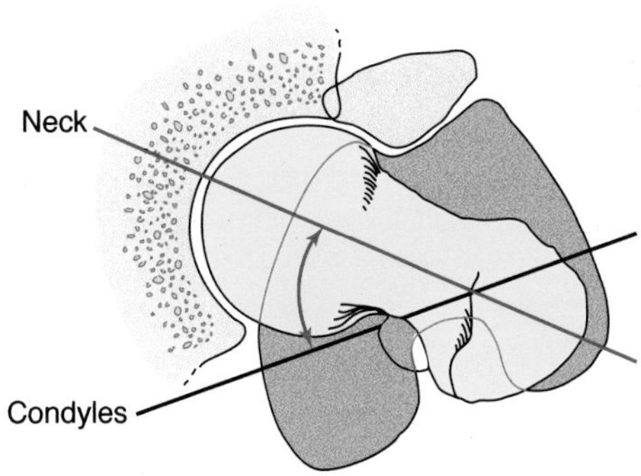

B

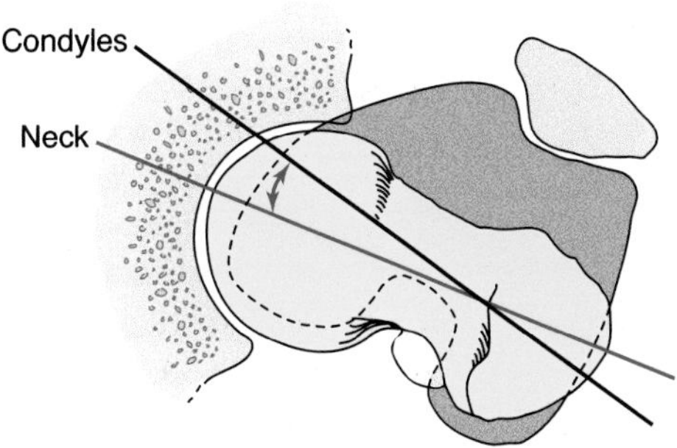

C

Figure 18-34. Superior view. **(A)** Angle of torsion normally has the head and neck rotated outward from the shaft approximately 15 to 25 degrees. An increase in this angle is called *anteversion* **(B)**, and a decrease in this angle is called *retroversion* **(C)**.

and bicyclists. This syndrome is believed to result from repeated friction of the band that slides over the lateral femoral epicondyle during knee motion. It is caused by such factors as muscle tightness, worn-down shoes, and running on uneven surfaces. Because many muscles insert at the greater trochanter, there are many bursae providing a friction-reducing cushion between the muscles and bone. **Trochanteric bursitis** is the result of either acute trauma or overuse. It can be seen in runners or bicyclists or in someone with a leg length discrepancy, or it can be caused by other factors that put repeated stress on the greater trochanter. A **hamstring strain,** also called *pulled hamstring,* is probably the most common muscle problem in the body. Unfortunately, it is often recurrent. It may result from an overload of the muscle or trying to move the muscle too fast. Therefore, this is a common injury among sprinters and in sports that require bursts of speed or rapid acceleration, such as soccer, track and field, football, baseball, and rugby. Hamstring strains can occur at one of the attachment sites or at any point along the length of the muscle.

Hip pointer is a misnomer because it occurs at the pelvis, not the hip joint. It is a severe bruise caused by direct trauma to the iliac crest of the pelvis. It is most commonly associated with football but can be seen in almost any contact sport. Spearing the hip/pelvis with a helmet while tackling may be the most common cause.

Summary of Muscle Action

Table 18-4 summarizes the actions of the prime movers of the hip joint.

Table 18-4 Action of Hip Prime Movers

Action	Muscle
Combination of flexion and abduction	Tensor fascia lata
Combination of flexion, abduction, and lateral rotation	Sartorius
Flexion	Rectus femoris, iliopsoas, pectineus
Extension	Gluteus maximus, semitendinosus, semimembranosus, biceps femoris (long head)
Hyperextension	Gluteus maximus
Abduction	Gluteus medius, gluteus minimus
Adduction	Pectineus, adductor longus, adductor brevis, adductor magnus, gracilis
Medial rotation	Gluteus minimus
Lateral rotation	Gluteus maximus, deep rotators

Summary of Muscle Innervation

Generally speaking, the femoral nerve innervates muscles on the anterior surface of the hip and thigh region (hip flexors). The obturator nerve innervates hip adductors on the medial side. The superior gluteal nerve supplies the hip abductors on the lateral side. The hamstring muscles, which are hip extensors and are located posteriorly, receive innervation from the tibial portion of the sciatic nerve.

There are, of course, exceptions to all generalizations. The gluteus maximus, a posterior muscle, receives innervation from the inferior gluteal nerve. The deep rotators do not fit neatly into any sort of category; therefore, they are included individually in the summary of hip joint muscle innervation in Table 18-3 and 18-5 instead of as a group. The deep rotators are included here as a group. Table 18-6 summarizes the segmental innervation. As has been stated in previous chapters, there is variation among sources regarding some segmental innervation.

Table 18-5 Innervation of the Muscles of the Hip

Muscle	Nerve	Spinal Segment
Iliopsoas		
Psoas part	Anterior rami	L1, L2
Iliacus part	Femoral	L2, L3
Rectus femoris	Femoral	L2, L3, L4
Sartorius	Femoral	L2, L3
Pectineus	Femoral	L2, L3
Gracilis	Obturator	L2, L3
Adductor longus	Obturator	L2, L3, L4
Adductor brevis	Obturator	L2, L3
Adductor magnus	Obturator/Sciatic – tibial division	L2, L3, L4
Gluteus maximus	Inferior gluteal	L5, S1, S2
Gluteus medius	Superior gluteal	L4, L5, S1
Gluteus minimus	Superior gluteal	L4, L5, S1
Tensor fascia lata	Superior gluteal	L4, L5, S1
Semitendinosus	Sciatic – tibial division	L5, S1, S2
Semimembranosus	Sciatic – tibial division	L5, S1, S2
Biceps femoris (long head)	Sciatic – tibial division	L5, S1, S2
Obturator externus	Obturator	L3, L4
Obturator internus	Nerve to the obturator internus	L5, S1
Gemellus superior	Nerve to the obturator internus	L5, S1, S2
Quadratus femoris	Nerve to the quadratus femoris	L5, S1
Gemellus inferior	Nerve to the quadratus femoris	L4, L5, S1
Piriformis	Anterior rami	L5, S1, S2

Table 18-6 Segmental Innervation of Hip Muscles

Spinal Cord Level	L2	L3	L4	L5	S1	S2	S3
Iliopsoas	X	X					
Sartorius	X	X					
Gracilis	X	X					
Rectus femoris	X	X	X				
Pectineus	X	X					
Adductor longus	X	X	X				
Adductor brevis	X	X					
Adductor magnus	X	X	X				
Tensor fascia lata			X	X			
Gluteus maximus				X	X	X	
Gluteus medius			X	X	X		
Gluteus minimus			X	X	X		
Semitendinosus				X	X	X	
Semimembranosus				X	X	X	
Biceps femoris (long head)				X	X	X	
Deep rotators		X	X	X	X	X	

Points to Remember

- In determining the leverage, the muscle's point of attachment to the bone is used.
- With a second-class lever, resistance is between the axis and the force. With a third-class lever, force is in the middle.
- End feel is the quality of the feel when applying slight pressure at the end of the joint's passive range.
- A closed kinetic chain requires that the distal segment is fixed and the proximal segment(s) move.
- To stretch a one-joint muscle, it is necessary to put any two-joint muscles on a slack over the joint not crossed by the one-joint muscle.
- To contract a two-joint muscle most effectively, start with it being stretched over both joints.
- When determining whether a concentric or eccentric contraction is occurring, decide
  - if the activity is accelerating against gravity or slowing down gravity, or
  - if a weight greater than the pull of gravity is affecting the activity.

Review Questions

General Anatomy Questions

1. List the bones that make up the:
   a. pelvis
   b. innominate
   c. hip joint
   d. acetabulum
   e. obturator foramen
   f. greater sciatic notch
2. If you were handed an unattached innominate bone, what landmarks would you use to determine whether it was a right or left bone?
3. How would you determine whether an unattached femur is a right or left one?
4. Describe the hip joint:
   a. Number of axes:
   b. Shape of joint:
   c. Type of motion allowed:

(continued on next page)

Review Questions—cont'd

5. What hip motions occur in:
   a. the transverse plane around the vertical axis?
   b. the sagittal plane around the frontal axis?
   c. the frontal plane around the sagittal axis?
6. What is referred to as the *Y ligament*? Why?
7. Regarding the statement "hanging on the Y ligaments":
   a. What position are the hips in relative to the shoulders?
   b. Where does the line of gravity fall relative to the hip joint axis of rotation?
   c. Gravity exerts a force that wants to move the hip into ___________.
   d. This strategy is most helpful when the hip ___________ muscles group is weak.
8. Why is the hip joint not prone to dislocation?
9. What is the direction of the line of attachment of the hip ligaments—vertical, horizontal, or spiral? What does this line of attachment allow for?
10. Which two-joint hip muscles attach below the knee?
11. Which hip joint muscles are not prime movers in any single action but are effective in a combination of movements? List the movements.
12. What muscles keep your pelvis from dropping on one side when you lift one foot off the floor? Describe what happens.
13. Does the femoral head surface glide in the same or opposite direction as the thigh during hip flexion/extension?
14. If hip lateral rotation was limited, the femoral head is restricted from gliding in the _________ direction.
15. What is the end feel of hip flexion? Hip extension?

Functional Activity Questions

1. A right-handed tennis player strikes a ball with a forehand swing and follows through. The left hip is moving into what positions (Fig. 18-35)?

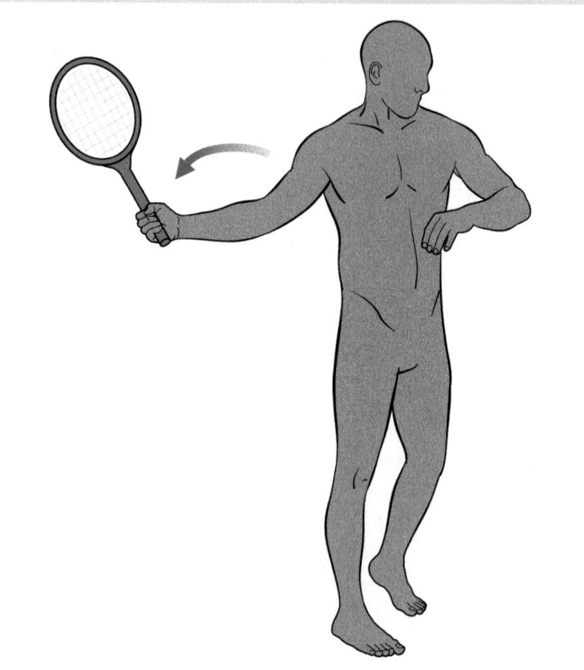

Figure 18-35. Position of tennis player when hitting a forehand swing.

2. a. How is hip flexion affected by sitting on a low surface versus a higher one (e.g., a regular versus a raised toilet seat)?
   b. What accompanying hip motions or positions may occur if a person has her feet apart, knees together,

Review Questions—cont'd

and hands on her knees, and she pushes down to assist when standing (Fig. 18-36)?

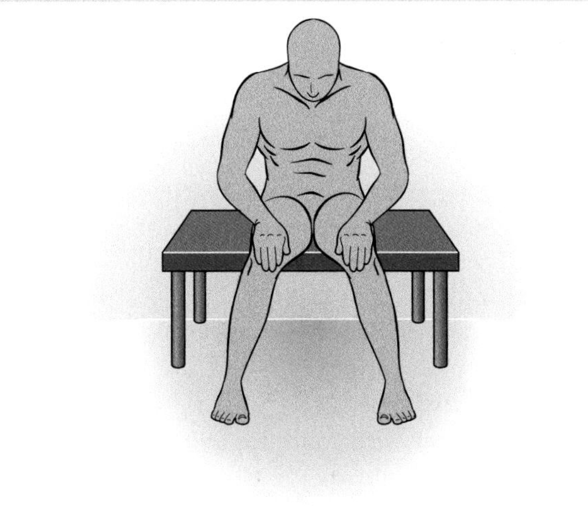

Figure 18-36. Position of hips when beginning to stand.

3. Standing in anatomical position and keeping your pelvis fairly level, shift your weight to your right foot.
   a. What hip joint motion has occurred at your right hip?
   b. What muscle group initiates this action?
   c. Is this an open- or closed-chain activity?
4. While weight-bearing on the left leg, note the motions of your right hip as you swing your right leg in the following activities:
   a. Walking
   b. Stepping up onto a curb
   c. Getting into a car
   d. Getting on what is commonly called a boy's bicycle (bar between handlebars and seat)
5. When an assistive device is used as a result of hip pain, which hand should the cane be held in, and why?
6. Lie supine on a table with your knees bent and feet flat. Note the position of your pelvis and determine whether you can put your hand on the small of your back.
   a. If you cannot, what is the position of your pelvis?
   b. If you can, what is the position of your pelvis and lumbar spine?
7. From the position described in question 5, slowly slide your feet down the table until your hips and knees are extended. Again, note the position of your pelvis and determine whether you can put your hand on the small of your back. Repeat this again, keeping your right knee and hip flexed with your foot flat while you move your left foot down until your left hip and knee are extended.
   a. What is accomplished at the pelvis by keeping your right hip and knee flexed?
   b. What can be said about left hip muscle length if you cannot rest your left thigh completely on the table? In other words, why would you not be able to extend your left hip?
   c. What is the one-joint hip muscle attaching on the pelvis and lumbar spine that may be responsible for this limitation?
   d. What difference does the position of the pelvis have on anterior hip muscle length?
8. Pretend that you cannot completely extend your hip due to tight hip flexors. How might you compensate for this when standing?
9. You are seated at a table. Stand up while turning to the right. Stop halfway through this motion (before you move your feet).
   a. The right hip is in what positions? (1) flexed/extended, (2) abducted/adducted, or (3) medially rotated/laterally rotated
   b. The left hip is in what positions? (1) flexed/extended, (2) abducted/adducted, or (3) medially rotated/laterally rotated

(continued on next page)

Review Questions—cont'd

10. When a tennis player hits the ball (see Fig. 18-35), what type of kinetic chain activity is occurring at the hip? At the shoulder?

Clinical Exercise Questions

1. While lying prone with your right knee flexed, raise your right leg straight up, keeping your pelvis flat on the table. Describe what has occurred in terms of:
   a. hip joint motion
   b. whether stretching or strengthening is occurring
   c. muscle(s) involved
2. In the position shown in Figure 18-37, move your right leg forward until your right knee is directly over your right ankle. Your left hip is hyperextended and your left knee is flexed and resting on the floor. Rock your weight forward onto the front (right) leg without moving your right foot. Describe what has occurred at the left hip in terms of:
   a. joint motion
   b. whether stretching or strengthening is occurring
   c. muscle(s) involved

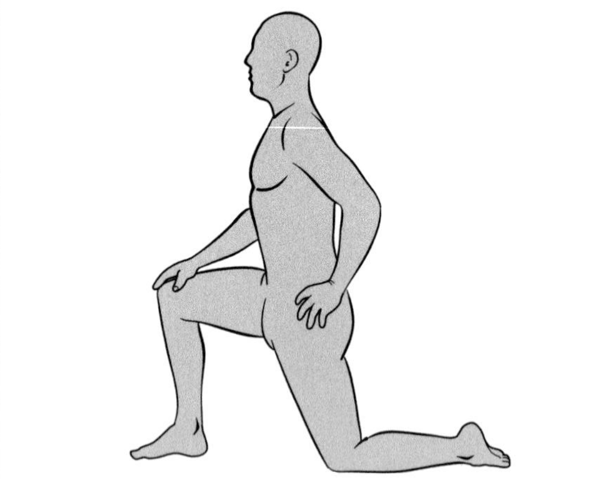

Figure 18-37. Starting position.

3. If the position in Figure 18-37 was changed by holding the left knee in more flexion (difficult to achieve comfortably, but pretend), do you think this is a good position in which to stretch the rectus femoris? Why?
4. Lying on your right side with your left hip and knee in extension, raise your left leg toward the ceiling about 2 feet. Describe what has occurred in terms of:
   a. joint motion
   b. whether stretching or strengthening is occurring
   c. muscle(s) involved
5. Repeat the exercise in question 4 with your left hip in approximately 30 degrees of flexion. Describe what has occurred in terms of:
   a. joint motion
   b. whether stretching or strengthening is occurring
   c. muscle(s) involved
6. Lie on your back with your hips and knees in extension. Raise your right leg toward the ceiling.
   a. Is a concentric or eccentric contraction occurring at the hip?
   b. The hip flexors are demonstrating what class of lever?
   c. What force do the hip flexors want to exert at the pelvis?
   d. What muscle group needs to contract to prevent the motion in (c)?
7. While lying prone with your left knee flexed, raise your left leg straight up, keeping your pelvis flat on the table.
   a. Are the hamstrings contracting at their strongest?
   b. Why or why not?
8. Sitting on the floor with your legs far apart, lean forward from the hips while keeping your back straight. Describe what has occurred in terms of:
   a. hip joint motion
   b. whether stretching or strengthening is occurring
   c. muscle(s) involved

Review Questions—cont'd

9. Figure 18-38 shows an individual doing hip flexion exercises two different ways. The starting position in both exercises is hip extension and knee extension. In exercise *A,* the person flexes the hips with the knees flexed. In exercise *B,* the person performs the same hip flexion motion but with the knees extended.
   a. Which exercise is more difficult?
   b. Why?
   c. In which exercise is an anterior pelvic tilt more likely to occur, and why?

10. Starting in a supine position with the knees flexed, move into the position shown in Figure 18-39.
    a. What type of kinetic chain activity is this?
    b. What hip motion is occurring?
    c. What type of contraction is occurring?
    d. What hip muscle group is the agonist?
    e. If this motion could not be completed because a muscle was passively insufficient, what muscle would that be?

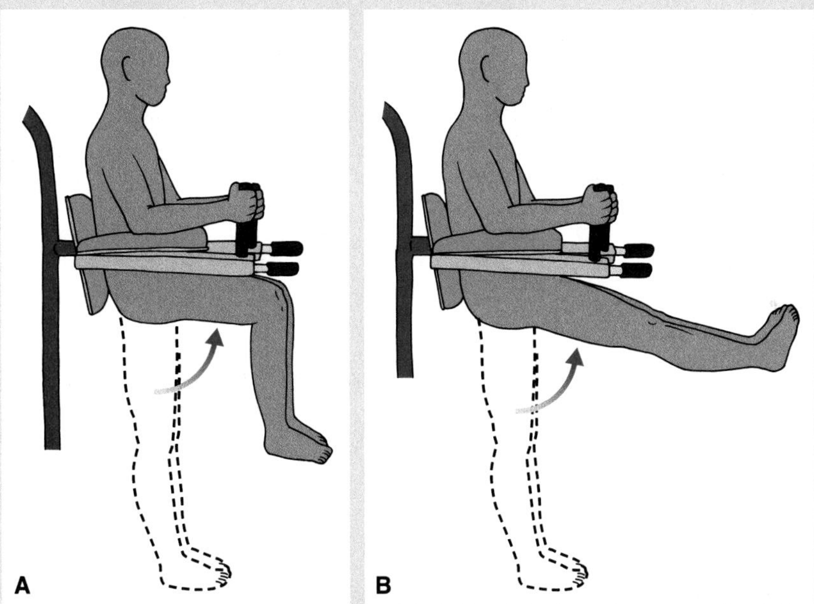

Figure 18-38. Hip flexion exercise.

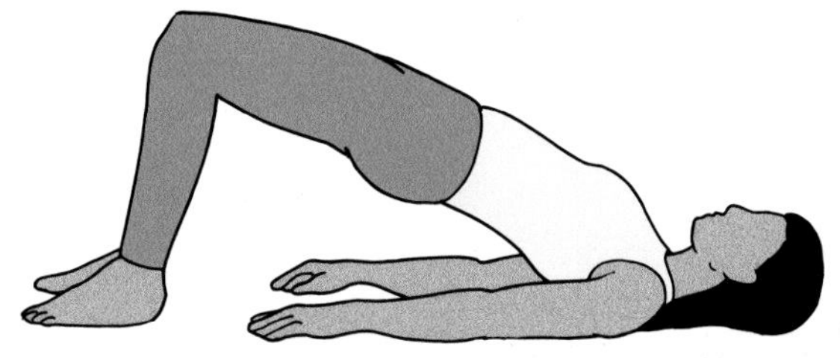

Figure 18-39. Ending position.

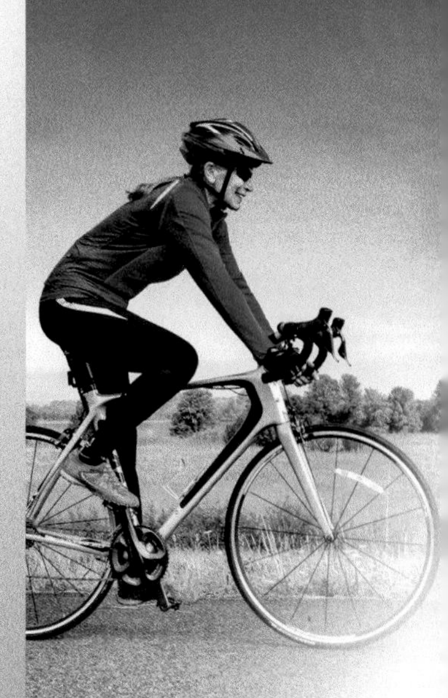

CHAPTER 19
Knee Joint

Joint Structure and Motions
Bones and Landmarks
Ligaments and Other Structures
Muscles of the Knee
Anterior Muscles
Posterior Muscles
Anatomical Relationships
Summary of Muscle Action
Summary of Muscle Innervation
Common Knee Pathologies
Points to Remember
Review Questions
General Anatomy Questions
Functional Activity Questions
Clinical Exercise Questions

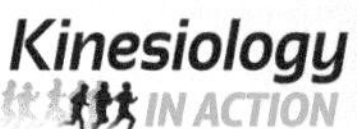

For additional practice activities and videos, please visit www.kinesiologyinaction.com

Joint Structure and Motions

At first glance, the knee joint appears to be relatively simple. However, it is one of the more complex joints in the body. The knee is supported and maintained entirely by muscles and ligaments with no bony stability, and it frequently is exposed to severe stresses and strains. Therefore, it should be no surprise that it is one of the most frequently injured joints in the body.

The knee joint is the largest joint in the body, and it is classified as a synovial hinge joint (Fig. 19-1). The motions possible at the knee are flexion and extension (Fig. 19-2). From 0 degrees of extension, there are approximately 120 to 135 degrees of flexion. Due to some ligament laxity, the knee may have a few degrees of hyperextension beyond 0; beyond 5 degrees of hyperextension is considered genu recurvatum. Unlike the elbow, the knee joint is not a true hinge, because it has a rotational component. This rotation is not a free motion but rather an accessory motion that accompanies flexion and extension.

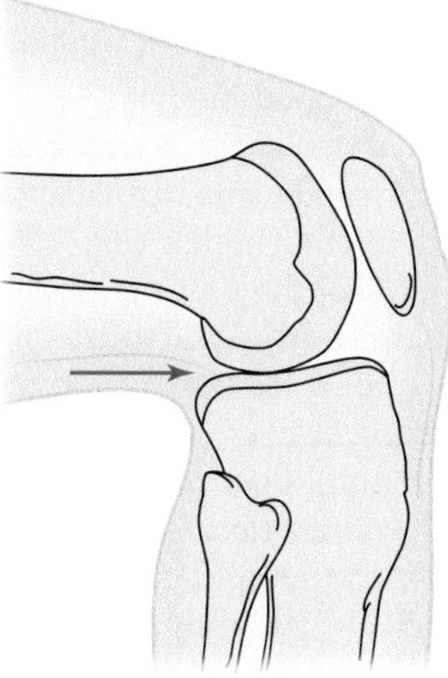

Figure 19-1. Knee joint (lateral view).

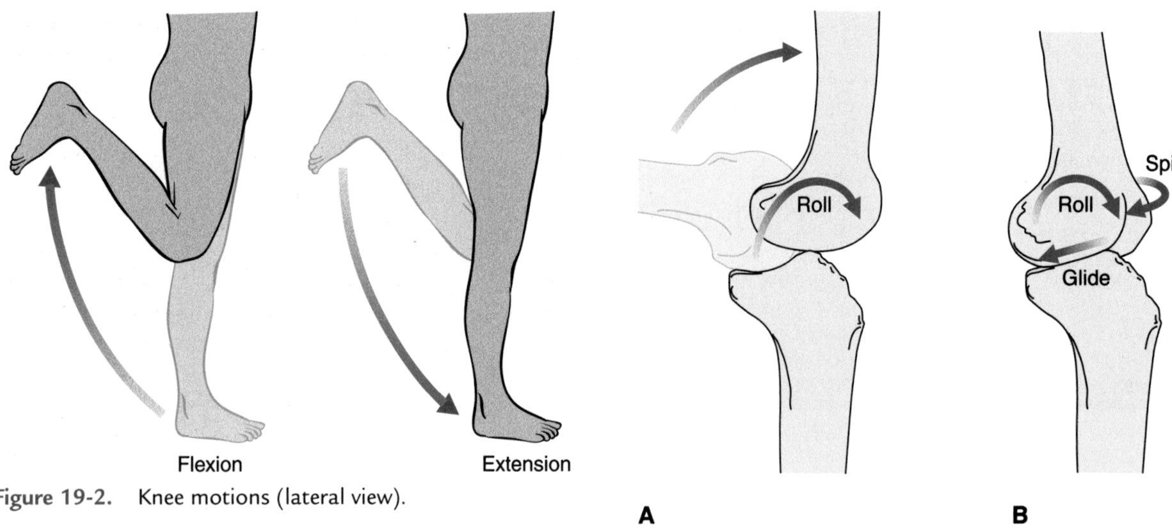

Figure 19-2. Knee motions (lateral view).

Figure 19-3. Arthrokinematic movements of the knee joint surfaces in a closed-chain activity of knee extension in which the femur moves on the tibia (medial view). **(A)** Pure rolling of the femur would cause it to roll off the tibia as the knee extends. **(B)** Normal motion of the knee demonstrates a combination of rolling, gliding (posteriorly), and spinning (medially) in the last 20 degrees of extension.

There are two types of end feel at the knee joint. With knee flexion, the end feel is soft (soft tissue approximation) due to the contact between the muscle bellies of the thigh and leg. With knee extension, the end feel is firm (soft tissue stretch) due to tension of the joint capsule and ligaments.

Arthrokinematics

All three types of arthrokinematic motion occur during knee flexion and extension. The convex femoral condyles move on the concave tibial condyles or vice versa, depending on whether it is an open- or closed-chain activity. The articular surface of the femoral condyles is much greater than that of the tibial condyles. If the femur rolled on the tibia from flexion to extension, the femur would roll off the tibia before the motion was complete (Fig. 19-3A). Therefore, the femur must **glide** posteriorly on the tibia as it **rolls** into extension (Fig. 19-3B). It should also be noted that the articular surface of the medial femoral condyle is longer than that of the lateral femoral condyle (Fig. 19-4A). As extension occurs, the articular surface of the lateral femoral condyle is used up while some articular surface remains on the medial femoral condyle (Fig. 19-4B). Therefore, the medial condyle of the femur must also glide posteriorly to use its entire articular surface (Fig. 19-4C). It is this posterior gliding of the medial femoral condyle during the last few degrees of weight-bearing extension (closed-chain action) that causes the femur to **spin** (rotate medially) on the tibia (see Fig. 19-3B).

Looking at the same spin, or rotational, movement during non-weight-bearing extension (open-chain action), note that the tibia rotates laterally on the femur. These last few degrees of motion lock the knee in extension; this is sometimes called the *screw-home mechanism* of the knee. With the knee fully extended, an individual can stand for a long time without using muscles. For knee flexion to occur, the knee must be "unlocked" by laterally rotating the femur on the tibia. This small amount of rotation of the femur on the tibia, or vice versa, keeps the knee from being a true hinge joint. Because this rotation is not an independent motion, it will not be considered a knee motion.

As described above, the knee has a convex-on-concave relationship in the closed chain, but this is reversed when non-weight-bearing. In the open chain, the knee has a concave-on-convex relationship where the concave tibial condyles glide posteriorly with flexion, and anteriorly with extension, while the distal end of the tibia moves in the same direction. The knee is in the open-packed position when it is flexed to 25 degrees, that is the position where most joint play is available. A mobilizing force applied to the proximal tibia in an anterior direction will facilitate knee extension, whereas a posterior glide will promote flexion.

The articulation between the femur and patella is referred to as the **patellofemoral joint** (Fig. 19-5). The smooth, posterior surface of the patella glides over the patellar surface of the femur. The main functions of the patella involve increasing the mechanical advantage of the quadriceps muscle and protecting the knee joint.

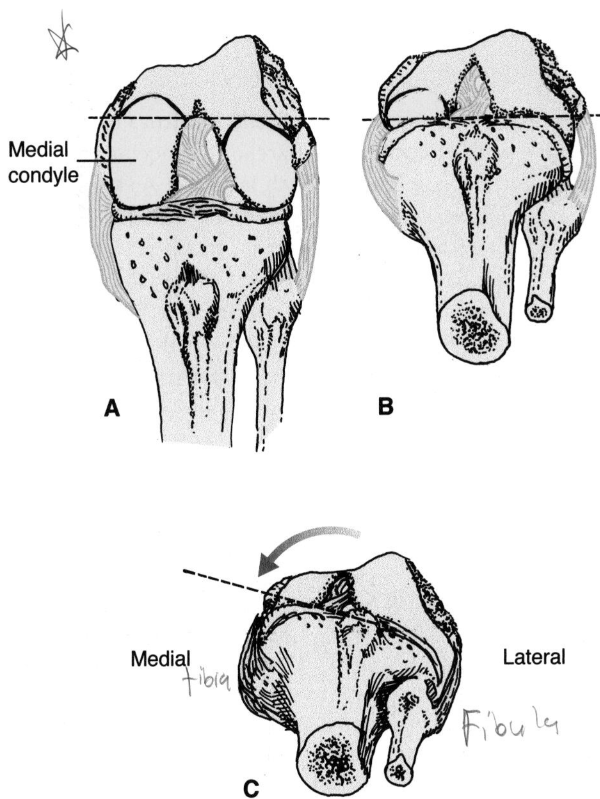

Figure 19-4. Screw-home motion of the left knee. In the weight-bearing position (closed-chain activity), the femur rotates medially on the tibia as the knee moves into the last few degrees of extension.

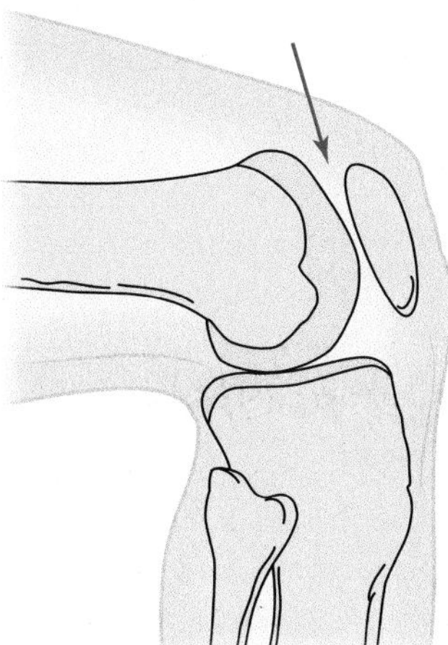

Figure 19-5. Patellofemoral joint (lateral view).

An increased mechanical advantage is achieved by lengthening the quadriceps moment arm. As discussed in Chapter 8 (in the "Torque" section), moment arm is the perpendicular distance between the muscle's line of action and the center of the joint (axis). By placing the patella between the quadriceps, or patellar tendon, and the femur, the action line of the quadriceps muscles is farther away (Fig. 19-6). Hence, the moment arm lengthens, allowing the muscle to have greater angular force. Without the patella, the moment arm would be shorter and much of the muscle's force would be a stabilizing force directed back into the joint.

The **Q angle,** or *patellofemoral angle,* is the angle between the quadriceps muscle (primarily the rectus femoris muscle) and the patellar tendon. It is determined by drawing a line from the anterior superior iliac spine (ASIS) to the midpoint of the patella, and from the tibial tuberosity to the midpoint of the patella. Although the rectus femoris attaches to the anterior inferior iliac spine (AIIS), the ASIS lies just above the AIIS and is easier to palpate. The angle formed by the intersection of these lines represents the Q angle (Fig. 19-7). In knee extension, this angle ranges from 13 to 19 degrees in normal individuals. The angle tends to be greater in females because the pelvis is generally wider in women. Many different knee and patellar problems, such as patellofemoral pain syndrome, are associated with Q angles greater or smaller than this range.

Bones and Landmarks

The knee is composed of the distal end of the femur articulating with the proximal end of the tibia. The landmarks of the **femur** significant to the knee are listed below (Fig. 19-8).

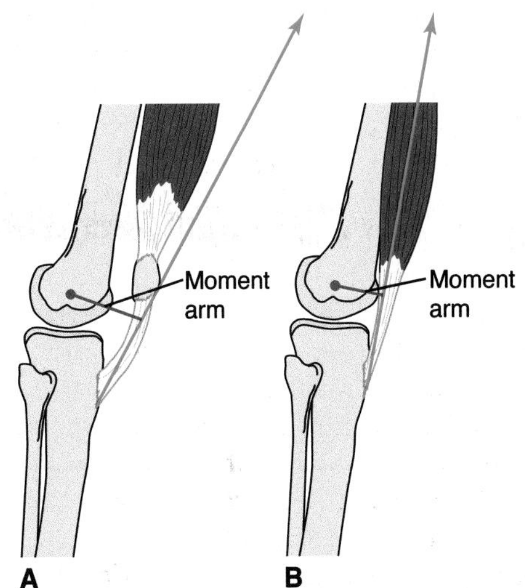

Figure 19-6. Moment arm of the quadriceps muscles is greater with a patella **(A),** than without a patella **(B)** (lateral view).

Clinical Application 19-1

Patellofemoral Compressive Forces During Flexion and Extension

When the knee is fully extended, the patella lies in its uppermost position, in the shallowest portion of the patellar surface of the femur. This is the open packed position for the patellofemoral joint. With the knee extended and the leg muscles relaxed, it should be easy to manually glide the patella side-to side (Fig. A). As the knee flexes, the patella is pulled downward by the patellar tendon through its attachment to the tibial tuberosity. In this lower position, the patella becomes quite stable as the depth of the patellar surface and amount of bony contact both increase. As knee flexion increases, manual glide of the patella side-to side is no longer possible (Fig. B). In activities like a deep knee bend, the knee is flexing and the quadriceps are eccentrically contracting. This compresses the patella tightly against the femur due to tension in the quadriceps and patellar tendons. Chronic compression can lead to patellofemoral pain.

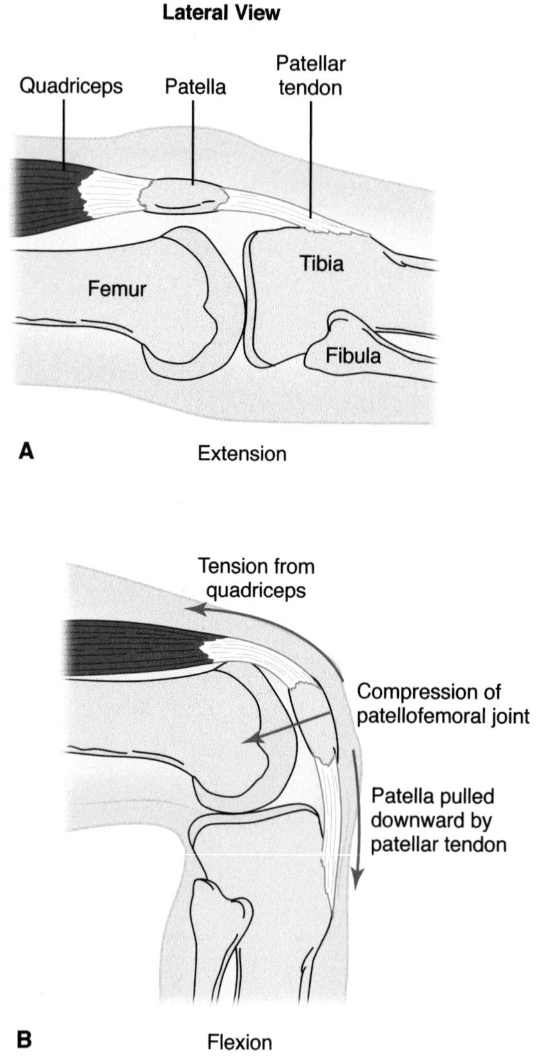

Patella mobility during knee flexion/extension. **(A)** with knee extended, patella can be moved side-to-side. **(B)** With knee flexed, side-to-side motion of patella is not possible.

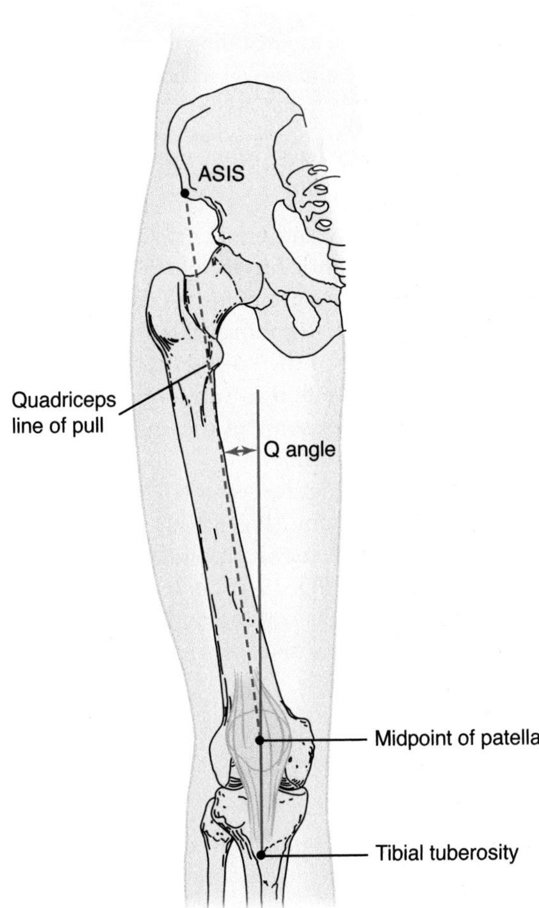

Figure 19-7. Q angle of the knee (anterior view).

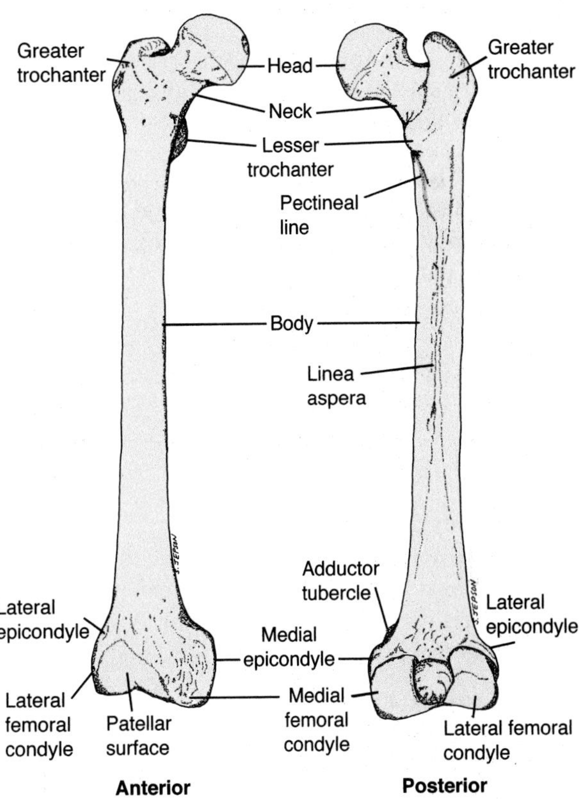

Figure 19-8. Right femur.

Important Bony Landmarks of the Femur

Head
The rounded portion articulating with the acetabulum.

Neck
The narrower portion located between the head and the trochanters.

Greater Trochanter
Large projection located laterally between the neck and the body of the femur, providing attachment for the gluteus medius and minimus and for most deep rotator muscles.

Lesser Trochanter
A smaller projection located medially and posteriorly, just distal to the greater trochanter; it provides attachment for the iliopsoas muscle.

Body
The long, cylindrical portion between the bone ends; also called the *shaft*. It is bowed slightly anteriorly.

Medial Femoral Condyle
Distal medial end

Lateral Femoral Condyle
Distal lateral end

Lateral Epicondyle
Projection proximal to the lateral condyle

Medial Epicondyle
Projection proximal to the medial condyle

Adductor Tubercle
Small projection proximal to the medial epicondyle to which a portion of the adductor magnus muscle attaches

Linea Aspera
Prominent longitudinal ridge or crest running most of the posterior length

Pectineal Line
Runs from below the lesser trochanter diagonally toward the linea aspera. It provides attachment for the adductor brevis.

Patellar Surface
Located between the medial and lateral condyle anteriorly. It articulates with the posterior surface of the patella.

The landmarks of the **tibia** significant to the knee are listed below (Fig. 19-9).

Important Bony Landmarks of the Tibia

Intercondylar Eminence
A double-pointed prominence on the proximal surface at about the midpoint, which extends up into the intercondylar fossa of the femur

Medial Tibial Condyle
Proximal medial end

Lateral Tibial Condyle
Proximal lateral end

Tibial Plateau
Enlarged proximal end, including the medial and lateral condyles and the intercondylar eminence

Tibial Tuberosity
Large projection at the proximal end on the anterior surface in the midline

The **fibula** is lateral to, and smaller than, the tibia. It is set back from the anterior surface of the tibia, allowing a large space for muscle attachment (Fig. 19-10). This feature gives the lower leg its rounded circumference. The fibula is not part of the knee joint because it does not articulate with the femur. Although it provides a point of attachment for some of the knee structures, it has a larger role at the ankle.

The **patella** is a triangular sesamoid bone within the quadriceps muscle tendon (Fig. 19-11). It has a broad, superior border and a somewhat pointed distal portion.

The **calcaneus** (see Fig. 19-10) is the most posterior of the tarsal bones and is commonly known as the *heel.* It is identified here because it provides attachment for the gastrocnemius muscle.

Ligaments and Other Structures

As stated earlier, the knee is held together not by its bony structure but by ligaments and muscles. The cruciate

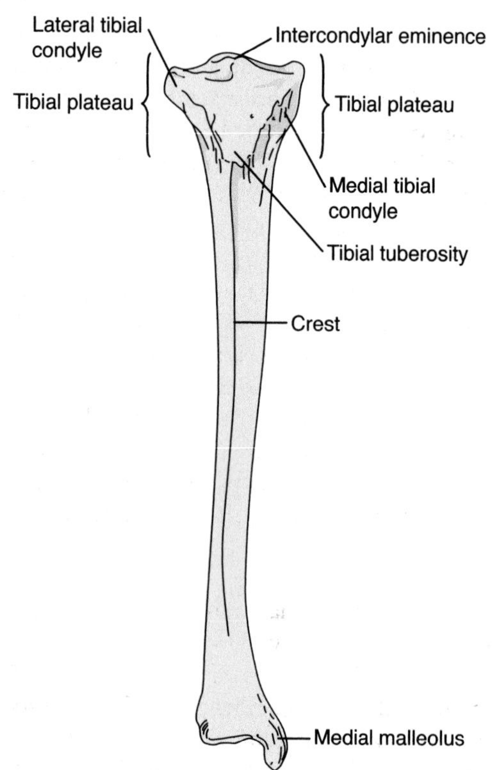

Figure 19-9. Right tibia (anterior view).

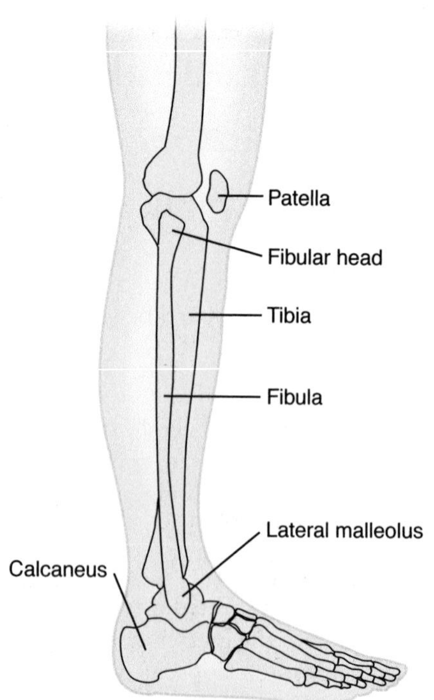

Figure 19-10. Right leg (lateral view).

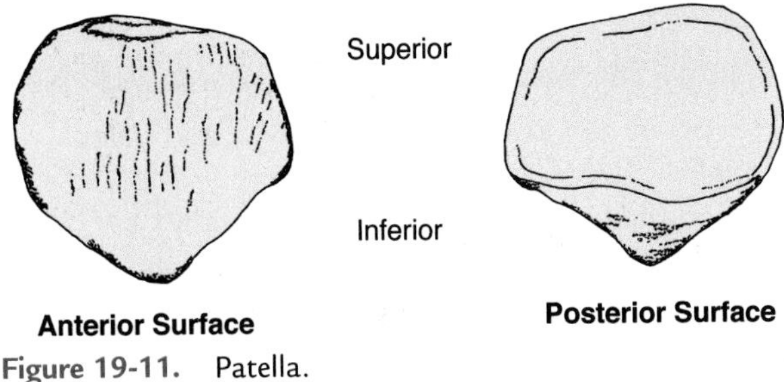

Figure 19-11. Patella.

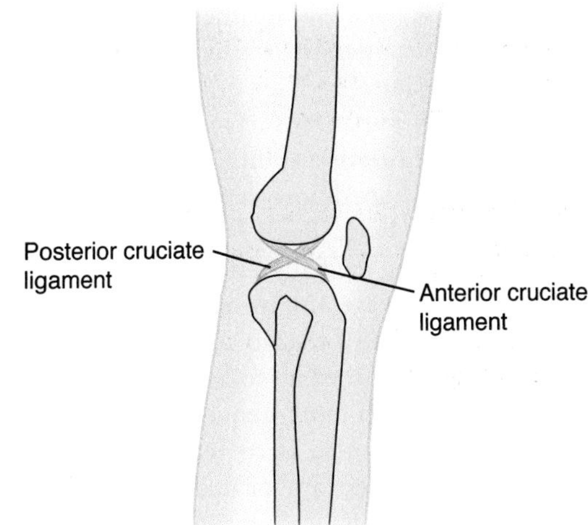

Figure 19-13. Cruciate ligaments are named for their attachment on the tibia (lateral view).

and collateral ligaments are the two main sets of ligaments for this task (Fig. 19-12). The cruciates are located within the joint capsule and are therefore called *intracapsular ligaments.* Situated between the medial and lateral condyles, the cruciates cross each other obliquely (*cruciate* means "resembling a cross" in Latin). They are named for their attachment on the *tibia* (Fig. 19-13). The **anterior cruciate ligament** attaches to the anterior surface of the tibia in the intercondylar area just medial to the medial meniscus. It spans the knee lateral to the posterior cruciate ligament, and it runs in a superior and posterior direction to attach posteriorly on the lateral condyle of the femur. The **posterior cruciate ligament** attaches to the posterior tibia in the intercondylar area, and it runs in a superior and anterior direction on the medial side of the anterior cruciate ligament. It attaches to the anterior femur on the medial condyle. In summary, the anterior cruciate runs from the anterior tibia to the posterior femur, and the posterior cruciate runs from the posterior tibia to the anterior femur.

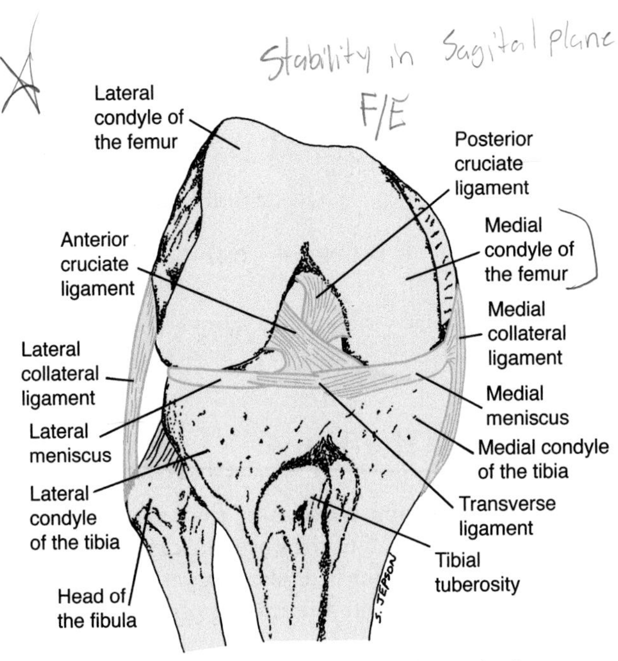

Figure 19-12. Right knee in flexion (anterior view).

The cruciates provide stability in the sagittal plane. The anterior cruciate ligament keeps the femur from being displaced posteriorly on the tibia. Conversely, it keeps the tibia from being displaced anteriorly on the femur. It tightens during extension, preventing excessive hyperextension of the knee. When the knee is partly flexed, the anterior cruciate keeps the tibia from moving anteriorly. Conversely, the posterior cruciate ligament keeps the femur from displacing anteriorly on the tibia or the tibia from displacing posteriorly on the femur. It tightens during flexion and is injured much less frequently than the anterior cruciate ligament.

Located on the sides of the knee are the collateral ligaments (see Fig. 19-12). The **medial collateral ligament,** or tibial collateral ligament, is a flat, broad ligament attaching to the medial condyles of the femur and tibia. Fibers of the medial meniscus are attached to this ligament, which contributes to frequent tearing of the medial meniscus during excessive stress to the medial collateral ligament. On the lateral side is the **lateral collateral ligament,** or fibular collateral ligament. This round, cordlike ligament attaches to the lateral condyle of the femur and runs down to the head of the fibula, independent of any attachment to the lateral meniscus. It provides stability to the lateral side of the knee against medial-to-lateral forces (varus force).

The collateral ligaments supply stability in the frontal plane. The medial collateral ligament provides medial stability and prevents excessive motion if there is a blow to the lateral side of the knee (valgus force). The lateral collateral ligament provides lateral stability and prevents excessive motion if there is a blow to the medial side of the knee (varus force). Because their attachments are offset posteriorly and superiorly to the knee joint axis, the collateral ligaments tighten during extension, contributing to the stability of the knee, and slacken during flexion.

Located on the superior surface of the tibia, the **medial** and **lateral menisci** (plural of *meniscus*) are two half-moon, wedge-shaped fibrocartilage disks. They are designed to absorb shock (Fig. 19-14). Because they are thicker laterally than medially and because the proximal surfaces are concave, the menisci deepen the relatively flat joint surface of the tibia. Perhaps because of its attachment to the medial collateral ligament, the medial meniscus is torn more frequently.

The purpose of a bursa is to reduce friction, and approximately 13 of them are located at the knee joint. They are needed because the many tendons located around the knee have a relatively vertical line of pull against bony areas or other tendons. Figure 19-15 illustrates many of the bursae around the knee as viewed from the medial side. Table 19-1 summarizes the most commonly discussed bursae.

The **popliteal space** is the area behind the knee, and it contains important nerves (tibial and common fibular) and blood vessels (popliteal artery and vein). This diamond-shaped fossa is bound superiorly on the medial side by the semitendinosus and semimembranosus muscles and by the biceps femoris muscle on the lateral side (Fig. 19-16). The inferior boundaries are the medial and lateral heads of the gastrocnemius muscle.

The **pes anserine** (Latin for "goose foot") **muscle group** is made up of the sartorius, gracilis, and semitendinosus (Fig. 19-17) muscles. Each muscle has a different proximal attachment. The sartorius muscle arises anteriorly from the iliac spine, the gracilis muscle arises medially from the pubis, and the semitendinosus muscle arises posteriorly from the ischial tuberosity. They all cross the knee posteriorly and medially, then join together to attach distally on the anterior medial surface of the proximal tibia. This arrangement can also be seen in Figure 18-29.

Orthopedic surgeons sometimes alter this common attachment to provide medial stability to the knee.

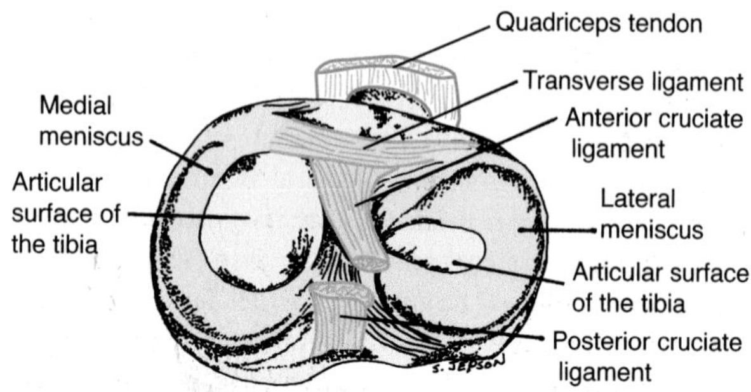

Figure 19-14. Right knee (superior view).

Clinical Application 19-2

Forces on the Knee Joint with Varus and Valgus Angles

When the lower limb is aligned neutrally (Fig. B), the weight-bearing force passes through the midline of the knee joints. With genu varus (Fig. A), the weight-bearing line shifts medial to the knee, which compresses the articular surfaces on the medial side of the knee joint. With genu valgus (Fig. C), the compressive force moves to the lateral knee joint. Once the weight-bearing force shifts medially or laterally, the constant sideward force causes the varus or valgus angle to worsen over time. Greater angles lead to greater compressive forces, which can damage the articular cartilage. Abnormal stresses to the knees will also alter the stresses placed upon the ankle and hip joints.

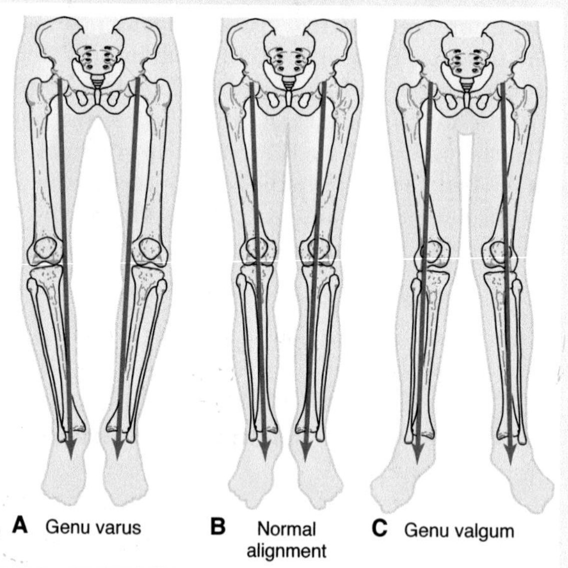

Forces on knee joint with varus and valgus angles.

Muscles of the Knee

Many of the two-joint muscles of the knee were discussed with the hip. All of the knee muscles, except the popliteus, cross the joint in a relatively vertical fashion. Anterior muscles extend the knee, posterior muscles flex the knee, and muscles crossing the medial and lateral sides help provide medial and lateral stability.

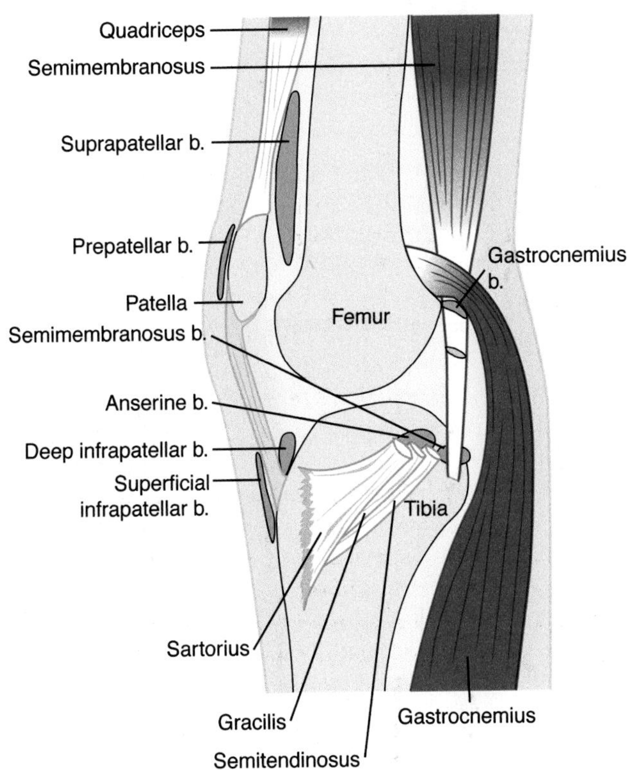

Figure 19-15. Bursae around the knee joint (medial view).

Table 19-1 Bursae of the Knee

Name	Location
Anterior	
Prepatellar	Between patella and skin
Deep infrapatellar	Between proximal tibia and patellar ligament
Superficial infrapatellar	Between tibial tuberosity and skin
Suprapatellar*	Between distal femur and quadriceps tendon
Posterior	
Gastrocnemius*	Between lateral head of gastrocnemius muscle and capsule
Biceps	Between fibular collateral ligament and biceps tendon
Popliteal*	Between popliteus tendon and lateral femoral condyle
Gastrocnemius*	Between medial head of gastrocnemius muscle and capsule
Semimembranosus	Between tendon of semimembranosus muscle and tibia
Lateral	
Iliotibial	Deep to iliotibial band at its distal attachment
Fibular collateral ligament	Deep to fibular collateral ligament, next to the bone
Medial	
Anserine	Deep to sartorius, gracilis, and semitendinosus tendons

*Communicates with knee joint.

However, further clarification of these muscles does need to be made. Table 19-2 shows the muscles that cross the knee, although not all have a major function.

Anterior Muscles

The quadriceps muscles are comprised of four muscles that cross the anterior surface of the knee (Fig. 19-18). The **rectus femoris muscle** is the only one of this group to cross the hip. Its proximal attachment is on the AIIS. It runs almost straight down the thigh, where it is joined by the three vasti muscles and blends into the quadriceps tendon (also called the *patellar tendon*). This tendon encases the patella, crosses the knee joint, and attaches to the tibial tuberosity. Some sources refer to the quadriceps tendon as that tendinous portion above the patella and the patellar tendon as that portion between the patella and the tibial tuberosity. There is not universal agreement, and that distinction will not be made here. The rectus femoris muscle is a prime mover in hip flexion and knee extension.

The three vasti muscles are one-joint muscles, which come together with the rectus femoris in the lower part of the thigh to form a single, very strong, quadriceps tendon before crossing the knee to attach to the tibial tuberosity. The **vastus lateralis muscle** is located lateral to the rectus femoris muscle. It originates from the linea aspera of the femur and spans the thigh laterally to join the other quadriceps muscles at the patella. The **vastus medialis muscle** also comes from the linea aspera, but it spans the thigh medially. Both the vastus lateralis and medialis "wrap around" the femur on their respective sides. Located deep to the rectus femoris muscle is the **vastus intermedialis muscle.** It arises from the anterior surface of the femur and spans the thigh anteriorly in a very vertical direction. It blends together with the other vasti muscles along its length. All four quadriceps muscles attach to the base of the patella and the tibial tuberosity via the patellar tendon.

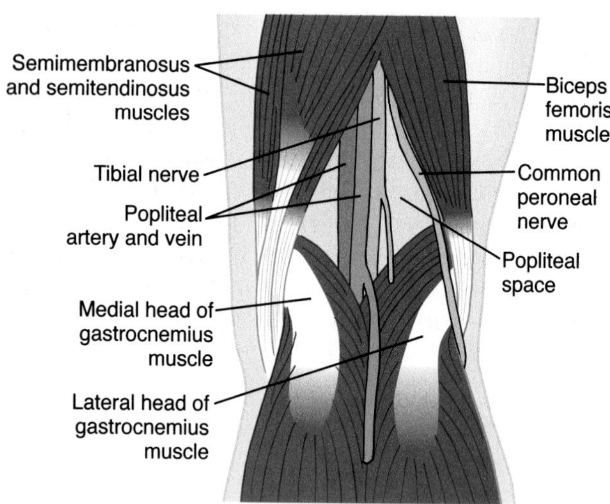

Figure 19-16. Muscular boundaries of the right popliteal space (posterior view).

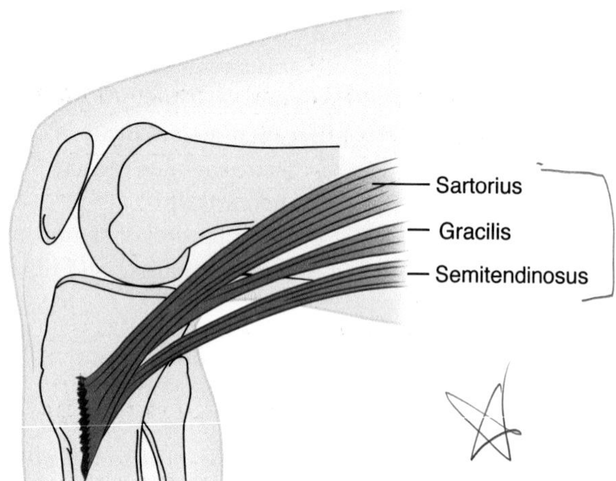

Figure 19-17. Three muscle attachments of pes anserine (medial view).

Table 19-2 Muscles of the Knee

Area	One-Joint Muscle	Two-Joint Muscle
Anterior	Vastus lateralis Vastus medialis Vastus intermedialis	Rectus femoris
Posterior	Biceps femoris (short) Popliteus	Biceps femoris (long) Semimembranosus Semitendinosus Sartorius Gracilis Gastrocnemius
Lateral		Tensor fascia lata

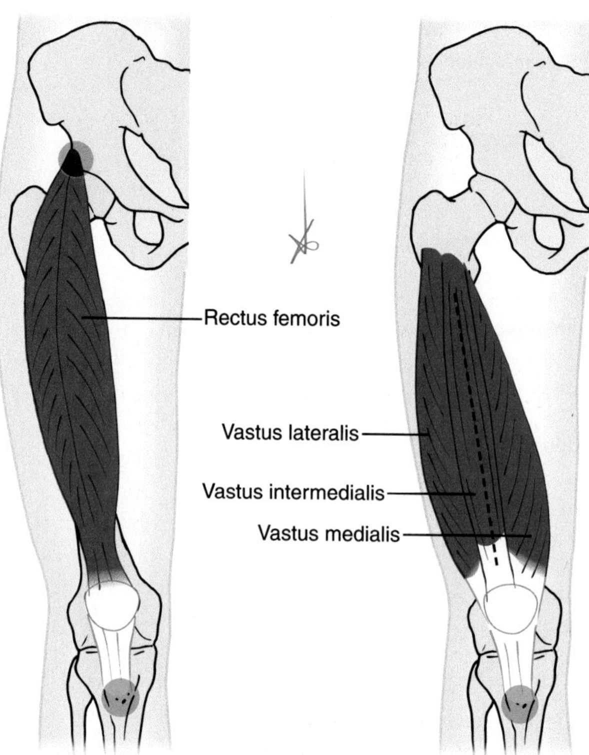

Figure 19-18. Quadriceps muscle group (anterior view). The three vasti muscles lie deep to the rectus femoris. The vastus medialis and lateralis attach proximally on the posterior femur but join the other two muscles to cross the knee anteriorly.

All four muscles span the knee anteriorly, and all extend the knee. Because the rectus femoris muscle also spans the hip anteriorly, it also flexes the hip.

Rectus Femoris Muscle

O	AIIS
I	Tibial tuberosity via patellar tendon
A	Hip flexion and knee extension
N	Femoral nerve (L2, L3, L4)

Vastus Lateralis Muscle

O	Linea aspera
I	Tibial tuberosity via patellar tendon
A	Knee extension
N	Femoral nerve (L2, L3, L4)

Vastus Medialis Muscle

O	Linea aspera
I	Tibial tuberosity via patellar tendon
A	Knee extension
N	Femoral nerve (L2, L3, L4)

	Vastus Intermedialis Muscle
O	Anterior femur
I	Tibial tuberosity via patellar tendon
A	Knee extension
N	Femoral nerve (L2, L3, L4)

Posterior Muscles

Three muscles that are known collectively as the *hamstring muscles* cover the posterior thigh. They consist of the semimembranosus, the semitendinosus, and the biceps femoris muscles (Fig. 19-19). They have a common site of origin on the ischial tuberosity.

The **semimembranosus muscle** runs down the medial side of the thigh deep to the semitendinosus muscle and inserts on the posterior surface of the medial condyle of the tibia. The **semitendinosus muscle** has a much longer and narrower distal tendon that moves anteriorly after spanning the knee joint posteriorly. It attaches to the anteromedial surface of the tibia with the gracilis and sartorius muscles. The **biceps femoris muscle** has two heads and runs laterally down the thigh on the posterior side. The long head arises with the other two hamstring muscles on the ischial tuberosity, but the short head arises from the lateral lip of the linea aspera. Both heads join together, spanning the knee posteriorly to attach laterally on the head of the fibula and, by a small slip, to the lateral condyle of the tibia. The short head of the biceps femoris is the only part of the hamstring muscle group that has a function only at the knee. The other parts have a function at both the hip and the knee.

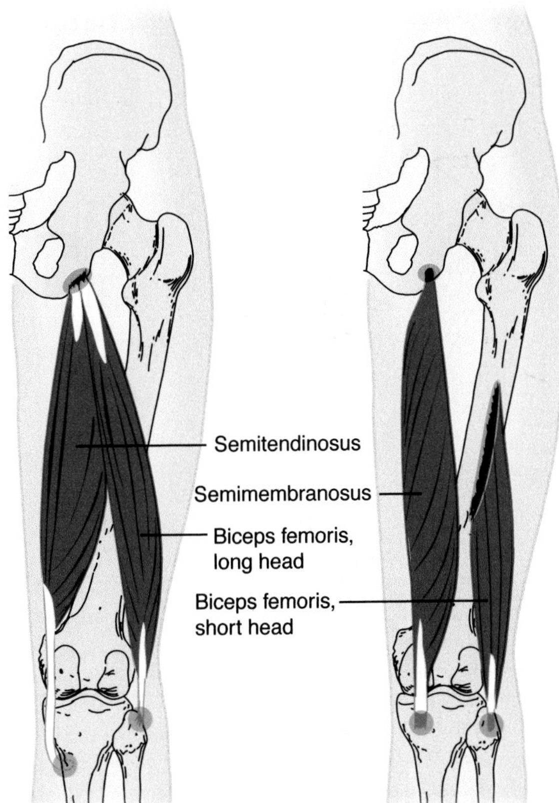

Figure 19-19. Hamstring muscle group (posterior view).

	Semimembranosus Muscle
O	Ischial tuberosity
I	Posterior surface of medial condyle of tibia
A	Hip extension and knee flexion
N	Sciatic nerve (L5, S1, S2)

	Semitendinosus Muscle
O	Ischial tuberosity
I	Anteromedial surface of proximal tibia
A	Extend hip and flex knee
N	Sciatic nerve (L5, S1, S2)

	Biceps Femoris Muscle
O	Long head: ischial tuberosity Short head: lateral lip of linea aspera
I	Fibular head
A	Long head: hip extension and knee flexion Short head: knee flexion
N	Long head: sciatic nerve (S1, S2, S3) Short head: common fibular nerve (L5, S1, S2)

The **popliteus muscle** is a one-joint muscle located posteriorly at the knee in the popliteal space, deep to the two heads of the gastrocnemius muscle (Fig. 19-20). It originates on the lateral side of the lateral condyle of the femur and crosses the knee posteriorly at an oblique angle to insert medially on the posterior proximal tibia. Because it spans the knee posteriorly, it flexes the knee. Because it has an oblique line of pull, it creates the rotational pull needed to "unlock" the knee as it initiates knee flexion.

	Popliteus Muscle
O	Lateral condyle of femur
I	Posterior medial condyle of tibia
A	Initiates knee flexion
N	Tibial nerve (L4, L5, S1)

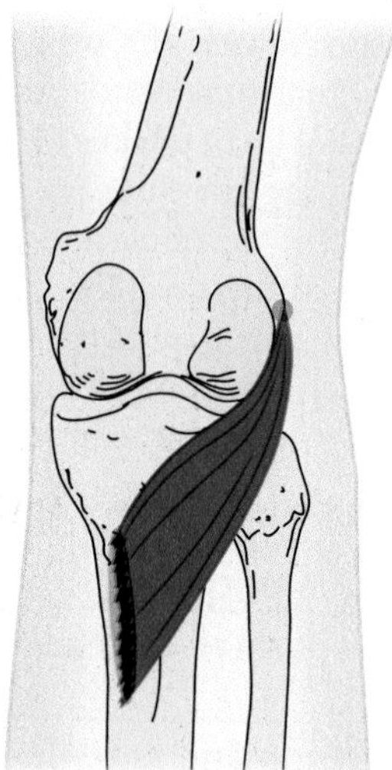

Figure 19-20. Popliteus muscle (posterior view).

The **gastrocnemius muscle** is a two-joint muscle that crosses the knee and the ankle (Fig. 19-21). It is an extremely strong ankle plantar flexor but also has a significant role at the knee. It attaches by two heads to the posterior surface of the medial and lateral condyles of the femur. After descending the posterior leg superficially, it forms a common *Achilles tendon* (often called the *heel cord* by laypersons) with the soleus muscle and attaches to the posterior surface of the calcaneus. Although its major function is at the ankle, it does span the knee posteriorly, has a good angle of pull, and is a large muscle. Therefore, its contribution as a knee flexor cannot be overlooked. In addition, its unusual contribution to knee *extension* has been demonstrated in individuals with no quadriceps muscle function (Fig. 19-22). In a closed kinetic chain action with the foot planted on the ground so that the distal segment (leg) is stationary, the proximal segment (thigh) becomes the movable part. This is also a reversal of muscle action in which the femur is pulled posteriorly, or into knee extension. This feature of the gastrocnemius muscle makes it possible for a person to stand upright without the use of the quadriceps muscles.

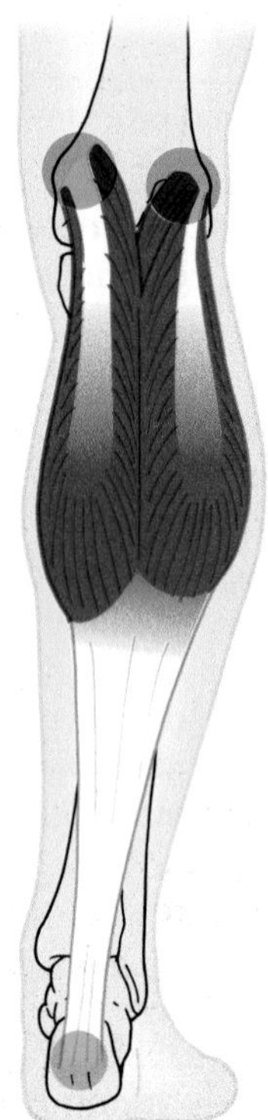

Figure 19-21. Gastrocnemius muscle (posterior view).

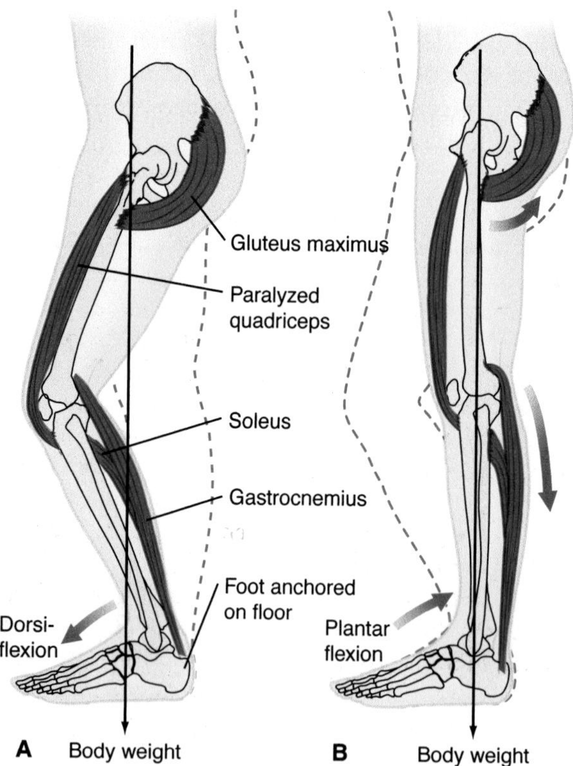

Figure 19-22. Lateral view. **(A)** With a paralyzed quadriceps unable to pull the knee into extension, the body weight line falls behind the knee, causing flexion. However, a combined reverse muscle action of the gluteus maximus and gastrocnemius muscles makes knee extension possible during stance. **(B)** In the closed-chain position, they pull the knee into extension. The soleus assists by plantar flexing the dorsiflexed ankle into a neutral ankle position. This puts the body weight line in front of the knee and ankle axes and allows the knee to remain extended.

Gastrocnemius Muscle

O	Medial and lateral condyles of femur
I	Posterior calcaneus
A	Knee flexion and ankle plantar flexion
N	Tibial nerve (S1, S2)

The gracilis, sartorius, and tensor fascia lata muscles span the knee joint posteriorly, but because of their angle of pull, their size in relation to other muscles, and other factors, they do not have a prime mover function. However, they do provide stability to the joint.

The **tensor fascia lata muscle** spans the knee laterally, essentially in the middle of the joint axis for flexion and extension. It contributes greatly to lateral stability. The **gracilis** and **sartorius muscles** span the knee medially, contributing greatly to medial stability. The gastrocnemius and hamstring muscles provide posterior stability both medially and laterally, and the quadriceps muscles provide anterior stability.

Anatomical Relationships

Muscles cross the knee either anteriorly or posteriorly. The rectus femoris is the most superficial muscle of the anterior group. At the mid- and lower thigh, the vastus lateralis and the vastus medialis are superficial on either side of the rectus femoris (Fig. 19-23). Deep to the rectus femoris and between the two vasti muscles is the vastus intermedialis (Fig. 19-24).

The hamstring muscles are on the posterior thigh. Superficially, the biceps femoris (long head) is on the lateral side, and the semitendinosus is on the medial side. Deep to these muscles is the short head of the biceps femoris (laterally) and the semimembranosus (medially). The deepest muscle at the distal end of the thigh is the popliteus. It lies deep to the proximal heads of the gastrocnemius.

The sartorius crosses the knee on the medial side, anterior to the gracilis, followed more posteriorly by the semitendinosus (pes anserine; see Fig. 19-17). The tensor fascia lata crosses the knee joint laterally by way of the iliotibial band.

Summary of Muscle Action

Table 19-3 summarizes the actions of the prime movers of the knee.

Summary of Muscle Innervation

The femoral and sciatic nerves play a major part in the innervation of the knee joint. The femoral nerve innervates the quadriceps muscle group, and the sciatic nerve innervates the hamstring muscle group.

The other two knee flexors, the popliteus and gastrocnemius muscles, receive innervation from the tibial nerve. (Not included in this discussion or in Table 19-4 are the two-joint hip muscles that span the knee but do not act as prime movers at the knee—the sartorius, gracilis, and tensor fascia lata muscles.) The knee extensors receive innervation from the femoral nerve, which

Clinical Application 19-3

Biomechanical Analysis of Wall Slide Exercise

From a starting position (Fig. A) sliding down a wall moves the knee axis further away from the line of gravity for the body (Fig. B). This increases the resistance arm created by the weight of the body, requiring the quadriceps to produce more force to prevent excessive knee flexion. To meet this demand, the rectus femoris maintains a constant length-tension relationship by shortening at the hip and lengthening at the knee while the one-joint vasti muscles are lengthened over the knee. This brings the entire quadriceps group to optimal length where they can create a large amount of force.

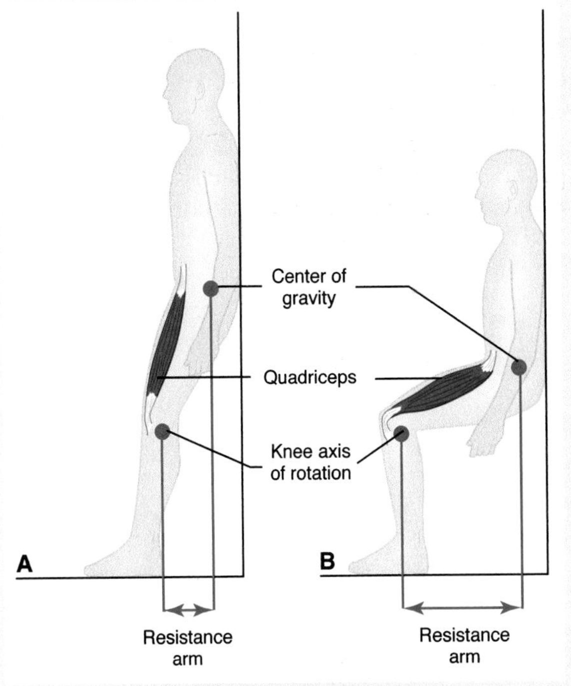

Biomechanical analysis of wall slide exercise

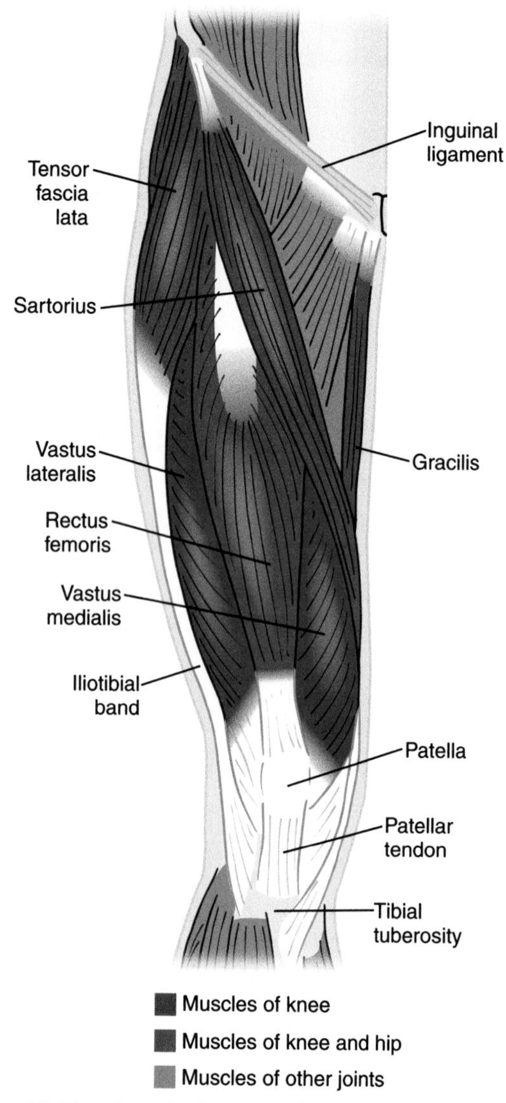

Figure 19-23. Anterior knee muscles (superficial view).

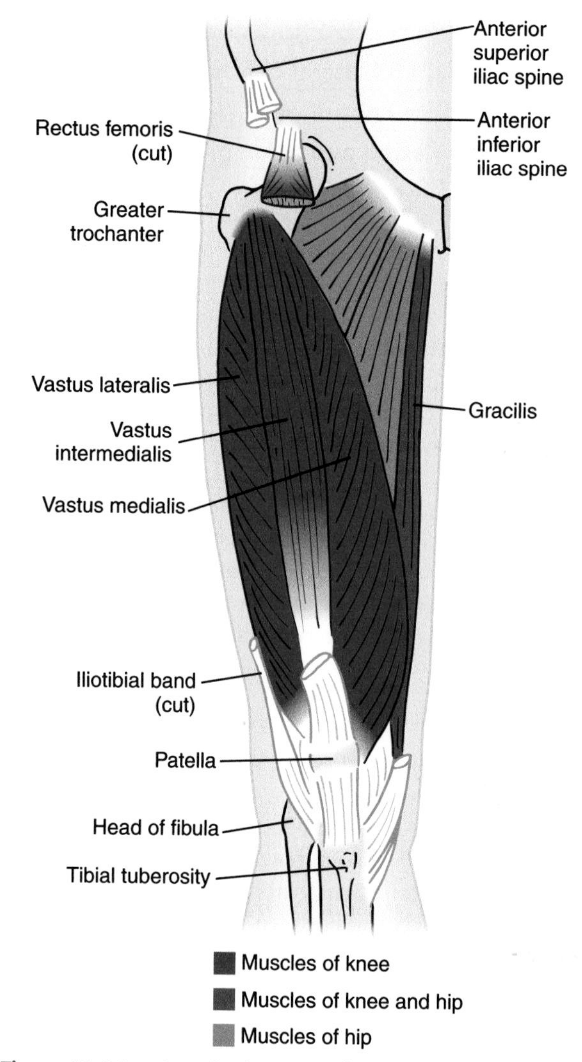

Figure 19-24. Anterior knee muscles (deep view).

comes off the spinal cord at a higher level than does innervation of the knee flexors. This is significant when dealing with individuals with spinal cord injuries. Tables 19-4 and 19-5 summarize the innervation to the knee. It should be noted that there is some discrepancy among various sources regarding spinal cord level of innervation.

Common Knee Pathologies

As shown on page 330, Figure C, **Genu valgum,** also called "knock knees," is a malalignment of the lower extremity in which the distal segments (ankles) are positioned more laterally than normal. The knees tend to touch while the ankles are apart. As shown on page 330, Figure A, **Genu varum** (bowlegs) is the opposite malalignment

Table 19-3 Prime Movers of the Knee

Action	Muscle
Extension	Quadriceps group Rectus femoris Vastus medialis Vastus intermedialis Vastus lateralis
Flexion	Hamstring group Semimembranosus Semitendinosus Biceps femoris Popliteus Gastrocnemius

Table 19-4 Innervation of the Muscles of the Knee

Muscle	Nerve	Spinal Segment
Quadriceps		
Rectus femoris	Femoral	L2, L3, L4
Vastus lateralis	Femoral	L2, L3, L4
Vastus intermedialis	Femoral	L2, L3, L4
Vastus medialis	Femoral	L2, L3, L4
Hamstrings		
Semimembranosus	Sciatic (tibial division)	L5, S1, S2
Semitendinosus	Sciatic (tibial division)	L5, S1, S2
Biceps femoris—long head	Sciatic (tibial division)	S1, S2, S3
Biceps femoris—short head	Sciatic (common fibular division)	L5, S1, S2
Others		
Popliteus	Tibial	L4, L5, S1
Gastrocnemius	Tibial	S1, S2

Table 19-5 Segmental Innervation of the Knee

Spinal Cord Level	L2	L3	L4	L5	S1	S2	S3
Knee Extensors							
Rectus femoris	X	X	X				
Vastus lateralis	X	X	X				
Vastus intermedialis	X	X	X				
Vastus medialis	X	X	X				
Knee Flexors							
Popliteus			X	X	X		
Semitendinosus				X	X	X	
Semimembranosus				X	X	X	
Biceps femoris					X	X	X
Gastrocnemius					X	X	

problem in which the distal segments are positioned more medially than normal. The ankles tend to touch while the knees are apart. Malalignment at one joint often affects alignment at an adjacent joint. Therefore, coxa varus is seen in conjunction with genu valgus, whereas coxa valgus may be seen in conjunction with genu varus. **Genu recurvatum,** also called "back knees," is the positioning of the tibiofemoral joint in which range of motion goes beyond 0 degrees of extension.

Patellar tendonitis, or jumper's knee, is characterized by tenderness at the patellar tendon and results from the overuse stress or sudden impact overloading associated with jumping. It is commonly seen in basketball players, high jumpers, and hurdlers. **Osgood-Schlatter disease** is a common overuse injury among growing adolescents. It is an inflammation involving the traction-type epiphysis (growth plate) on the tibial tuberosity of growing bone where the tendon of the quadriceps muscle attaches. A **popliteal cyst,** or Baker's cyst, is actually misnamed as a "cyst." This general term refers to any synovial hernia or bursitis involving the posterior aspect of the knee.

Although there is no universal agreement on terminology and causation, **patellofemoral pain syndrome** generally refers to a common problem causing diffuse anterior knee pain. It is generally considered the result of a variety of alignment factors, such as increased Q angle, patella alta (high-riding patella), quadriceps weakness or tightness, weakness of hip lateral rotators, and excessive foot pronation. **Chondromalacia patella** is the softening and degeneration of the cartilage on the posterior aspect of the patella, causing anterior knee pain. Abnormal tracking of the patella within the patellofemoral groove causes the patellar articular cartilage to become inflamed, leading to its degeneration. **Prepatellar bursitis** (housemaid's knee) occurs when there is constant pressure between the skin and the patella. It is commonly seen in carpet layers and is the result of repeated direct blows or sheering stresses on the knee.

Terrible triad is a knee injury caused by a single blow to the knee and involves tears to the anterior cruciate ligament, the medial collateral ligament, and the medial meniscus. **Miserable malalignment syndrome** is an alignment problem of the lower extremity involving increased anteversion of the femoral head and is associated with genu valgus, increased tibial torsion, and a pronated flat foot.

Points to Remember

- The body commonly experiences forces such as traction, approximation, shear, bending, and rotation. These forces also have other names.
- The muscle's point of attachment to the bone is used to determine leverage. With a second-class lever, resistance occurs between the axis and the force. With a third-class lever, force is in the middle.
- The longer the force arm, the easier it is to move the part. Conversely, the longer the resistance arm, the harder it is to move the part.
- End feel is the quality of the feel when slight pressure is applied at the end of the joint's passive range.
- An open kinetic chain requires that the distal segment is free to move and the proximal segment(s) remains stationary.
- To stretch a one-joint muscle, it is necessary to put any two-joint muscles on slack over the joint not crossed by the one-joint muscle.
- To contract a two-joint muscle most effectively, start with it being stretched over both joints.
- A muscle becomes actively insufficient when it contracts over all its joints as the same time.
- When determining whether a concentric or eccentric contraction is occurring, decide
  - if the activity is accelerating against gravity or slowing down gravity, or
  - if a weight greater than the pull of gravity is affecting the activity.
- Reversal of muscle action occurs when the origin moves toward the insertion.

Review Questions

General Anatomy Questions

1. Describe the knee joints:
   a. Number of axes:
      Knee ________________
      Patellofemoral ________________
   b. Shape of joint:
      Knee ________________
      Patellofemoral ________________
   c. Type of motion allowed:
      Knee ________________
      Patellofemoral ________________
2. Describe knee joint motion in terms of planes and axes.
3. What is the "Q angle"? Why is it important?
4. Which bones make up the knee joint?
5. Why is the action of the popliteus muscle often described as "unlocking" the joint?
6. What is the pes anserine?
7. An individual with a spinal cord injury at L3 would be expected to have what knee motion?
8. In Figure 19-22:
   a. What type of kinetic chain activity is demonstrated?
   b. Is it possible for the muscles to perform this function in either an open or closed kinetic chain?
   c. Is either the gastrocnemius or gluteus maximus muscle working in a reversal of muscle action role?

Review Questions—cont'd

9. A snowboarder catches an edge and falls. His board twists in one direction as his body twists in the opposite direction. What is the most likely type of force experienced at the knee?
10. When assessing the knee collateral ligaments, the examiner pulls laterally on your ankle while pushing medially on your knee.
    a. What type of load is placed on your lower extremity?
    b. Which side of your knee undergoes a tensile stress?
    c. Which side of your knee undergoes a compressive stress?
11. In the open chain:
    a. The tibia rotates in a (an) ___lateral___ direction during the last few degree of knee extension.
    b. This happens because the ___lateral___ femoral condyle is shorter and runs out of articular surface before the tibia reaches full extension.
    c. If this extension was happening in the closed chain, rather than seeing tibial rotation, the femur would instead rotate in a (an) ___medial___ direction.

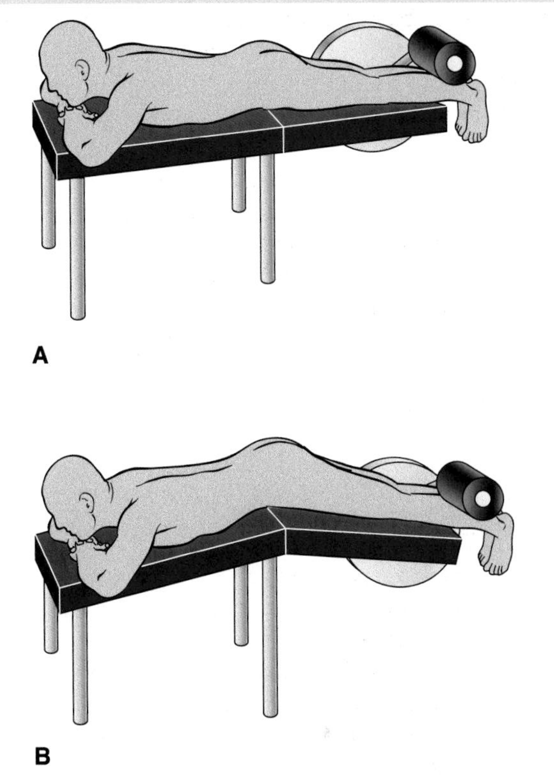

Figure 19-25. Bench positions for hamstring curl exercise.

Functional Activity Questions

1. Analyze the person's position lying on the two benches illustrated in Figure 19-25 to determine whether one is more advantageous than the other for strengthening the hamstrings by doing leg curls. Note that the knees remain extended in both positions.
    a. What is the hamstring action at the hip and at the knee?
    b. What is the position of the hips in Figure 19-25A?
    c. What is the position of the hips in Figure 19-25B?
    d. In what position would the hamstrings be actively insufficient?
    e. Which person's position on the bench will more effectively work the hamstrings?
    f. Why?
2. Analyze the person's sitting positions illustrated in Figure 19-26 to determine whether one is more advantageous than the other for strengthening the knee extensors. Knee extension is the motion being performed.
    a. What are the hip positions in Figures 19-26A and 19-26B?
    b. What are the names of the one-joint muscles performing the knee extension?
    c. What is the name of the two-joint muscle, and what hip and knee motions does it perform?
    d. Describe the length-tension effect on these muscles in each position.
    e. Which person's position will more effectively work the rectus femoris?
    f. Which person's position will more effectively work the vasti muscles?
3. What is the sequence of right-knee motions when stepping up onto a curb leading with the right foot, starting with the right knee extended?
    a. Placing right foot up on curb
    b. Bringing left foot up on curb
4. Identify the sequence of knee motions (starting with the knee in extension) for kicking a ball, and identify the activity of the rectus femoris during each phase.
    a. What is the knee motion when preparing to kick?
    b. Over what joints is the rectus femoris being elongated?
    c. What is the knee motion when making ball contact?

(continued on next page)

Review Questions—cont'd

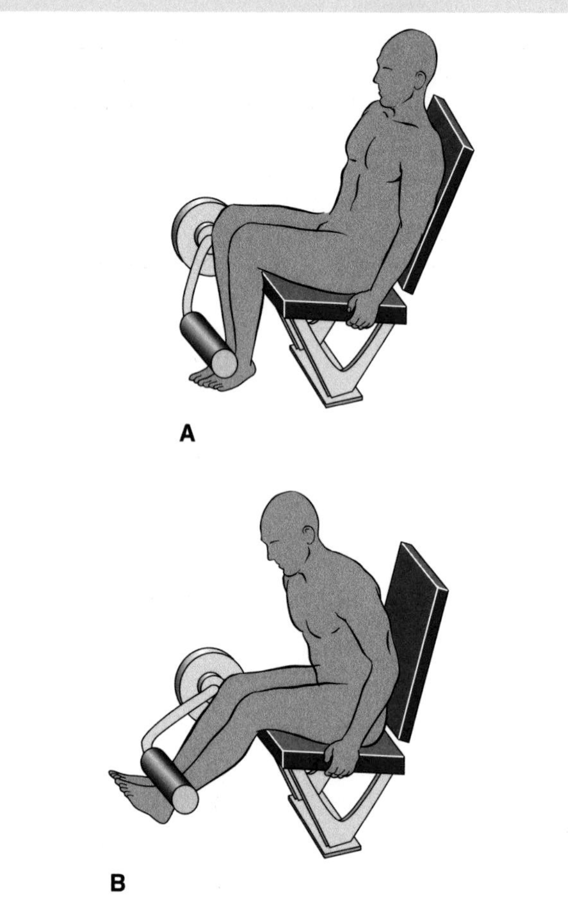

Figure 19-26. Starting positions for knee extension exercise.

d. What is happening to the rectus femoris at the knee during ball contact?
e. What is the knee motion during follow-through?
f. What is happening to the rectus femoris during follow-through?

5. What compensatory motions may occur when stepping up onto a curb if your right leg were in a long leg cast?
   a. Which would be the leading leg?
   b. What pelvic motion would assist in getting the right leg up onto the curb?

Clinical Exercise Questions

1. What types of exercises are occurring during a "wall sit"? Keeping the head, shoulders, and back against the wall with your feet shoulder-width apart, slowly slide down the wall until the thighs are almost parallel to the floor. Hold that position for the count of five. Return to the starting position.

   During the slide-down phase:
   a. What is the knee motion?
   b. What type of contraction (isometric, concentric, or eccentric) is occurring?
   c. What muscles are performing this action?
   d. Is this an open- or closed-chain activity?

   During the holding phase:
   a. What type of contraction (isometric, concentric, or eccentric) is occurring?
   b. What muscles are performing this action?

   During the return phase:
   a. What is the knee motion?
   b. What type of contraction (isometric, concentric, or eccentric) is occurring?
   c. What muscles are performing this action?

2. Sit on the edge of a table with your right leg resting on the table and your left leg over the side with your left foot on the floor. Keeping the back and right leg straight, lean forward at the right hip. See Figure 19-27 for the starting position.
   a. What are the right hip and knee motions?
   b. Is stretching or strengthening occurring?
   c. What muscles are involved?

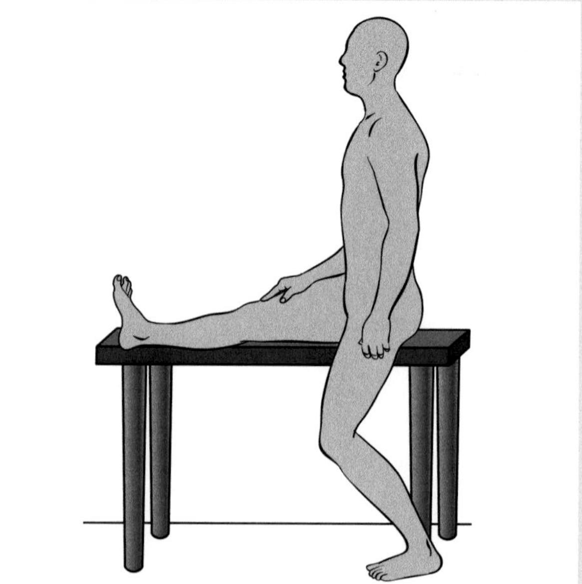

Figure 19-27. Starting position.

Review Questions—cont'd

3. Lying supine, raise your right leg up toward the ceiling about 24 inches, keeping your right knee straight.
   a. What are the right hip and knee motions?
   b. Is stretching or strengthening occurring?
   c. What muscles are involved?
   d. Is this an open- or closed-chain activity?
4. Standing on your left leg and holding on to something for balance, bend your right knee and grasp your right foot. Slowly pull your right heel toward your right buttock.
   a. What are the right hip and knee motions?
   b. Is stretching or strengthening occurring?
   c. What muscles are involved?
5. When performing passive range of motion (PROM) on an individual's knee, the end feel for flexion should be ____________ and ______________ for extension.
6. Sit on the edge of a table with a 10-pound weight on your ankle. Hold each of the following positions for 30 seconds:
   - Knee fully extended (position A)
   - Knee flexed 30 degrees (position B)
   - Knee flexed 60 degrees (position C)

   a. Which position is easiest to hold? Which is most difficult?
   b. Identify the force, resistance, axis, and lever class.
   c. How does the resistance arm length change as you move from position A to position C?
   d. How does the force arm length change as you switch positions?
7. In a standing position, loop an elastic band around the back of your knee and anchor the other end around a heavy table leg or in a doorjamb. You may want to pad the back of the knee with a small towel. Face the anchor point and be far enough away so that there is sufficient tension in the elastic band (Fig. 19-28). From a partly flexed position, slowly straighten the knee, and keep the foot on the floor.

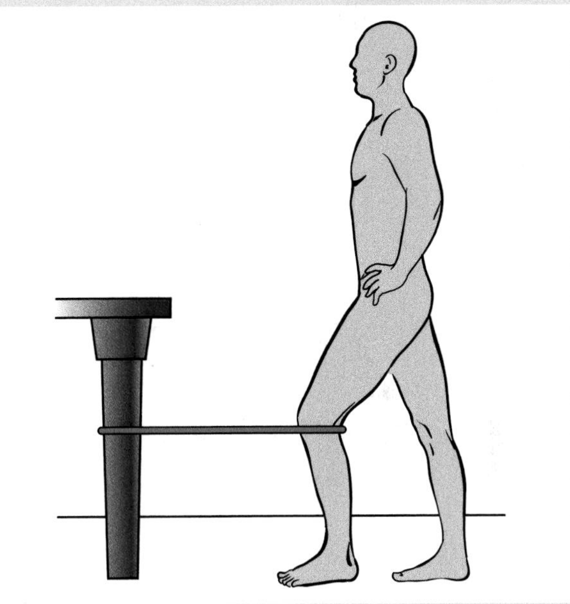

Figure 19-28. Starting position.

(continued on next page)

Review Questions—cont'd

Hold for the count of five, and then bend it (returning to starting position).

Straighten phase:

a. What knee motion is occurring?
b. What type of contraction is occurring?
c. What muscles are involved?
d. Is this an open- or closed-chain activity?

Holding phase:

a. What is the position of the knee?
b. What type of contraction is occurring?
c. What muscles are involved?

Bending phase:

a. What knee motion is occurring?
b. What type of contraction is occurring?
c. What muscles are involved?

8. A clinician is applying force to the lower leg of a patient who is trying to extend the knee (Fig. 19-29). Can the clinician apply more force to the patient's leg by pushing down just below the knee (A) or just above the ankle (B)? Why?

Just above the ankle
Resistance is further away from axis

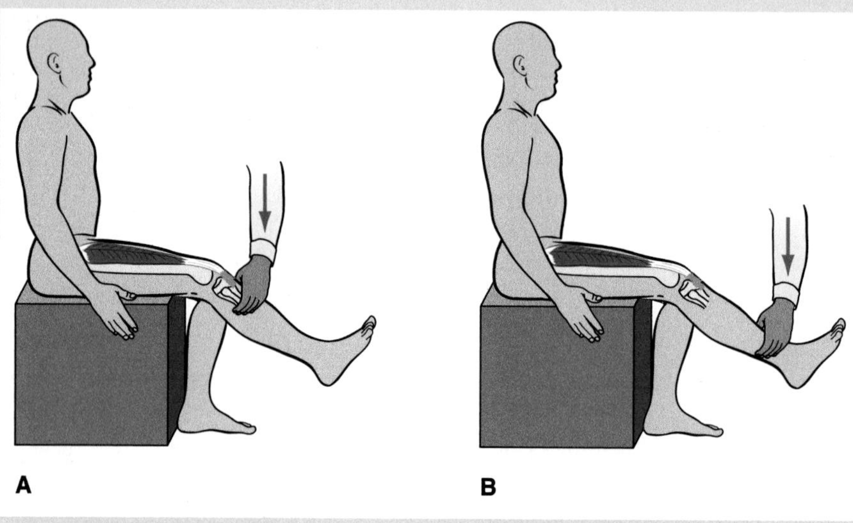

Figure 19-29. Point of applied force.

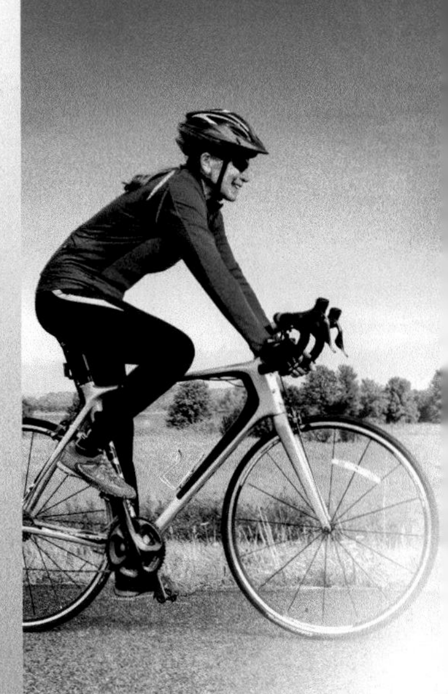

CHAPTER 20
Ankle Joint and Foot

Bones and Landmarks
Functional Aspects of the Foot
Joints and Motions
Terminology
Ankle Joints
Motion at the Ankle Joint
Foot Joints
Ligaments and Other Structures
Arches
Muscles of the Ankle and Foot
Extrinsic Muscles
Intrinsic Muscles
Anatomical Relationships
Summary of Muscle Innervation
Common Ankle Pathologies
Points to Remember
Review Questions
General Anatomy Questions
Functional Activity Questions
Clinical Exercise Questions

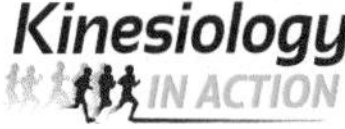

For additional practice activities and videos, please visit www.kinesiologyinaction.com

The leg (the portion of the lower extremity extending from the knee to the ankle) consists of the tibia and fibula. A strong interosseous membrane keeps the two bones together and provides a greater surface area for muscle attachment (Fig. 20-1).

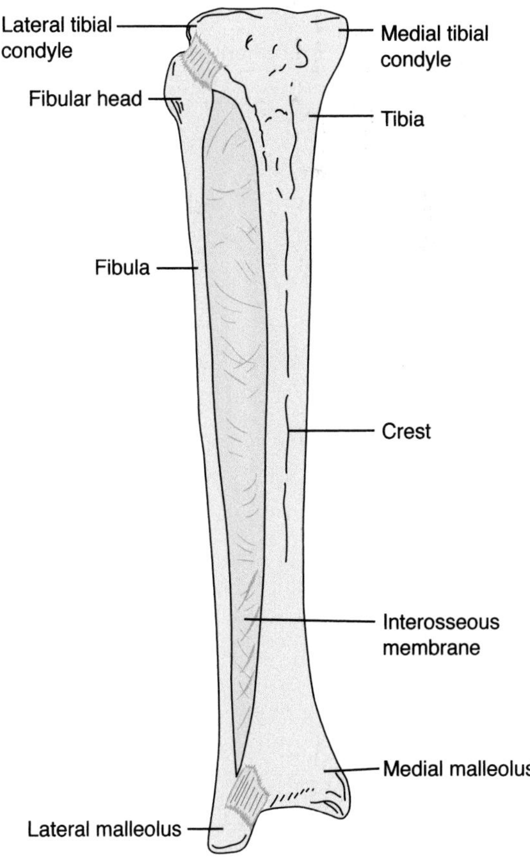

Figure 20-1. Leg bones and interosseous membrane (anterior view).

Bones and Landmarks

The tibia, the larger of the two bones, is the only true weight-bearing bone of the leg. Triangular in shape, the tibia's apex (crest) is located anteriorly. The long, thin fibula is set back in line with the posterior surface of the tibia (Fig. 20-2). Lateral to the tibia, the fibula forms a channel, with the interosseous membrane as the floor; this permits attachment of several muscles without distorting the shape of the leg. Landmarks of the **tibia** and fibula pertaining to the ankle are listed below (see Fig. 20-1).

Important Bony Landmarks of the Tibia and Fibula

Medial Condyle (Tibia)
Proximal medial end

Lateral Condyle (Tibia)
Proximal lateral end

Crest (Tibia)
Anterior and most prominent of the three borders

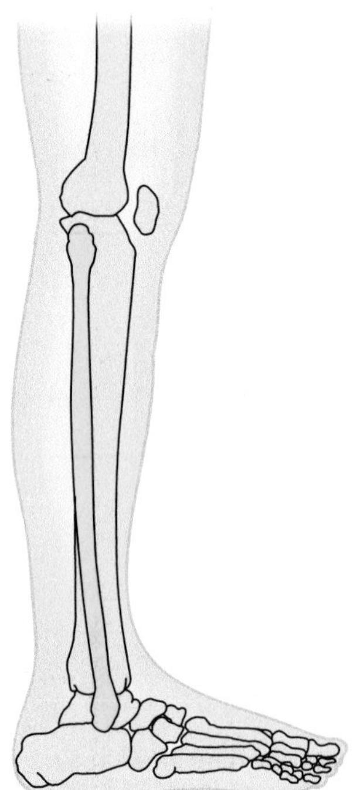

Figure 20-2. Right leg (lateral view). Note the posterior position of the fibula.

Medial Malleolus (Tibia)
Enlarged distal medial surface

Head (Fibula)
Enlarged proximal end

Lateral Malleolus (Fibula)
Enlarged distal end

The bones of the foot include the tarsals, metatarsals, and phalanges. The seven **tarsal bones** and their landmarks are listed below (Fig. 20-3).

Important Bony Landmarks of the Tarsal Bones

Calcaneus
Largest and most posterior tarsal bone

Calcaneal Tuberosity
Projection on the posterior inferior surface of the calcaneus

Sustentaculum Tali
Medial superior part projecting out from the rest of the calcaneus, supporting the medial side of the talus. Three tendons loop around this projection, changing directions from the posterior leg to the plantar foot.

Talus
Sitting on the calcaneus, it is the second largest tarsal

Navicular
On the medial side, in front of the talus and proximal to the three cuneiforms

Tuberosity of Navicular
Projection on the medial side of the navicular; easily seen on the medial border of the foot

Cuboid
On the lateral side of the foot, proximal (superior) to the fourth and fifth metatarsals and distal (inferior) to the calcaneus

Cuneiforms
Three in number and named the first through third, going from the medial toward the lateral side in line with the metatarsals. The first is the largest of the three.

The **metatarsals** (see Fig. 20-3) are numbered 1 through 5, starting medially. Normally, the first and fifth metatarsals are weight-bearing bones, and the second, third, and fourth are not. We tend to stand on a triangle. Weight is borne from the base of the calcaneus to the heads of the

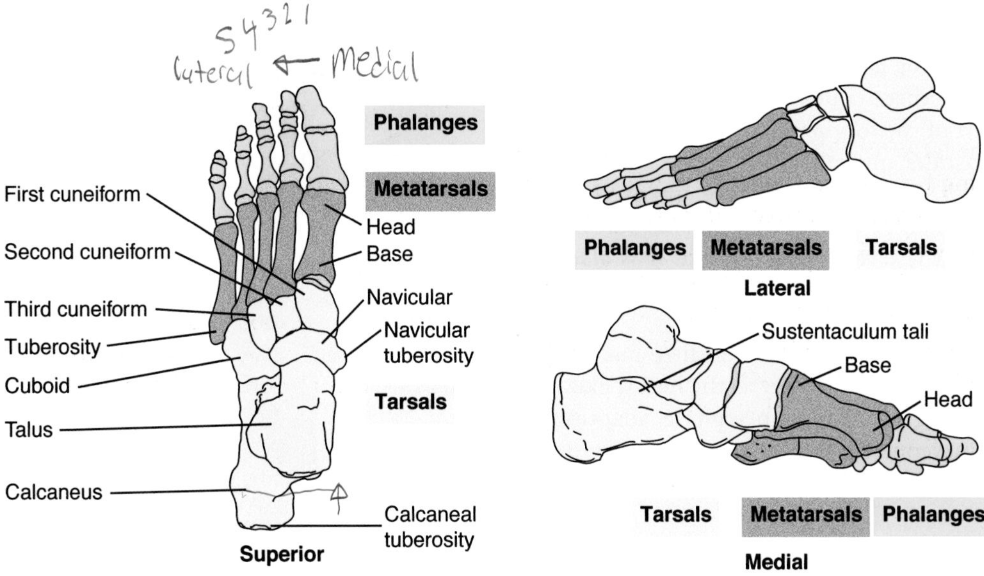

Figure 20-3. Bones of the left foot (superior, lateral, and medial views).

first and fifth metatarsals. The significant features and landmarks of the metatarsals are listed below.

Important Bony Landmarks of the Metatarsals

Base
Proximal end of each metatarsal

Head
Distal end of each bone

First
Thickest and shortest metatarsal; located on the medial side of the foot; articulates with the first cuneiform

Second
Longest; articulates with the second cuneiform

Third
Articulates with the third cuneiform

Fourth
Together with the fifth metatarsal, articulates with the cuboid

Fifth
Has prominent tuberosity located on the lateral side of its base

The **phalanges** of the foot have the same composition as those of the hand (see Fig. 20-3). The first digit, the **great toe,** has a proximal and distal phalanx but no middle phalanx. The second through fifth digits, also called the four **lesser toes,** each have a proximal, middle, and distal phalanx.

Functional Aspects of the Foot

The foot can be divided into three parts (Fig. 20-4). The hindfoot is made up of the talus and calcaneus. In the gait cycle, the hindfoot is the first part of the foot that makes contact with the ground, thus influencing the function and movement of the other two

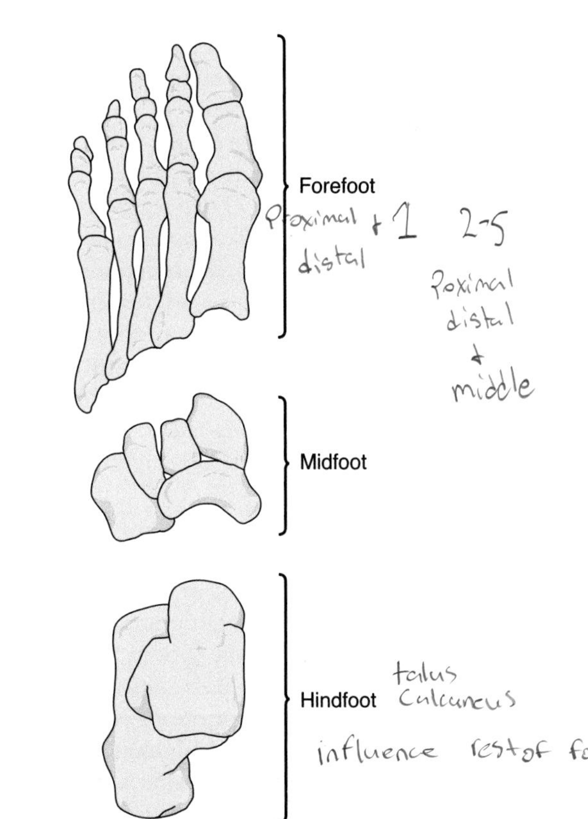

Figure 20-4. Functional areas of the foot (superior view).

parts. The midfoot is made up of the navicular, the cuboid, and the three cuneiform bones. The mechanics of this part of the foot provide stability and mobility as it transmits movement from the hindfoot to the forefoot. The forefoot is made up of the five metatarsals and all of the phalanges. This part of the foot adapts to the level of the ground. It is also the last part of the foot to make contact with the ground during stance phase.

The ankle joint and foot perform three main functions: acting as a shock absorber as the heel strikes the ground at the beginning of stance phase, adapting to the level (or unevenness) of the ground, and providing a stable base of support from which to propel the body forward.

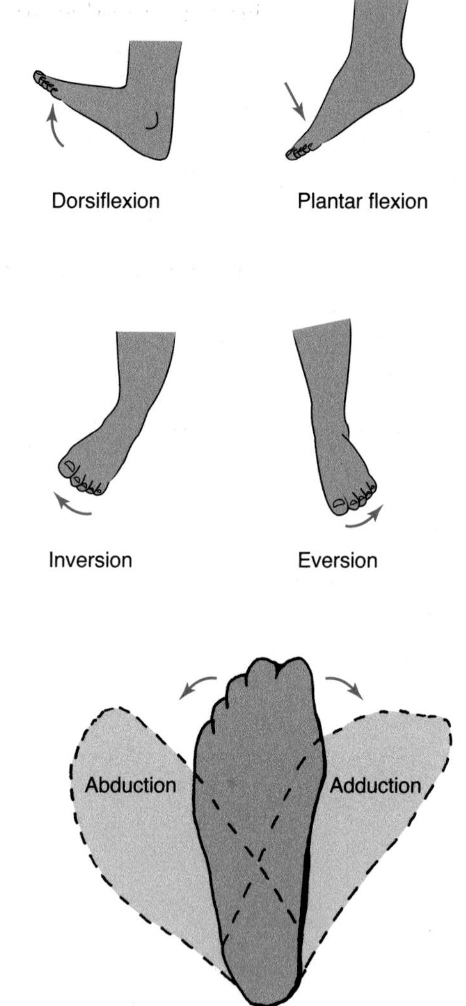

Figure 20-5. Ankle joint and foot motions.

Joints and Motions

Terminology

Motions of the ankle joint and foot need to be defined because there is not uniform agreement among authors (Fig. 20-5). **Plantar flexion** is movement toward the plantar surface of the foot, whereas **dorsiflexion** occurs when the dorsal surface of the foot moves toward the anterior surface of the leg. These motions occur in the *sagittal plane around the frontal axis.* Due to conflicting definitions, the terms **flexion** and **extension** should not be used. As a case in point, functionally speaking, plantar flexion is the same as extension in that it is part of the general extension movement of the hip, knee, and ankle. Anatomically speaking, plantar flexion is not a true flexion because there is no approximation of two segments.

Movements in the *frontal plane around the sagittal axis* are called *inversion* and *eversion.* **Inversion** is the raising of the medial border of the foot, turning the forefoot inward. **Eversion,** the opposite motion, is the raising of the lateral border of the foot, turning the forefoot outward. Movements in the transverse plane are called **adduction** and **abduction.** These motions occur primarily in the forefoot and accompany inversion and eversion, respectively.

Although the cardinal plane motions above offer a nice description of ankle and foot motion, in reality, the axis of motion for each joint in the ankle region is oriented at an angle. Therefore, motion at any given joint happens in an oblique plane (not in a cardinal plane). Because the axis is said to pass somewhere *between* the three cardinal planes of motion, the axis and resulting motion can be described as **triplanar** (see Fig. 20-9). To better define the triplanar motion that occurs, clinicians have begun using the terms *supination* and *pronation.* Depending on the particular joint, and the exact orientation of its axis, some of the cardinal plane component motions will predominate more than other. This will be covered in the sections below.

In recent years, clinicians have begun using *supination* and *pronation* to describe ankle joint and foot motion. **Supination** describes a combination of plantar flexion, inversion, and adduction, and **pronation** describes a combination of dorsiflexion, eversion, and abduction. In summary, the terminology commonly used by clinicians to describe ankle and foot motions are *dorsiflexion, plantar flexion, supination* (a combination of plantar flexion, inversion, and forefoot adduction), and *pronation* (a combination of dorsiflexion, eversion, and forefoot abduction). However, when describing muscle action, *dorsiflexion/plantar flexion* and *inversion/eversion* will be used. These motions are illustrated in Figure 20-5.

To avoid further confusion of terms, *valgus* and *varus* must be defined. These terms are more commonly used to describe a *position,* usually an abnormal one. **Valgus** refers to a position in which the distal segment is situated away from the midline. Conversely, **varus** refers to a position in which the distal segment is located toward the midline. Therefore, a calcaneal valgus is a position in which the distal (inferior) part of the calcaneus is angled away from the midline (Fig. 20-6). These terms will not be used here because *motion,* not *position,* is the emphasis.

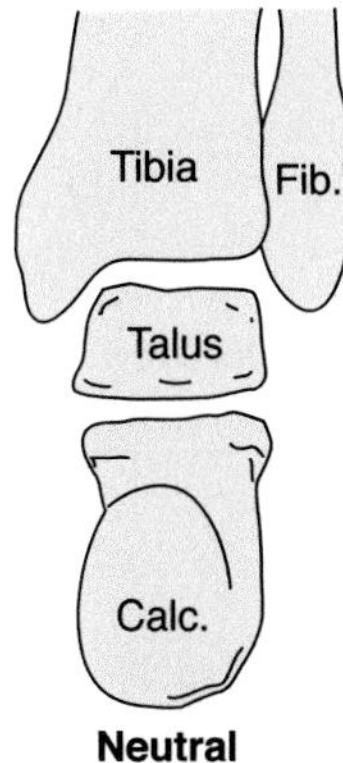

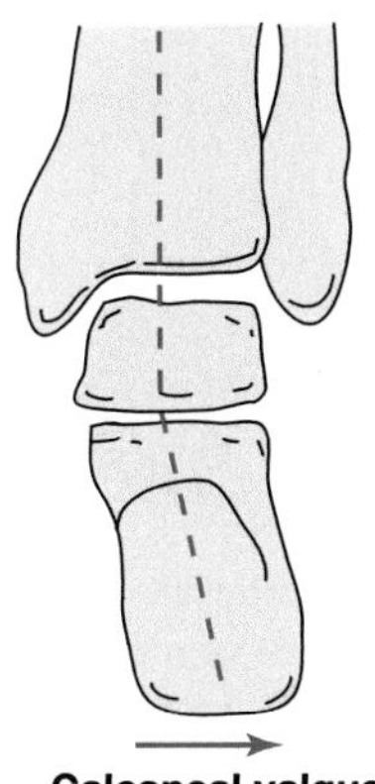

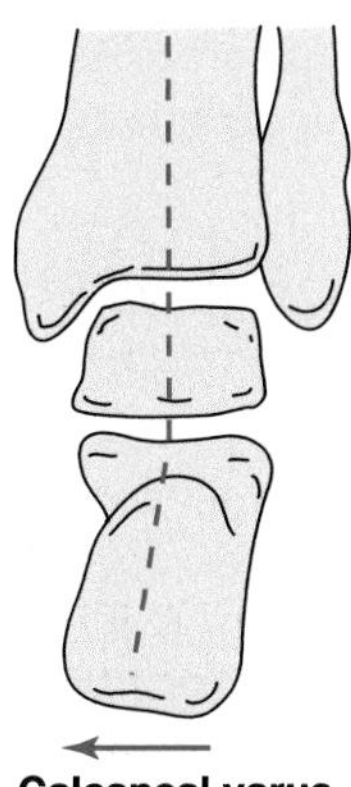

Figure 20-6. Calcaneal positions.

Ankle Joints

Joints of the Leg

Two joints, with little motion, that are not part of the true ankle joint but that play a small role in the proper function of the ankle are the tibiofibular joints (Fig. 20-7). The **superior tibiofibular joint** is the articulation between the head of the fibula and the posterior lateral aspect of the proximal tibia. It is a plane joint that allows a relatively small amount of gliding and rotation of the fibula on the tibia. Being a synovial joint, it has a joint capsule. Ligaments reinforce the capsule, and the joint functions to dissipate the torsional stresses applied at the ankle joint. The **inferior tibiofibular joint** is a syndesmosis (fibrous union) between the concave distal tibia and the convex distal fibula. Because it is not a synovial joint, there is no joint capsule. However, fibrous tissue separates the bones and several ligaments that hold the joint together. Much of the ankle joint's strength depends on a strong union at this joint. The ligaments holding the inferior tibiofibular joint together allow slight movement to accommodate the motion of the talus.

Talocrural Joint

The true **ankle joint** (*talocrural joint* or *talotibial joint*) is made up of the distal tibia, which sits on the talus with

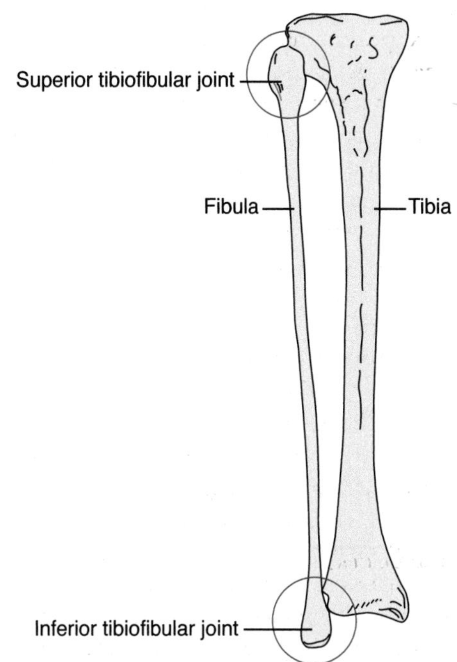

Figure 20-7. The two tibiofibular joints (anterior view).

the medial malleolus of the tibia fitting down around the medial aspect of the talus, and the lateral malleolus of the fibula, which fits down around the lateral aspect of the talus. This type of joint is often described using a carpentry term: *tenon and mortise joint.* A mortise is a notch that is cut in a piece of wood to receive a projecting piece (tenon) shaped to fit. Therefore, the malleoli of the tibia and fibula would be the mortise, and the talus would be the tenon (Fig. 20-8). This joint connects the leg and foot and is responsible for controlling the majority of foot motion relative to the leg.

In summary, the ankle is a uniaxial hinge joint consisting of an articulation of the talus with the distal end and medial malleolus of the tibia and the lateral malleolus of the fibula. The ankle joint allows approximately 30 to 50 degrees of plantar flexion and 20 degrees of dorsiflexion. In the anatomical position, the ankle is in a neutral position. Because the axis of rotation is at an angle, it is considered **triplanar** (Fig. 20-9), a term used to describe motion around an obliquely oriented axis that passes through all three planes. The lateral malleolus extends more distally and lies more posteriorly than the medial malleolus. To visualize the triplanar axis place the ends of your index fingers at the distal ends of the malleoli on your left ankle (Fig. 20-9). Notice that when viewed from above, the finger on the lateral malleolus side is more posterior. When viewed from the front, the finger over the lateral mallelous is more distal. Imagine the fingers as a straight rod passing through the joint. Notice that the fingers do not line up in a pure side-to-side direction. The left finger is slightly posterior and inferior while the right finger is slightly anterior and superior. This line essentially represents the axis of the ankle joint. It tips approximately 8 degrees from the transverse plane, 82 degrees from sagittal plane, and 20 to 30 degrees from the frontal plane. During ankle dorsiflexion, the foot not only comes up but also moves out slightly (abduction). During ankle plantar flexion, the foot moves down and in (adduction).

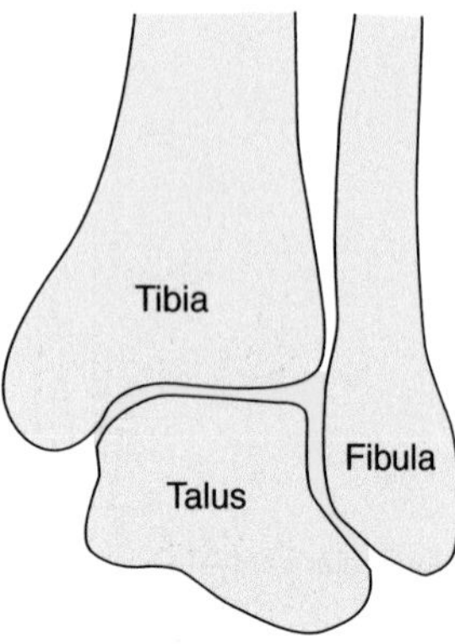

Figure 20-8. Ankle joint (posterior view).

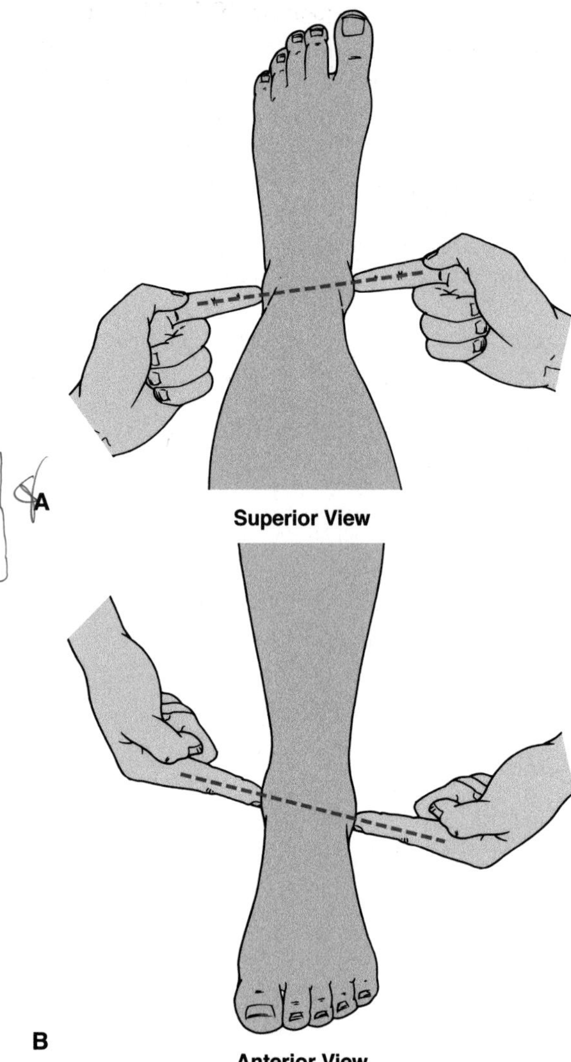

Figure 20-9. Triplanar axis of motion for the left ankle joint. **(A)** Superior view. **(B)** Anterior view.

The end feel of both dorsiflexion and plantar flexion is firm and is classified as soft tissue stretch. This is due to the tension of the joint capsule, ligaments, and tendons.

Motion at the Ankle Joint

In an open kinetic chain, with the leg fixed and the foot free to move, the angle of the joint axis causes the foot to abduct during dorsiflexion and adduct during plantar flexion. The opposite action occurs with a closed chain. With the foot fixed and the leg moving over it, the angle of the joint axis causes the leg to medially rotate on the foot. During ankle plantar flexion when the foot is fixed on the ground, the leg laterally rotates on the foot. This rotation is allowed because of the slight movement that is possible at the tibiofibular joints. It is an accessory movement much like the rotation of the CMC joint of the thumb. This rotation is not possible to do in an open chain. Table 20-1 summarizes the motions of the ankle and foot.

Arthrokinematics

In terms of arthrokinematic motion, the convex talus glides posteriorly on the concave tibia during ankle dorsiflexion and glides anteriorly during ankle plantar flexion. This is illustrated in Figure 20-10.

Subtalar and Transverse Tarsal Joints

The **subtalar,** or talocalcaneal, **joint** consists of the inferior surface of the talus articulating with the superior surface of the calcaneus (Fig. 20-11). It is a plane synovial joint with 1 degree of freedom. The motions of inversion and eversion occur around an oblique axis.

Table 20-1 Ankle and Foot Motions

	Ankle Dorsiflexion	Ankle Plantar Flexion
Open Kinetic Chain		
Leg fixed		
Foot moves	Foot abducts	Foot adducts
Closed Kinetic Chain		
Foot fixed		
Leg moves	Leg medially rotates	Leg laterally rotates

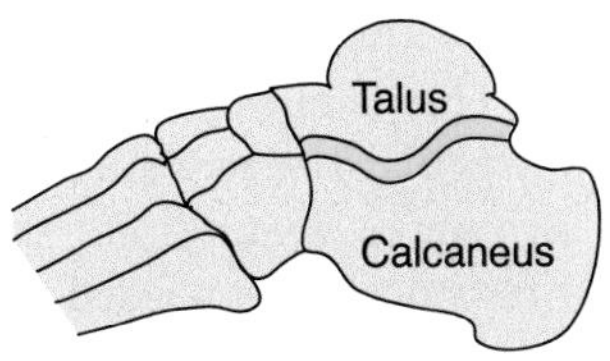

Figure 20-11. Subtalar joint (lateral view).

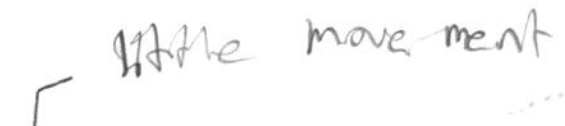

The **transverse tarsal joint** (midtarsal joint; Fig. 20-12) is made up of the anterior surfaces of the talus and calcaneus articulating with the posterior surfaces of the navicular and the cuboid, respectively. Although they lie next to each other, very little movement occurs between the navicular and the cuboid. The motions of the transverse tarsal joint link the hindfoot and forefoot in inversion and eversion.

Because the motions of these two joints occur on an oblique axis (triplanar), they are combinations of movements. Functionally, the subtalar and transverse tarsal joints cannot be separated. For the sake of simplicity, *inversion/eversion* will be used to describe motions occurring at both the subtalar and transtarsal joints. **Inversion** will include a combination of adduction, supination, and plantar flexion, whereas **eversion** will include a combination of abduction, pronation, and dorsiflexion. Therefore, plantar flexion and dorsiflexion occur primarily at the talocrural joint. Inversion and eversion occur primarily at the subtalar and transverse tarsal joints. The combined motions of

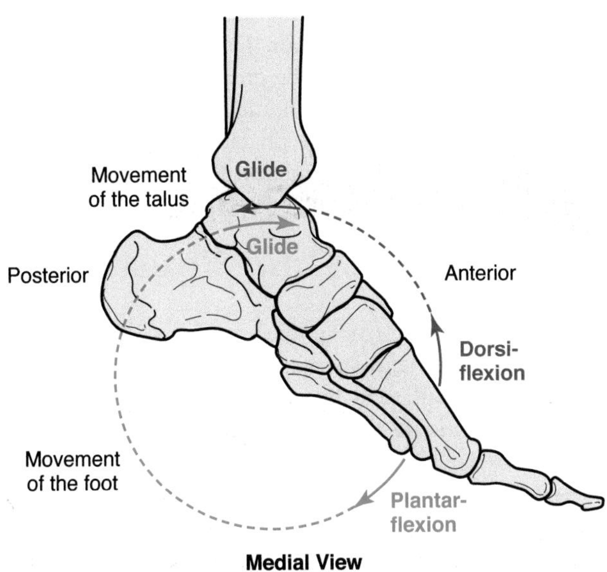

Figure 20-10. Arthrokinematic motion for ankle dorsiflexion/plantar flexion.

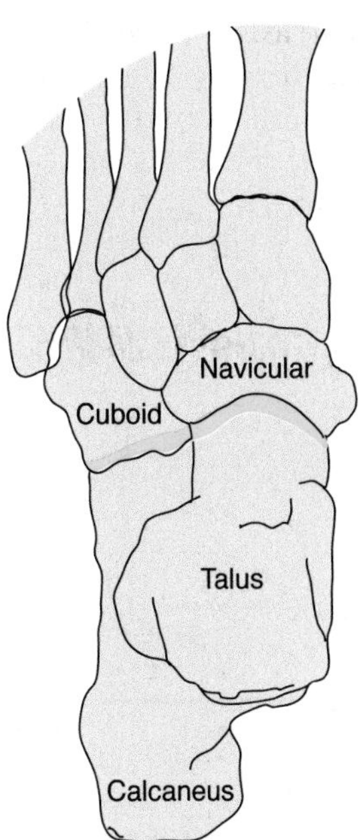

Figure 20-12. Transverse tarsal joint (superior view).

all these joints allow the foot to assume almost any position in space. This is quite useful in allowing the foot to adapt to irregular surfaces such as those found when walking on uneven ground. For example, think about the many foot positions needed when climbing on rocks at the beach or in the mountains.

Foot Joints

The **metatarsophalangeal (MTP)** joints consist of the metatarsal heads articulating with the proximal phalanges (Fig. 20-13). Like the metacarpophalangeal joints of the hand, there are five joints allowing flexion, extension, hyperextension, abduction, and adduction (Fig. 20-14). The first MTP joint is the most mobile. It allows approximately 45 degrees of flexion and extension and 90 degrees of hyperextension. The second through fifth MTP joints allow about 40 degrees of flexion and extension and only about 45 degrees of hyperextension. Hyperextension is very important during the toe-off phase of walking. The point of reference for abduction and adduction is the second toe. Like the middle finger, the second toe abducts in both directions but adducts only as a return motion from abduction.

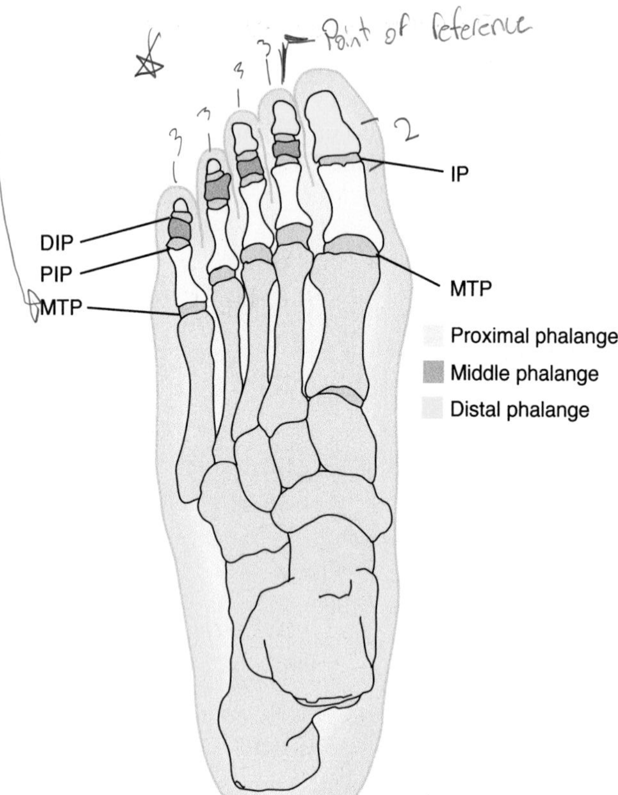

Figure 20-13. Joints of the phalanges of the foot (superior view). Note that the great toe has only two joints, whereas the four lesser toes have three.

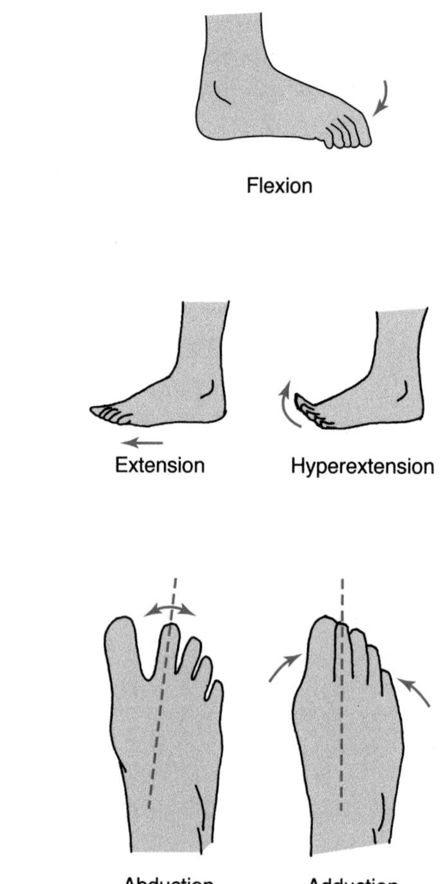

Figure 20-14. Toe motions.

Also like the hand, each of the lesser toes (2 through 5) has a **proximal interphalangeal (PIP)** and a **distal interphalangeal (DIP) joint.** Individually, these joints are not as significant as they are in the hand because the foot requires less dexterity. The great toe has a proximal and distal phalanx but no middle phalange. Therefore, like the thumb, it has only one phalangeal joint, the **interphalangeal (IP) joint** (see Fig. 20-13).

Ligaments and Other Structures

The ankle joint, a synovial joint, has a joint capsule. This **capsule** is rather thin anteriorly and posteriorly but is reinforced by collateral ligaments on the sides. These collateral ligaments are actually groups of several ligaments. The collateral ligament on the medial side is a triangular **deltoid ligament** whose apex is located along the tip of the medial malleolus. Its broad base spreads out to attach to the talus, navicular, and calcaneus in four parts (Fig. 20-15). The anterior fibers attach to the navicular (tibionavicular ligament). The middle fibers (tibiocalcaneal ligament) descend directly

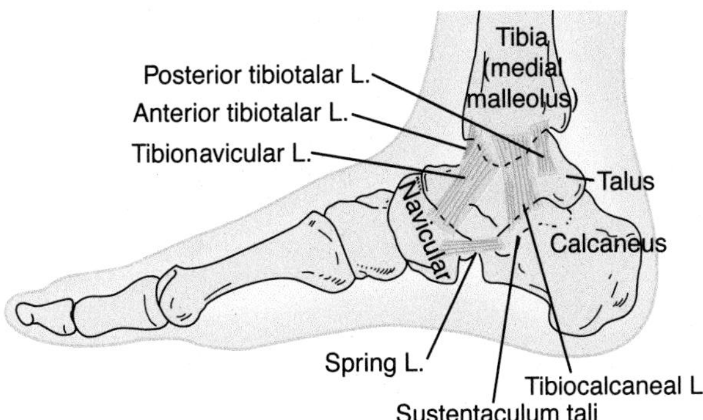

Figure 20-15. Ligaments of the right medial ankle. The four parts of the deltoid ligament. Note that the dotted lines show the outline of the talus under the ligaments.

to the sustentaculum tali of the calcaneus. The posterior fibers (posterior tibiotalar ligament) run backward to the talus. The deep fibers (anterior tibiotalar ligament) can barely be seen from the medial side because they are deep to the tibionavicular portion. The deltoid ligament strengthens the medial side of the ankle joint, holds the calcaneus and navicular against the talus, and helps maintain the medial longitudinal arch.

On the lateral side of the ankle joint is a group of three ligaments commonly and collectively referred to as the **lateral ligament** (Fig. 20-16). The three parts of this ligament connect the lateral malleolus to the talus and calcaneus. The rather weak anterior talofibular ligament attaches the lateral malleolus to the talus. Posteriorly, the fairly strong posterior talofibular ligament runs almost horizontally to connect the lateral malleolus to the talus. In the middle is the long and fairly vertical calcaneofibular ligament that attaches the malleolus to the calcaneus. Numerous other ligaments attach the various tarsals to each other, to the metatarsals, and so on. They tend to be named for the bones to which they attach. Their individual names and locations will not be discussed here.

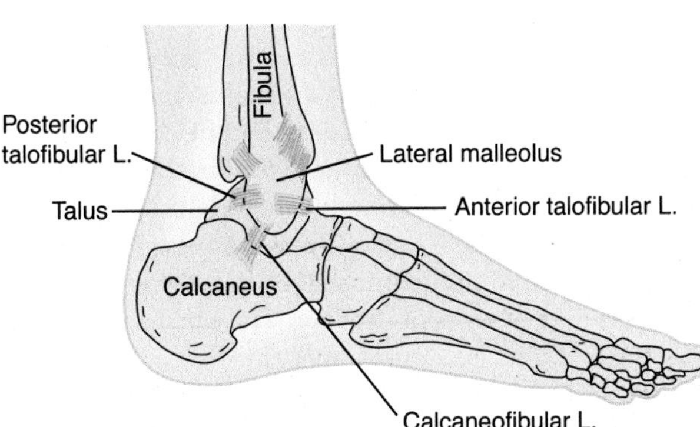

Figure 20-16. Ligaments of the right lateral ankle. The three parts of the lateral ligament.

Arches

Because the foot is the usual point of impact with the ground, it must be able to absorb a great deal of shock, adjust to changes in terrain, and propel the body forward. To allow these actions to occur, the bones of the foot are arranged in arches. We stand on a triangle that distributes weight-bearing from the base of the calcaneus to the heads of the first and fifth metatarsals (Fig. 20-17). Between these three points are two arches (medial and lateral longitudinal; Fig. 20-18) at right angles to the third (transverse) arch (Fig. 20-19).

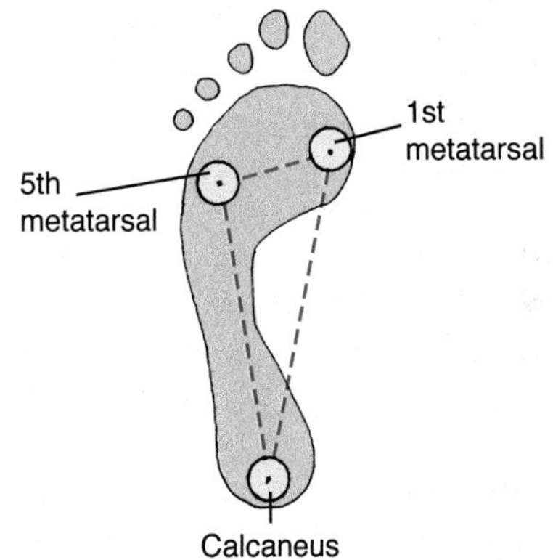

Figure 20-17. The main weight-bearing surfaces of the right foot (plantar view).

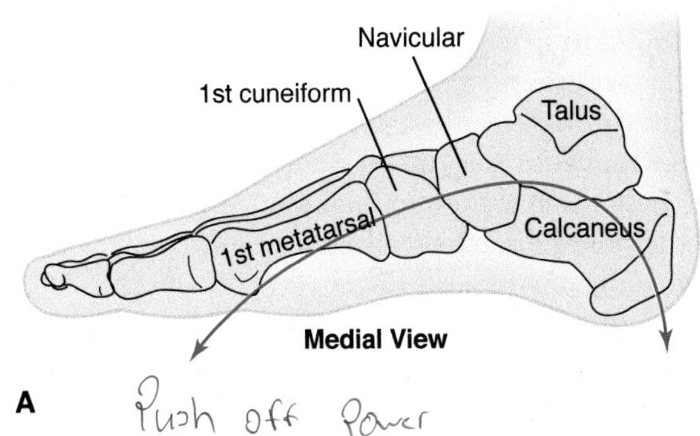

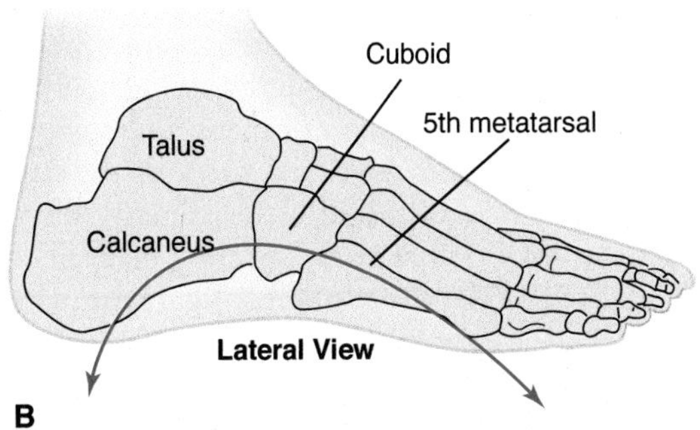

Figure 20-18. The two longitudinal arches of the right foot: **(A)** Medial longitudinal arch. **(B)** Lateral longitudinal arch.

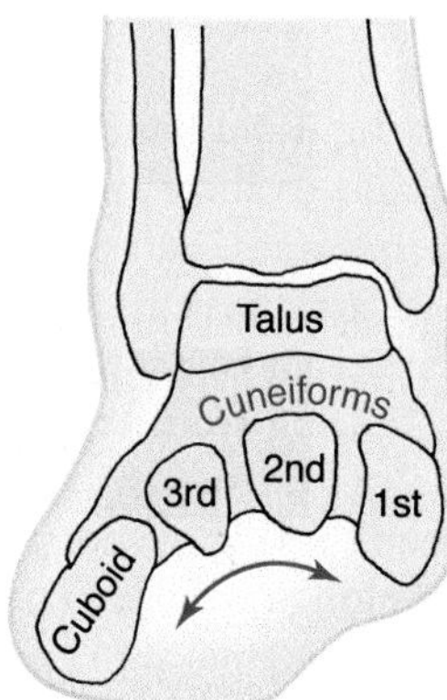

Figure 20-19. Transverse arch of the foot (frontal view).

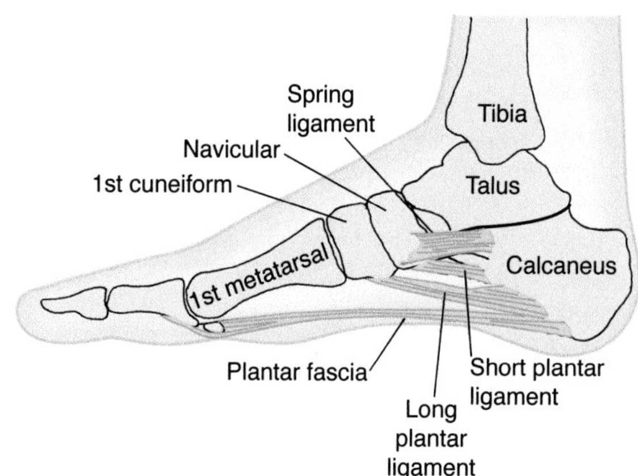

Figure 20-20. Support structures of the right foot and arches (medial view).

The **medial longitudinal arch** makes up the medial border of the foot, running from the calcaneus anteriorly through the talus, navicular, and three cuneiforms anteriorly to the first three metatarsals (Fig. 20-18A). The talus is at the top of the arch; it is often referred to as the *keystone* because it receives the weight of the body. An essential part of an arch, the keystone is usually the central, or topmost, part. The arch depresses somewhat during weight-bearing and then recoils when the weight is removed. Normally, it never flattens or touches the ground. touches ground w/ bearing weight

The **lateral longitudinal arch** runs from the calcaneus anteriorly through the cuboid to the fourth and fifth metatarsals (Fig. 20-18B). It normally rests on the ground during weight-bearing.

The **transverse arch** (see Fig. 20-19) runs from side to side through the three cuneiforms to the cuboid. The second cuneiform is the keystone of this arch.

These three arches are maintained by (1) the shape of the bones and their relation to each other, (2) the plantar ligaments and fascia (Figs. 20-20 and 20-21), and (3) the muscles. The ligaments and fascia are perhaps the most important features. The **spring ligament** (plantar calcaneonavicular ligament) attaches to the calcaneus and runs forward to the navicular (See Fig. 20-15). It is short and wide, and it is most important because it supports the medial side of the longitudinal arch.

The **long plantar ligament,** the longest of the tarsal ligaments, is more superficial than the spring ligament. It attaches posteriorly to the calcaneus and runs forward to attach on the cuboid and bases of the third, fourth, and fifth metatarsals. It is the primary support of the lateral longitudinal arch. The long plantar ligament is assisted by the **short plantar ligament,** which also attaches the calcaneus to the cuboid. It mostly lies deep to the long plantar ligament. Both longitudinal arches are supported by the superficially located **plantar fascia,** which runs from the calcaneus forward to the proximal phalanges. It acts as a tie-rod, keeping the posterior segments (calcaneus and talus) from separating from the anterior portion (anterior tarsals and metatarsal heads). The plantar fascia increases the stability of the foot and arches during weight-bearing and walking (Fig. 20-22; see also Clinical Application 20-1).

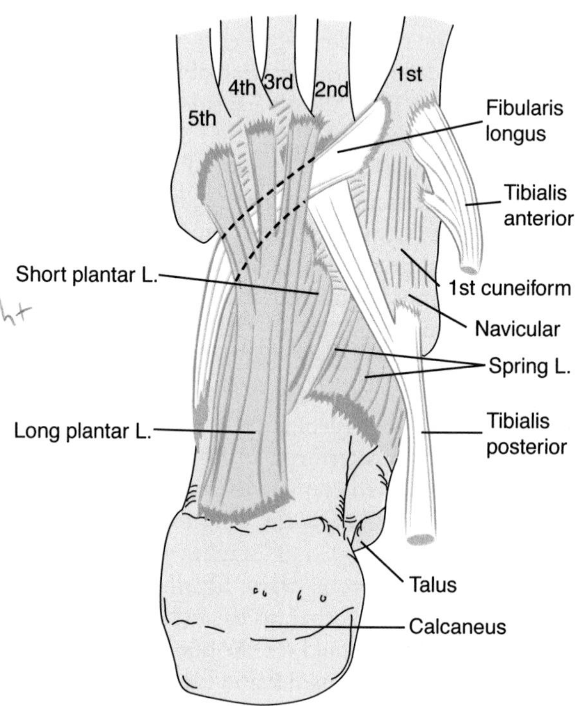

Figure 20-21. Support structures of the right foot and arches (inferior view).

The arches are also supported by muscles, mainly the invertors and evertors of the foot. The tibialis posterior, the flexor hallucis longus, and the flexor digitorum longus muscles all span the ankle posteriorly on the medial side, passing under the sustentaculum tali of the calcaneus. Thus, they give some support to the medial

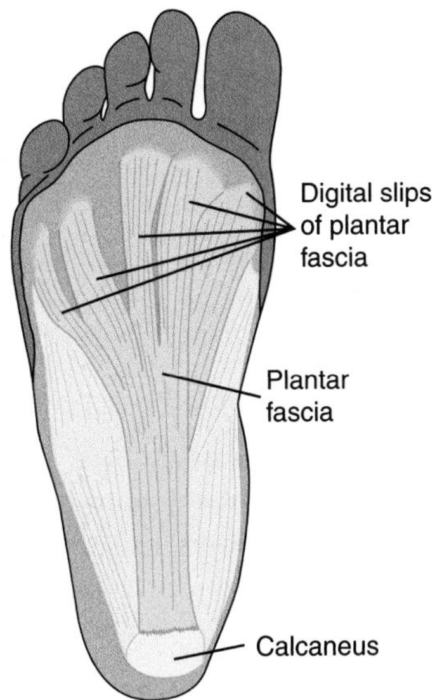

Figure 20-22. Plantar fascia (plantar view).

Clinical Application 20-1

Role of the Plantar Fascia in Supporting the Arch of the Foot

When the foot is pushing off for the next step, the ankle plantar flexors lift the calcaneus upward, pulling the ankle into plantar flexion while simultaneously extending the metatarsophalangeal (MTP) joints. The resulting increased tension on the plantar fascia causes the arch to rise (see figure). As the arch rises, it mechanically forces the foot into supination. The result of the foot being in supination creates the rigid lever necessary for push-off. This is known as the "windlass effect." "Windlass" is a sailing term for a winch mechanism in which a rope is wound around a drum. In the foot, the plantar fascia is being wound around the metatarsal head.

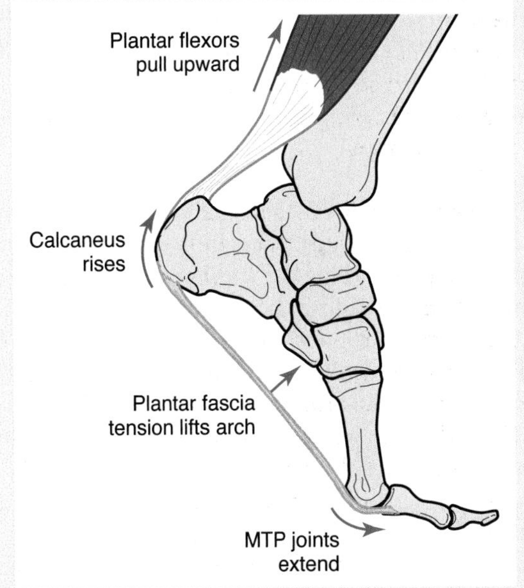

Plantar fascia and the windlass effect.

side of the foot. The flexor hallucis longus and flexor digitorum longus muscles span the medial longitudinal arch and help support it. The fibularis (aka peroneus) longus muscle spans the foot from the lateral to the medial side, providing support to the transverse and lateral longitudinal arches. The intrinsic muscles provide more support than the extrinsics, because any motion will involve them. However, the total muscular support to the arches has been estimated to bear only about 15% to 20% of the total stress to the arches.

Muscles of the Ankle and Foot

Extrinsic Muscles

As in the wrist and hand, there are extrinsic and intrinsic muscles in the ankle and foot. The extrinsic muscles originate on the leg, and the intrinsic muscles originate on the tarsal bones. The extrinsic muscles have vertical lines of pull in the leg, but the foot acts as a pulley to change their line of pull distally. Muscles that cross the ankle anteriorly will dorsiflex the ankle and possibly extend the toes. Those that cross the ankle posteriorly will plantar flex the ankle and possibly flex the toes. The medial muscles will invert the ankle, and the lateral ones will evert.

The extrinsic muscles of the leg are found in groups of three or combinations of three and are located in four anatomical areas. Those four anatomical areas also represent the four compartments of the leg, separated by heavy fascia. Within each compartment is a group of muscles that have a common function(s). They are the (1) superficial posterior, (2) deep posterior, (3) anterior, and (4) lateral groups/compartments (see Figs. 20-34 through 20-38). All have proximal attachments on the femur, tibia, or fibula, and all cross the ankle joint. Table 20-2 summarizes these muscles. Assistive movers are the muscles indicated in parentheses. All other muscles listed are prime movers.

Superficial Posterior Group

The superficial posterior group includes the gastrocnemius, soleus, and plantaris muscles. The **gastrocnemius muscle** is a two-joint muscle that crosses the knee

Table 20-2 Extrinsic Muscles of the Ankle and Foot

Muscle	Joint Crossing	Possible Actions
	Posterior Group	
Superficial Posterior Group		
Gastrocnemius	Posterior	Plantar flexion
Soleus	Posterior	Plantar flexion
(Plantaris)	Posterior	Plantar flexion
Deep Posterior Group		
Tibialis posterior	Posterior, medial	Plantar flexion, inversion
Flexor digitorum longus	Posterior, medial	Plantar flexion, inversion, lesser toe flexion
Flexor hallucis longus	Posterior, medial	Plantar flexion, inversion, great toe flexion
	Anterior Group	
Tibialis anterior	Anterior, medial	Dorsiflexion, inversion
Extensor hallucis longus	Anterior, medial	Dorsiflexion, inversion, great toe extension
Extensor digitorum longus	Anterior	Dorsiflexion, lesser toe extension
	Lateral Group	
Fibularis longus	Posterior, lateral	Eversion, plantar flexion
Fibularis brevis	Posterior, lateral	Eversion, plantar flexion
(Fibularis tertius)	Anterior	Eversion, dorsiflexion

and the ankle (Fig. 20-23). It is an extremely strong ankle plantar flexor. It attaches by two heads to the posterior surface of the medial and lateral condyles of the femur. After descending the posterior leg superficially, it forms a common *Achilles tendon* (often called the *heel cord* by laypersons) with the soleus muscle and attaches to the posterior surface of the calcaneus. Although its major function is at the ankle, it does span the knee posteriorly and has a significant role at the knee.

Gastrocnemius Muscle

O	Medial and lateral condyles of femur
I	Posterior calcaneus
A	Knee flexion and ankle plantar flexion
N	Tibial nerve (S1, S2)

The **soleus muscle** is a large, one-joint muscle located deep to the gastrocnemius muscle (Fig. 20-24). Originating on the posterior tibia and fibula, it spans the posterior leg, blending with the gastrocnemius muscle to form the large, strong Achilles tendon that inserts on the posterior calcaneus. Because the soleus muscle spans the ankle in the midline, its only function is to plantar flex the ankle. The two heads of the gastrocnemius and soleus muscles make up what is sometimes referred to as the **triceps surae,** meaning "three-headed calf" muscle.

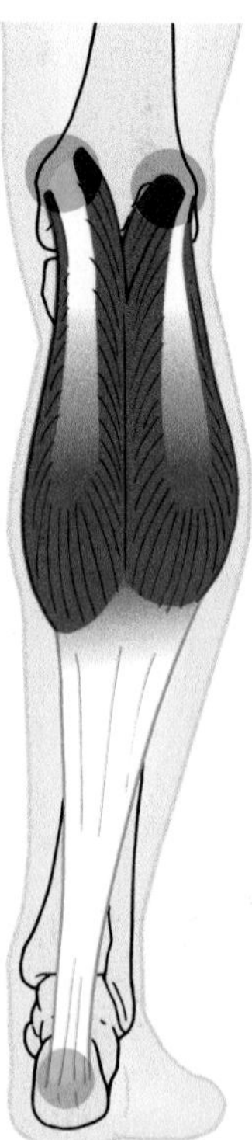

Figure 20-23. The gastrocnemius muscle (posterior view).

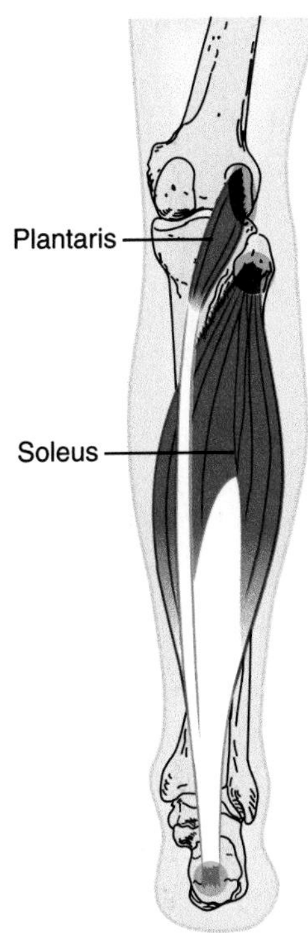

Figure 20-24. The soleus and plantaris muscles (posterior view).

Soleus Muscle

O	Posterior tibia and fibula
I	Posterior calcaneus
A	Ankle plantar flexion
N	Tibial nerve (S1, S2)

The **plantaris muscle** is a long, thin, two-joint muscle with no significant function (see Fig. 20-24). It originates on the posterior surface of the lateral epicondyle of the femur, spans the posterior leg medially, and blends with the gastrocnemius and soleus muscles in the Achilles tendon. Theoretically, it should flex the knee and plantar flex the ankle. However, because of its size in relation to the prime movers of those actions, it is assistive at best. It is absent in one or both legs in some individuals. Similar to the palmaris longus in the hand, its long tendon is sometimes harvested when there is need for a tendon transplant for some other muscle. Its absence does not affect function.

Clinical Application 20-2

Biomechanical Impact of a Heel Lift

Wearing a heeled shoe causes the calcaneus to be elevated during weight-bearing compared with the rest of the foot. This causes the gastrocnemius and soleus to be put on slack. Individuals who regularly wear high-heeled shoes can develop adaptive shortening of these muscles as a result.

Plantaris Muscle

O	Posterior lateral condyle of femur
I	Posterior calcaneus
A	Very weak assist in knee flexion and ankle plantar flexion
N	Tibial nerve (L4, L5, S1)

Deep Posterior Group

The deep posterior group is made up of the tibialis posterior, the flexor hallucis longus, and the flexor digitorum longus muscles. They all attach to the posterior tibia and/or fibula and all terminate in the foot. Because they all cross the ankle posteriorly, they can plantar flex it. However, because of their size in relation to the soleus and gastrocnemius muscles, their role is only assistive in ankle plantar flexion.

The **tibialis posterior muscle** is the deepest-lying posterior muscle. Its proximal attachment is on the interosseous membrane and adjacent portions of the tibia and fibula (Fig. 20-25). It descends on the posterior aspect of the leg, looping around the medial malleolus to attach on the navicular with fibrous expansions to the cuboid, the three cuneiforms, the sustentaculum tali of the calcaneus, and the bases of the second through fourth metatarsals. Because the tibialis posterior muscle crosses the ankle medially and posteriorly, it can invert and plantar flex the ankle. As mentioned above, because of its size in relation to the other plantar flexors, it is only assistive in plantar flexion.

Tibialis Posterior Muscle

O	Interosseous membrane, adjacent tibia and fibula
I	Navicular and most tarsals and metatarsals
A	Ankle inversion; assists in plantar flexion
N	Tibial nerve (L5, S1)

Situated mostly on the lateral side of the leg, the **flexor hallucis longus muscle** arises from the posterior fibula and interosseous membrane. It descends the leg posteriorly, loops around the medial malleolus through a groove in the posterior talus, and goes under the sustentaculum tali of the calcaneus. This muscle travels down the foot through the two heads of the flexor hallucis

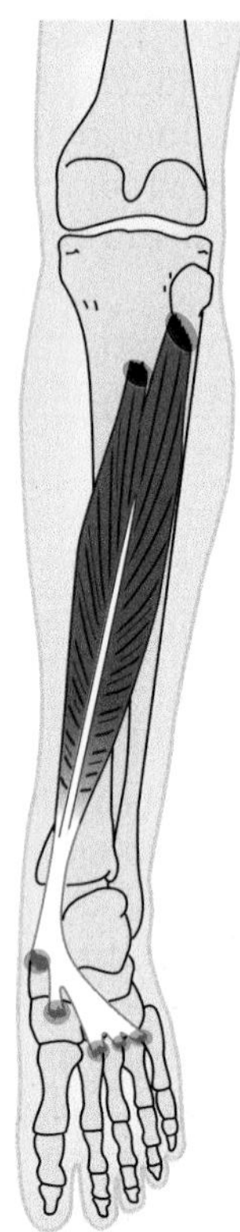

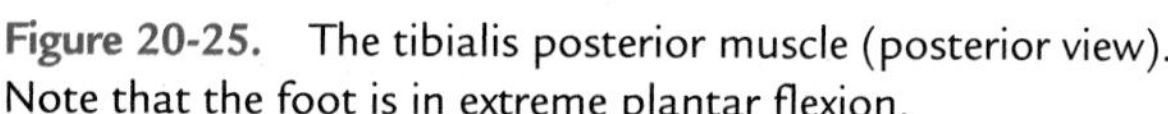

Figure 20-25. The tibialis posterior muscle (posterior view). Note that the foot is in extreme plantar flexion.

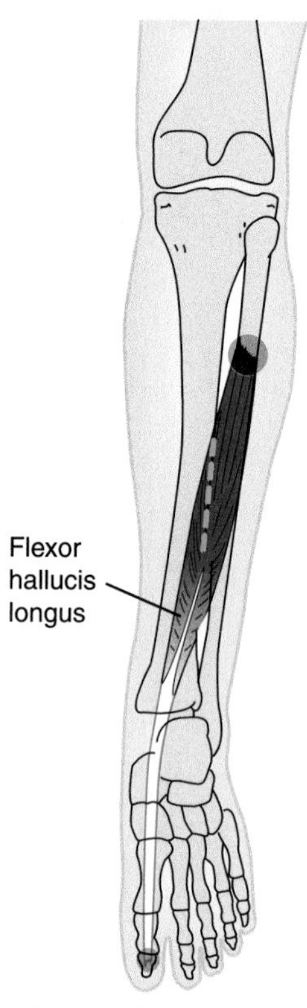

Figure 20-26. The flexor hallucis longus muscle (posterior view). Note that the foot is in extreme plantar flexion. Dotted line denotes attachment along interosseous membrane.

brevis muscle to attach at the base of the distal phalanx of the great toe (Fig. 20-26). This distal attachment is similar to the flexor digitorum profundus and superficialis muscles in the hand. The flexor hallucis longus muscle flexes the great toe and assists in inversion and, to a lesser degree, assists in plantar flexion of the ankle.

Flexor Hallucis Longus Muscle

O	Posterior fibula and interosseous membrane
I	Distal phalanx of the great toe
A	Flexes great toe; assists in inversion and plantar flexion of the ankle
N	Tibial nerve (L5, S1, S2)

Situated mostly on the medial side of the leg, the **flexor digitorum longus muscle** arises from the posterior tibia (Fig. 20-27). It descends the leg posteriorly, loops around the medial malleolus, and runs down the foot, splitting into four tendons and inserting into the distal phalanx of the second through fifth toes. This muscle passes through the split in the flexor digitorum brevis tendon in a fashion similar to the flexor digitorum profundus muscle, which goes through the split in the flexor digitorum superficialis muscle in the hand. It flexes the four lesser toes and assists in inversion and plantar flexion of the ankle.

Flexor Digitorum Longus Muscle

O	Posterior tibia
I	Distal phalanx of four lesser toes
A	Flexes the four lesser toes; assists in ankle inversion and plantar flexion of the ankle
N	Tibial nerve (L5, S1)

The relationships among the deep posterior muscles are interesting, as they cross and intertwine with one another from their proximal to distal attachments (Fig. 20-28). Table 20-3 summarizes this changing relationship. Note that at their origins, the tibialis posterior muscle is in the middle of these three muscles. Where they loop around the medial malleolus, the flexor digitorum longus is in the middle. At their insertions, the flexor hallucis longus is in the middle. The flexor digitorum longus is on the opposite side from where it was at the origin. This feature of changing relationship provides added strength, much like a braided rope that is stronger than a rope in which the individual fibers run parallel to one another.

Anterior Group

The anterior muscle group is made up of the tibialis anterior, the extensor hallucis longus, and the

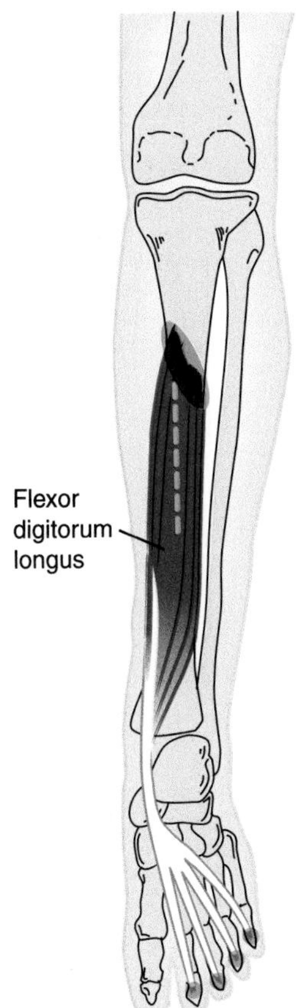

Figure 20-27. The flexor digitorum longus muscle (posterior view). Note that the foot is in extreme plantar flexion. Dotted line denotes attachment along tibia.

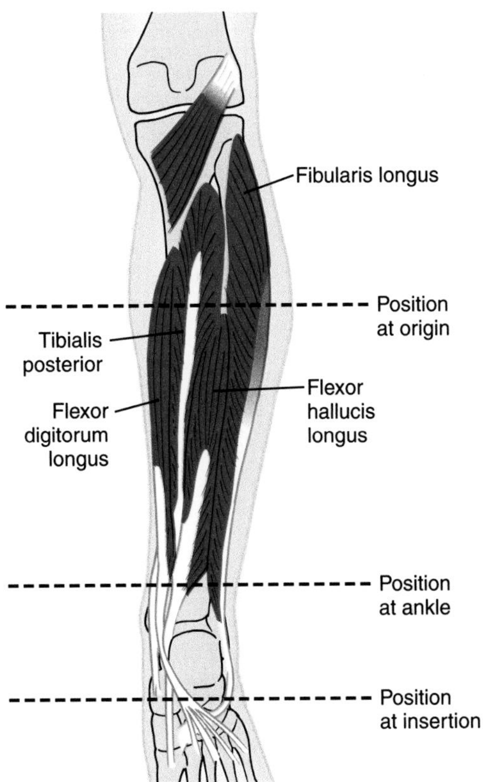

Figure 20-28. From origin to insertion, the changing positions of the flexor digitorum longus, the tibialis posterior, and the flexor hallucis longus provide added strength (posterior and plantar views of leg and foot).

extensor digitorum longus muscles. They all attach proximally on the anterior lateral leg and cross the ankle anteriorly.

The **tibialis anterior muscle** originates on the lateral side of the tibia and interosseous membrane, then descends the leg to insert medially on the first cuneiform and the base of the first metatarsal (Fig. 20-29). It makes up most of the anterior lateral leg's bulk. Because the tibialis anterior muscle spans the ankle anteriorly and medially, it dorsiflexes and inverts the ankle.

Tibialis Anterior Muscle	
O	Lateral tibia and interosseous membrane
I	First cuneiform and first metatarsal
A	Ankle inversion and dorsiflexion
N	Deep fibular nerve (L4, L5, S1)

The **extensor hallucis longus muscle,** a thin muscle lying deep to and between the tibialis anterior and the extensor digitorum longus muscles, originates on the fibula and interosseous membrane and inserts into the base of the distal phalanx of the great toe (Fig. 20-30). Its primary function is to extend the great toe at the IP

Table 20-3 Deep Posterior Group

Location	Relationship		
Origin (medial to lateral)	Flexor digitorum longus (FDL)	Tibialis posterior (TP) FDL	Flexor hallucis longus (FHL)
Medial malleolus (superior to inferior)	TP	FHL	FHL
Insertion (medial to lateral)	TP		FDL

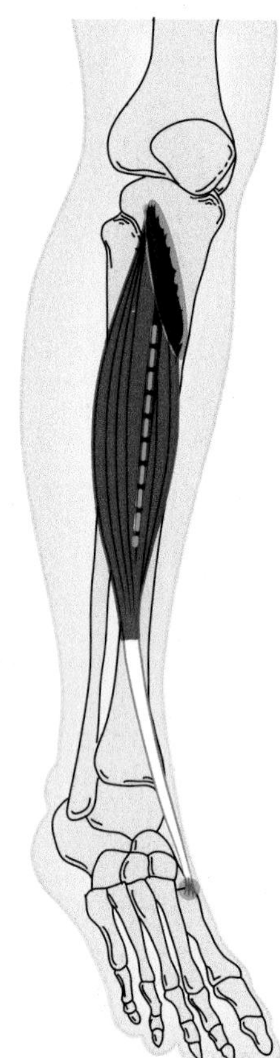

Figure 20-29. The tibialis anterior muscle (anterolateral view). Dotted line denotes attachment along interosseous membrane.

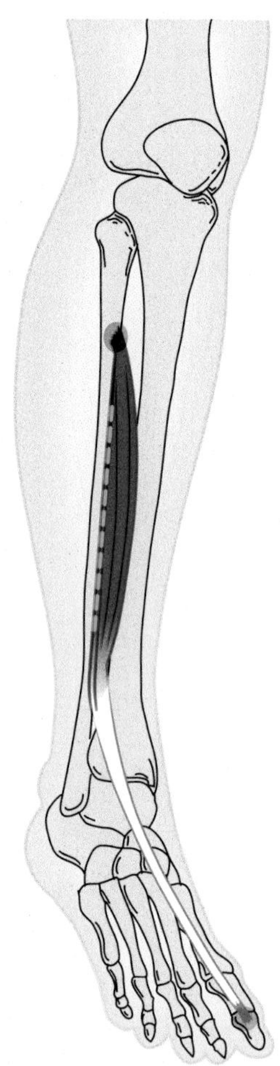

Figure 20-30. The extensor hallucis longus muscle (anterolateral view). Dotted line denotes attachment along interosseous membrane.

and then the MTP joints, but this muscle also assists in dorsiflexing and inverting the ankle.

Extensor Hallucis Longus Muscle

O	Fibula and interosseous membrane
I	Distal phalanx of great toe
A	Extends first toe IP and MTP joints; assists in ankle inversion and dorsiflexion
N	Deep fibular nerve (L4, L5, S1)

The **extensor digitorum longus muscle** is the most lateral of the anterior muscles. It attaches to most of the anterior fibula, the interosseous membrane, and the lateral condyle of the tibia. It descends the leg to attach to the distal phalanx of the four lesser toes (Fig. 20-31). The extensor digitorum longus muscle functions primarily to extend the second through fifth toes, but it also assists in dorsiflexing the ankle. It does not have an inversion/eversion role because it crosses the joint through the middle of that axis.

Extensor Digitorum Longus Muscle

O	Fibula, interosseous membrane, tibia
I	Distal phalanx of four lesser toes
A	Extends four lesser toes, assists in ankle dorsiflexion
N	Deep fibular nerve (L4, L5, S1)

Lateral Group

The lateral group of muscles consists of the fibularis longus, fibularis brevis, and fibularis tertius muscles. They all originate proximally on the fibula and run distally to the foot. Two cross the ankle joint posteriorly, and one crosses the ankle anteriorly. In recent years, the *Terminologi Anatomica,* the international standard on human anatomic terminology, began using the term "fibularis" and "fibular" instead of "peroneus" and "peroneal." "Fibularis" more accurately described the anatomical locations of these muscles and nerves and will be used here. The reader should be familiar with both terms, as usage is not universal.

The **fibularis longus muscle** is the most superficial of the fibular muscles. Arising from the proximal end of the fibula and interosseous membrane, it descends the lateral leg and loops behind the lateral malleolus along

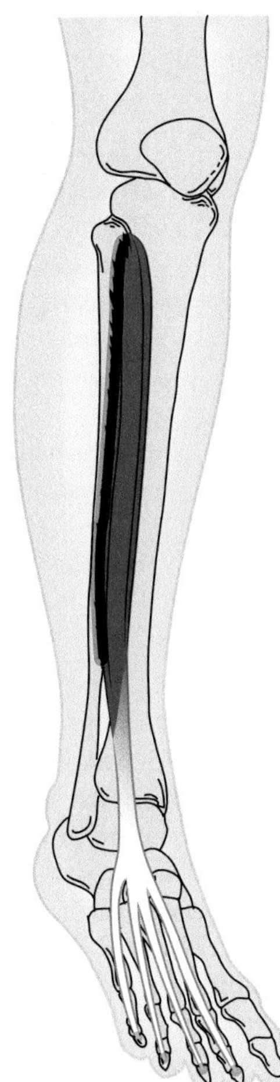

Figure 20-31. The extensor digitorum longus muscle (anterolateral view).

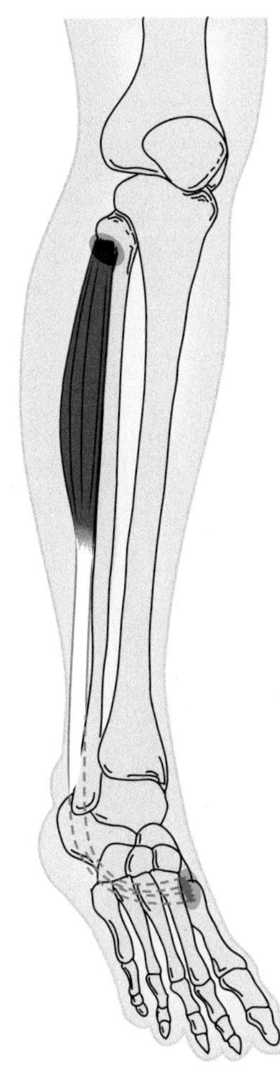

Figure 20-32. The fibularis longus muscle (anterolateral view). Dotted lines indicate location on plantar surface.

with the fibularis brevis muscle. At this point, the fibularis longus muscle goes deep, crossing the foot obliquely from the lateral to the medial side and inserting into the plantar surface of the first metatarsal and first cuneiform (Fig. 20-32). This distal attachment is very close to the attachment of the tibialis anterior muscle. Together, the fibularis longus and tibialis anterior muscles are sometimes referred to as the **stirrup of the foot** because the fibularis longus muscle descends the leg laterally before crossing the foot medially to join the tibialis anterior muscle. The tibialis anterior muscle descends the leg medially to meet the fibularis longus muscle, forming a *U*, or stirrup (see Fig. 20-21). Crossing the foot as it does, the fibularis longus muscle provides some support to the lateral longitudinal and transverse arches of the foot. Its prime function is to evert the ankle, although this muscle can assist somewhat in ankle plantar flexion.

Fibularis Longus Muscle

O	Lateral proximal fibula and interosseous membrane
I	Plantar surface of first cuneiform and metatarsal
A	Ankle eversion; assists in ankle plantar flexion
N	Superficial fibular nerve (L4, L5, S1)

Deep to the fibularis longus muscle is the smaller, shorter **fibularis brevis muscle.** It attaches laterally on the distal fibula, descends the leg, and loops behind the lateral malleolus before coming forward to attach on the tuberosity on the base of the fifth metatarsal (Fig. 20-33). The fibularis brevis muscle is superficial from the lateral malleolus forward. Like the fibularis longus muscle, the primary function of this muscle is to evert the ankle, although it can assist somewhat in plantar flexion.

Fibularis Brevis Muscle

O	Lateral distal fibula
I	Tuberosity on base of fifth metatarsal
A	Ankle eversion; assists in plantar flexion
N	Superficial fibular nerve (L4, L5, S1)

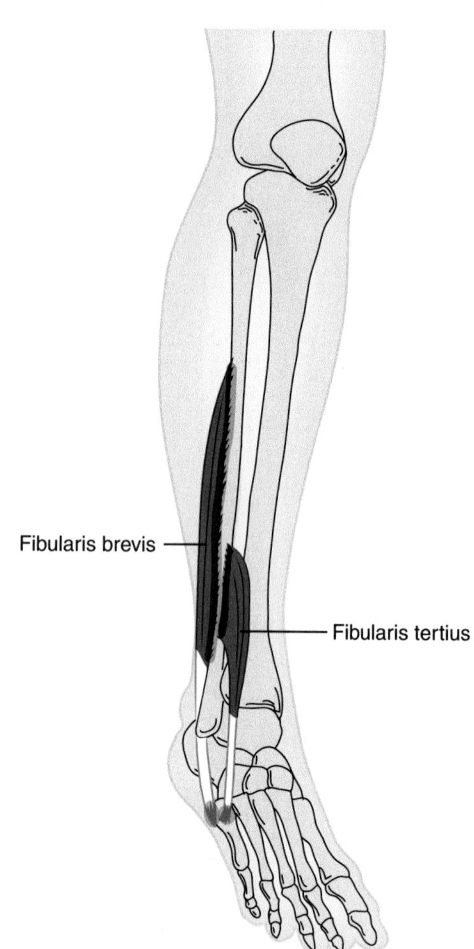

Figure 20-33. The fibularis brevis and tertius muscles (anterolateral view).

The **fibularis tertius muscle,** which is not present in all people, is difficult to identify and often is confused as part of the extensor digitorum longus muscle. This muscle arises from the distal medial fibula and interosseous membrane. It crosses the ankle anteriorly to insert on the dorsal surface of the base of the fifth metatarsal, near the fibularis brevis muscle (see Fig. 20-33). Theoretically, this muscle should dorsiflex and evert the ankle, but due to its size, it is assistive at best.

Fibularis Tertius Muscle

O	Distal medial fibula
I	Tuberosity on base of fifth metatarsal
A	Assists somewhat in ankle eversion and dorsiflexion
N	Deep fibular nerve (L4, L5, S1)

Table 20-4 summarizes the actions of the prime movers of the ankle.

Table 20-4 Actions of Ankle Prime Movers

Action	Muscle
Plantar flexion	Gastrocnemius, soleus
Dorsiflexion	Tibialis anterior
Inversion	Tibialis anterior, tibialis posterior
Eversion	Fibularis longus, fibularis brevis
Flexion of second through fifth toes	Flexor digitorum longus
Flexion of first toe	Flexor hallucis longus
Extension of second through fifth toes	Extensor digitorum longus
Extension of first toe	Extensor hallucis longus
No prime mover action	Plantaris, fibularis tertius

Intrinsic Muscles

Intrinsic muscles have both attachments distal to the ankle joint. Because we do not use these muscles in the foot to perform intricate actions, they tend not to be as well developed as their counterparts in the hand. Their names tell a great deal about their location and action. All intrinsic muscles are located on the plantar surface, essentially in layers; the exceptions to this are the extensor digitorum brevis, the extensor hallucis brevis, and the dorsal interossei, which are between the metatarsals and dorsal to the plantar interossei (See Figs. 20-39 through 20-43). Table 20-5 summarizes the intrinsic muscles according to surface location, depth location, function, and similar structure in the hand. Table 20-6 summarizes the innervation of the intrinsic muscles.

Anatomical Relationships

To appreciate the relationships between muscles of the ankle and foot, they should be put into anterior, lateral, and posterior groups, with superficial and deep subgroups. The posterior group has six muscles arranged in three layers. The gastrocnemius is the only superficial muscle that is located posteriorly (Fig. 20-34). Deep to it are the very long, thin plantaris muscle and the large, one-joint soleus muscle (Fig. 20-35). The deepest layer has the flexor digitorum longus, the tibialis posterior, and the flexor hallucis longus arranged from medial to lateral (Fig. 20-36). As noted earlier, the interrelationship of these muscles changes two more times before they reach their insertions (see Table 20-3).

Of the lateral group, the fibularis longus is superficial and the fibularis brevis lies deep to it. Just above the lateral malleolus, the fibularis brevis can be palpated just anterior to the fibularis longus (Fig. 20-37). Below the

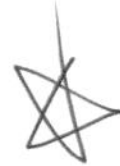

Table 20-5 Intrinsic Muscles of the Foot

Muscle	Action	Comparable Hand Muscle
Dorsal Surface		
Extensor digitorum brevis	Extends PIP joints of second through fourth digits	None
Extensor hallucis brevis	Extends IP joint of first digit	None
Plantar Surface		
First Layer (most superficial)		
Abductor hallucis	Abducts; flexes IP of first toe	Abductor pollicis brevis
Flexor digitorum brevis	Flexes PIP of digits second through fifth digits	Flexor digitorum superficialis
Abductor digiti minimi	Flexes; abducts fifth digit	Same name
Second Layer		
Quadratus plantae	Straightens diagonal line of pull of flexor digitorum longus	None
Lumbricals	Flexes MPs; extends PIPs and DIPs	Same name
Third Layer		
Flexor hallucis brevis	Flexes MP of first digit	Flexor pollicis brevis
Adductor hallucis	Adducts; flexes first digit	Adductor pollicis
Flexor digiti minimi	Flexes PIP of fifth digit	Same name
Dorsal Surface		
Fourth Layer (deepest)		
Dorsal interossei	Abducts second through fourth digits	Same name
Plantar interossei	Adducts third through fifth digits	Palmar interossei

Table 20-6 Innervation of the Intrinsic Foot Muscles

Muscle	Nerve
Dorsal Surface	
Extensor digitorum brevis	Deep fibular
Extensor hallucis brevis	Deep fibular
Plantar Surface	
Abductor hallucis	Tibial
Flexor digitorum brevis	Tibial
Abductor digiti minimi	Tibial
Quadratus plantae	Tibial
Lumbricals	Tibial
Flexor hallucis brevis	Tibial
Adductor hallucis	Tibial
Flexor digiti minimi	Tibial
Dorsal interossei	Tibial
Plantar interossei	Tibial

malleolus, the fibularis longus cannot be seen or palpated because it goes deep to cross the plantar surface of the foot. However, at the base of the fifth metatarsal, the tendon of the fibularis brevis should be seen coming from behind the malleolus and the tendon of the fibularis tertius should be seen coming in front of the malleolus. Do not confuse it as a tendon of the extensor digitorum longus. Note that it does not go to the fifth toe.

The tibialis anterior muscle comes from the proximal lateral tibia and is superficial as it runs the entire distance to the medial side of the ankle. Just above the ankle, the tendons of the tibialis anterior, the extensor hallucis longus, and the extensor digitorum longus can be seen from medial to lateral (Fig. 20-38). Note that the extensor digitorum longus has a tendon running to the second, third, fourth, and fifth toes. Be sure to note, too, the difference between the tendon of the extensor digitorum longus going to the fifth toe and the tendon of the fibularis tertius going only to the base of the fifth metatarsal.

The intrinsic muscles of the foot are arranged in essentially four layers on the plantar surface. The first muscular layer lies deep to the plantar fascia (see Fig. 20-22). The flexor digitorum brevis lies in the midline, with tendons going to the second through the fifth toes. On the medial side lies the abductor hallucis, and on the lateral side is the abductor digiti minimi (Fig. 20-39). The second layer has two intrinsic muscles and tendons of two extrinsic muscles (flexor digitorum longus and flexor hallucis longus) (Fig. 20-40). The quadratus plantae runs from the

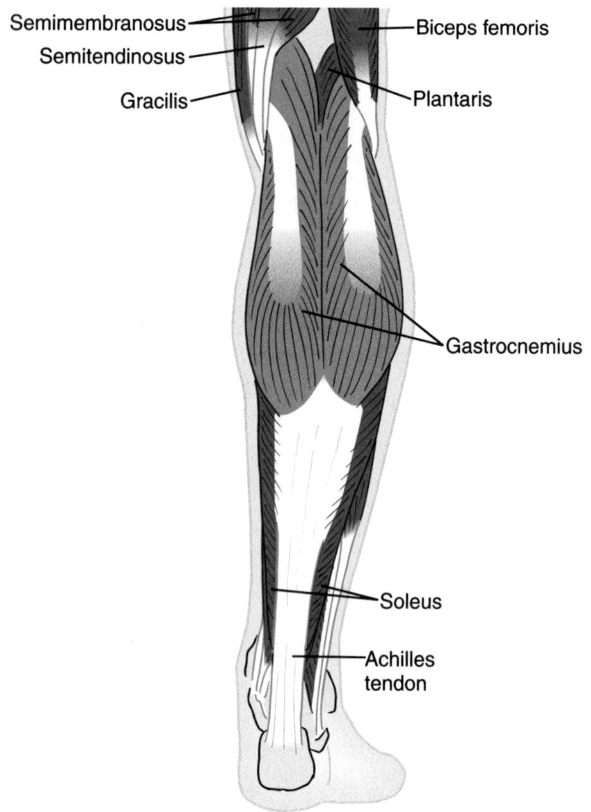

Figure 20-34. Muscles of the posterior leg, superficial layer (posterior view, right leg).

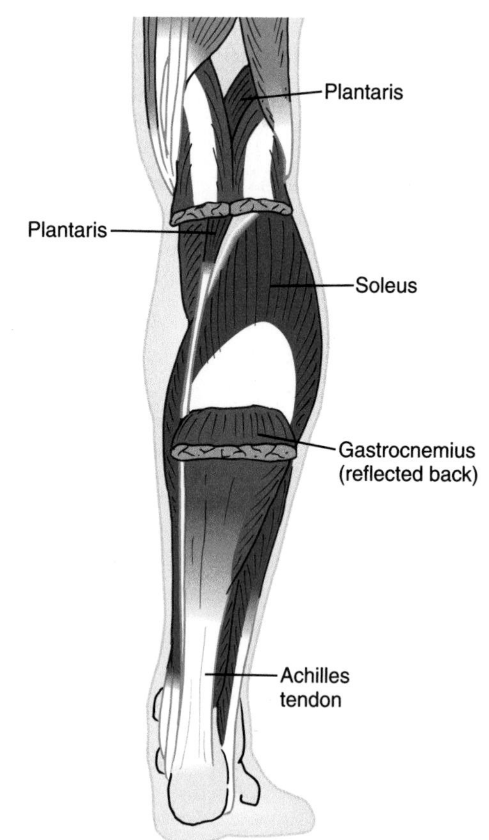

Figure 20-35. Middle layer of the posterior group. The middle section of the gastrocnemius muscle has been removed.

calcaneus toward the tendon of the flexor digitorum longus, where it attaches just before the flexor digitorum longus splits into four tendons that go to the second through fifth toes. When it contracts, the quadratus plantae straightens the long toe flexor's line of pull. The tendon of the flexor hallucis longus can also be seen in this layer. The lumbricals are four intrinsic muscles that arise from the tendons of the flexor digitorum longus, pass on the medial side of the four lesser toes, and attach on the tendons of the extensor digitorum longus on the dorsal surface. The third layer has the two heads of the flexor hallucis brevis medially, the two heads of the adductor hallucis in the middle, and the flexor digiti minimi laterally (Fig. 20-41). The fourth and deepest layer includes the interossei muscles. As their names imply, they lie between the bones (metatarsals) on the plantar and dorsal sides (Fig. 20-42). They have the same function as their counterparts in the hand and have very similar attachments (see Figs. 13-25 and 13-26 for a comparison). Unlike their counterparts in the hand, the second toe is the one from which the other toes either abduct or adduct.

The intrinsic muscles on the dorsum of the foot lie underneath or next to their counterpart extrinsic muscles (Fig. 20-43). The extensor hallucis brevis is just lateral to the extensor hallucis longus. The three tendons of the extensor digitorum brevis are deep to the extensor

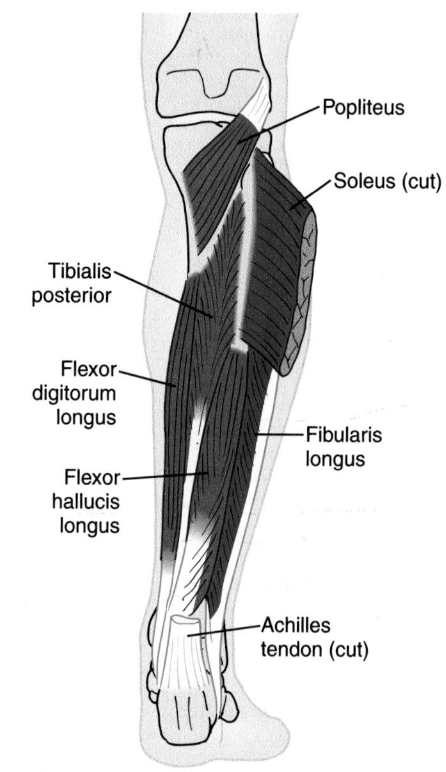

Figure 20-36. Deep layer of the posterior group.

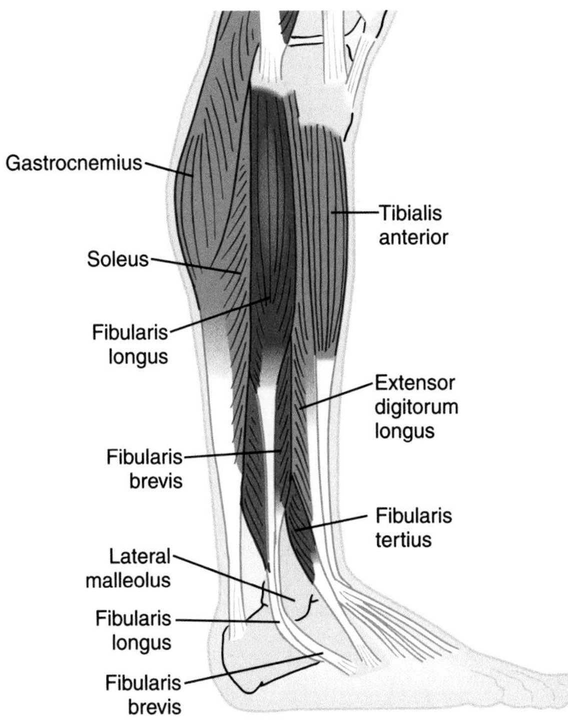

Figure 20-37. Muscles of the right lateral group (lateral view).

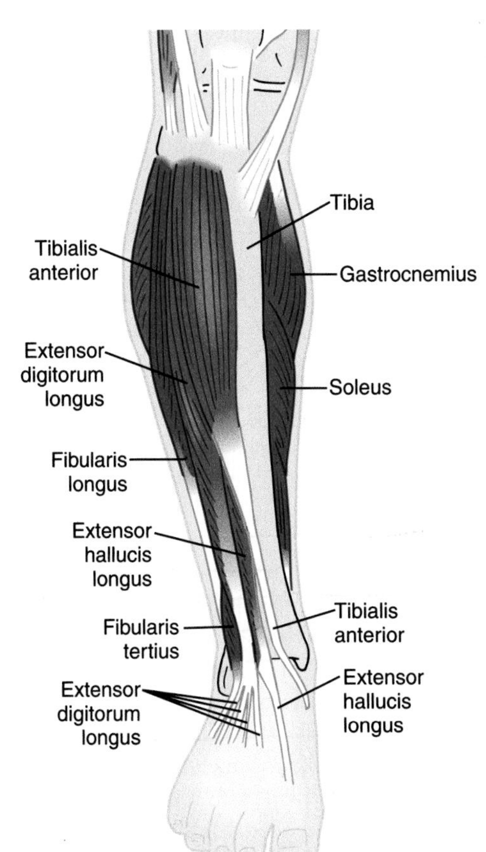

Figure 20-38. Muscles of the right anterior group (anterior view).

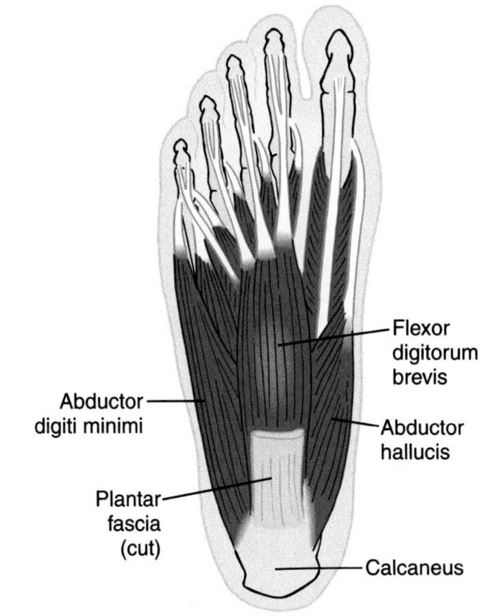

Figure 20-39. Muscles of the plantar surface of the foot—first (superficial) layer (plantar view).

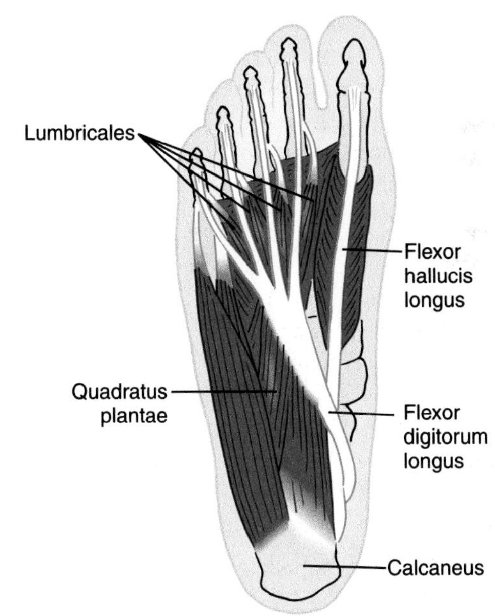

Figure 20-40. Muscles of the plantar surface of the foot—second layer (plantar view).

digitorum longus and attach laterally to its distal attachment on the second, third, and fourth toes.

Summary of Muscle Innervation

The ankle and foot muscles fall into relatively tidy groupings according to innervation. Those muscles located on the posterior leg and plantar surface of the foot receive innervation from the **tibial nerve.** Similar to the hand, the plantar foot muscles divide into two groups. The lateral plantar branch of the tibial nerve innervates

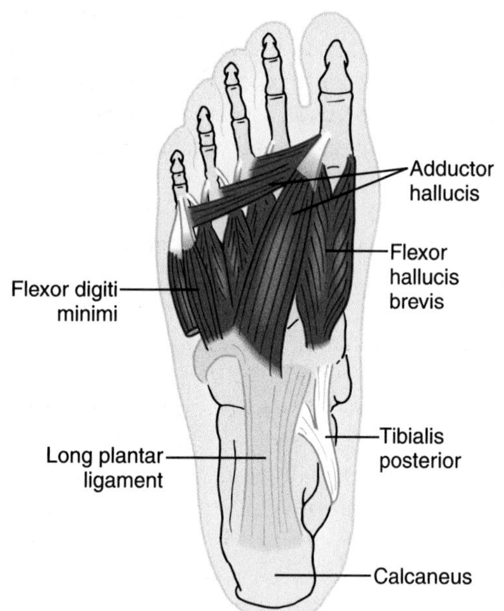

Figure 20-41. Muscles of the plantar surface of the foot—third layer (plantar view).

muscles located on the lateral side, and the medial plantar branch innervates those on the medial side.

The **superficial fibular nerve** innervates muscles on the lateral side of the leg. The fibularis tertius muscle is the exception because it crosses the ankle anteriorly and receives innervation with the other anterior muscles from the **deep fibular nerve.**

Tables 20-6, 20-7, and 20-8 summarize ankle and foot innervation according to nerve and spinal segment. As has been noted in previous chapters, there is some variation among sources regarding spinal cord level. *Gray's Anatomy,* 40th edition, is used as the reference source when discrepancies occur.

Common Ankle Pathologies

Shin splints is a general term given to exercise-induced pain along the medial edge of the tibia, usually a few inches above the ankle to midway up the tibia. Most commonly, inflammation of the periosteum causes the pain. Shin splints are an overuse injury that can result from running on hard surfaces, running on tiptoes, and playing sports that involve a lot of jumping. **Medial tibial stress syndrome** is a more specific term that includes anterior leg pain not associated with a stress fracture.

Deformities of the feet and toes often affect other joints of the lower extremity and trunk, especially during walking or running. A normal foot is defined as **plantigrade,** in that the sole is at right angles to the leg when a person is standing. **Equinus foot** (horse's foot) means that the hindfoot is fixed in plantar flexion. A **calcaneus foot** is one that is fixed in dorsiflexion. **Pes cavus** refers

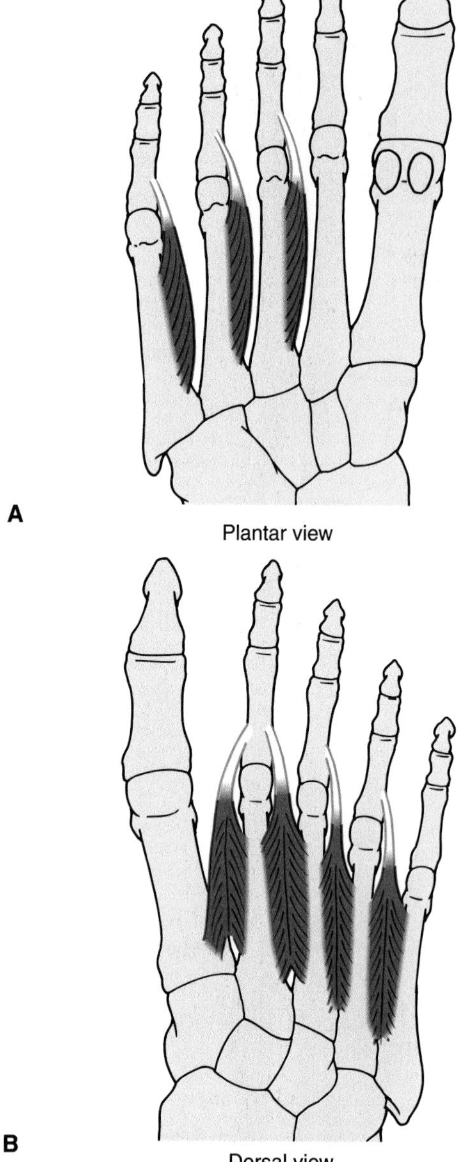

Figure 20-42. Muscles of the plantar surface of the right foot—fourth (deepest) layer. **(A)** Plantar interossei. **(B)** Dorsal interossei.

to an abnormally high arch, whereas **pes planus** (flat foot) is the loss of the medial longitudinal arch. **Hallux valgus** is caused by pathological changes in which the great toe develops a valgus deformity (distal end pointed laterally). **Hallux rigidus** is a degenerative condition of the first MTP joint associated with pain and diminished range of motion. In the following lesser toe deformities, all MTP joints are hyperextended: In **hammer toe,** the PIP is flexed and the DIP is extended. **Mallet toe** is just the opposite; it has an extended PIP joint and a flexed DIP joint. **Claw toe** has a flexed PIP joint and a flexed DIP joint.

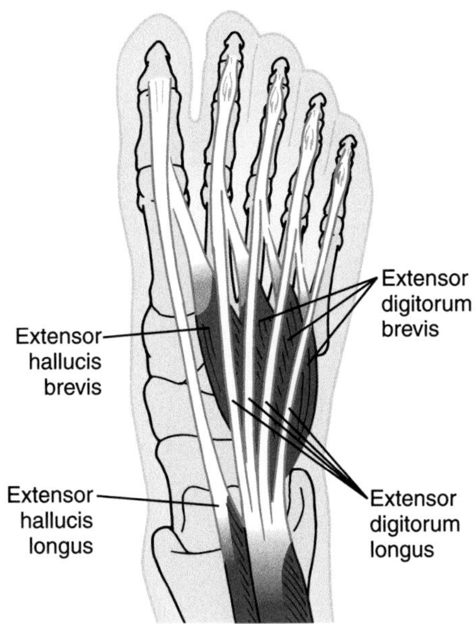

Figure 20-43. Intrinsic muscles of the dorsum of the foot.

Metatarsalgia is a general term referring to pain around the metatarsal heads. The individual often describes the pain as a bruise, or "like walking on pebbles." The pain usually becomes worse with increased activity. **Morton's neuroma** is caused by abnormal pressure on the plantar digital nerves commonly at the web space between the third and fourth metatarsals. This pressure can result in pain and numbness in the toe area that gets worse with activity such as running. **Turf toe** is caused by forced hyperextension of the great toe at the MTP joint. It is commonly seen in football, baseball, and soccer players.

The ankle is considered the most frequently injured joint in the body. **Ankle sprains** are probably the most common injury among recreational and competitive athletes, and the lateral ligament is the most frequently injured ligament in these groups. Lateral or inversion sprains occur when the foot lands in a plantar-flexed and inverted position. One or more of the lateral ligament's three parts may be stretched or torn.

An **ankle fracture** often occurs when a person trips over an unexpected obstacle or falls from a height, and it usually involves a twisting component to the ankle. The lateral malleolus is most commonly involved. A

Table 20-7 Innervation of the Muscles of the Leg and Foot

Muscle	Nerve	Spinal Segment
Gastrocnemius	Tibial	S1, S2
Soleus	Tibial	S1, S2
Plantaris	Tibial	L4, L5, S1
Tibialis posterior	Tibial	L5, S1
Flexor digitorum longus	Tibial	L5, S1
Flexor hallucis longus	Tibial	L5, S1, S2
Fibularis longus	Superficial fibular	L4, L5, S1
Fibularis brevis	Superficial fibular	L4, L5, S1
Fibularis tertius	Deep fibular	L4, L5, S1
Extensor digitorum longus	Deep fibular	L4, L5, S1
Extensor digitorum brevis	Deep fibular	L5, S1
Extensor hallucis longus	Deep fibular	L4, L5, S1
Extensor hallucis brevis	Deep fibular	L5, S1
Tibialis anterior	Deep fibular	L4, L5, S1
Abductor hallucis	Medial plantar (tibial)	L4, L5, S1, S2
Flexor hallucis brevis	Medial plantar (tibial)	L4, L5, S1, S2
Flexor digitorum brevis	Medial plantar (tibial)	L4, L5, S1, S2
Lumbricals (medial 1)	Medial plantar (tibial)	L4, L5
Lumbricals (lateral 3)	Lateral plantar (tibial)	S1, S2, S3
Abductor digiti minimi	Lateral plantar (tibial)	S1, S2, S3
Quadratus plantae	Lateral plantar (tibial)	S1, S2, S3
Adductor hallucis	Lateral plantar (tibial)	S1, S2, S3
Flexor digiti minimi	Lateral plantar (tibial)	S1, S2, S3
Dorsal interossei	Lateral plantar (tibial)	S1, S2, S3
Plantar interossei	Lateral plantar (tibial)	S1, S2, S3

Table 20-8 Segmental Innervation of the Ankle Joint and Foot

Spinal Cord Level	L4	L5	S1	S2	S3
Gastrocnemius			X	X	
Soleus			X	X	
Plantaris	X	X	X		
Tibialis posterior		X	X		
Flexor digitorum longus		X	X		
Flexor hallucis longus		X	X	X	
Fibularis longus	X	X	X		
Fibularis brevis	X	X	X		
Fibularis tertius	X	X	X		
Extensor digitorum longus	X	X	X		
Extensor digitorum brevis		X	X		
Extensor hallucis longus	X	X	X		
Extensor hallucis brevis		X	X		
Tibialis anterior	X	X	X		
Abductor hallucis	X	X	X	X	
Flexor hallucis brevis	X	X	X	X	
Flexor digitorum brevis	X	X	X	X	
Lumbricales	X	X	X	X	X
Abductor digiti minimi			X	X	X
Quadratus plantae			X	X	X
Adductor hallucis			X	X	X
Flexor digiti minimi			X	X	X
Dorsal interossei			X	X	X
Plantar interossei			X	X	X

bimalleolar fracture involves both malleoli, whereas a **trimalleolar fractures** involves both malleoli and the posterior lip of the tibia.

Plantar fasciitis is a common overuse injury, resulting in pain in the heel. The plantar fascia helps to maintain the medial longitudinal arch and acts as a shock absorber during weight-bearing. The pain is usually located at the point where the fascia attaches to the calcaneus on the plantar surface. **Achilles tendonitis,** an inflammation of the gastrocnemius-soleus tendon, is sometimes a precursor to a **ruptured Achilles tendon.** With a complete rupture, the individual loses the ability to plantar flex the ankle. To determine whether the tendon is intact, have an individual lie prone with the feet off the edge of the table. Squeeze on the muscle belly of the gastrocnemius muscle. If the tendon is intact, slight plantar flexion will occur, but no motion will occur if the tendon is ruptured.

A **triple arthrodesis** is a surgical procedure that fuses the talocalcaneal, calcaneocuboid, and talonavicular joints. It provides medial-lateral stability of the foot and relieves pain at the subtalar joint, but inversion and eversion at the ankle are lost. Ankle dorsiflexion and plantar flexion remain because the talotibial joint has not been involved.

Points to Remember

- Stretching is performed on *relaxed* muscles; and strengthening occurs when muscles contract.
- To stretch a two-joint muscle, stretch it over both joints at the same time within pain limits of that muscle.
- To stretch a one-joint muscle when a two-joint muscle crosses the same joint, select a joint position that stretches a two-joint muscle over only one joint.
- The excursion of a one-joint muscle being stretched will be greater than the range allowed by the joint.
- The excursion of a two-joint muscle is less than the combined range allowed by both joints.
- A muscle contraction is strongest if the muscle is stretched before it contracts.
- A muscle loses power quickly as it shortens.
- Two-joint muscles maintain their force of contraction for a longer period than a one-joint muscle. This is because they are able to elongate over one joint while shortening over the other joint.

Review Questions

General Anatomy Questions

1. Describe the ankle (talotibial) joint:
   a. Number of axes:
   b. Shape of joint:
   c. Type of muscle action allowed:
   d. Bones involved:
2. a. What bones are involved in the subtalar joint?
   b. What bones are involved in the transverse tarsal joint?
   c. What muscle actions are predominantly allowed by these joints?
3. What are the functions of the interosseous membrane?
4. What ligaments provide medial stability to the ankle? What is their collective name?
5. What ligaments provide lateral stability to the ankle? What is their collective name?
6. What are the names of the two longitudinal arches?
7. List the bones involved in each longitudinal arch.
8. List the bones involved in the transverse arch.
9. What is the function of the arches?
10. Which muscles pass behind the medial malleolus?
11. Which extrinsic muscles attach on the medial side of the foot?
12. Which muscles pass behind the lateral malleolus?
13. Which extrinsic muscles attach on the lateral side of the foot?
14. Which muscles form the "stirrup" of the foot? Describe how the stirrup is formed.
15. Would an individual with a spinal cord injury at L4 be able to actively do ankle plantar flexion?
16. Muscles that cross the plantar aspect of the toes will contribute toward _________, whereas muscles that cross the dorsal aspect of the toes will contribute toward ________.
17. What cardinal plane motions combine to contribute toward pronation and supination?

Functional Activity Questions

Identify the main ankle joint action or position in the following activities:

1. Pushing your foot down on the accelerator pedal while driving
2. Standing in high heels
3. Walking up a steep slope
4. Walking down a steep slope
5. Foot on floor with the heel as the pivot point, creating a "windshield wiper" motion of the foot
6. Walking on your heels
7. Taking off when jumping, hopping, or skipping
8. Your ankle begins to roll outward as if to sustain a lateral sprain. Name the muscle group that is primarily responsible for preventing this motion.

Clinical Exercise Questions

1. Answer the following questions about each muscle:
   Gastrocnemius
   a. Number of joints crossed?
   b. Knee motion?
   c. Ankle motion?
   Soleus
   a. Number of joints crossed?
   b. Knee motion?
   c. Ankle motion?
2. Place your hands on the wall at shoulder level. Stand with your left foot 24 inches from the wall and your right foot about 12 inches from the wall (Fig. 20-44).

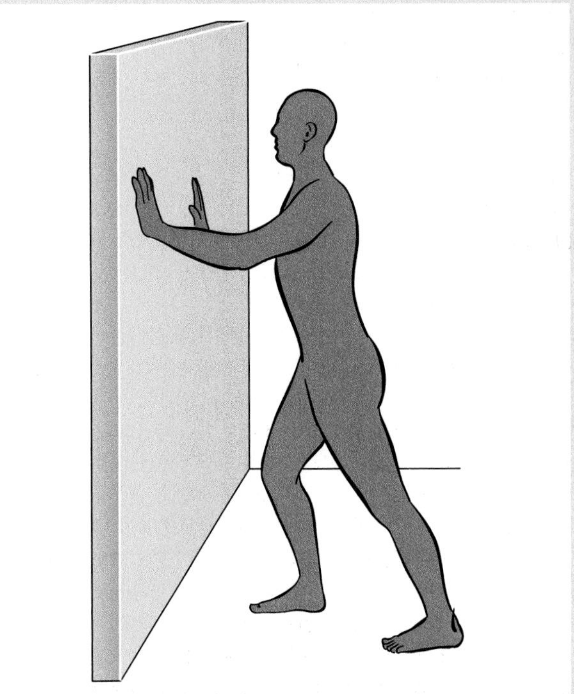

Figure 20-44. Starting position.

(continued on next page)

Review Questions—cont'd

Keeping your left leg straight and your right foot flat on the floor, lean in toward the wall, leading with your pelvis and allowing your right knee to bend. In terms of what is occurring at the left knee and ankle, answer the following questions:

a. What are the joint positions or motions that are occurring:
   at the left knee? ____________
   at the left ankle? ____________
b. To be in the above position, is the left gastrocnemius contracting or stretching?
c. To be in the above position, is the left soleus contracting or stretching?
d. Which of these two muscles is being stretched more than the other?
e. Why?

3. Repeat the position of the exercise in question 2, except this time bend your left knee as you lean into the wall.
   a. What are the joint positions or motions that are occurring:
      at the left knee? __________
      at the left ankle? __________
   b. In this new position, is the left gastrocnemius stretched or slack at the knee?
   c. In this new position, is the left gastrocnemius stretched or slack at the ankle?
   d. In this new position, is the left soleus stretched at the knee?
   e. In this new position, is the left soleus stretched at the ankle?
   f. Which of these two muscles is stretched more?
   g. Why?
4. Standing upright and holding on to the back of a chair for balance, rise up on your toes as high as possible.
   a. What are the joint positions or motions that are occurring:
      at the knee? _________
      at the ankle? _________
   b. Is the gastrocnemius shortening or elongating over the knee?
   c. Is the gastrocnemius shortening or elongating over the ankle?
   d. Does the soleus have an action at the knee?
   e. Is the soleus shortening or elongating over the ankle?
   f. Why is the gastrocnemius stronger than the soleus in this position?
5. Sitting with your knees bent, roll your feet and legs until the soles of your feet are together (Fig. 20-45).
   a. Is inversion or eversion the joint motion (or attempted joint motion) at the ankle?
   b. What type of muscle contraction (isometric, concentric, or eccentric) is occurring?
   c. What are the prime movers of this action?
6. Sitting on the floor with knee extended, loop an elastic band around the midfoot with the ankle plantar flexed and anchor the other end around a heavy table leg. Be far enough away to create sufficient tension in the elastic band. Bring your toes up toward your knees as much as possible. Hold for the count of five. Return to the starting position.
   a. What motion is occurring in each of the three phases?
   b. What type of contraction is occurring in each phase?
   c. What muscles are involved as prime movers?
   d. Is this an open or closed kinetic chain?

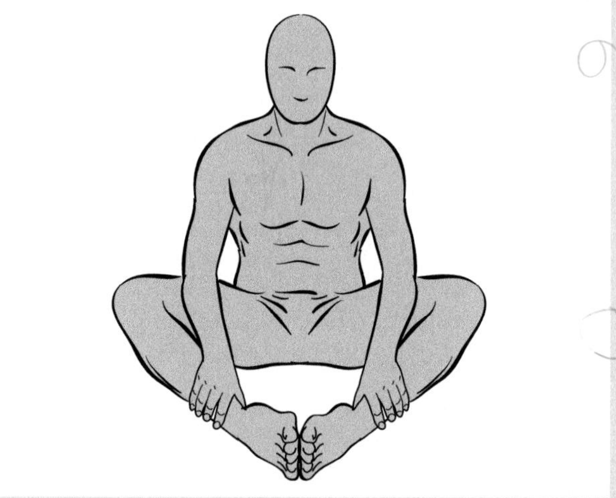

Figure 20-45. Starting position.

7. When measuring ankle dorsiflexion range of motion, the knee should be placed in flexion. Why?

PART V

Clinical Kinesiology and Anatomy of the Body

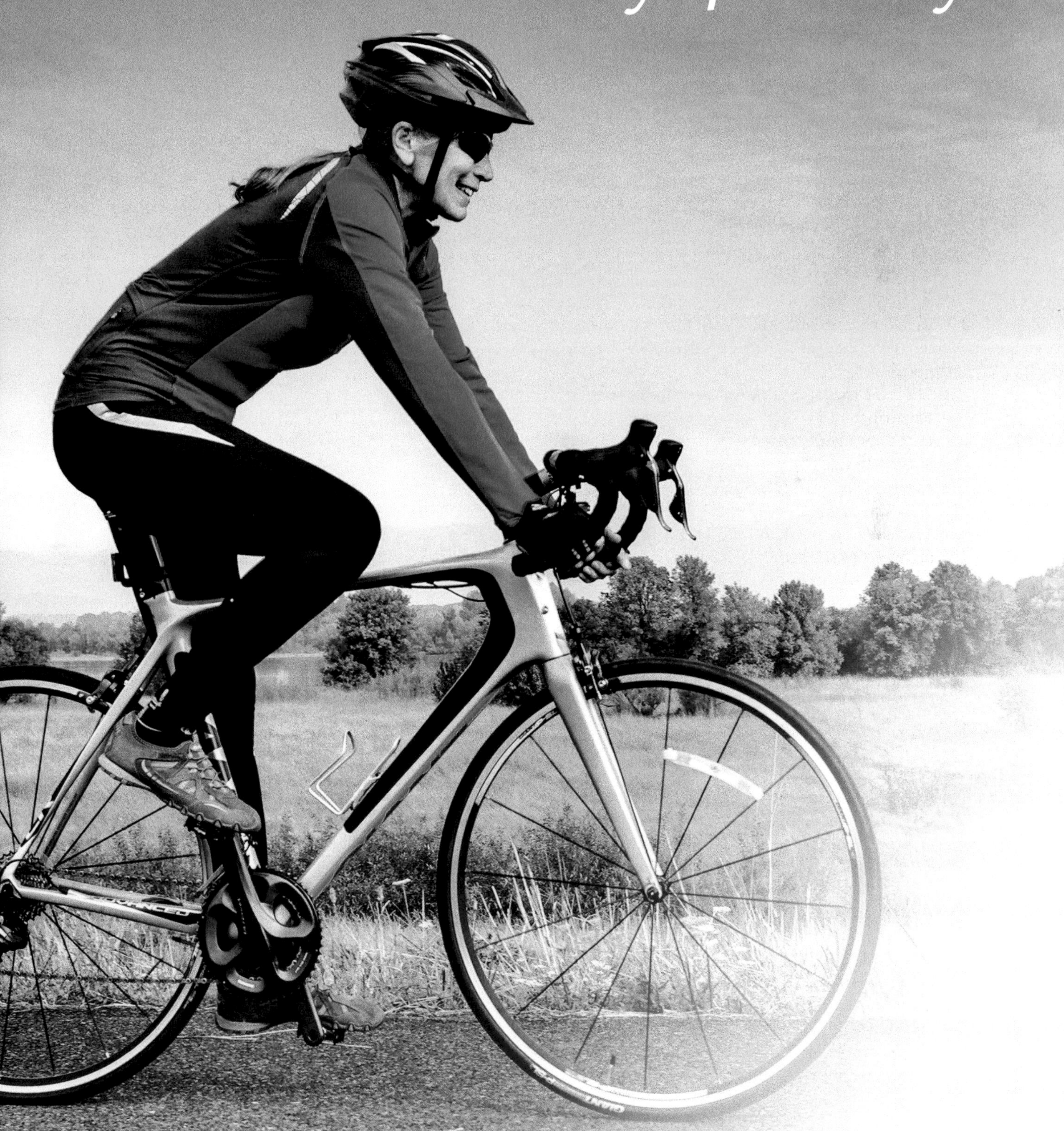

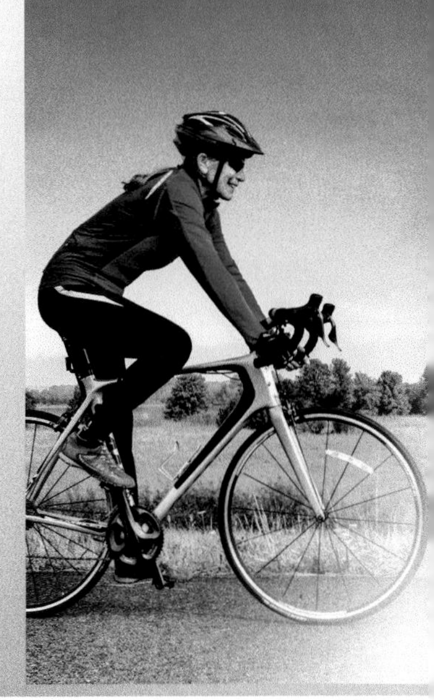

CHAPTER 21 Posture

Vertebral Alignment

Development of Postural Curves

Standing Posture

Lateral View

Anterior View

Posterior View

Sitting Posture

Supine Posture

Common Postural Deviations

Review Questions

General Anatomy Questions

Functional Activity Questions

Clinical Exercise Questions

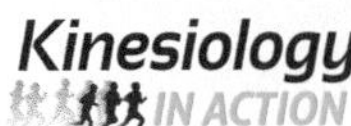

For additional practice activities and videos, please visit www.kinesiologyinaction.com

In general, posture is the position of your body parts in relation to each other at any given time. Posture can be static, as in a stationary position such as standing, sitting, or lying. It can be dynamic as the body moves from one position to another. Posture deals with alignment of the various body segments. These body segments can be compared with blocks. If you start stacking blocks, one directly on top of the other, the column will remain relatively stable. However, if you stack them off center from each other, the column will remain upright only if the block (or blocks) above offsets the block(s) below and remain(s) within the base of support. In the human body, each joint involved with weight-bearing can be considered a postural segment.

Vertebral Alignment

The vertebral column can be compared with the column of blocks. It is not completely straight but has a series of counterbalancing anterior-posterior curves. These curves, which must be maintained during rest and activity, act as shock absorbers and reduce the amount of injury. The thoracic and sacral curves offset the cervical and lumbar curves (Fig. 21-1). The thoracic and sacral curves are concave anteriorly and convex posteriorly and are seen when viewed in the sagittal plane. Conversely, the lumbar and cervical curves are just the opposite—convex anteriorly and concave posteriorly. Remember that a curve has two sides to it: a concave side and a convex side. Therefore, whether a curve is concave or convex depends on the side to which you are referring.

When one or more of these vertebral curves either increases or decreases significantly from what is considered good posture, poor posture results. For example, a "sway back" is an increased lumbar curve, whereas a "flat back" is a decreased lumbar curve. In most cases, if there is an increased lumbar curve, there is also an increased thoracic curve. No lateral curves should exist.

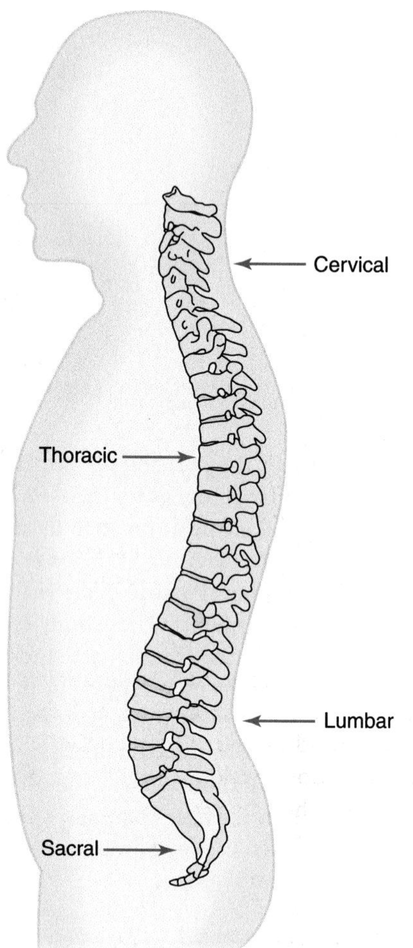

Figure 21-1. The four major curves of the vertebral column (lateral view).

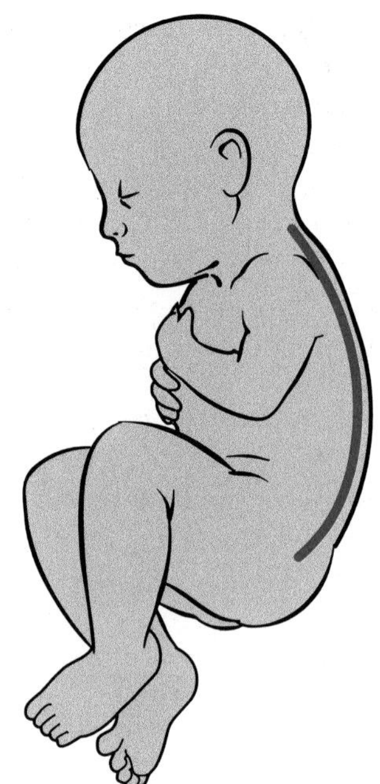

Figure 21-2. The primary curve of a newborn (lateral view).

Any lateral curvature of the spine is a pathological condition called *scoliosis.*

Development of Postural Curves

At birth, the entire vertebral column is flexed. When viewed from the sagittal plane, it is anteriorly concave. This concave curve is called a **primary curve** (Fig. 21-2). The thoracic and sacral curves are considered primary curves for this reason. When lying in a prone position, a 2- to 4-month-old infant begins to lift its head; at approximately 5 to 6 months of age, a prone infant begins bilateral lifting of its lower extremities. These two antigravity extension actions create the **secondary curves.** These are the anteriorly convex curves of the cervical and lumbar regions.

Think of the pelvis in the upright position as a bowl of water. If the bowl is level, it will hold water. If the bowl is tipped forward or backward, water will spill out. Similarly, the position of the pelvis has great influence on the vertebral column, especially the lumbar region. The pelvis should maintain a neutral position. A position is neutral when (1) the anterior superior iliac spine (ASIS) and the posterior superior iliac spine (PSIS) are level with each other in the transverse plane and (2) the ASIS is in the same vertical plane as the symphysis pubis. When the pelvis is in a neutral position, the lumbar curve has the desired amount of curvature. When the pelvis tilts anteriorly, lumbar curvature increases **(lordosis).** When the pelvis tilts posteriorly, lumbar curvature decreases (flat back). Figure 17-13 illustrates these positions.

With weight evenly distributed on both legs, the pelvis should remain level from side to side, with both ASISs being at the same level. During walking, however, the pelvis dips from side to side as weight shifts from stance to swing phase. This **lateral pelvic tilt** is controlled by the hip abductors, mainly the gluteus medius and gluteus minimus, and by the trunk lateral benders, mainly the erector spinae and quadratus lumborum. If you bend your left knee and lift your foot off the ground, your pelvis on the left side becomes unsupported and will drop. Force couple action of the hip abductors and trunk lateral benders hold the pelvis level. The right hip abductors on the opposite side contract to pull the pelvis down on the right side, while trunk lateral benders on the left (same side) contract to pull the pelvis up on the left side. These motions are illustrated in Figure 17-21. An abnormal lateral pelvic tilt can also occur if both legs are not of equal length. This will result in a lateral curvature, or scoliosis.

Muscle contractions are primarily responsible for keeping the body in the upright position in both static and dynamic posture. The muscles most involved are called **antigravity muscles** (Fig. 21-3). These are the hip and knee extensors and the trunk and neck extensors. Other muscles involved (perhaps to a lesser extent but also important in maintaining the upright position) are the trunk and neck flexors and lateral benders, the hip abductors and adductors, and the ankle pronators and supinators. If all of these muscles were to relax, the body would collapse.

The ankle plantar flexors and dorsiflexors are important in controlling postural sway (Fig. 21-4). **Postural sway** is anterior-posterior motion of the upright body caused by motion occurring primarily at the ankles. This sway is the result of constant displacement and correction of the center of gravity within the base of support.

To demonstrate this, stand upright with your feet slightly apart. Lean your entire body slowly forward by bending at the ankles. You will reach a point where you will need to either correct the forward lean or you will lose your balance. Notice that your ankle plantar flexors contract to bring you back to an upright position. Next, lean backward and notice what happens. Again, you will reach a point where you either need to correct the lean or lose your balance. Notice that your ankle dorsiflexors contract to bring you back to an upright position.

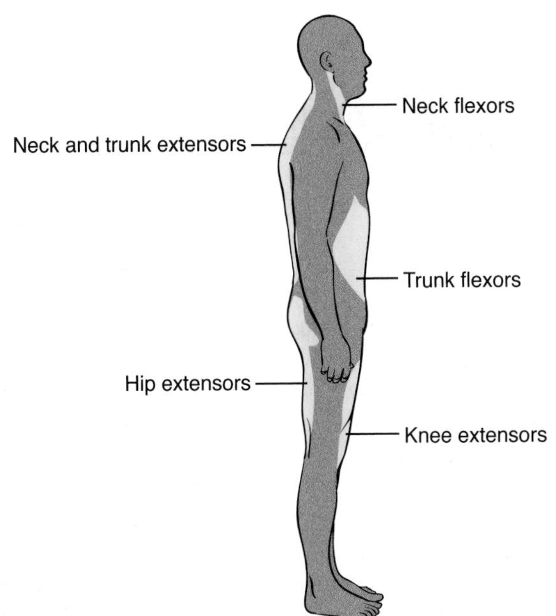

Figure 21-3. Antigravity muscles (lateral view).

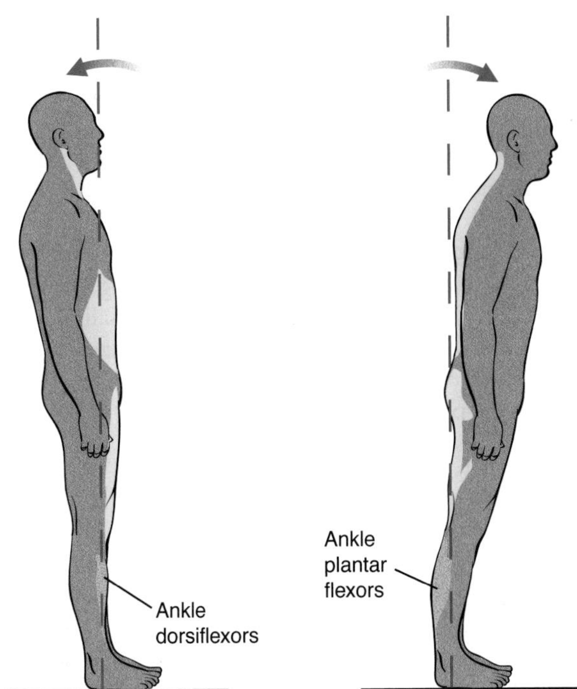

Figure 21-4. Postural sway.

A high center of gravity and small base of support tend to increase the amount of postural sway. To again demonstrate this, stand upright with your feet slightly apart. Notice how much your body tends to move back and forth. Next, observe the amount of sway when you stand on your toes in the upright position with your feet close together. You should notice much more motion in the latter position, because you have raised your center of gravity higher and made your base of support smaller.

Good posture, which means good alignment, is important because it decreases the amount of stress placed on bones, ligaments, muscles, and tendons. Good alignment also improves function and decreases the amount of muscle energy needed to keep the body upright. For example, if the knee is in full extension, little muscle contraction is needed to keep the knee from buckling. However, when the knee is partially flexed, the muscles at that joint (knee extensors) must contract to keep the knee from collapsing. Because standing is a closed-chain activity, muscles at the hip and ankle must also contract to keep the body's center of gravity over its base of support.

To watch a ballet dancer move is to watch good posture in motion. Ballet aspires to show motion in an aesthetically beautiful manner. What is most beautiful is also most functional. Maintaining good postural alignment and keeping one's center of gravity well within one's base of support places less stress on body parts and allows for better balance. Ballet dancers learn the basic elements of good posture from the very beginning of their training. They are instructed in various ways to get taller, tighten their knee muscles, tighten their abdominal muscles to flatten the abdomen "like a pancake," and hold their buttocks "like a rock." In other words, dancers assume and maintain good alignment. The dancer in Figure 21-5 is maintaining good body alignment while balancing over a fairly small base of support. She is maintaining this posture dynamically as she turns (pirouette) on pointe (toes extended and ankle in extreme plantar flexion).

Standing Posture

Posture is easier to describe in a static standing position because, except for a slight amount of sway when standing, the body is not moving. However, many of the guidelines for static posture can be applied to dynamic posture. Assessing a person's posture can be done most accurately with the use of a plumb line suspended from the ceiling or a posture grid behind the person as a point of reference. A plumb line is a string or cord with a weight attached to the lower end. Because the string is weighted, it makes a perfectly straight vertical line of gravity.

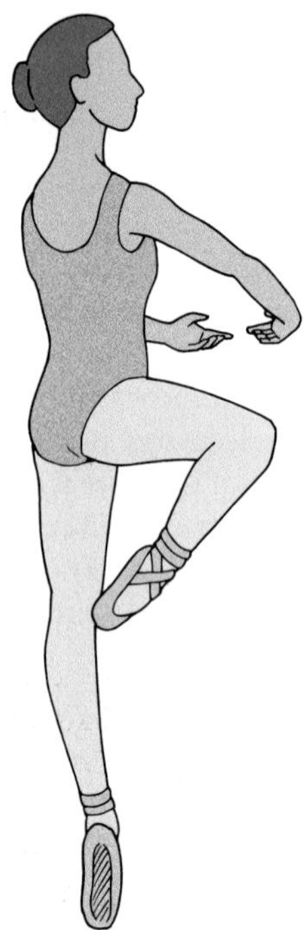

Figure 21-5. A ballet dancer must maintain good posture during motion.

Lateral View

In the standing position and viewed from the **lateral position,** the plumb line should be aligned so that it passes slightly in front of the lateral malleolus (Fig. 21-6). For ideal posture, the body segments should be aligned so that the plumb line passes through the landmarks in the order listed.

Head
Through the earlobe

Shoulder
Through the tip of the acromion process

Thoracic Spine
Anterior to the vertebral bodies

Lumbar Spine
Through the vertebral bodies

Pelvis
Level

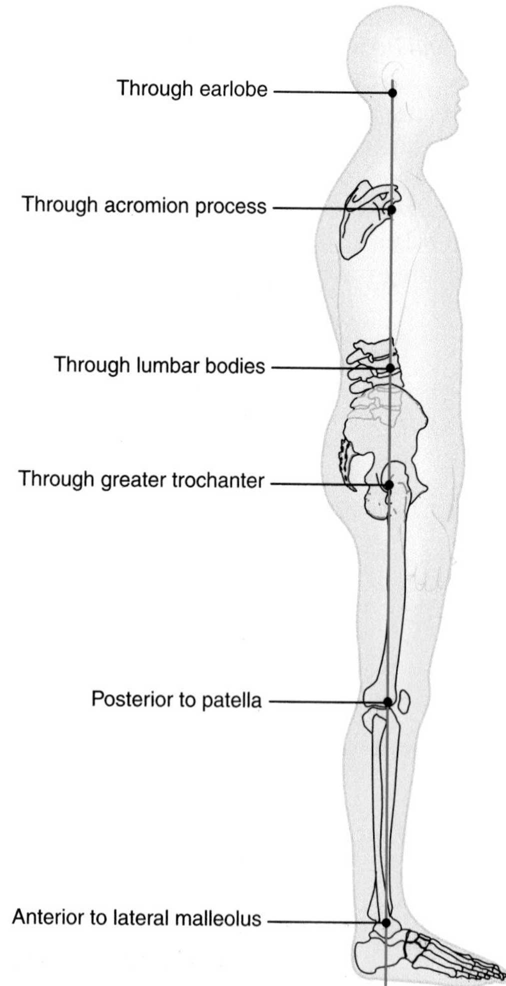

Figure 21-6. Posture (lateral view).

Hip
Through the greater trochanter (slightly posterior to the hip joint axis)

Knee
Slightly posterior to the patella (slightly anterior to the knee joint axis) with the knees in extension

Ankle
Slightly anterior to the lateral malleolus, with the ankle joint in a neutral position between dorsiflexion and plantar flexion

Table 21-1 summarizes common postural deviations that can be detected from the lateral view. Because standing is a closed kinetic chain activity, the position or motion of one joint will affect the positions or motions of other joints.

Anterior View

In the standing position and viewed from the **anterior position,** the plumb line should be aligned to pass through the midsagittal plane of the body, thus dividing the body into two equal halves (Fig. 21-7). The body segments listed below should be aligned in the following order:

Head
Extended and level, not flexed or hyperextended

Shoulders
Level and not elevated or depressed

Sternum
Centered in the midline

Hips
Level, with both ASISs in the same plane

Legs
Slightly apart

Knees
Level and not bowed or knock-kneed

Ankles
Normal arch in feet; foot not inverted or pronated

Feet
Slight outward toeing

Table 21-1 Summary of Common Postural Deviations

	Lateral View	Posterior View	Anterior View
Head	Forward	Tilted Rotated	Tilted Rotated Mandible asymmetrical
Cervical spine	Exaggerated curve Flattened curve		
Shoulders	Rounded	Elevated Depressed	Elevated Depressed
Scapulae		Abducted Adducted Winged	
Thoracic spine	Exaggerated curve	Lateral deviation	
Lumbar spine	Exaggerated curve Flattened curve	Lateral deviation	
Pelvis	Anterior pelvic tilt Posterior pelvic tilt	Lateral pelvic tilt Pelvis rotated	
Hip			Medially rotated Laterally rotated
Knee	Genu recurvatum Flexed knee	Genu varum Genu valgum	External tibial torsion Internal tibial torsion
Ankle/foot	Forward posture Flattened longitudinal arch Exaggerated longitudinal arch	Pes planus Pes cavus	Hallux valgus Claw toe Hammertoe Mallet toe

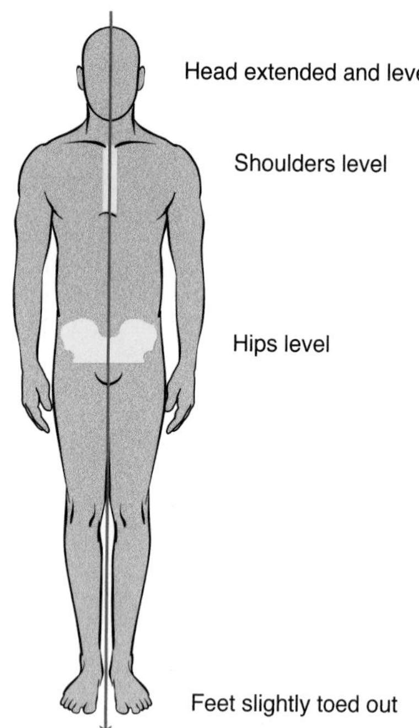

Figure 21-7. Posture (anterior view).

Posterior View

In the standing position and viewed from the **posterior position,** the plumb line should also be aligned to pass through the midsagittal plane of the body, dividing the body into two equal halves (Fig. 21-8). The following body segments should be aligned in the order listed below:

Head
Extended, not flexed or hyperextended

Shoulders
Level and not elevated or depressed

Spinous Processes
Centered in the midline

Hips
Level, with both PSISs in the same plane

Legs
Slightly apart

Knees
Level and not bowed or knock-kneed

Ankles
Calcaneus should be straight.

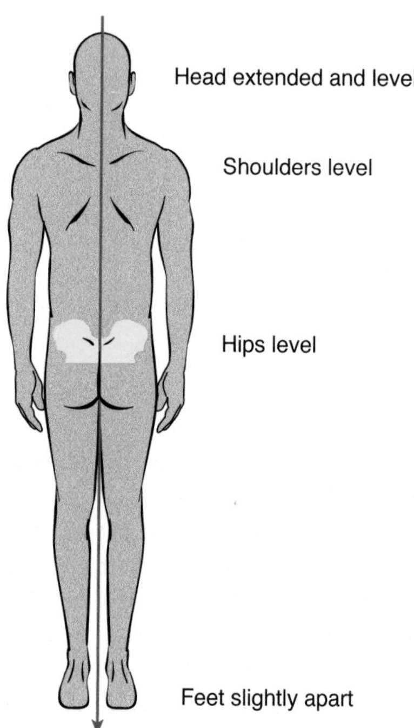

Figure 21-8. Posture (posterior view).

Sitting Posture

Good postural alignment while sitting is important, because sitting can place a great deal of pressure on the intervertebral disks. Studies have shown that disk pressure in the sitting position increases by slightly less than half of the amount of disk pressure in the standing position. To state the obvious, shifting weight onto the front part of the vertebrae will increase the amount of pressure placed on the intervertebral disks. As the person leans forward, disk pressure increases. As a person reaches forward or picks up a weight, disk pressure further increases as the weight or length of the lever arm increases. Figure 21-9 illustrates disk pressure in various positions. Disk pressure is least when you are lying supine. It increases as you stand and increases more as you sit. Leaning forward in these positions increases the disk pressure, and leaning forward with an object in your hand obviously increases it even more.

If the lumbar curve decreases, as often happens when sitting with the back unsupported (Fig. 21-10), the pressure on the intervertebral disks and posterior structures increases. A chair with the seat inclined anteriorly, such as the kneeling stool (Fig. 21-11), can decrease disk pressure by tilting the pelvis forward slightly. This helps to maintain the lumbar curve. However, because the back is unsupported, increased and sustained muscle contraction is required to keep the body upright.

Shifting weight onto the front part of the vertebra is not always a problem. Although disk pressure increases in this position, the stresses placed on the posterior part of the vertebra (the facet joints) decreases. Therefore, if a

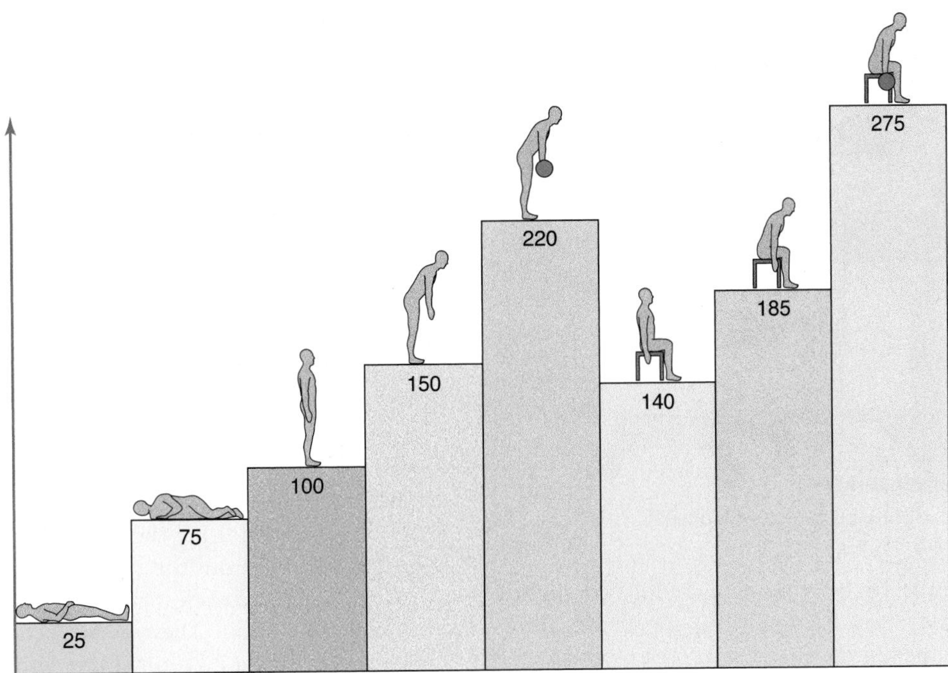

Figure 21-9. Disk pressures in various positions.

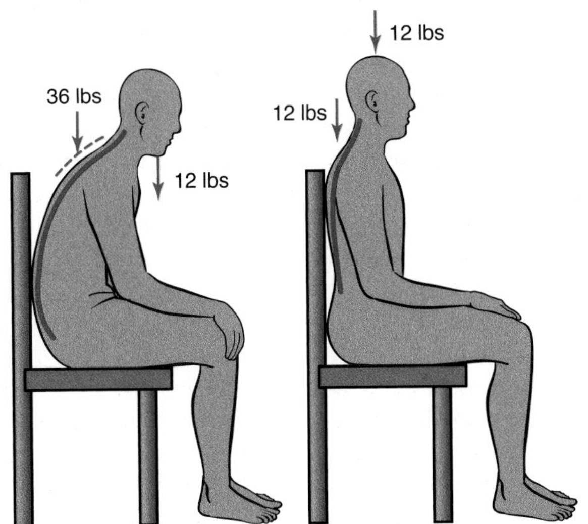

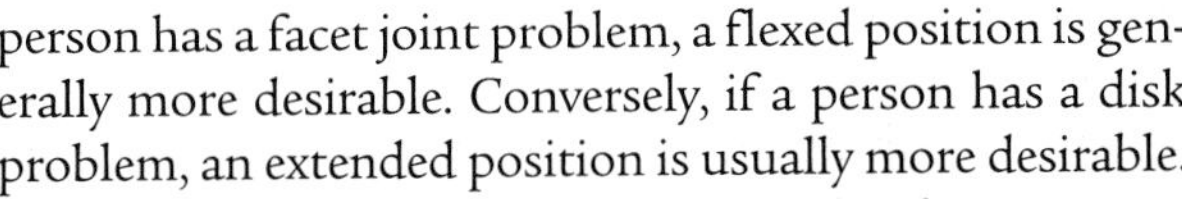

Figure 21-10. Slouched posture increases disk pressure.

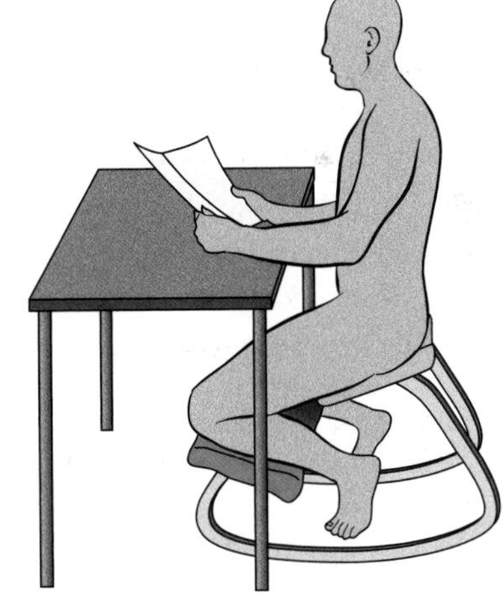

Figure 21-11. Kneeling stool posture reduces disk pressure.

person has a facet joint problem, a flexed position is generally more desirable. Conversely, if a person has a disk problem, an extended position is usually more desirable.

In sitting postures, a chair with lumbar support and/or a slight forward angle to the seat helps maintain lumbar lordosis and minimize pressure on the disks. It is also helpful to have adjustable height work station and computer monitor, a keyboard tray, and a chair with adjustable height armrests. Maintaining the vertebral curves, keeping the feet flat on the floor, having the low back supported, and keeping the upper body in good alignment are key elements of good sitting posture. Figure 21-12 demonstrates good posture while working at a computer. The neck and trunk are upright, the trunk is supported, and the lumbar spine has a support. The top of the monitor is at eye level. A person should not have to hyperextend or flex the head to view the screen (see Clinical Application 21-1). The shoulders are relaxed. The elbows are flexed and close to the body and supported by armrests. The hands, wrists, and forearms are straight and parallel to the ground. The chair should allow the hips and knees to be flexed so that the

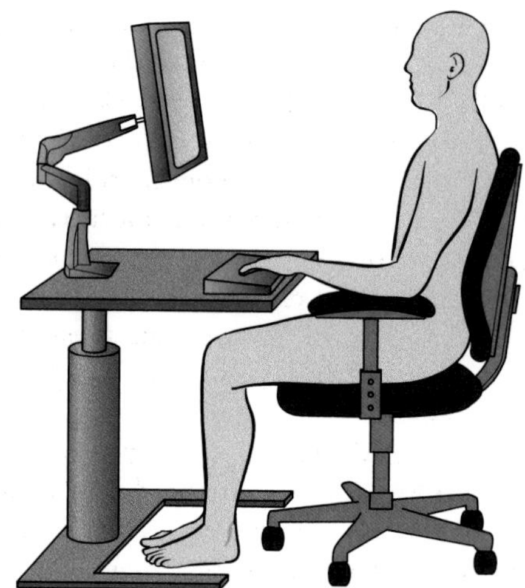

Figure 21-12. Sitting posture at computer.

thighs are parallel to the ground, or the hips are slightly higher than the knees. The lower legs are vertical, allowing the feet to be flat on the floor or on a footrest.

Supine Posture

Lying down is considered a resting position (Fig. 21-13). The least amount of intervertebral disk pressure occurs while lying supine (see Fig. 21-9). If you could run a plumb line horizontally, it would intersect many of the same landmarks as in the standing position. Good alignment in this position is also important. A good resting surface should be firm enough to avoid loss of the lumbar curve, yet soft enough to conform and give support to the normal curves of the body. In the side-lying position, the bottom leg is extended and the top leg is flexed. Placing a pillow between the legs can increase comfort by keeping the hips in good alignment. Lying prone is usually not recommended because of the increased pressure placed on the neck. In this position, using a pillow only increases the stresses on the neck.

When actively moving about and changing positions, whether vacuuming the rug, picking up a box from the floor, or raking leaves, keeping the body (especially the trunk) in good postural alignment is important. Most principles of good body mechanics involve avoiding stress to the trunk and maintaining the spinal curves, which involve maintaining good posture.

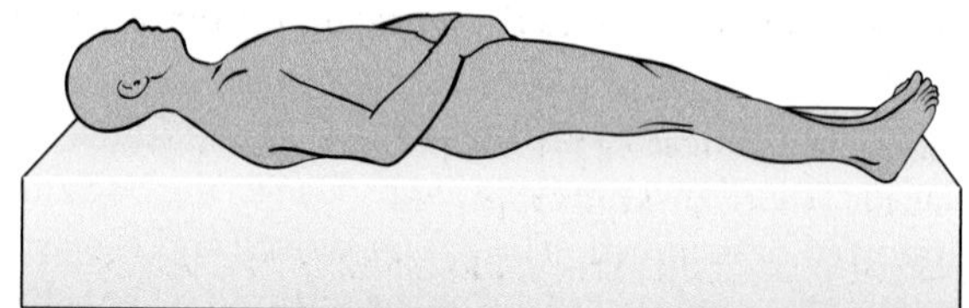

Figure 21-13. Lying posture.

Common Postural Deviations

Table 21-1 summarizes the common postural deviations seen when assessing posture. It is not within the

Clinical Application 21-1

Text Neck

Smart phones are wonderful inventions but may come at a musculoskeletal price. Looking at and using them for long periods of time throughout the day puts a great deal of stress on the neck, hence the common name "text neck." The typical posture while texting or looking at our smart phones is one of extreme neck flexion. The problem is that the more the neck is flexed, the more weight is placed on the cervical spine. When you are in good postural alignment, the line of gravity passes through the earlobe (see Fig. 21-6). In that position, the weight on the cervical spine is approximately 10 pounds. Flexing the neck to 45 degrees (Fig. A) can increase the stress on the cervical spine five times to approximately 50 pounds. If you use your phone 2 to 3 hours per day, that is a lot a strain on the cervical disks, extensor muscles, and posterior ligaments. A simple change of holding the phone higher and looking down with your eyes can significantly decrease the stress on the neck (Fig. B).

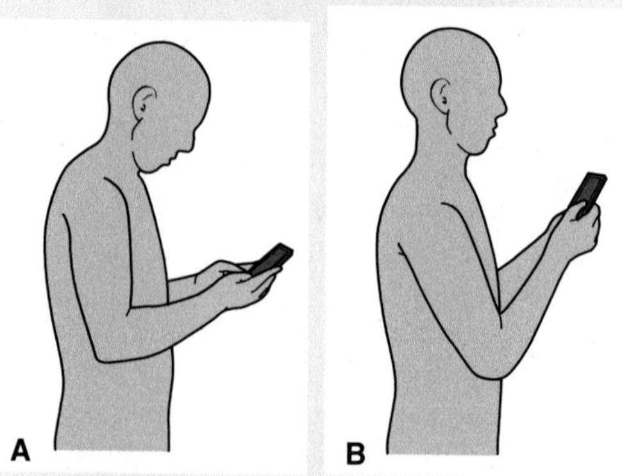

Text neck. **(A)** Flexed neck - greater stress. **(B)** Extended neck - less stress.

scope of this book to describe the individual causes and effects of postural problems. However, some general statements regarding cause and effect should be made.

Deviation from "good" posture is considered "poor" or "bad" posture. Causes of poor posture can be the result of structural problems. These structural problems may result from a congenital malformation such as a hemivertebra. The deviation may be an acquired deformity caused by trauma such as a compression fracture. Postural deviations also may result from neurological conditions that cause paralysis or spasticity. In addition, postural problems may be functional, or nonstructural, in nature. A person who sits or stands for long periods of time will tend to slouch. This can result in muscle imbalance.

Generally, if a person tends to maintain a posture in which a curve is increased, the muscles on the concave side will tend to tighten (adaptive shortening) while the muscles on the convex side tend to weaken (adaptive lengthening). For example, you would expect a person with a lumbar lordosis to have tight back extensors and weak abdominal muscles. Also, postures that tend to increase the lordotic curves (cervical and lumbar) will increase pressure on the more posterior facet joints and decrease pressure on the more anterior intervertebral disks. Conversely, an increase in the kyphotic curves (thoracic and sacral) will increase the pressure on the intervertebral disks while decreasing the pressure on the facet joints.

It should be noted that the terms *kyphotic* and *lordotic* can lead to confusion. They are used to describe both the normal amount of curvature and the abnormal or excessive amount of curvature of the thoracic and lumbar spine, respectively. *Scoliosis* is a term that refers to a lateral curvature. However, any amount of scoliosis is considered abnormal.

Review Questions

General Anatomy Questions

1. If a person had an excessive cervical lordosis, would you expect the cervical extensors or flexors to be tight?
2. Which position–side, front, or back–would be best to assess the condition in question 1?
3. If a person had an anterior tilt of the pelvis, would you expect the hip flexors or hip extensors to be tight?
4. To assess the condition in question 3, which position–the side, front, or back–would be best?
5. What position should the shoulders be in relation to each other?
6. Which position–side, front, or back–would be best to assess the position of the shoulders in relation to each other?
7. When using a plumb line to assess a person's posture in the lateral standing position, you should begin by lining up the plumb line with what body structure?
8. For ideal posture (when viewed laterally), where should the plumb line pass on the following structures:
   a. Knee
   b. Hip
   c. Shoulder
   d. Head

Functional Activity Questions

1. Sitting in a chair with a back and armrests, put your hands together, resting them between your thighs near your knees. Your shoulder girdles are in what position?
2. Sitting in the same position as in question 1, move from that position to one with your forearms resting on the arms of the chair. How does the position of your shoulder girdles change from their position in question 1?
3. Sitting slouched down in the chair, keep your back in contact with the back of the chair and slide your buttocks forward. What position does your head assume?
4. Carry a heavy book bag on your right shoulder. By changing posture, how do you keep the strap from sliding off your shoulder?

For questions 5 through 9, consider the posture of a woman during pregnancy.

5. In what direction does the woman's center of gravity shift?
6. There is a tendency for the pelvis to tilt in which direction in the sagittal plane?
7. What type of change would occur in the lumbar spine?

(continued on next page)

Review Questions—cont'd

8. Those changes in the pelvic and lumbar positions could lead to:
   a. which trunk muscle group becoming tight?
   b. which trunk muscle group becoming stretched?
9. As a compensatory posture, would you expect the hip flexors or extensors to become tight?

Clinical Exercise Questions

1. Sit in front of a computer. Pretend (if necessary) that you are wearing bifocals that require you to look through the bottom of the lenses for close-up work. This can be simulated by wrapping plastic wrap on the top half of a pair of eyeglasses or sunglasses. To read the screen, what position do the head and neck assume?
2. If the position in the exercise in question 1 became a chronic posture:
   a. muscle groups on which side of the neck would become tighter?
   b. muscle groups on which side of the neck would become stretched?
3. Stand upright with equal weight on both feet and a 1- to 3-inch block under your left foot (depending on your height). Does your pelvis remain level? If not, which side of the pelvis is higher?
4. If the posture in the exercise in question 3 became a permanent condition:
   a. muscle groups on which side of the trunk would become tighter?
   b. muscle groups on which side of the trunk would become stretched?
5. Continuing with the exercise in question 3:
   a. Which side of the intervertebral disk would be compressed? Distracted?
   b. Which side of the intervertebral disk would be distracted?
   c. The intervertebral foramen on which side would be opened more?
   d. The intervertebral foramen on which side would be made smaller?
6. Lie supine, hug your knees to your chest, and bring your knees and forehead together. Hug the knees close to your chest (Fig. 21-14).
   a. What trunk muscle group is being stretched?
   b. Which part of the intervertebral disk is being compressed?
7. Lie prone with your hips and knees extended. Rise up and rest on your elbows (Fig. 21-15).
   a. What trunk muscles are being stretched?
   b. Which part of the intervertebral disk is being compressed?

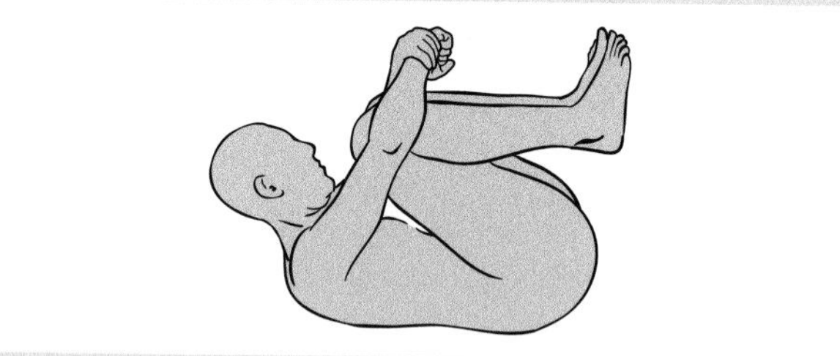

Figure 21-14. Exercise position. Lie supine, hugging knees to chest.

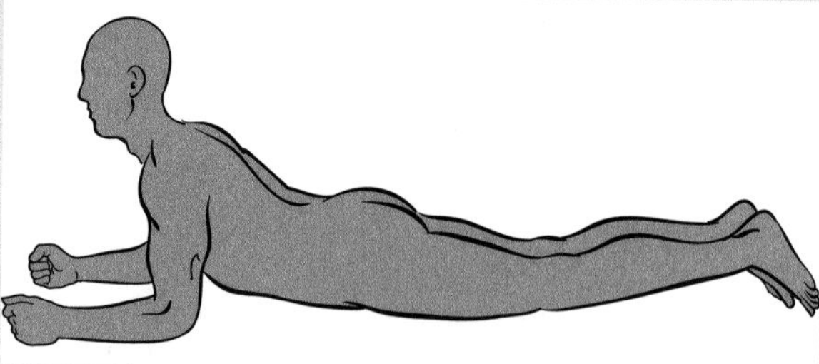

Figure 21-15. Exercise position. Lie prone, resting on elbows.

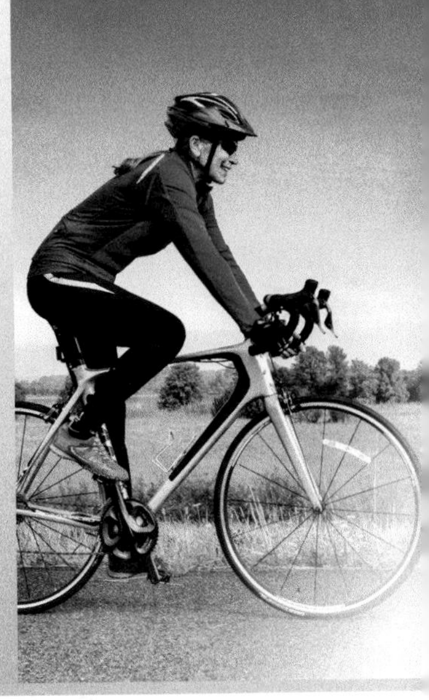

CHAPTER 22 Gait

Definitions
Analysis of Stance Phase
Analysis of Swing Phase
Additional Determinants of Gait
Age-Related Gait Patterns
Abnormal (Atypical) Gait
Muscular Weakness/Paralysis
Joint/Muscle Range-of-Motion Limitation
Neurological Involvement
Pain
Leg Length Discrepancy
Points to Remember
Review Questions
General Anatomy Questions
Functional Activity Questions
Clinical Exercise Questions

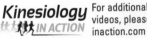

Kinesiology IN ACTION For additional practice activities and videos, please visit www.kinesiologyinaction.com

Walking is the manner or way in which you move from place to place with your feet. *Gait* is the process or components of walking. Each person has a unique style, and this style may change slightly with mood. When you are happy, your step is lighter, and there may be a "bounce" in your walk. Conversely, when you are sad or depressed, your step may be heavy. For some people, their walking pattern is so unique that they can be identified from a distance even before their face can clearly be seen. Regardless of the numerous different styles, the components of normal gait are the same.

In the most basic sense, walking requires balancing on one leg while the other leg moves forward. This requires movement not only of the legs but also of the trunk and arms. To analyze gait, you must first determine what joint motions occur. Then, based upon that information, you must decide which muscles or muscle groups are acting.

Definitions

Certain definitions must be made to describe gait. **Gait cycle,** also called **stride,** is the activity that occurs between the time one foot touches the floor and the time the same foot touches the floor again (Fig. 22-1). A **stride length** is the distance traveled during the gait cycle.

A **step** is basically one-half of a stride. It takes two steps (a right one and a left one) to complete a stride or gait cycle. These steps should be equal. A **step length** is that distance between the heel strike of one foot and the heel strike of the other foot (see Fig. 22-1). With an increased or decreased walking speed, the step length will increase or decrease, respectively. Regardless of speed, the step length of the two legs should remain equal.

Walking speed, or **cadence,** is the number of steps taken per minute. It can vary greatly. Slow walking may be as slow as 70 steps per minute. However, students on

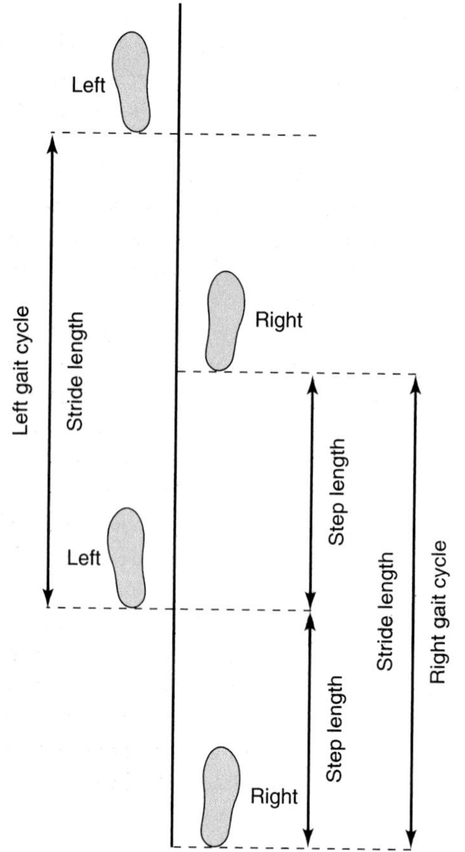

Figure 22-1. Gait cycle terminology. A right and left step make up a gait cycle (also called *stride*).

their way to an examination have been clocked at much slower speeds. Fast walking may be as fast as 130 steps per minute, although race walkers will walk much faster. Regardless of speed, the gait cycle is the same; all parts occur in their proper place at the proper time.

There are two phases of the gait cycle (Fig. 22-2). **Stance phase** is the activity that occurs when the foot is in contact with the ground. It begins with the heel strike of one foot and ends when that foot leaves the ground. This phase accounts for about 60% of the gait cycle. **Swing phase** occurs when the foot is not in contact with the ground. It begins as soon as the foot leaves the floor and ends when the heel of the same foot touches the floor again. The swing phase makes up about 40% of the gait cycle.

Perry (1992) identifies three tasks that need to be accomplished during these phases of the gait cycle: (1) weight acceptance, (2) single-leg support, and (3) leg advancement. Figure 22-2 shows the phases of the gait cycle. **Weight acceptance** occurs at the very beginning of stance phase when the foot touches the ground and the body weight begins to shift onto that leg. **Single-leg support** occurs next, as the body weight shifts completely onto the stance leg so that the opposite leg can swing forward. The task of **leg advancement** occurs during swing phase.

The gait cycle has two periods of double support and two periods of single support (see Fig. 22-2). When both feet are in contact with the ground at the same time,

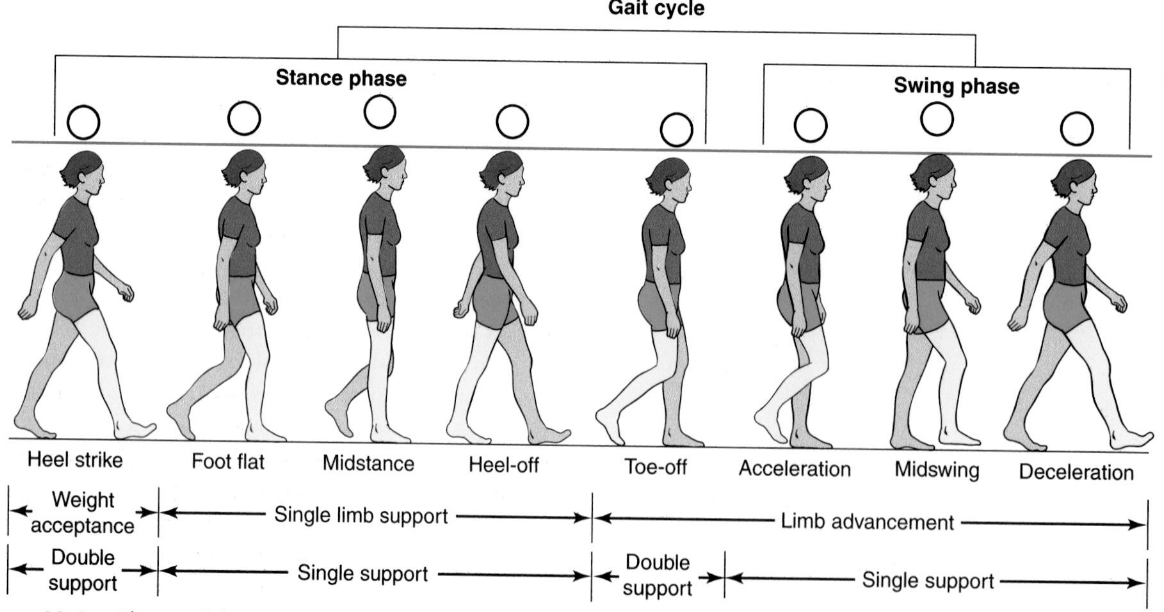

Figure 22-2. Phases of the gait cycle.

this is a period of **double support.** This occurs as one leg is beginning its stance phase and the other leg is ending its stance phase. For example, the first period of double support occurs as the right leg is beginning stance phase and the left leg is ending stance phase. The second period of double support occurs as the right leg is ending its stance phase and the left leg is beginning its stance phase. Each period of double support takes up about 10% of the gait cycle at an average walking speed. If you increase your walking speed, you spend less time with both feet on the ground. Conversely, when you walk slowly, you spend more time in double support.

A period of **nonsupport**—that is, a time during which neither foot is in contact with the ground—does not occur during walking. However, nonsupport does occur during running. Other than speed, this may be the biggest difference between running and walking. Other activities, such as hopping, skipping, and jumping, have a period of nonsupport but lose the order of progression that walking and running have. In other words, these activities do not include all the parts of stance and swing phase that walking and running have.

The period of **single support** occurs when only one foot is in contact with the ground (see Fig. 22-2). Thus, two periods of single support occur in a gait cycle: once when the right foot is on the ground as the left foot is swinging forward, then again when the left foot bears weight and the right leg swings forward. Each single-support period takes up about 40% of the gait cycle.

Many sets of terms have been developed from the original, or traditional, terminology to describe the components of walking. In many cases, although the terminology may be accurate, it is often cumbersome. However, terminology developed by the Gait Laboratory at Rancho Los Amigos (RLA) Medical Center has been gaining acceptance. Perhaps the biggest difference between the two sets of terms is that the traditional terms refer to *points in time,* whereas RLA terms refer to *periods of time.* Traditional terminology accurately reflects key points within the gait cycle, whereas RLA periods accurately reflect the moving or dynamic nature of gait. It is best to be familiar with both sets of terms because both terminologies will be seen in the literature. Table 22-1 compares traditional terminology with RLA terms. One can see that they are similar, with a few exceptions. Table 22-2 describes the activities of each phase and the key points to observe. The table reiterates the slight differences between the two sets of terms. However, the key points are in the same sequence of the gait cycle, regardless of which terminology is used.

Table 22-1 Comparison of Gait Terminology

Traditional		Rancho Los Amigos	
Term	**Definition**	**Term**	**Definition**
Stance Phase			
Heel strike	Heel contacts the ground	Initial contact	Same
Foot flat	Plantar surface of the foot in contact with ground	Loading response	Beginning: Just after initial contact when body weight is being transferred onto leg and entire foot makes contact with the ground Ending: Opposite foot leaves the ground
Midstance	Point at which the body passes over the weight-bearing leg	Midstance	Beginning: Opposite foot leaves the ground Ending: Body is directly over the weight-bearing limb
Heel-off	Heel leaves the ground while ball of the foot and toes remain in contact with the ground	Terminal stance	Beginning: As the heel of weight-bearing leg rises Ending: Initial contact of the opposite foot; the body has moved in front of the weight-bearing leg

Continued

Table 22-1 Comparison of Gait Terminology—cont'd

Traditional		Rancho Los Amigos	
Term	**Definition**	**Term**	**Definition**
Toe-off	Toes leave the ground, ending stance phase	Preswing	Beginning: Initial contact and weight shifted onto the opposite leg Ending: Just before toes of weight-bearing leg leave the ground
Swing Phase			
Acceleration	The swing leg begins to move forward	Initial swing	Beginning: The toes leave the ground Ending: The swing foot is opposite the weight-bearing foot, and the knee is in maximum flexion
Midswing	The swing (non–weight-bearing) leg is directly under the body	Midswing	Beginning: The swing foot is opposite the weight-bearing foot Ending: The swing leg has moved in front of the body and the tibia is in a vertical position
Deceleration	The leg is slowing down in preparation for heel strike	Terminal swing	Beginning: The tibia is in a vertical position Ending: Just before initial contact

Table 22-2 Key Events of Normal Gait Cycle

Traditional Terminology	RLA Terminology	Activity	Key Points to Observe
Stance Phase (indicated here as right leg to coincide with Figures 22-3 through 22-8)			
Heel strike* Stance (right) foot touches the ground	*Initial contact* Stance (right) foot touches the ground	• Stance phase begins • Task of weight acceptance begins • Double leg support begins • Center of gravity (COG) at lowest point in cycle	• Head and trunk are upright throughout cycle • Right ankle dorsiflexed to neutral • Right knee extended • Right hip flexed • Right leg in front of body • Pelvis rotated forward–ipsilateral side • Ipsilateral (right) arm back, contralateral (left) arm forward
Foot flat Entire stance (right) foot in contact with ground	*Loading response* Begins with stance (right) foot touching the ground, continues until opposite (left) foot leaves the ground	• Weight shift onto stance leg continues • Double leg support ends	• Right ankle plantar flexes putting foot on the ground • Right knee partially flexed, absorbing shock • Right hip moving into extension • Body catching up with leg • Ipsilateral (right) arm swinging forward

Table 22-2 Key Events of Normal Gait Cycle—cont'd

Traditional Terminology	RLA Terminology	Activity	Key Points to Observe
Midstance Body passes over stance (right) leg	*Midstance* Begins with other leg (left) leaving the ground, continues until body is over stance (right) leg	• COG at highest point in cycle • Single leg support begins	• Right ankle slightly dorsiflexed • Right knee and hip continue extending • Body passes over right foot • Pelvis in neutral position • Both arms parallel with body
Heel-off Right heel rises off the ground, beginning of push-off	*Terminal stance* Begins with right heel rising, continues until other foot (left) touches the ground	• Body moves ahead of foot • Single-leg support ends	• Right ankle slightly dorsiflexed, then begins plantar flexion • Right knee extending, then beginning slight flexion • Right hip hyperextending • Body ahead of stance (right) leg • Pelvis rotating back—ipsilateral (right) side • Ipsilateral arm (right) swinging forward
Toe-off Right toe leaves the ground	*Preswing* Begins with other foot touching the ground, continues until toes leave the ground	• Task of leg advancement begins • Double-leg support begins and ends	• Right ankle plantar flexed • Right knee and hip are flexing • Lateral pelvic tilt to right side • Ipsilateral (right) arm forward
Swing Phase (indicated here as right leg to coincide with Figures 22-9 through 22-12)			
Acceleration Swing leg is behind body, moving forward to catch up	*Initial swing* Begins with right foot leaving the ground, ends with swinging foot opposite (left) stance foot	• Swing phase (non–weight-bearing) begins • Single leg support begins on contralateral (left) side	• Right ankle beginning to dorsiflex • Right knee and hip continue flexing • Right leg is behind body but moving forward • Pelvis beginning to rotate forward • Ipsilateral (right) arm swinging backward
Midswing Right foot swings under and past body	*Midswing* Begins with foot opposite stance foot (left), ends with tibia in vertical position	• Leg shortens to clear the ground • Single-leg support on contralateral (left) side continues	• Right ankle dorsiflexed • Right knee at maximum flexion and begins to extend • Right hip at maximum flexion • Right leg passing under and moving in front of body • Pelvis in neutral position • Arms parallel with body and moving in opposite directions
Deceleration Right leg slowing down, preparing to touch the ground	*Terminal swing* Begins with vertical tibia (right), ends when right foot touches the ground	• Leg advancement task ends • Single support ends	• Right ankle continuing in dorsiflexion • Right knee extended • Right hip flexed • Right leg ahead of body • Pelvis rotated forward—ipsilateral (right) side • Ipsilateral arm (right) back, contralateral arm (left) forward

*__Bold__ indicates traditional terminology. *Italics* indicates Rancho Los Amigos (RLA) terminology.

Analysis of Stance Phase

As defined earlier, *stance* is that period in which the foot is in contact with the floor. Traditionally, the stance phase has been broken down into five components: (1) heel strike, (2) foot flat, (3) midstance, (4) heel-off, and (5) toe-off (Fig. 22-3). Some sources give stance phase only four components by combining heel-off and toe-off into one and calling it *push-off*. Because significantly different activities occur during these two periods, it is best to keep them separated.

Heel strike signals the beginning of stance phase, the moment the heel comes in contact with the ground (Fig. 22-4). At this point, the ankle is in a neutral position between dorsiflexion and plantar flexion, and the knee begins to flex. This slight knee flexion provides some shock absorption as the foot hits the ground. The hip is in about 25 degrees of flexion. The trunk is erect and remains so throughout the entire gait cycle. The trunk is rotated toward the opposite (contralateral) side, the opposite arm is forward, and the same-side (ipsilateral) arm is back in shoulder hyperextension. At this point, body weight begins to shift onto the stance leg. In RLA, this is the period of *initial contact.*

The ankle dorsiflexors are active in putting the ankle in its neutral position. The quadriceps, which have been contracting concentrically, switch to contracting eccentrically to minimize the amount of knee flexion. The hip flexors have been active. However, the hip extensors are beginning to contract, keeping the hip from flexing more. The erector spinae are active in keeping the trunk from flexing. The force of the foot hitting the ground transmits up through the ankle, knee, and hip to the trunk. This would cause the pelvis to rotate anteriorly, flexing the trunk somewhat, if it were not for the erector spinae counteracting this force.

Foot flat, when the entire foot is in contact with the ground, occurs shortly after heel strike (Fig. 22-5). The ankle moves into about 15 degrees of plantar flexion with the dorsiflexors contracting eccentrically to keep the foot from "slapping" down on the floor. The knee moves into about 20 degrees of flexion. The hip is moving into extension, allowing the rest of the body to begin catching up with the leg. Weight shift onto the stance leg continues. Foot flat is roughly comparable to the RLA period called *loading response,* which is that period between the end of heel strike and the end of foot flat.

The point at which the body passes over the weight-bearing foot is called **midstance** (Fig. 22-6). In this phase, the ankle moves into slight dorsiflexion. However, the dorsiflexors become inactive. The plantar flexors begin to contract, controlling the rate at which the leg moves over the ankle. The knee and hip continue to extend; both arms are in shoulder extension, essentially parallel with the body; and the trunk is in a neutral position of rotation. In RLA, *midstance* is the period between the end of foot flat and the end of midstance.

Following midstance is **heel-off,** in which the heel rises off the floor (Fig. 22-7). The ankle will dorsiflex slightly (approximately 15 degrees) and then begin to plantar flex. This is the beginning of the **push-off** phase, sometimes called the *propulsion phase,* because the ankle plantar flexors are actively pushing the body forward. The knee is in nearly full extension, and the hip has moved into hyperextension. The leg is now behind the body. The trunk has begun to rotate to the same side, and the arm is swinging forward into shoulder flexion. In RLA, *terminal stance* is that period between the end of midstance and the end of heel-off.

The end of the push-off portion of stance is **toe-off** (Fig. 22-8). The toes are in extreme hyperextension at the metatarsophalangeal joints. The ankle moves into about 10 degrees of plantar flexion, and the knee and

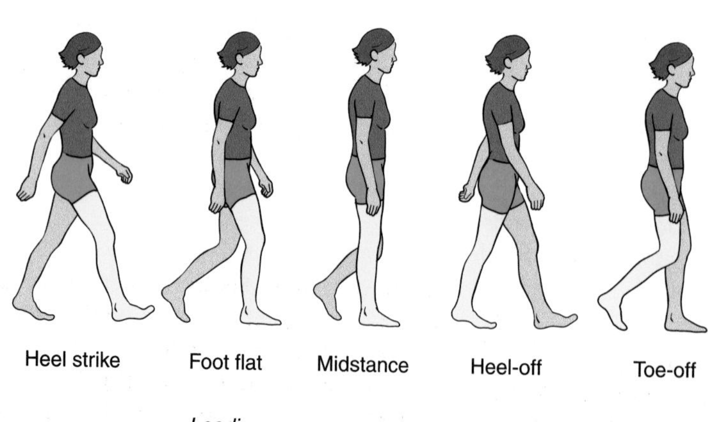

Figure 22-3. The five components of stance phase.

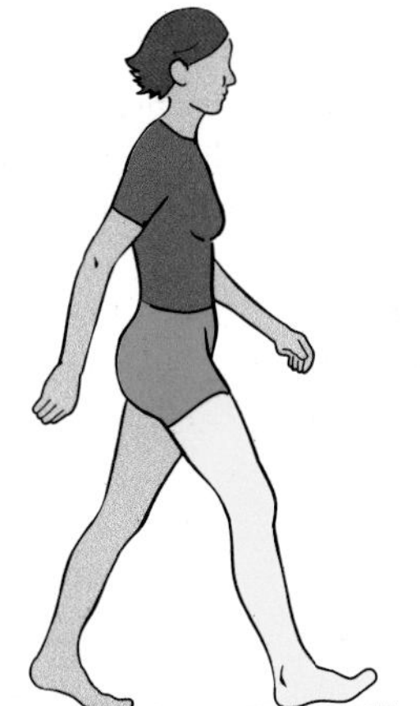

Figure 22-4. Heel strike (*initial contact – RLA*).

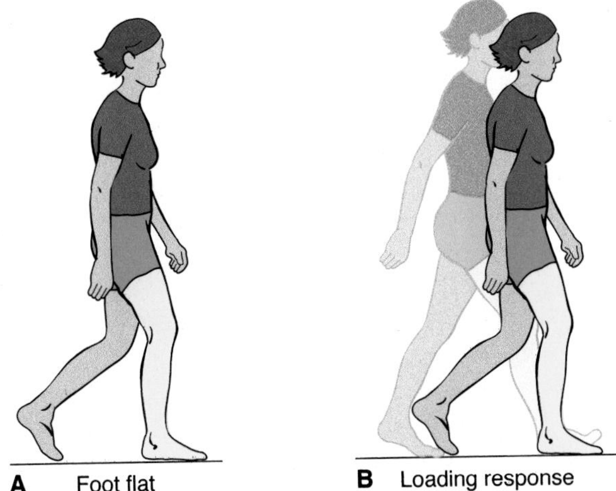

Figure 22-5. **(A)** Foot flat. **(B)** Loading response period (RLA). The lighter tone shows the beginning of the loading response, and the darker tone shows the ending of this period.

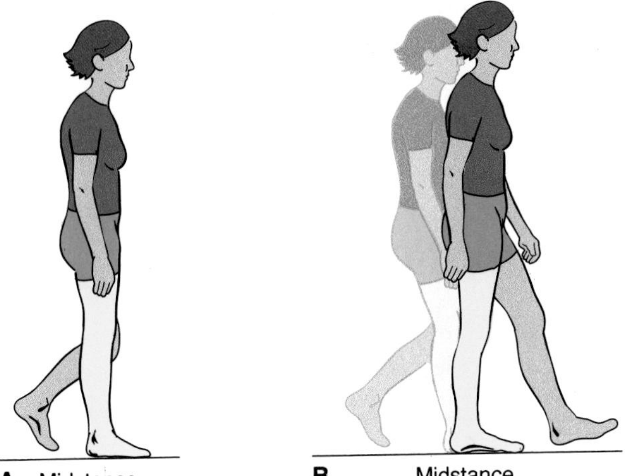

Figure 22-6. **(A)** Midstance. **(B)** Midstance period (RLA). The lighter tone shows the beginning of the loading response, and the darker tone shows the ending of this period.

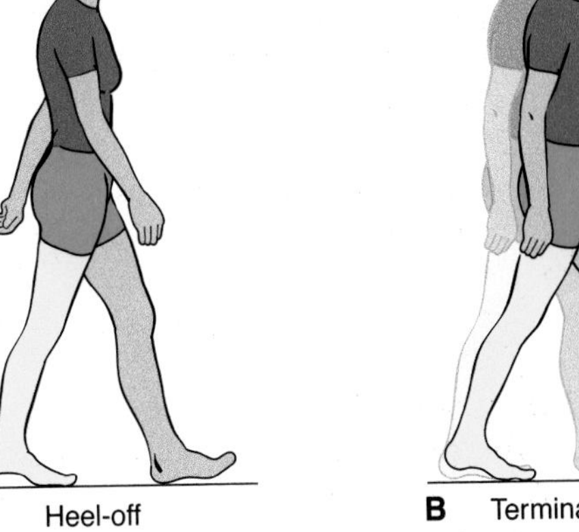

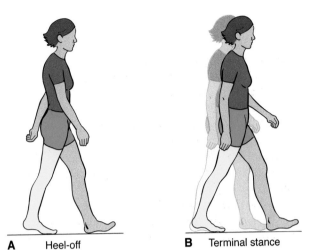

Figure 22-7. **(A)** Heel-off. **(B)** Terminal stance period (RLA). The lighter tone shows the beginning and the darker tone shows the ending of this period.

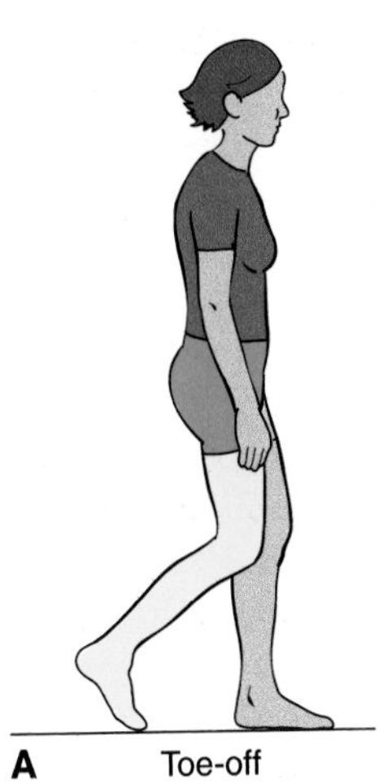

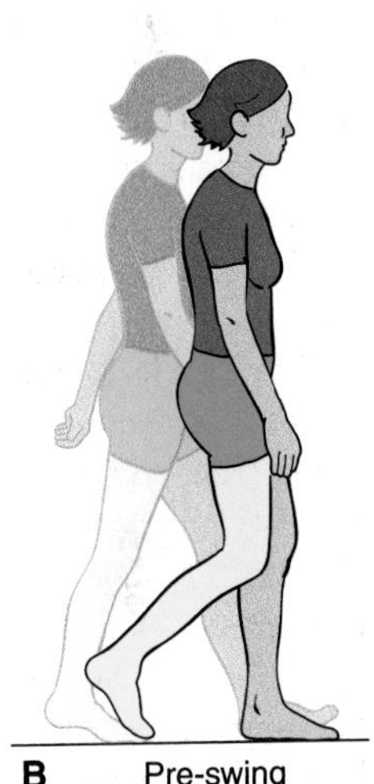

Figure 22-8. **(A)** Toe-off. **(B)** Preswing period (RLA). The lighter tone shows the beginning and the darker tone shows the ending of this period.

hip are flexing. The thigh is perpendicular to the ground. In RLA, *preswing* is the period just before and including when the toes leave the ground, signaling the end of stance phase and the beginning of swing phase.

Analysis of Swing Phase

The swing phase consists of three components: acceleration, midswing, and deceleration (Fig. 22-9). These components are all non–weight-bearing activities. The first part is **acceleration** (Fig. 22-10). The leg is behind the body and moving to catch up. The ankle is dorsiflexing, and the knee and hip continue to flex, which is moving

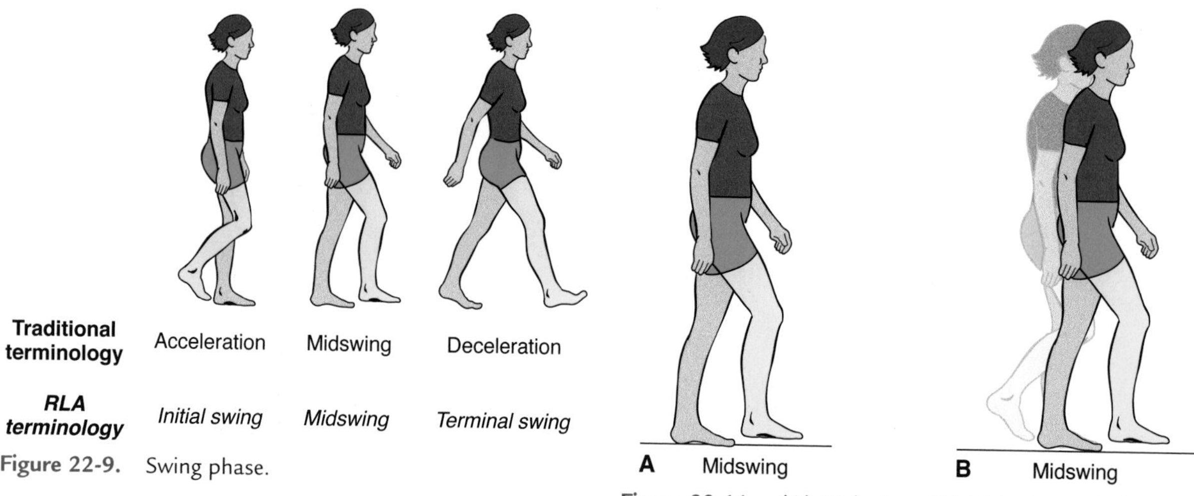

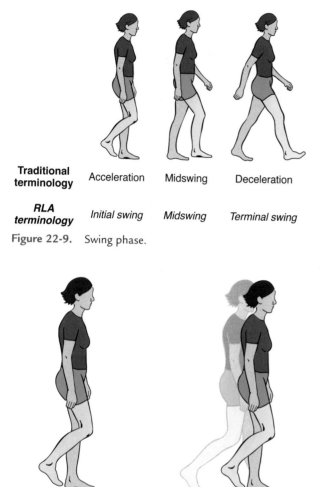

Figure 22-9. Swing phase.

Figure 22-11. **(A)** Midswing. **(B)** Midswing period (RLA). The lighter tone shows the beginning and the darker tone shows the ending of this period.

A Acceleration

B Initial swing

Figure 22-10. **(A)** Acceleration. **(B)** Initial swing period (RLA). The lighter tone shows the beginning and the darker tone shows the ending of this period.

the leg forward. In RLA, *initial swing* is that period between the end of toe-off and the end of acceleration.

At **midswing,** the ankle dorsiflexors have brought the ankle to a neutral position. The knee is at its maximum flexion (approximately 65 degrees), as is the hip (at about 25 degrees of flexion). These motions act to shorten the leg, allowing the foot to clear the ground as it swings through (Fig. 22-11). Further hip flexion moves the leg in front of the body and puts the lower leg in a vertical position. In RLA, *midswing* is that period between the end of acceleration and the end of midswing.

In **deceleration,** the ankle dorsiflexors are active to keep the ankle in a neutral position in preparation for heel strike (Fig. 22-12). The knee is extending, and the hamstring muscles are contracting eccentrically to slow down the leg, keeping it from snapping into extension. The leg has swung as far forward as it is going to swing.

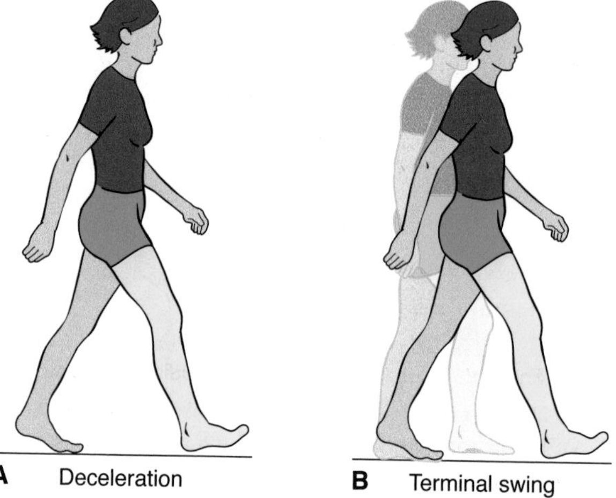

Figure 22-12. **(A)** Deceleration. **(B)** Terminal swing (RLA). The lighter tone shows the beginning and the darker tone shows the ending of this period.

The hip remains in flexion. In RLA, *terminal swing* is that period between the end of midswing and the end of deceleration.

Additional Determinants of Gait

To this point, the description of gait has centered mostly on the lower legs. However, other events are occurring in the rest of the body that must also be considered.

If you held a piece of chalk against the blackboard and walked the board's length, you would see that the line drawn bobs up and down in wavelike fashion. This is described as the **vertical displacement** of the center of gravity (Fig. 22-13). The normal amount of this

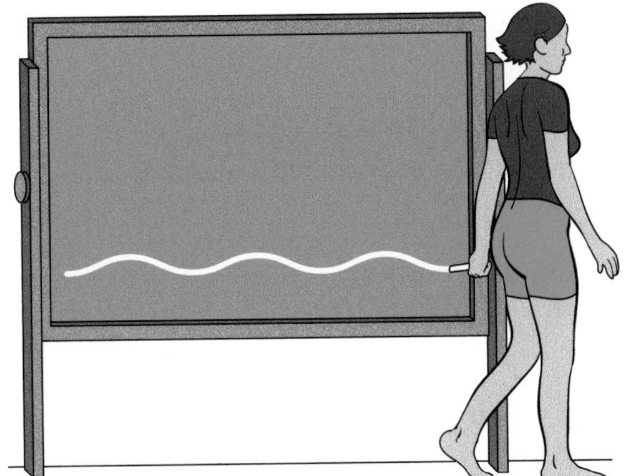

Figure 22-13. Vertical displacement of the body's center of gravity during the gait cycle.

displacement is approximately 2 inches, being highest at midstance and lowest at heel strike *(initial contact)*. There is also an equal amount of **horizontal displacement** of the center of gravity as the body weight shifts from side to side. This displacement is greatest during the single-support phase at midstance. In other words, this represents the distance the body's center of gravity must shift horizontally onto one foot so that the other foot can swing forward. This side-to-side displacement is usually about 2 inches.

When you walk, you do not place your feet one step in front of the other but slightly apart. If lines were drawn through the successive midpoints of heel contact *(initial contact)* on each foot, this distance would range from 2 to 4 inches. This is described as the **width of walking base** (Fig. 22-14).

If you walked across the room with your hands on your hips, you would notice that they move up and down as your pelvis on each side drops down slightly. As shown in Figure 22-15, this **lateral pelvic tilt** occurs when weight is removed from the leg at toe-off *(preswing)*. This slight drop is sometimes referred to as the *Trendelenburg sign*. The dip would be greater if it were not for the hip abductors on the opposite side (weight-bearing) and the erector spinae on the same side working together, keeping the pelvis essentially level. When the pelvis drops on the right side (the non-weight-bearing side), the left hip (the weight-bearing side) is forced into adduction. To keep the pelvis level, although it actually dips slightly, the left hip abductors contract to prevent hip adduction. At the same time, the right erector spinae muscle, which has attachments on the pelvis, contracts and "pulls up" on the side of the pelvis that wants to drop (Fig. 22-16).

In addition, step length should normally be equal in both distance and time. The arm should swing with the opposite leg. The trunk rotates forward as the leg progresses through the swing phase. Arms swinging in opposition to trunk rotation controls the amount of trunk rotation by providing counterrotation. The head should be erect, shoulders level, and trunk in extension.

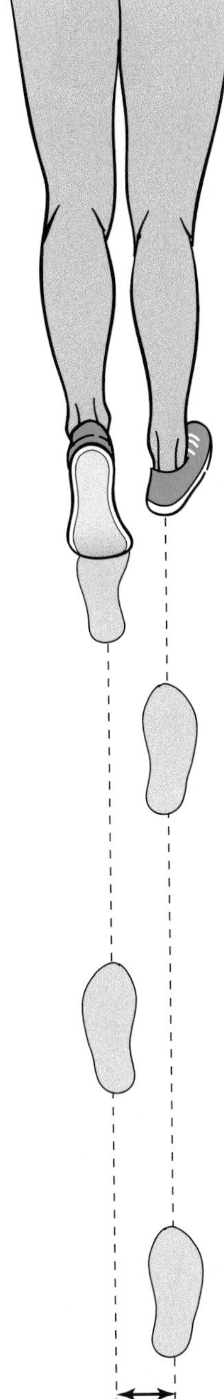

Figure 22-14. Walking base width.

When analyzing someone's gait, it is best to view the person from both the side and the front (and sometimes the back). Step length, arm swing, position of head and trunk, and the activities of the lower leg are usually best

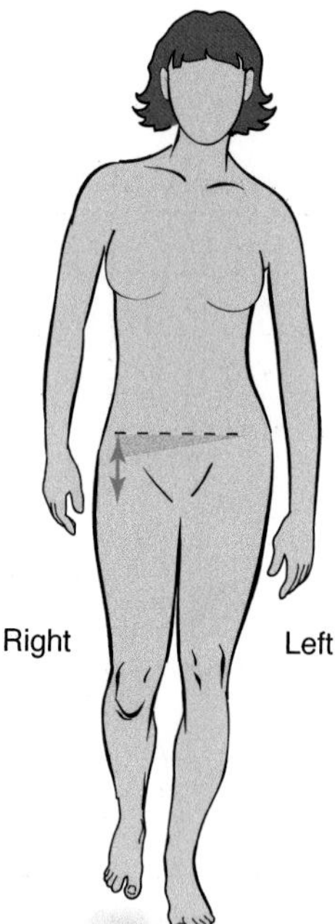

Figure 22-15. Lateral pelvic tilt.

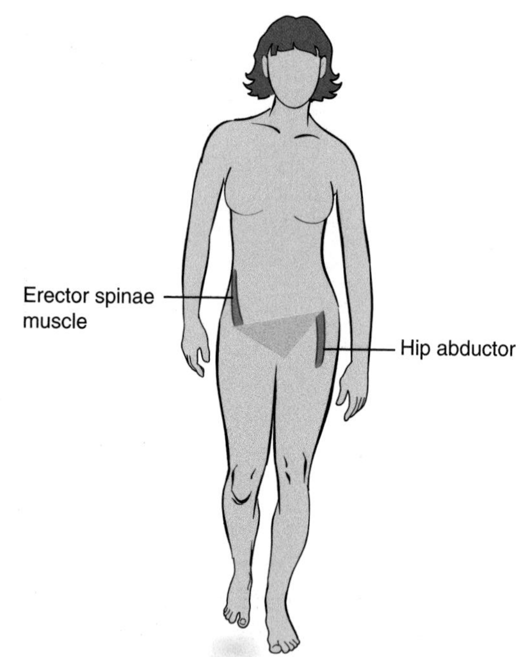

Figure 22-16. Muscles working to minimize lateral pelvic tilt. (A) Hip abductors. (B) Erector spinae muscles.

viewed from the side. Width of walking base, dip of the pelvis, and position of the shoulders and head should be viewed from the front or back. To learn about the difference between walking and running, see Clinical Application 22-1.

Age-Related Gait Patterns

Not all gait patterns that do not comply with "normal" gait characteristics are the result of pathology. The walking patterns of young children and elderly adults have characteristic differences from the walking pattern of younger adults. These are considered age-related, not pathological, changes. The differences seen in young children tend to disappear as they get older. Young children tend to walk with a wider walking base, their cadence is faster, and their stride length is shorter. Initial contact with the floor is with a flat foot, as opposed to heel strike. Their knees remain mostly extended during stance phase. In other words, they tend to take more steps that are short and choppy in a faster period of time. They also have little or no reciprocal arm swing. This is easy to observe as a child walks with an adult.

Even in the absence of pathology, an elderly adult's walking pattern undergoes change. Although there is not universal agreement on the reasons for these changes, it is generally thought that security and fear of falling are major contributors. Typically, older adults lose muscle mass, are less active, and often have poorer hearing and vision. It should be recognized that the effects of age are relative to many factors such as health, activity level, and even attitude. Some 70-year-old people may appear "older" than others who are 10 or more years their senior. Given all of these qualifiers, some general statements can be made regarding the changes in the walking pattern of elderly individuals. They tend to walk slower, spending more time in stance phase. Therefore, there are longer periods of double support. Because they take shorter steps, vertical displacement is less. They walk with a wider base, and so have greater horizontal displacement. There are fewer and slower automatic movements, which may increase the chance of stumbling or falling. In turn, these factors may contribute to decreased toe-floor clearance.

Abnormal (Atypical) Gait

The causes of an abnormal gait are numerous. It may be temporary, such as a sprained ankle, or it may be permanent, such as after a stroke. There can be great variation, depending on the severity of the problem. If a muscle is weak, how weak is it? If joint motion is limited, how limited is it? As with all causes of abnormal motion, severity or degree of involvement will always result in a range of variations from minor ones to major ones. There are many methods of classifying abnormal gait. The following is a listing of the causes for abnormal gait:

Muscular weakness/paralysis
Joint/muscle range-of-motion (ROM) limitation

Clinical Application 22-1

Comparison of Running and Walking

When gait velocity increases to a certain point, it actually takes less energy to run than to "speed walk." When comparing walking and running, each individual leg progresses through the stance and swing phases the same way, but time spent in each phase differs. During running, each leg completes its entire stance phase while the other leg is in swing phase. There is a period of nonsupport, which does not occur during walking. Unlike running, walking has a period of double support. With running, the amount of time spent in stance phase decreases while the amount of time spent in swing phase increases. This causes the right and left swing phases to overlap, creating periods of nonsupport (see Table).

To conserve energy and minimize demand on supporting muscles, both vertical and horizontal displacement of the body is reduced during running. This is achieved by: (1) keeping the hips and knees in more flexion throughout the gait cycle, which minimizes the peak height of the center of gravity, and (2) narrowing the width of the walking base, thus minimizing the body's need to shift laterally during single-limb stance. There are, however, increased demands on the body with running. Without periods of double support, and with a narrower walking base, the body is less stable, so good balance and coordination is necessary. Due to the increased velocity of movement, there are also more forces to absorb and a demand for stronger eccentric muscle contractions.

The Walking Gait Cycle

Right Leg	Left Leg	Period of Support
Heel strike	Heel-off	Double support
Foot flat	Toe-off	
Midstance	Acceleration	Single support
	Midswing	
	Deceleration	
Heel-off	Heel strike	Double support
Toe-off	Foot flat	
Acceleration	Midstance	Single support
Midswing		
Deceleration		

The Running Gait Cycle

Right Leg	Left Leg	Period of Support
Heel strike	Acceleration	Single support
Foot flat		
Midstance	Midswing	
Heel-off	Deceleration	
Toe-off		
--------	--------	Non-support
Acceleration	Heel strike	Single support
	Foot flat	
Midswing	Midstance	
Deceleration	Heel-off	
	Toe-off	

Stance phase   Swing phase

Neurological involvement
Pain
Leg length discrepancy

Muscular Weakness/Paralysis

Depending on the cause or severity of the condition, muscle weakness can range from slight weakness to complete paralysis, in which there is no strength at all. Generally speaking, with muscle weakness, the body tends to compensate by shifting the center of gravity over, or toward, the part that is involved. Basically, this reduces the moment of force (torque) on the joint, lessening the muscle strength required. Obviously, the portion of the gait cycle affected will be that portion in which the muscles or joints have a major role. Traditional terminology will be used with RLA terms in italics when there is a difference in terms.

In the case of the **gluteus maximus gait,** the trunk quickly shifts posteriorly at heel strike *(initial contact)*. This will shift the body's center of gravity posteriorly over the gluteus maximus, moving the line of force posterior to the hip joints (Fig. 22-17). With the foot in contact with the floor, this requires less muscle strength to maintain the hip in extension during stance

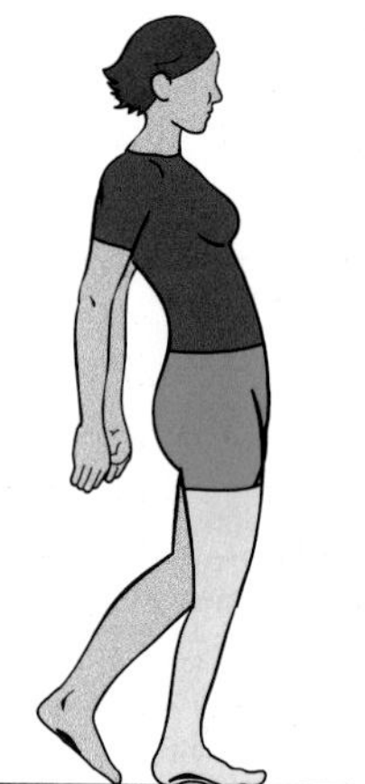

Figure 22-17. Gluteus maximus gait due to muscle weakness/paralysis on right side.

phase. This shifting is sometimes referred to as a *rocking horse gait* because of the extreme backward-forward movement of the trunk.

With a **gluteus medius gait,** the individual shifts the trunk over the affected side during stance phase. In Figure 22-18, the left gluteus medius, or hip abductor, is weak, causing two things to happen: (1) the body leans over the left leg during that leg's stance phase, and (2) the right side of the pelvis drops when the right leg leaves the ground and begins swing phase. This gait is also referred to as a *Trendelenburg gait.* Do not confuse it with the normal amount of dipping of the pelvis. Shifting the trunk over the affected side is an attempt to reduce the amount of strength required by the gluteus medius to stabilize the pelvis.

When there is weakness in the **quadriceps** muscle group, several different compensatory mechanisms may be used. Depending on whether only the quadriceps muscles are weak or if there are additional weaknesses in the extremity, various compensatory maneuvers may be used. With quadriceps weakness, the individual may lean the body forward over the quadriceps muscles at the early part of stance phase, as weight is being shifted onto the stance leg. Normally at this time, the line of force falls behind the knee, requiring quadriceps action to keep the knee from buckling. By leaning forward at the hip, the center of gravity is shifted forward and the line of force now falls in front of the knee. This will force the knee backward into extension. Another compensatory maneuver is using the hip extensors and ankle plantar flexors in a closed-chain action to pull the knee into extension at heel strike *(initial contact).* This reversal of muscle action can be seen in Figure 19-22. In addition, the person may physically push on the anterior thigh during stance phase, holding the knee in extension (Fig. 22-19).

If the **hamstrings** are weak, two things may happen. During stance phase, the knee will go into excessive hyperextension, sometimes referred to as *genu recurvatum gait* (Fig. 22-20). Without the hamstrings to slow the forward swing of the lower leg during the deceleration *(terminal swing)* part of swing phase, the knee will snap into extension.

The amount of weakness of the **ankle dorsiflexors** will determine how an individual may compensate. If there is insufficient strength to move the ankle into dorsiflexion at the beginning of stance phase, the foot will land with a fairly flat foot. However, if there is no ankle dorsiflexion, the toes will strike first, which is commonly referred to as an **equinus gait** (Fig. 22-21A). Next, weak ankle dorsiflexors may not be able to support the body weight after heel strike and will thus move toward foot flat *(loading response)* as they ineffectively eccentrically contract. The result is **foot slap.** With the dorsiflexors

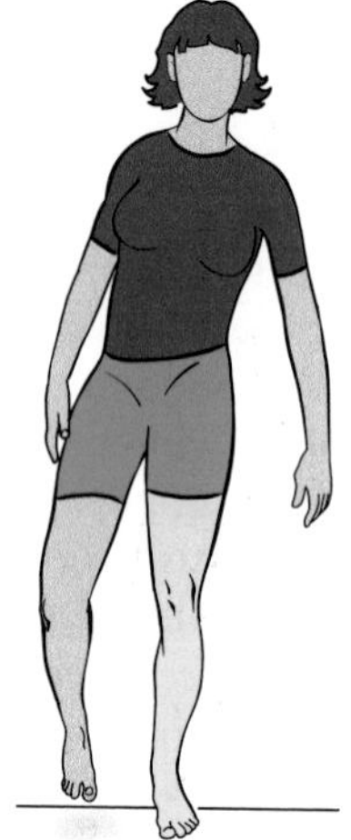

Figure 22-18. Gluteus medius gait.

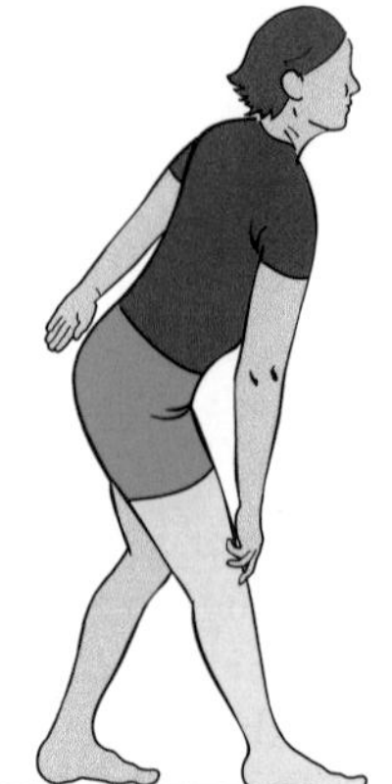

Figure 22-19. Gait resulting from quadriceps weakness/paralysis.

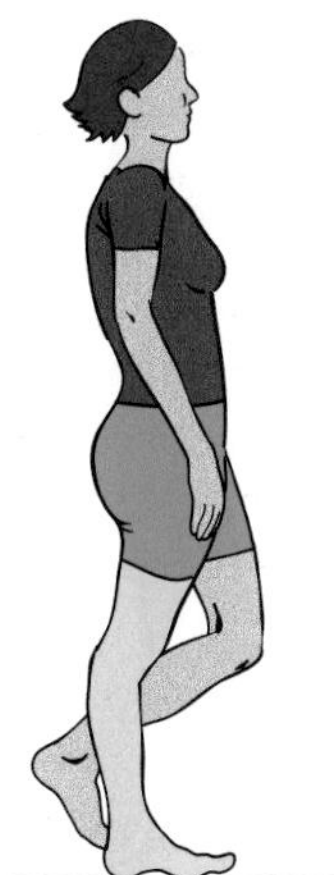

Figure 22-20. Genu recurvatum gait.

not being able to slow the descent of the foot, the foot slaps into plantar flexion as more weight is put on the leg. During swing phase, they may not be able to dorsiflex the ankle. Gravity will cause the foot to fall into plantar flexion when it is off the ground. This is called **drop foot.** As a result, the knee will need to be lifted higher for the dropped foot to clear the floor and **steppage gait** will result (Fig. 22-21B). The drum major in a marching band will utilize the elements of this gait when performing.

When the **triceps surae group** (the gastrocnemius and soleus) is weak, there is no heel rise at push-off *(terminal stance),* resulting in a shortened step length on the unaffected side. This is sometimes referred to as a *sore foot limp.* Although this gait is noticeable on level ground, it becomes most pronounced when walking up an incline.

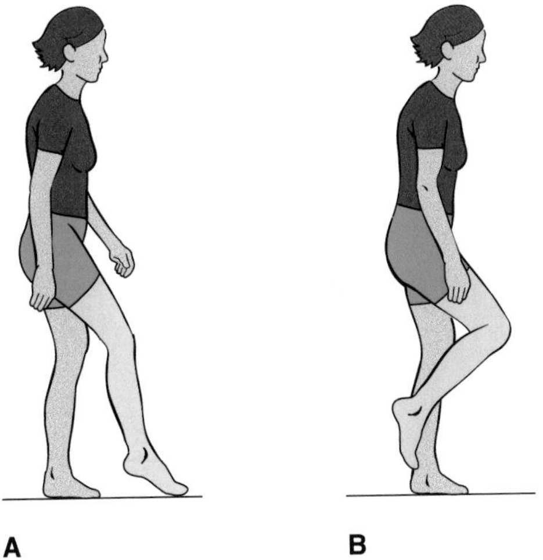

Figure 22-21. Weakness, paralysis, or absence of ankle dorsiflexors results in **(A)** equinus gait at heel strike *(initial contact – RLA)* and **(B)** steppage gait during swing phase.

A **waddling gait** is commonly seen with muscular and other types of dystrophies, because there is diffuse weakness of many muscle groups. The person stands with the shoulders behind the hips, much like a person with paraplegia would balance resting on the iliofemoral ligament of the hips (Fig. 22-22). There is an increased lumbar lordosis, pelvic instability, and Trendelenburg gait. Little or no reciprocal pelvis and trunk rotation occur. To swing the leg forward, the entire side of the body must swing forward. For example, normally, as the right leg swings forward, the right arm swings backward. In this case, the right arm and leg swing forward together. Add this to the excessive trunk lean of Trendelenburg gait bilaterally, and one can see the waddling nature of the gait. A steppage gait is often also present.

Joint/Muscle Range-of-Motion Limitation

In this grouping, the joint is unable to go through its normal range of motion because there is either bony fusion or soft tissue limitation. This limitation can be the result of contractures of muscle, capsule, or skin.

When a person has a **hip flexion contracture,** the involved hip is unable to go into hip extension and hyperextension during the midstance and push-off phases *(terminal stance).* To compensate, the person will commonly assume the salutation or greeting position in which the hip is flexed and the person's trunk leans forward as if bowing (Fig. 22-23). The involved leg may also simultaneously flex the knee when it normally would be extended.

With a **fused hip,** increased motion of the lumbar spine and pelvis can greatly compensate for hip motion. A decreased lordosis and posterior pelvic tilt will allow the leg to swing forward (Fig. 22-24A), whereas an increased lordosis and anterior pelvic tilt will swing the leg posteriorly (Fig. 22-24B). This is sometimes referred

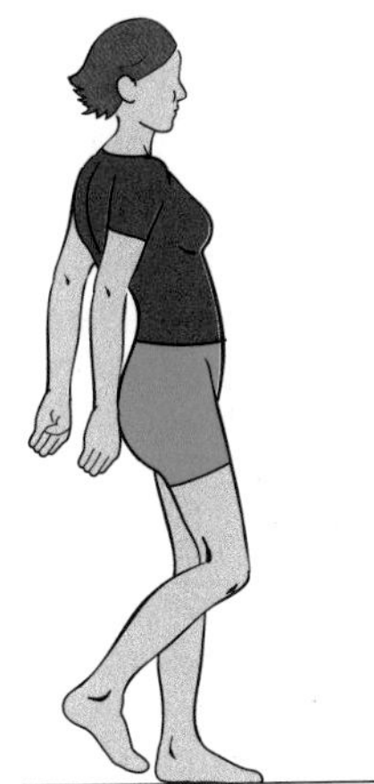

Figure 22-22. Waddling gait.

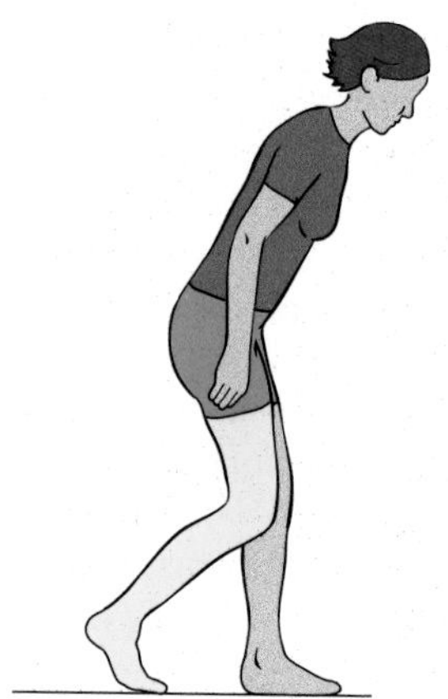

Figure 22-23. Salutation greeting resulting from hip flexion contracture.

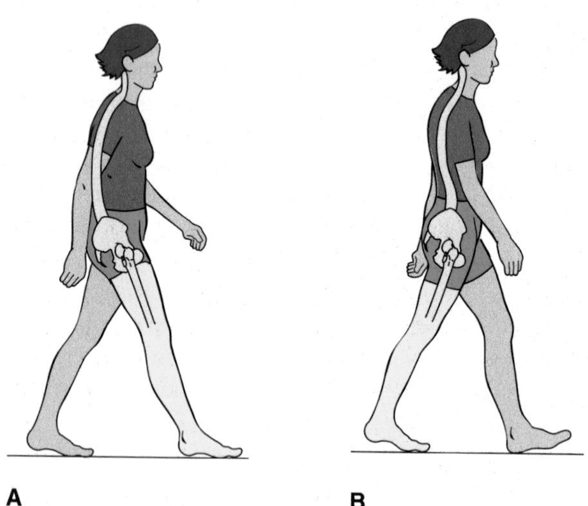

Figure 22-24. Bell-clapper gait resulting from a fused hip. In **(A)** the leg swings forward by flattening the lumbar lordosis and tilting the pelvis posteriorly. In **(B)** the leg swings backward by increasing the lumbar lordosis and tilting the pelvis anteriorly.

to as a *bell-clapper gait.* A bell swings back and forth, causing the clapper inside to also move back and forth.

A **knee flexion contracture** will result in excessive dorsiflexion during midstance and an early heel rise during push-off *(terminal stance).* There is also a shortened step length of the unaffected side. If a **knee fusion** is present, the lower leg will be at a fixed length. That length will depend on the position of the joint. If the knee is fused in extension, the leg will be unable to shorten during swing phase. To compensate, the person must (1) rise up on the toes of the uninvolved leg in a **vaulting gait** (Fig. 22-25), (2) hike the hip of the involved side, (3) swing the leg out to the side, or (4) do some variation of the three methods. With a **circumducted gait,** the leg begins near the midline at push-off *(terminal stance),* swings out to the side during swing phase, then returns to the midline for heel strike (Fig. 22-26). It is called an **abducted gait** if the leg remains in an abducted position throughout the gait cycle.

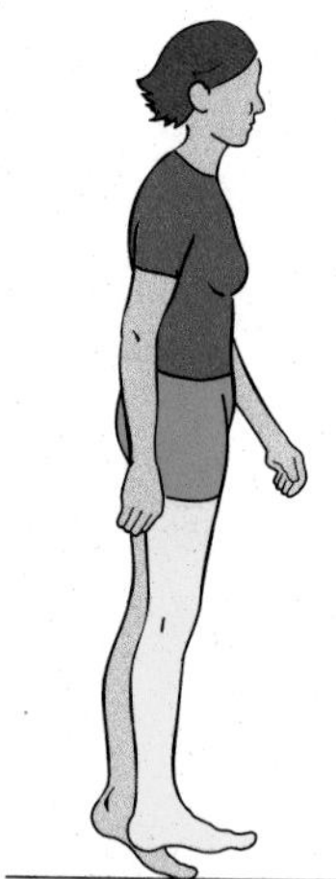

Figure 22-25. Vaulting gait resulting from a right knee fused in extension. The person must rise up on her toes on the left side to allow the involved right leg to swing through.

Depending on the severity of a **triceps surae contracture,** several things may result. The knee can be forced into excessive extension during midstance, because there is insufficient length of the plantar flexors to allow dorsiflexion. If the gastrocnemius does not have enough extensibility to be stretched over both the

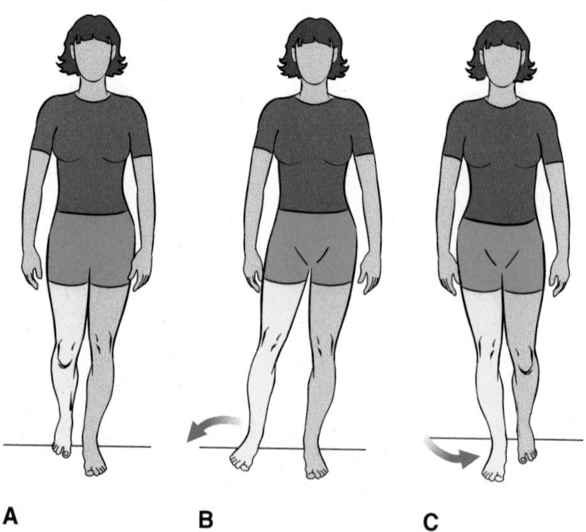

Figure 22-26. Circumducted gait. **(A)** The leg is in the normal position at the end of stance phase. The leg then swings out and around during swing phase **(B)**, returning to the normal position for the beginning of stance phase **(C)**.

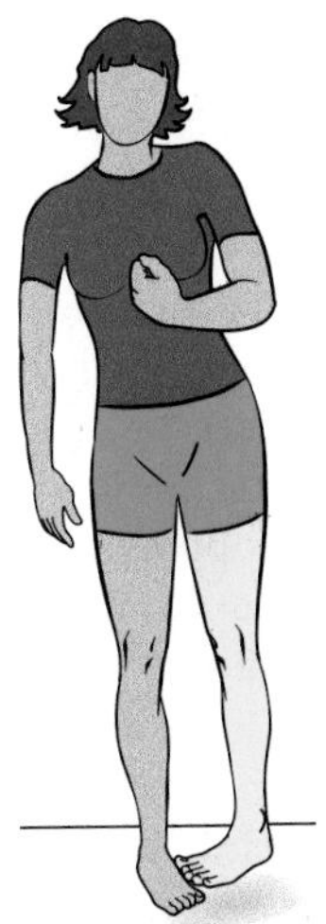

Figure 22-27. Hemiplegic gait.

ankle and knee, something must give. There will be either limited ankle dorsiflexion or the knee will be pulled into extreme extension. Remember that the gastrocnemius is a two-joint muscle that plantar flexes the ankle and flexes the knee. In weight-bearing, body weight may force a certain amount of dorsiflexion, thus forcing a tight gastrocnemius to pull the knee into extension. In addition, an early heel rise will occur during push-off *(terminal stance),* the knee will be lifted higher during swing phase, and the toes will land first during heel strike *(initial contact).* The latter is called a *steppage gait.*

An **ankle fusion** is commonly called a *triple arthrodesis* because of fusion of the subtalar joint and the two articulations making up the transtarsal joint. This will result in loss of ankle pronation and supination. Plantar flexion and dorsiflexion will remain but will be limited. Usually, there is a shortened stride length. The person will have more difficulty walking on uneven ground because the ability to pronate and supinate the foot has been lost.

Neurological Involvement

The amount of gait disturbance depends on the severity of neurological involvement. For example, spasticity of the hip flexors affects moving the leg forward in midstance and terminal stance. Hamstring spasticity can keep the knee in a flexed position, which can interfere with moving the leg forward during stance phase and limit the effectiveness of straightening the leg at the end of the swing. Spasticity of the triceps surae can keep the ankle plantar flexed, creating problems during both stance and swing phase. Spasticity tends to put the foot in a varus position, and flaccidity tends to put the foot in a valgus position.

A **hemiplegic gait** will vary depending on the severity of neurological involvement and the presence and amount of spasticity. Generally speaking, with spasticity there is an extension synergy in the involved lower extremity. The hip goes into extension, adduction, and medial rotation. The knee is in extension, though often unstable. The ankle demonstrates a drop foot with ankle plantar flexion and inversion (equinovarus), which is present during both stance phase and swing phase. The involved upper extremity may typically be in a flexion synergy (Fig. 22-27). Usually, there will be no reciprocal arm swing. Step length tends to be lengthened on the involved side and shortened on the uninvolved side.

Cerebellar involvement often results in an **ataxic gait.** Lack of coordination leads to jerky, uneven movements. Balance tends to be poor, and the person walks with a wide base of support (abducted gait). The person usually has difficulty walking in a straight line and tends to stagger. Reciprocal arm motion also appears to be jerky and uneven. All movements appear exaggerated.

A **parkinsonian gait,** in which one has tremors, demonstrates diminished movement. The posture of the lower extremities and trunk tends to be flexed. The elbows are partially flexed, and there is little or no reciprocal arm swing. Stride length is greatly diminished, and the forward heel does not swing beyond the rear foot. The person walks with a shuffling gait, with the feet flat and weight mostly forward on the toes (Fig. 22-28). The person has difficulty initiating movements. This shuffling gait tends to start slowly and increase in speed, and the person often has difficulty stopping. It gives the appearance that the person's feet are trying to catch up to the forward-leaning trunk. This is called a **festinating gait.**

Spasticity in the hip adductors results in a **scissors gait.** This gait is most evident during the swing phase,

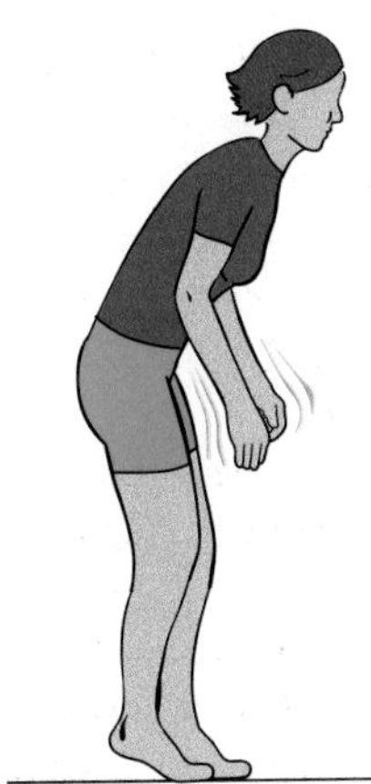

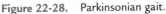

Figure 22-28. Parkinsonian gait.

when the unsupported leg swings against or across the stance leg. Needless to say, the walking base is narrowed. The trunk may lean over the stance leg as the swing phase leg attempts to swing past it (Fig. 22-29).

A **crouch gait** describes the bilateral lower extremity involvement seen in the spastic diplegia associated with cerebral palsy. There is often great variation in the gait from what is considered "typical." There is excessive flexion, adduction, and medial rotation at the hips and flexion at the knees. The ankles are plantar flexed. The pelvis maintains an anterior pelvic tilt, and there is an increased lumbar lordosis. To compensate, the reciprocal arm swing and horizontal displacement are exaggerated.

Pain

When a person has pain in any of the lower extremity joints, the tendency is to shorten the stance phase. In other words, if it hurts to stand on it, do not stand on it. A shortened, often abducted stance phase on the involved side results in a rapid and shortened step length on the uninvolved side. Compensation in the reciprocal arm swing is also evident. Reciprocal arm swinging shortens as the step length is shortened, exaggerated, and often abducted. This gait is often referred to as **antalgic gait.** If the pain is caused by a hip problem, the person will lean over that hip during weight-bearing. This will decrease the torque placed on the joint and the amount of pressure placed on the femoral head. Magee (1987) stated that the amount of pressure will be decreased from more than twice the body weight to approximately that of the person's body weight.

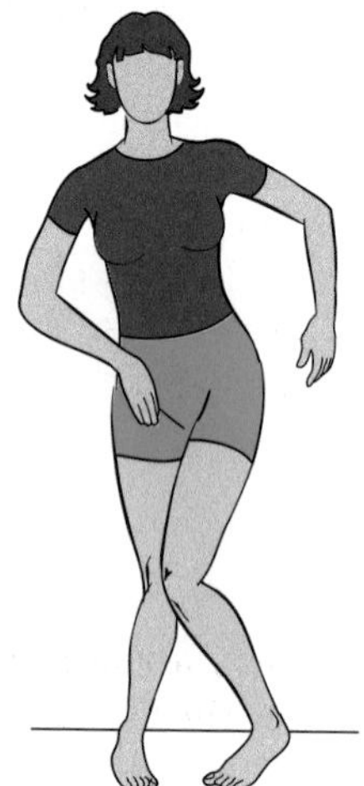

Figure 22-29. Scissors gait.

Leg Length Discrepancy

We all have legs of unequal length. Often the discrepancy is as much as approximately one-quarter inch between the right and left legs. Because both feet need to be in contact with the ground while in standing posture, how does the body adjust to the difference in leg length? Clinically, these smaller discrepancies are often corrected by inserting heel lifts of various thicknesses into the shoe. Without any other correction, dropping the pelvis on the shorter leg side (affected side) can compensate for a minimal leg length discrepancy. Although this may not look abnormal, it does place added stress on the lower back, hips, and knees. In addition to increased lateral pelvic tilt, the person may compensate by leaning over the shorter leg. This would result in greater lateral leaning of the upper body. These techniques can accommodate leg length discrepancies of up to approximately 3 inches.

When there is **moderate discrepancy,** between approximately 3 and 5 inches (depending on one's height), dropping the pelvis on the affected side will no longer be effective. The person needs to either shorten the uninvolved leg or make the involved leg functionally longer. A longer leg is needed, so the person usually walks on the ball of the foot on the involved (shorter) side. This is called an **equinus gait.** The most obvious change in the gait pattern would be loss of heel strike *(initial contact)* and foot flat *(loading response).*

A person can compensate for severe leg length discrepancy (e.g., any discrepancy more than 5 inches, again, depending on one's height) by using a variety of techniques. In addition to dropping the pelvis and walking in an equinus gait, the person could flex the knee on the uninvolved side. In this case, stance phase would tend to begin with flat foot rather than with heel strike. The knee would remain in a flexed position for the entire gait cycle. To gain an appreciation for how this may feel or look, walk down the street with one leg in the street and the other on the sidewalk.

When a person has a leg length discrepancy beyond what can be accommodated with heel lifts, it is usually the result of some sort of pathology. For example, a person with a fractured femur that healed in an overriding position would have a shorter leg. If a child who is still growing sustains damage to the epiphyseal plate of one or more long bones of the leg, it could result in arrested growth in that leg. Premature growth stoppage would result in a significant leg length discrepancy if the child had not nearly finished growing. These pathologies are not common, but they can result in significant changes in gait.

Points to Remember

- Stance and swing are the two phases of the gait cycle.
- Using traditional terminology, there are five periods in stance phase: heel strike, foot flat, midstance, heel-off, and toe-off.
- In swing phase, there are acceleration, midswing, and deceleration.
- Using RLA terminology, stance phase also has five periods: initial contact, loading response, midstance, terminal stance, and preswing.
- RLA terms for the swing phase periods are *initial swing, midswing,* and *terminal swing.*
- Additional determinants of gait are vertical and horizontal displacement, walking base width, lateral pelvic tilt, equal step length, and opposite and equal arm swing.

Review Questions

General Anatomy Questions

1. Describe how running differs from walking with respect to:
   a. Periods of support
   b. Vertical displacement of center of gravity
   c. Degree of hip and knee flexion
   d. Horizontal displacement of center of gravity
   e. Width of walking base
2. What are the main differences between the traditional terminology and terminology developed by Rancho Los Amigos?
3. What is the phase used for the period that occurs between heel strike and toe-off?
4. What is the time period called when both feet are in contact with the ground? What part of stance phase is each foot in during this period?
5. At what period of stance phase is a person's overall vertical height the greatest?
6. During which phase is the person's foot *not* in contact with the ground?
7. What will happen to the step length and cadence when a person increases his or her walking speed?
8. If unsteady, how does a person tend to adjust his or her walking?
9. If "foot drop" is present, which parts of the swing and stance phases of the person's gait will be altered?
10. If a person has an unrepaired ruptured Achilles tendon, which phase of the gait will be altered?
11. When the left leg steps forward, the __________ arm swings forward at the same time. This prevents the vertebral column from continuing to rotate to the __________.

Functional Activity Questions

Identify the parts of gait that will change during the following:

1. Walking across ice
2. Walking on a beam that is 4 inches wide
3. Walking down a railroad track with one foot on each side of the track (no train is coming!)
4. Walking in soft, dry sand (similar to running hard uphill)
5. Walking by taking long steps
6. Walking with a long leg brace (also known as a knee-ankle-foot orthosis, or KAFO)
7. The vertical displacement that occurs during walking demonstrates what type of motion?

Clinical Exercise Questions

1. Stand upright as though you had bilateral knee flexion contractures of approximately 45 degrees. Identify how positions of other joints must change to maintain an upright posture.
   a. Ankle
   b. Hip
   c. Pelvis
   d. Lumbar spine
2. Identify the type of muscle contraction and muscle group involved during the following phases of walking:
   a. At the knee going into heel strike
      Type of contraction __________________
      Muscle group involved __________________

(continued on next page)

Review Questions—cont'd

b. At the ankle during foot flat
   Type of contraction ________________
   Muscle group involved ________________
c. At the hip as the leg is moving into midstance
   Type of contraction ________________
   Muscle group involved ________________
d. At the hip (in the frontal plane) during toe-off
   Type of contraction ________________
   Muscle group involved ________________
e. At the knee during deceleration
   Type of contraction ________________
   Muscle group involved ________________

3. List the functional changes in gait that a person may use to compensate for a leg length discrepancy. Start with a minimal discrepancy and end with a severe discrepancy.
4. Explain why the body tends to shift toward the weak area during gait.
5. a. Name two muscle groups that can help create knee extension during the stance phase of gait if the quadriceps muscles are weak.
   b. Does this occur in an open- or closed-chain activity, or both?
   c. Name the term that describes these muscle groups' action.
6. Name at least two compensations that a person will use when they cannot bend the knee enough to clear the toes from the floor during the swing phase of gait.
7. Describe the part of the gait cycle that will be most impacted with a hip flexion contracture? Why?
8. After a stroke, what happens to the step length on the uninvolved side? Why?
9. Spasticity in what muscle group will cause a scissors gait?
10. a. When pain is present, will the painful or nonpainful leg have a shorter stance time?
    b. Which leg will have a shorter step length?

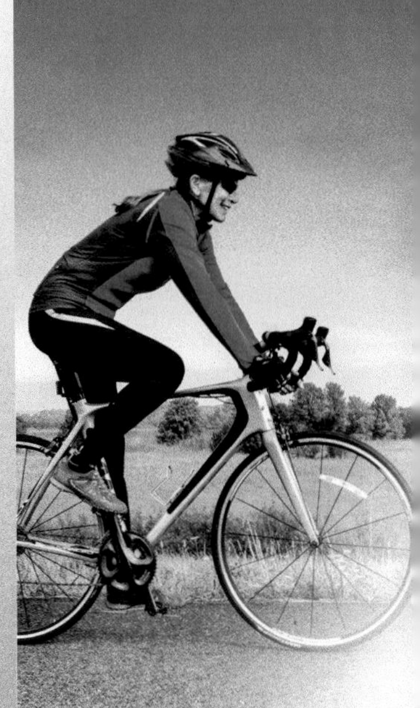

Bibliography

Abrahams, P, Craven, J, and Lumley, J: Illustrated Clinical Anatomy. Oxford University Press, New York, 2005.

Anderson, MK: Fundamentals of Sports Injury Management. Lippincott Williams & Wilkins, Philadelphia, 2002.

Anderson, MK, Hall, SJ, and Martin, M: Sports Injury Management, ed 2. Lippincott Williams & Wilkins, Philadelphia, 2002.

Beachey, W: Respiratory Care Anatomy and Physiology: Foundations for Clinical Practice, Mosby, St. Louis, MO, 1998.

Bertoti, DB: Functional Neurorehabilitation Through the Life Span. FA Davis, Philadelphia, 2004.

Brunnstrom, S: Clinical Kinesiology, ed 3. FA Davis, Philadelphia, 1972.

Burt, J and White, G: Lymphedema: A Breast Cancer Patient's Guide to Prevention and Healing. Hunter House, Berkeley, 2005.

Cael, C: Functional Anatomy: Musculoskeletal Anatomy, Kinesiology, and Palpation for Manual Therapists, revised. Lippincott Williams & Wilkins, Philadelphia, 2010.

Calais-Germain, B: Anatomy of Movement, revised. Eastland Press, Seattle, 2007.

DesJardins, T: Cardiopulmonary Anatomy and Physiology, ed 4. Thomson Delmar Learning, Clifton Park, NY, 2002.

Donatelli, RA: The Biomechanics of the Foot and Ankle, ed 2. FA Davis, Philadelphia, 1996.

Drake, RL, Vogl, AW, Mitchell, AWM, Tibbitts, RM, and Richardson, PE: Gray's Atlas of Anatomy, ed 2. Churchill Livingstone Elsevier, Philadelphia, 2015.

Dufort, A: Ballet Steps: Practice for Performance. Hodder Arnold, London, 1993.

Ellis, H: Clinical Anatomy: A Revision and Applied Anatomy for Clinical Students, ed 10. Blackwell, Malden, MA, 2002.

Gilman, S and Newman, SW: Essentials of Clinical Neuroanatomy and Neurophysiology, ed 10. FA Davis, Philadelphia, 2003.

Gilroy, AM, MacPherson, BR, and Ross, LM (eds): Atlas of Anatomy. Thieme Medical Publishers, New York, 2008.

Goodman, CC and Fuller, KS: Pathology: Implications for the Physical Therapist, ed 3. Saunders-Elsevier, St. Louis, MO, 2009.

Goss, CM (ed): Gray's Anatomy of the Human Body, American, ed 29. Lea & Febiger, Philadelphia, 1973.

Grimshaw, P, Lees, A, Fowler, N, and Burden A: Sport and Exercise Biomechanics, Taylor & Francis, New York, 2006.

Hall, SJ: Basic Biomechanics, ed 3. McGraw-Hill, Boston, 1999.

Hamill, J and Knutzen, KM: Biomechanical Basis of Human Movement, ed 2. Lippincott Williams & Wilkins, Philadelphia, 2003.

Hislop, HJ and Montgomery, J: Daniels and Worthingham's Muscle Testing: Techniques of Manual Examination, ed 8. Saunders Elsevier, St. Louis, 2007.

Houglum, PA and Betoti, DB: Clinical Kinesiology, ed 6. FA Davis, Philadelphia, 2012.

Jenkins, DB: Hollinshead's Functional Anatomy of the Limbs and Back, ed 7. WB Saunders, Philadelphia, 1998.

Jenkins, DB: Hollinshead's Functional Anatomy of the Limbs and Back, ed 8. WB Saunders, Philadelphia, 2002.

Jones, K and Barker, K: Human Movement Explained. Butterworth-Heinemann, Oxford, 1996.

Kendall, FP, McCreary, EK, and Provance, PG: Muscles: Testing and Function, ed 4. Williams & Wilkins, Baltimore, 1993.

Kingston, B: Understanding Joints: A Practical Guide to Their Structure and Function. Stanley Thornes Ltd, Cheltenham, UK, 2000.

Kisner, C and Colby, LA: Therapeutic Exercise: Foundations and Techniques, ed 6. FA Davis, Philadelphia, 2007.

Lamport, NK, Coffey, MS, and Hersch, GI: Activity Analysis and Application, ed 4. Slack, Thorofare, NJ, 2001.

Lesh, SG: Clinical Orthopedics for the Physical Therapist Assistant, ed 1. FA Davis, Philadelphia, 2000.

Levangie, PK and Norkin, CC: Joint Structure and Function, ed 5. FA Davis, Philadelphia, 2011.

Loudon, JK, Manske, RC, and Reiman MP: Clinical Mechanics and Kinesiology, Human Kinetics, Champaign, IL, 2013.

Low, J and Reed, A: Basic Biomechanics Explained. Butterworth-Heinemann, Oxford, 1996.

Marieb, EN and Mitchell, SJ: Human Anatomy and Physiology Laboratory Manual, ed 9. Pearson Benjamin Cummings, San Francisco, 2008.

Martini, FH: Fundamentals of Anatomy and Physiology, ed 7. Pearson Benjamin Cummings, San Francisco, 2006.

McKinnis, LN: Fundamentals of Musculoskeletal Imaging, ed 2. FA Davis, Philadelphia, 2005.

McMillan, B: The Illustrated Atlas of the Human Body, Weldon Owen Pty Ltd, Sydney, 2008.

Moore, K: Clinically Oriented Anatomy, ed 4. Williams & Wilkins, Baltimore, 2004.

Moore, K and Agur, A: Essential Clinical Anatomy, ed 2. Lippincott Williams & Wilkins, Philadelphia, 2002.

Muscolino, JE: Kinesiology: The Skeletal System and Muscle Function. Elsevier, 2005.

Netter, FH: Atlas of Human Anatomy. Ciba-Geigy Corporation, Summit, NJ, 1989.

Netter, FH: Atlas of Human Anatomy, ed 5. Saunders Elsevier, Philadelphia, 2011.

Neumann, DA: Kinesiology of the Musculoskeletal System: Foundations for Physical Rehabilitation, ed 2. Mosby, St. Louis, MO, 2010.

Nolan, MF: Clinical Applications of Human Anatomy: A Laboratory Guide, ed l. Slack, Thorofare, 2003.

Nordin, M and Frankel, VH: Basic Biomechanics of the Musculoskeletal System, ed 3. Lippincott Williams & Wilkins, Baltimore, 2001.

Norkin, C and White, D: Measurement of Joint Motion: A Guide of Goniometry, ed 4. FA Davis, Philadelphia, 2009.

Oatis, CA: Kinesiology: The Mechanics and Pathomechanics of Human Movement, ed 2. Lippincott Williams & Wilkins, Philadelphia, 2009.

Olson, TR: ADAM: Student Atlas of Anatomy. Williams & Wilkins, Baltimore, 1996.

Ombregt, L, Bisschop, P, ter Veer, HJ, and Van de Velde, T: A System of Orthopedic Medicine. WB Saunders Company, London, 1995.

O'Sullivan, SB, Schmitz, TJ, and Fulk, GD: Physical Rehabilitation, ed 6. FA Davis, Philadelphia, 2014.

Palastanga, N, Field, D, and Soames, R: Anatomy and Human Movement: Structure and Function, ed 2. Butterworth-Heinemann, Oxford, 1994.

Palmer, M and Epler, M: Clinical Assessment Procedures in Physical Therapy, ed 2. JB Lippincott, Philadelphia, 1998.

Pedretti, LW and Early, MB: Occupational Therapy: Practice Skills for Physical Dysfunction, ed 5. CV Mosby, St. Louis, MO, 2001.

Perry J: Gait Analysis: Normal and Pathological Function. Slack, Thorofare, NJ, 1992.

Rolak, LA: Neurology Secrets, ed 4. Elsevier Mosby, St. Louis, MO, 2005.

Scanlon, VC and Sanders, T: Essentials of Anatomy and Physiology, ed 6. FA Davis, Philadelphia, 2011.

Snyder, DC, Conner, LM, and Lorenz, GF: Kinesiology Foundations for OTAs and PTAs, ed 5. Cengage, 2005.

Starkey, C and Ryan, J: Evaluation of Orthopedic and Athletic Injuries, ed 2. FA Davis, Philadelphia, 2002.

Steindler, A: Kinesiology of the Human Body: Under Normal and Pathological Conditions. Charles C. Thomas, Springfield, IL, 1955.

Strandring, S (ed): Gray's Anatomy: The Anatomical Basis of Clinical Practice, ed 40. Churchill Livingstone Elsevier, 2008.

Tovin, BJ and Greenfield, BH: Evaluation and Treatment of the Shoulder: An Integration of the Guide to Physical Therapist Practice. FA Davis, Philadelphia, 2001.

Vander, AJ, Sherman, JH, and Luciano, DS: Human Physiology: The Mechanisms of Body Function, ed 5. McGraw-Hill Publishing Company, New York, 1990.

Venes, D: Taber's Cyclopedic Medical Dictionary, ed 20. FA Davis, Philadelphia, 2005.

Whittle, MW: Gait Analysis: An Introduction, ed 4. Butterworth-Heinemann, Oxford, 1996.

Wise, CH, and Gulick, DT: Mobilization Notes: A Rehabilitation Specialist's Pocket Guide. FA Davis, Philadelphia, 2009.

Wise, CH: Orthopedic Manual Physical Therapy: From Art to Evidence. FA Davis, Philadelphia, 2015.

Journal Articles:

1. Cappellini G, Ivanenko Y. Motor patterns in human walking and running. *J Neurophysiol.* 2006;95:3426-3437. doi:10.1152/jn.00081.2006.

2. Chester R, Smith TO, Sweeting D, Dixon J, Wood S, Song F. The relative timing of VMO and VL in the aetiology of anterior knee pain: a systematic review and meta-analysis. *BMC Musculoskelet Disord.* 2008;9:64. doi:10.1186/1471-2474-9-64.
3. Cobb TK, Dalley BK, Posteraro RH, Lewis RC. Anatomy of the flexor retinaculum. *J Hand Surg Am.* 1993;18(3):91-99. doi:10.1016/0363-5023(93)90251-W.
4. Cronin NJ, Barrett RS, Carty CP. Long-term use of high-heeled shoes alters the neuromechanics of human walking. *J Appl Physiol.* 2012;112(9):1054-1058. doi:10.1152/japplphysiol.01402.2011.
5. Dal Maso F, Raison M, Lundberg A, Arndt A, Allard P, Begon M. Glenohumeral translations during range-of-motion movements, activities of daily living, and sports activities in healthy participants. *Clin Biomech.* 2015;30(9):1002-1007. doi:10.1016/j.clinbiomech.2015.06.016.
6. Dal Maso F, Raison M, Lundberg A, Arndt A, Begon M. Coupling between 3D displacements and rotations at the glenohumeral joint during dynamic tasks in healthy participants. *Clin Biomech.* 2014;29(9):1048-1055. doi:10.1016/j.clinbiomech.2014.08.006.
7. DeLeo AT, Dierks TA, Ferber R, Davis IS. Lower extremity joint coupling during running: A current update. *Clin Biomech.* 2004;19:983-991. doi:10.1016/j.clinbiomech.2004.07.005.
8. Dugan SA, Bhat KP. Biomechanics and analysis of running gait. *Phys Med Rehabil Clin N Am.* 2005;16:603-621. doi:10.1016/j.pmr.2005.02.007.
9. El-Rich M, Shirazi-Adl A, Arjmand N. Muscle activity, internal loads, and stability of the human spine in standing postures: combined model and in vivo studies. *Spine (Phila Pa 1976).* 2004;29(23):2633-2642. doi:10.1097/01.brs.0000146463.05288.0e.
10. Ettema GJC, Styles G, Kippers V. The moment arms of 23 muscle segments of the upper limb with varying elbow and forearm positions: Implications for motor control. *Hum Mov Sci.* 1998;17:201-220. doi:10.1016/S0167-9457(97)00030-4.
11. Farahmand F, Tahmasbi MN, Amis A. The contribution of the medial retinaculum and quadriceps muscles to patellar lateral stability - An in-vitro study. *Knee.* 2004;11:89-94. doi:10.1016/j.knee.2003.10.004.
12. Franklin ME, Chenier TC, Brauninger L, Cook H, Harris S. Effect of positive heel inclination on posture. *J Orthop Sports Phys Ther.* 1995;21(2):94-99. doi:10.2519/jospt.1995.21.2.94.
13. Greathouse D, Halle J, Dalley A. Terminologia anatomica: revised anatomical terminology. *J Orthop Sport Phys Ther.* 2004;34:363-367. doi:10.2519/jospt.2004.0107.
14. Jang J, Koh E, Han D. The effectiveness of passive knee extension exercise in the sitting position on stretching of the hamstring muscles of patients with lower back pain. *J Phys Ther Sci.* 2013;25:501-504. doi:10.1589/jpts.25.501.
15. Ji G, Wang F, Zhang Y, Chen B, Ma L, Dong J. Medial patella retinaculum plasty for treatment of habitual patellar dislocation in adolescents. *Int Orthop.* 2012;36:1819-1825. doi:10.1007/s00264-012-1544-3.
16. Kim M, Yi C, Kwon O, et al. Comparison of lumbopelvic rhythm and flexion-relaxation response between 2 different low back pain subtypes. *Spine (Phila Pa 1976).* 2013;38(15):1260-1267. doi:10.1097/BRS.0b013e318291b502.
17. Le Huec JC, Saddiki R, Franke J, Rigal J, Aunoble S. Equilibrium of the human body and the gravity line: the basics. *Eur Spine J.* 2011;20:1-6. doi:10.1007/s00586-011-1939-7.
18. Lee JC, Healy FJC. Anatomy of the wrist and hand. *Radiographics.* 2005;25:1577-1590. doi:10.1148/rg.256055028.
19. Merican AM, Amis AA. Anatomy of the lateral retinaculum of the knee. *J Bone Joint Surg Br.* 2008;90(4):527-534. doi:10.1302/0301-620X.90B4.20085.
20. Neumann DA. The convex-concave rules of arthrokinematics: flawed or perhaps just misinterpreted? *J Orthop Sports Phys Ther.* 2012;42(2):53-55. doi:10.2519/jospt.2012.0103.
21. Nicolella DP, O'Connor MI, Enoka RM, et al. Mechanical contributors to sex differences in idiopathic knee osteoarthritis. *Biol Sex Differ.* 2012;3(1):28. doi:10.1186/2042-6410-3-28.
22. Nishiihara R. The dilemmas of a scaphoid fracture: a difficult diagnosis for primary care physicians. *Hosp Physician.* 2000;(March):24-40.
23. Opila KA, Wagner SS, Schiowitz S, Chen J. Postural alignment in barefoot and high-heeled stance. *Spine (Phila Pa 1976).* 1988;13:542-547. doi:10.1097/00007632-198805000-00018.
24. Park S, Kong Y-S, Ko Y-M, Jang G-U, Park J-W. Differences in onset timing between the vastus medialis and lateralis during concentric knee contraction in individuals with genu varum or valgum. *J Phys Ther Sci.* 2015;27:1207-1210. doi:10.1589/jpts.27.1207.
25. Powers CM. Rehabilitation of patellofemoral joint disorders: a critical review. *J Orthop Sport Phys Ther.*

1998;28:345-354. http://www.ncbi.nlm.nih.gov/entrez/query.fcgi?cmd=Retrieve&db=PubMed&dopt=Citation&list_uids=9809282.

26. Rassier DE, MacIntosh BR, Herzog W. Length dependence of active force production in skeletal muscle. *J Appl Physiol.* 1999;86(5):1445-1457.
27. Sasaki K, Neptune RR. Muscle mechanical work and elastic energy utilization during walking and running near the preferred gait transition speed. *Gait Posture.* 2006;23:383-390. doi:10.1016/j.gaitpost.2005.05.002.
28. Schwab F, Lafage V, Boyce R, Skalli W, Farcy J-P. Gravity line analysis in adult volunteers: age-related correlation with spinal parameters, pelvic parameters, and foot position. *Spine (Phila Pa 1976).* 2006;31(25):E959-E967. doi:10.1097/01.brs.0000248126.96737.0f.
29. Shirazi-Adl a., El-Rich M, Pop DG, Parnianpour M. Spinal muscle forces, internal loads and stability in standing under various postures and loads - Application of kinematics-based algorithm. *Eur Spine J.* 2005;14:381-392. doi:10.1007/s00586-004-0779-0.
30. Stecco C, Macchi V, Lancerotto L, Tiengo C, Porzionato A, De Caro R. Comparison of transverse carpal ligament and flexor retinaculum terminology for the wrist. *J Hand Surg Am.* 2010;35(5):746-753. doi:10.1016/j.jhsa.2010.01.031.
31. Sullivan PBO, Grahamslaw KM, Ther MM, et al. The effect of different standing and sitting postures on trunk muscle activity in a pain-free population. *Spine.* 2002;27(11):1238-1244.
32. Thompson NW, Mockford BJ, Cran GW. Absence of the palmaris longus muscle: A population study. *Ulster Med J.* 2001;70(1):22-24.
33. Throckmorton GS, Finn RA, Bell WH. Biomechanics of differences in lower facial heights. *Am J Orthod Dentofac Orthop.* 1980;77(4):410-420.
34. Waligora AC, Johanson NA, Hirsch BE. Clinical anatomy of the quadriceps femoris and extensor apparatus of the knee. *Clin Orthop Relat Res.* 2009;467:3297-3306. doi:10.1007/s11999-009-1052-y.
35. Ward SR, Winters TM, Blemker SS. The architectural design of the gluteal muscle group: implications for movement and rehabilitation. *J Orthop Sports Phys Ther.* 2010;40(2):95-102. doi:10.2519/jospt.2010.3302.
36. Whalen RT, Carter DR, Giddings VL, E GSB. Calcaneal loading during walking and running. *Med Sci Sports Exerc.* 2000;32(3):627-634.
37. Williams DS, McClay IS, Hamill J, Buchanan TS. Lower extremity kinematic and kinetic differences in runners with high and low arches. *J Appl Biomech.* 2001;17:153-163.
38. Witvrouw E, Sneyers C, Lysens R, Victor J, Bellemans J. Reflex response times of vastus medialis oblique and vastus lateralis in normal subjects and in subjects with patellofemoral pain syndrome. *J Orthop Sports Phys Ther.* 1996;24(3):160-165. doi:10.2519/jospt.1996.24.3.160.

Answers to Review Questions

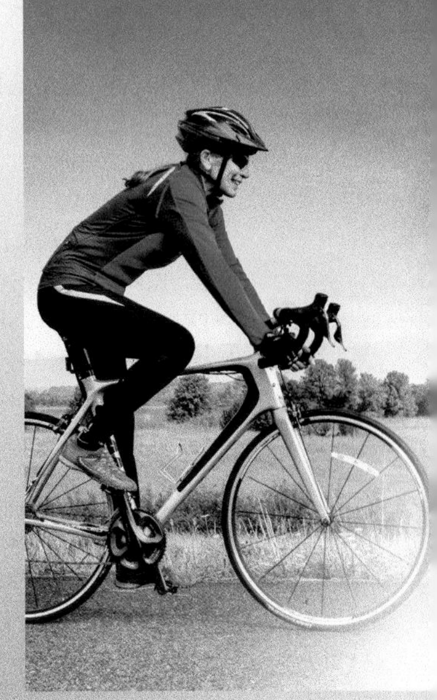

Chapter 1 Basic Information

1. a. Anterior
   b. Posterior
   c. Inferior
   d. Proximal
   e. Lateral
2. The football is demonstrating curvilinear motion, whereas the kicker's leg is demonstrating angular motion.
3. Neck hyperextension
4. Shoulder medial rotation
5. Trunk lateral bending
6. Hip lateral rotation
7. The forearms are in supination.
8. Dorsal surface of dog, posterior surface of person
9. Angular motion is being used by upper extremity joints—shoulders, elbows, wrists—to propel the wheelchair. Linear motion occurs as the person moves across the room in the wheelchair.
10. Supine
11. Ipsilateral
12. Left hip flexion (slight), adduction, lateral rotation
13. Left knee extension
14. Right forearm supination
15. Neck extension, rotation to the left

Chapter 2 Skeletal System

1. The axial skeleton contains no long or short bones, whereas the appendicular skeleton contains no irregular bones. The bones of the axial skeleton are particularly important in providing support and protection; the appendicular skeleton provides the framework for movement.
2. Compact bone is found in the diaphysis of long bones, and cancellous bone is found in the metaphysis and epiphysis. In other types of bone, cancellous bone is found sandwiched between layers of compact bone.
3. Compact bone is heavier than cancellous bone because it is less porous.
4. An individual's height growth occurs mainly in long bones. The growth occurs at the epiphysis of long bones.
5. Sesamoid bones protect tendons from excess wear. The patella has the additional function of increasing the angle of pull of the quadriceps muscle.
6. a. Foramen, fossa, groove, meatus, sinus
   b. Condyle, eminence, facet, head
   c. Crest, epicondyle, line, spine, trochanter, tuberosity, tubercle
7. Bicipital groove: ditchlike depression
8. Humeral head: rounded, articular projection that fits into a joint
9. Acetabulum: deep depression
10. Endosteum
11. Diaphysis
12. Pressure epiphysis
13. Appendicular skeleton
14. Appendicular skeleton
15. Axial skeleton

Chapter 3 Articular System

1. A joint that allows very little or no motion is referred to as a *fibrous joint.* The three types of fibrous joints are synarthrosis, syndesmosis, and gomphosis.
2. A joint that allows a great deal of motion is called a *synovial joint* or *diarthrosis.*

3. Diarthrodial joints can be described by:
   a. the number of axes.
   b. the shape of the joint.
   c. the joint motion involved.
4. Tendon
5. Bursa
6. Hyaline cartilage is located on the bone ends of synovial joints and provides a smooth articulating surface. Fibrocartilage is thicker and is located between bones. Fibrocartilage provides shock absorption and spacing. Examples of fibrocartilage are the menisci of the knee and the disks of the vertebrae.
7. The joint motion involved is elbow flexion; it occurs in the sagittal plane around the frontal axis.
8. The joint motions involved are forearm pronation (palm down) and supination (palm up); they occur in the transverse plane around the vertical axis.
9. The joint motion involved is finger (MP) adduction; it occurs in the frontal plane around the sagittal axis.
10. Shoulder = 3, elbow = 1, radioulnar = 1, wrist = 2, MCP = 2, PIP = 1, DIP = 1
11. Bones in the skull
12. Shoulder joint, yes, hip joint
13. CMC joint of thumb
14. Amphiarthrosis and cartilaginous
15. Joint capsule

Chapter 4 Arthrokinematics

1. Osteokinematic
2. Arthrokinematic
3. Soft end feel
4. a. Humerus is moving on scapula.
   b. Proximal end of humerus is convex.
   c. Glenoid fossa of scapula is concave.
   d. Convex surface is gliding on a fixed concave surface.
   e. Opposite direction
5. a. Compression or approximation
   b. Shear
   c. Traction or distraction
   d. Torsional
   e. Traction or distraction
6. Close-packed position of TMJ is when teeth are clenched.
7. a. Convex
   b. Concave
   c. Concave
   d. Convex
   e. Sellar
8. Roll
9. Glide (slide)
10. a. Yes
    b. Glide (slide)
11. Spin
12. Firm end feel
13. a. Compression
    b. Distraction
14. Torsional
15. Ovoid
16. This is an arthrokinematic movement because we are referring to the direction of movement of the "joint surfaces."
17. a. Distal end of humerus – convex , proximal end of radius and ulna – concave
    b. Radius and ulna
    c. Concave-on-convex
    d. The joint surfaces of the radius and ulna will glide in the same direction as the rest of the radius and ulna.
18. a. Anterior movement of the radius and ulna
    b. Anterior glide of the proximal ends (articular surfaces) of the radius and ulna

Chapter 5 Muscular System

1. a. Insertion
   b. Origin
2. Reversal of muscle action
3. a. Agonists in wrist flexion
   b. Antagonists in ulnar/radial deviation
4. a. Gluteus maximus and hamstrings
   b. Hip lateral rotation
   c. Gluteus minimus
5. Active insufficiency
6. Eccentric
7. a. Shoulder abduction
   b. Concentric
   c. Shoulder abductors
   d. Isometric
   e. Elbow extensors

8. a. Shoulder flexion
   b. Concentric
   c. Shoulder flexors during first 90 degrees
   d. Eccentric
   e. Shoulder extensors during second 90 degrees
9. a. Wheelchair push-ups: closed-chain activity
   b. Exercises with weight cuffs: open-chain activity
   c. Overhead wall pulleys: open-chain activity
10. Supine (or prone) lying
11. Anterior surface
12. The hip must be flexed to place the rectus femoris on slack, and the knee is flexed.
13. Oblique
14. Parallel
15. a. Contract
    b. Elasticity
16. The rectus femoris is lengthening over the anterior aspect of the hip and contracting (shortening) over the anterior aspect of the knee.

Chapter 6 Nervous System

1. L2
2. Gray matter is unmyelinated tissue, and white matter is myelinated tissue.
3. The brain is protected from trauma by (1) the bony outer layer called the *skull,* (2) the three layers of membrane called the *meninges,* and (3) the *cerebrospinal fluid,* which provides shock absorption.
4. Motor neurons that synapse above the level of the spinal cord's anterior horn are upper motor neurons. Those synapsing at the cell bodies or axons are lower motor neurons. Pathological conditions occurring to either upper or lower motor neurons have quite different clinical signs.
5. Thoracic nerves directly innervate the muscles near where they arise from the spinal cord. Cervical or lumbar nerves branch or divide, forming a plexus and innervating muscle quite distal to the level of the cord from which they originate.
6. Afferent nerve fibers transmit sensory impulses from the periphery toward the brain. Efferent fibers transmit motor impulses from the brain or spinal cord toward the periphery.
7. The involved nerve is the median nerve. The condition is referred to as *ape hand.*
8. The involved nerve is the fibular nerve. The condition is referred to as *foot drop.*
9. The muscle group involved with claw hand is the intrinsic group, which is mostly innervated by the ulnar nerve.
10. The hematoma would be deep to the dura, the outermost covering of the brain.
11. The intervertebral foramen made up of the inferior vertebral notch of the vertebra above and the superior vertebral notch of the vertebra below
12. Lower motor neuron lesion
13. More like a peripheral nerve lesion because the spinal cord ends at L2. Below that, the cord is made up of a collection of nerve roots.
14. From the spinal cord to the periphery

Chapter 7 Circulatory System

Cardiovascular System

1. Tricuspid valve
2. a. Bicuspid valve
   b. Mitral valve
3. Pulmonic valve, aortic valve
4. Pulmonary arteries, pulmonary veins
5. a. Deoxygenated
   b. Pulmonary veins
   c. Oxygenated
   d. Pulmonary arteries
6. a. AV valves
   b. SL valves
7. It will end up distal to its origin in a leg artery or an arteriole small enough in diameter to prevent its passage.
8. It will end up in one of the pulmonary arteries (or arterioles) in the lung because it will travel until reaching a vessel with a small enough diameter to prevent further passage.
9. External iliac artery and vein to femoral artery and vein
10. External and internal jugular
11. Common carotid artery
12. Major structures from left femoral vein to lung: (1) left femoral vein, (2) left external iliac vein, (3) left common iliac vein, (4) inferior vena cava, (5) right atrium, (6) right AV valve, (7) right ventricle, (8) pulmonic valve, (9) pulmonary arteries, and (10) lungs

13. a. Diastolic pressure (lowest) occurs when the heart relaxes between beats.
    b. Systolic pressure (highest) occurs while the heart contracts.

Lymphatic System

1. Afferent lymph vessel
2. Subclavian vein
3. (c) Muscle
4. Valves, lymph angion, squeezing action of muscles, movement of diaphragm, and good posture
5. Cervical, axillary, and inguinal regional nodes
6. Thoracic duct
7. Collect, filter, and return lymph to the bloodstream

Chapter 8 Basic Biomechanics

1. a. The wrist, because there is a longer resistance arm when the weight is around the wrist than when it is around the elbow.
2. b. The shorter person, who is not on stilts, has a lower COG.
3. a.

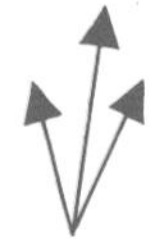

   b.

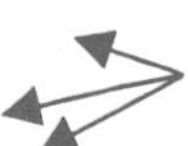

4. a. Scalar = 5 miles (magnitude only)
   b. Vector = 30 feet to the north (magnitude and direction)
5. More force is required when the hand truck is more horizontal. The force arm remains constant, while changing the angle of the hand truck lengthens or shortens the resistance arm. Lowering the load (angle becomes more horizontal) in effect lengthens the resistance arm and requires the person to exert more force. Raising the load (angle becomes more vertical) shortens the resistance arm and allows the person to use less force to move the hand truck.
6. This demonstrates the concept of the wheel and axle. The smaller push rim will require more force, but the distance the wheelchair will travel with a single push is greater.
7. No, the object will fall because the LOG (and COG) is outside the BOS.

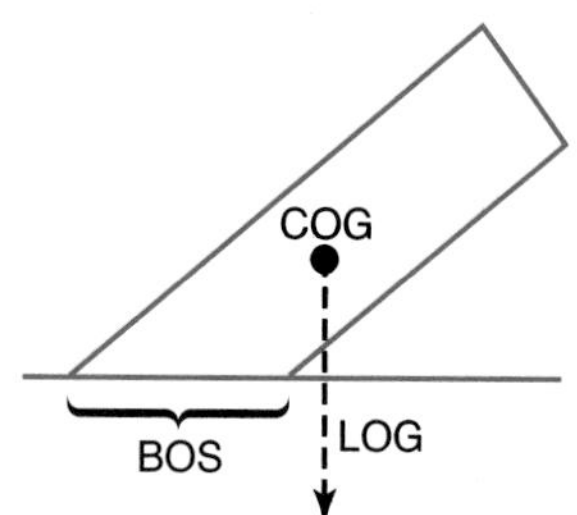

8. The BOS of a wheelchair during a "wheelie" is very narrow. To maintain balance, the person must keep the body's COG within that BOS. However, the BOS is very wide when the wheelchair is resting on all four wheels, and it is easy to keep the body's COG within it.
9. Linear force
10. People need to get as close to the bed as possible as this shortens their lever arms; they need to move their legs apart, especially in the A/P direction as this increases their BOS; they need to bend their knees slightly as this lowers their COG.
11. Putting the nut closer to the axis makes the resistance arm shorter, thus making it easier to crack the nut.
12. Parallel forces; the two people exert an upward force on the mats while the mats (and gravity) exert a downward force. The upward and downward forces are parallel.
13. The medial condyles of the tibia and femur increase the angle of pull of the gracilis. The patella and femoral condyles increase the angle of pull of the quadriceps.
14. Holding the suitcase on the left shifts her COG to the left. By leaning to the right, she is bringing her COG back over the BOS. With a very heavy suitcase, the person's COG shifts farther to the left, so besides leaning to the right, she might raise her right arm out to the side in an attempt to shift the COG more to the right.
15. To increase the amount of friction between the crutch tip and the ground to prevent slippage

16. In Figure 8-44, answer the following questions:
   a. F = person pulling luggage, R= luggage, A = wheels of luggage
   b.

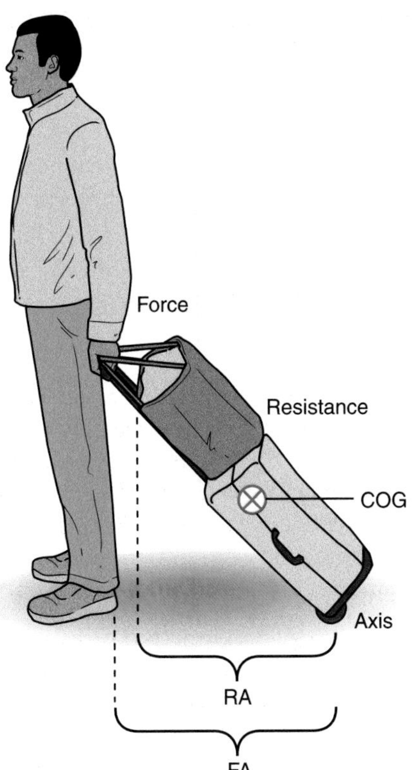

   c.

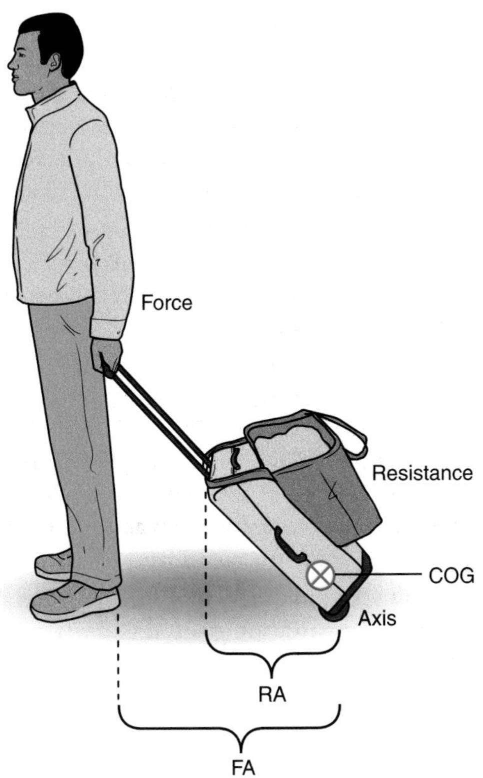

   d. Fig. A
   e. Force arm remains the same in both scenarios.
   f. Fig. B = putting the bag lower on the suitcase shortens the resistance arm, making the luggage easier to pull.

Chapter 9 Shoulder Girdle

General Anatomy Questions

1. The shoulder girdle includes the articulations between the scapula and clavicle. The shoulder joint includes the scapula and humerus. The shoulder complex includes the scapula, clavicle, humerus, sternum, and rib cage.
2. a. Use the inferior angle as a point of reference.
   b. When the scapula moves away from the vertebral column, the motion is scapular upward rotation. When it moves back toward the vertebral column to the starting position, the motion is scapular downward rotation.
3. Scapular elevation/depression and protraction/retraction are more linear.
4. Scapular upward and downward rotation are more angular.
5. Angular motions
6. Scapular upward rotation
7. Scapulohumeral rhythm is the movement relationship between the shoulder girdle and the shoulder joint. After the first 30 degrees, for every 2 degrees of shoulder joint flexion or abduction, the shoulder girdle rotates upwardly 1 degree.
8. Without this shoulder girdle movement, one cannot normally and completely raise the arm above the head.
9. a. Because the three different attachments of the trapezius muscle produce three different lines of pull, the three parts have different muscle actions.
   b. The rhomboid muscles, however, have the same line of pull and thus the same muscle action. There is no functional difference between the rhomboid muscles.
10. The serratus anterior plus the upper and lower trapezius muscles
11. Force couple: a situation in which two or more muscles pull in different, often opposite, directions to accomplish the same motion
12. SC joint, AC joint, and scapulothoracic articulation

13. The rhomboid muscles, the lower and middle trapezius muscles, the levator scapula muscle, and the upper trapezius muscle
14. Pectoralis major
15. Pectoralis major, latissimus dorsi

Functional Activity Questions

1. Downward rotation
2. Upward rotation
3. Elevation
4. Upward rotation and retraction
5. Protraction
6. (1) Concentric, (2) concentric, (3) isometric, (4) isometric, (5) concentric

Clinical Exercise Questions

1. a. Scapular retraction
   b. Middle trapezius, rhomboids
   c. Open
2. a. Scapular retraction
   b. Middle trapezius and rhomboids
   c. Concentric
3. a. Scapular depression; technically, there is a small amount of upward rotation due to the shoulder flexion from a hyperextended to extended position. This would result in some upward rotation of the scapula.
   b. Lower trapezius, pectoralis minor; upper trapezius, serratus anterior
   c. Concentric
4. a. Scapular protraction and upward rotation
   b. Serratus anterior, pectoralis minor, upper and lower trapezius
   c. Closed
5. a. Scapular retraction and downward rotation
   b. Middle trapezius, rhomboids, levator scapula, pectoralis minor
   c. Concentric contraction; the external weight is greater than the pull of gravity. Therefore, it is an accelerating force, not a decelerating one.
6. a. Upper trapezius and levator scapula contract concentrically.
   b. The upper trapezius and levator scapula contract eccentrically to control the rate and degree of depression.
7. Serratus anterior

Chapter 10 Shoulder Joint

General Anatomy Questions

1. a. In the frontal plane around the sagittal axis: shoulder abduction/adduction
   b. In the transverse plane around the vertical axis: shoulder medial/lateral rotation, horizontal abduction/adduction
   c. In the sagittal plane around the frontal axis: shoulder flexion/extension/hyperextension
2. The circular arc of the upper extremity formed by a combination of the shoulder motions–flexion, abduction, extension, and adduction
3. Subscapular fossa
4. The supraspinous and infraspinous fossas
5. With the humerus in the vertical position, the bicipital groove facing anteriorly, and the head facing medially, the right humeral head faces toward the left.
6. The **s**upraspinatus, **i**nfraspinatus, **t**eres minor, and **s**ubscapularis muscles; they hold the head of the humerus in toward the glenoid fossa as it moves within the socket.
7. The subscapularis and coracobrachialis muscles and the short head of the biceps brachii muscle
8. The teres major, teres minor, infraspinatus, supraspinatus, and posterior deltoid muscles
9. The anterior deltoid, pectoralis major, and latissimus dorsi muscles
10. a. Clavicular portion
    b. First part of range–to approximately 60 degrees
    c. Its vertical line of pull makes it more effective in the early part of the range and less so as it approaches a more horizontal line of pull.
11. Anterior deltoid: (1) is a larger muscle and (2) passes farther from the axis of rotation of the shoulder (it has a longer moment arm) and is therefore stronger.

Functional Activity Questions

1. a. Shoulder hyperextension and medial rotation
   b. Scapular tilt and protraction
2. a. Shoulder abduction and lateral rotation
   b. Scapular upward rotation and retraction
3. a. Shoulder adduction and medial rotation
   b. Scapular downward rotation and protraction
4. a. Shoulder flexion
   b. Scapular upward rotation and protraction

5. a. Shoulder adduction
   b. Scapular downward rotation
6. a. Shoulder abduction
   b. Scapular upward rotation
7. Circumduction

Clinical Exercise Questions

1. a. Shoulder horizontal abduction
   b. Concentric contraction of shoulder horizontal abductors
   c. Posterior deltoid, infraspinatus, teres minor
2. a. No
   b. Yes
   c. With a shortened resistance arm, there is less resistance that the force needs to move.
3. a. Shoulder flexion
   b. Eccentric contraction
   c. Latissimus dorsi, posterior deltoid, teres major, sternal part of pectoralis major
   d. Frontal axis
4. a. Shoulder hyperextension
   b. Concentric contraction of shoulder hyperextensors
   c. Latissimus dorsi, posterior deltoid
5. a. Shoulder flexion
   b. Eccentric contraction of shoulder hyperextensors
   c. Latissimus dorsi, posterior deltoid
6. a. Shoulder flexion
   b. Shoulder abduction
   c. Plane of the scapula
7. First part:
   a. Shoulder lateral rotation
   b. Concentric
   c. Shoulder lateral rotators: infraspinatus, teres minor, posterior deltoid

   Second part:
   a. Shoulder lateral rotation
   b. Isometric
   c. Shoulder lateral rotators

   Third part:
   a. Shoulder medial rotation
   b. Eccentric
   c. Shoulder lateral rotators
8. Shoulder adductors
9. a. Latissimus dorsi and pectoralis major
   b. Reverse muscle action
   c. Reverse muscle action of the lower trapezius and pectoralis minor

Chapter 11 Elbow Joint

General Anatomy Questions

1. a. *Bones in joint:*
      Forearm: radius, ulna
      Elbow: humerus, radius, ulna
   b. *Number of axes:*
      Forearm: 1
      Elbow: 1
   c. *Shape of joint:*
      Forearm: pivot
      Elbow: hinge
   d. *Joint motion allowed:*
      Forearm: supination/pronation
      Elbow: flexion/extension
2. The trochlear notch at the superior end faces anteriorly, the radial notch at the same end faces laterally, and the styloid process at the inferior end is on the medial side.
3. a. Lateral, or radial, collateral ligament
   b. Medial, or ulnar, collateral ligament
   c. Annular ligament
4. The biceps and long head of the triceps muscles
5. Radius, because it is the radius moving around the ulna that produces these motions.
6. The pronator quadratus, biceps, and long head of the triceps muscles
7. The biceps (to radius) and long head of the triceps (to ulna) muscles
8. Anconeus, triceps, and brachialis muscles
9. Long head of triceps
10. Flexion, flexion
11. a. Shoulder flexion, elbow flexion, forearm supination
    b. Shoulder hyperextension, elbow extension, forearm pronation
12. Opposite direction
13. a. Biceps
    b. Triceps
    c. Brachioradialis
    d. Contralateral
14. a. Annular ligament
    b. Joint capsule
    c. Prevents the joint capsule from getting pinched in the olecranon fossa during elbow extension
15. a. Supinator and biceps
    b. Neutralizer; the biceps flexes the elbow and supinates the forearm. The extension action of

the triceps neutralizes the flexion action of the biceps, maintaining the elbow in the partially flexed position.

Functional Activity Questions

1. a. Shoulder flexion
   b. Anterior deltoid, clavicular portion of pectoralis major, biceps
   c. Elbow extension
   d. Triceps
   e. Forearm supination
   f. Supinator, biceps
   g. Firm
   h. Open chain
2. a. Elbow flexion
   b. Forearm supination (or possibly midposition)
3. a. Elbow extension
   b. Becomes more taut, put on slack
   c. Hard
   d. Forearm pronation
   e. Hard
   f. Pronator teres, pronator quadratus
4. a. Open chain
   b. Elbow flexion
   c. Soft
   d. Biceps, brachialis, brachioradialis
   e. Forearm supination
   f. Proximal and distal radioulnar joints
5. a. Elbow extension
   b. At both the humeroradial and humeroulnar joints, there is a concave-on-convex articulation where the concave radial head and the concave trochlear notch glide posteriorly on their respective humeral articular surfaces—the convex capitulum and the convex trochlea.
   c. Forearm midposition
   d. The brachioradialis will always return the forearm to neutral from either positions of pronation or supination.

Clinical Exercise Questions

1. a. Forearm supination
   b. Pronator teres, pronator quadratus
2. a. Elbow extension
   b. Concentric
   c. Triceps
   d. Closed chain
3. a. Elbow flexion
   b. Triceps
4. a. Isometric
   b. Triceps
5. a. Elbow extension
   b. Eccentric
   c. Biceps, brachialis, brachioradialis
   d. Open chain
6. a. Elbow extension
   b. Triceps performs a concentric contraction
   c. Elbow flexion
   d. triceps perform an eccentric contraction
7. a. supinator and biceps are contracting concentrically
   b. pronator teres and pronator quadratus are contracting eccentrically

Chapter 12 Wrist Joint

General Anatomy Questions

1. Proximal row, lateral to medial: scaphoid, lunate, triquetrum, pisiform
   Distal row, lateral to medial: trapezium, trapezoid, capitate, hamate
2. a. Wrist flexion and extension
   b. Wrist radial and ulnar deviation
   c. No wrist motions occur in the transverse plane around the vertical axis.
3. a. *Number of axes:*
   Radiocarpal joint: 2
   Intercarpal joint: 0
   b. *Shape of joint:*
   Radiocarpal joint: ellipsoid
   Intercarpal joint: plane or irregular
   c. *Joint motion allowed:*
   Radiocarpal joint: flexion/extension, radial/ulnar deviation
   Intercarpal joint: gliding
4. Flexor carpi ulnaris, flexor carpi radialis, palmaris longus
5. Extensor carpi radialis longus and brevis, extension carpi ulnaris
6. If the pisiform bone and "hook" of the hamate bone are visible, it would be the anterior side.
7. Extensor carpi radialis longus and flexor carpi radialis
8. Extensor carpi ulnaris and flexor carpi ulnaris
9. The palmaris longus located on the anterior surface in the middle of the wrist

10. Flexor carpi ulnaris, palmaris longus (with flexor digitorum superficialis and profundus deep to it), flexor carpi radialis (abductor pollicis longus, extensor pollicis long and brevis, which are primarily thumb muscles but also cross the wrist), extensor carpi radialis longus and brevis (extensor digitorum, a finger extensor), and extensor carpi ulnaris
11. Because an articular disk is located between the ulna and the proximal row of carpals
12. You are using a longer lever arm and larger muscles.
13. You are working against gravity when hammering overhead and with gravity when hammering at waist level.
14. For wrist flexion, extension, and ulnar deviation, the end feel is soft. For wrist radial deviation, the end feel is hard.
15. Lateral supracondylar ridge

Functional Activity Questions

1. a. Ulnar deviation
   b. Extensor carpi radialis longus (ECRL), flexor carpi ulnaris (FCU)
   c. Flexion and extension
2. a. Flexion
   b. ECRL, extensor carpi radialis brevis (ECRB), and extensor carpi ulnaris (ECU)
   c. Radial and ulnar deviation
3. a. Radial deviation
   b. ECU, FCU
   c. Flexion and extension
4. a. Wrist hyperextension
   b. FCU, FCR
   c. Radial and ulnar deviation
5. a. Wrist hyperextension
   b. FCU, FCR

Clinical Exercise Questions

1. a. Wrist flexion
   b. Concentric
   c. Wrist flexors
   d. Posterior
2. a. Wrist extension
   b. Eccentric
   c. Wrist flexors
3. a. Wrist extension
   b. Palmar radiocarpal ligament
   c. Concentric
   d. Wrist extensors
4. a. Wrist flexion
   b. Eccentric
   c. Wrist extensors
5. a. Wrist ulnar deviation
   b. Concentric
   c. Wrist ulnar deviators
6. a. Wrist radial deviation
   b. Eccentric
   c. Elasticity of tubing would bring wrist back to neutral if ulnar deviators were not slowing down the motion.
   d. Wrist ulnar deviators
7. a. Wrist extension
   b. Anterior

Chapter 13 Hand

General Anatomy Questions

1. a. Finger: MCP abduction/adduction
   Thumb: CMC flexion/extension, MCP and IP flexion/extension
   b. Finger: MCP, PIP, DIP flexion/extension
   Thumb: CMC abduction/adduction
   c. Thumb: CMC opposition/reposition
2. Compare the thumb and fingers:
   a. *Number of bones:*
   Thumb: 4
   Finger: 5
   b. *Number of joints:*
   Thumb: 3
   Finger: 4
   c. *Names of the joints:*
   Thumb: CMC, MCP, IP
   Finger: CMC, MCP, PIP, DIP
3. CMC flexion, abduction, and rotation
4. Rotation
5. They hold the extrinsic tendons close to the wrist.
6. a. The floor of the carpal tunnel is made up of the carpal bones, and the ceiling is the transverse carpal ligament portion of the flexor retinaculum.
   b. The flexor digitorum superficialis and profundus and the flexor pollicis longus muscles and the median nerve run through the carpal tunnel.
7. a. An extrinsic muscle has its proximal attachment above the wrist and its distal attachment below the wrist.
   b. The extrinsic muscles include the flexor digitorum superficialis and profundus, extensor digitorum, extensor digiti minimi, and extensor indicis

muscles of the fingers. Extrinsic muscles of the thumb are the flexor pollicis longus, abductor pollicis longus, and extensor pollicis longus and brevis.

8. a. An intrinsic muscle has both attachments below the wrist.
   b. The nine intrinsic muscles include the flexor and abductor pollicis brevis, the opponens and adductor pollicis, the flexor/abductor/opponens digiti minimi, the interossei, and the lumbricals.
9. Thenar muscles are intrinsic muscles on the thumb (lateral) side of the hand; hypothenar muscles are on the little finger (medial) side. Any intrinsic muscle with *pollicis* in its name (i.e. flexor pollicis brevis) is a thenar muscle, whereas one with *digiti minimi* (i.e. flexor digiti minimi) is a hypothenar muscle.
10. The indentation formed between the tendons of the abductor pollicis longus and extensor pollicis brevis laterally and extensor pollicis longus medially is referred to as the *anatomical snuffbox*.
11. a. The lumbricals
    b. They attach proximally to the tendons of the flexor digitorum profundus muscle and distally to the tendons of the extensor digitorum muscle.
    c. MCP flexion and PIP/DIP extension
12. a. Concave
    b. Convex
    c. Same
    d. Medially
13. a. MCP joint
    b. CMC joint
14. The flexor digitorum superficialis, because it is superficial to the flexor digitorum profundus, and therefore crosses farther away from the MCP joint axis of rotation.
15. Convex, concave, posterior, medial

Functional Activity Questions

1. Holding the handle of a skillet: cylindrical grip
2. Pulling a little red wagon: hook grip
3. Turning pages of a book: pad-to-pad or pad-to-side prehension
4. Fastening snaps or buttons: tip-to-tip prehension
5. Carrying a coffee mug by its handle: lateral prehension
6. Holding a hand of playing cards: lumbrical grip
7. Holding an apple: spherical grip
8. Holding on to a barbell: cylindrical grip
9. Picking up a CD: pad-to-pad or pad-to-side prehension
10. a. Combination of cylindrical and lumbrical grips
    b. Held in neutral position by wrist flexors and radial deviators
    c. Flexor carpi ulnaris and radialis, extensor carpi radialis longus
    d. Elbow flexors
    e. Biceps, brachialis, and especially brachioradialis
    f. Shoulder flexors and adductors
    g. Anterior deltoid, pectoralis major, teres major, and latissimus dorsi
    h. Shoulder girdle upward rotation and protraction
    i. Upper and lower trapezius, serratus anterior, pectoralis minor
11. a. Pad-to-side grip
    b. Forearm supination

Clinical Exercise Questions

1. Joint motion: finger MCP abduction followed by MCP adduction
   Prime movers: dorsal interossei and abductor digiti minimi followed by palmar interossei
2. Joint motion: thumb abduction
   Prime movers: abductor pollicis brevis and longus
3. Joint motion: thumb and little finger opposition
   Prime movers: opponens pollicis, opponens digiti minimi
4. Joint motion: finger MP flexion and IP extension
   Prime movers: lumbricals
5. Joint motion: thumb CMC, MCP, and IP flexion
   Prime movers: flexor pollicis longus and brevis
6. Middle phalanx, posterior, posterior
7. Flexion at the DIP, PIP, MCP, and wrist joints
8. Flexors, passively, hyperextended
9. Actively, passively

Chapter 14 Temporomandibular Joint

General Anatomy Questions

1. Zygomatic and temporal bones
2. Synonymous terms are mandibular
   a. depression.
   b. elevation.
   c. retraction or retrusion.
   d. protraction or protrusion.
   e. lateral deviation.

3. Mandibular fossa of the temporal bone, condyle of the mandible
4. Temporalis
5. Masseter
6. Digastric and omohyoid
7. Fifth cranial (trigeminal) nerve
8. Anterior rotation of the mandibular condyle on the disk
9. The left condyle spins in the mandibular socket while the right condyle slides forward.
10. The thyroid cartilage

Functional Activity Questions

1. Mandibular depression, buccinator
2. a. Mandibular elevation
   b. Side opposite the bread
   c. Same side as the bread
   d. F = muscles, R = bread
   e. Third-class lever
   f. The force arm would stay the same as the muscle attachments, and joint axis has not moved. The resistance arm would increase as the distance between the joint axis and the resistance (point where teeth contact bread) has gotten longer.
   g. When biting with the front teeth (long resistance arm), more force must be generated to overcome the larger resistance
3. Side-to-side motion—lateral deviation
   Anterior-posterior motion—protraction/retraction
4. Motion: mandibular elevation
   Muscle: temporalis, masseter, medial pterygoid
5. The anterior fibers because they are oriented more vertically
6. All muscles of mandibular elevation (temporalis, masseter, and medial pterygoid) are contracting isometrically.

Clinical Exercise Questions

1. a. Mandibular lateral deviation
   b. Concentric
   c. Right temporalis and masseter, left medial and lateral pterygoid
2. a. Mandibular protraction
   b. Isometric
   c. Medial and lateral pterygoid
3. a. Mandibular depression
   b. Concentric
   c. Lateral pterygoid
   d. Lateral pterygoid, suprahyoid group
   e. The infrahyoid group contracts to stabilize the hyoid and prevent it from elevating when the suprahyoid group contracts.

Chapter 15 Neck and Trunk

General Anatomy Questions

1. a. Neck and trunk lateral bending
   b. Neck and trunk rotation
   c. Neck and trunk flexion, extension, and hyperextension
2. The cervical vertebra has a bifid spinous process, and there is a foramen in the transverse process. The thoracic vertebra has a long, slender, downward-pointing spinous process with rib facets on the body and transverse processes; the superior articular processes face posteriorly. The lumbar vertebra has a large spinous process pointing straight back; the superior articular processes face medially.
3. The frontal plane position of the superior and inferior articular processes
4. The sagittal plane position of the superior and inferior articular processes
5. From the occiput to C7: nuchal ligament
   From C7 to the sacrum: supraspinous ligament
6. Ligamentum flavum
7. a. Anterior and posterior longitudinal ligaments
   b. Anterior longitudinal ligament limits extension, posterior longitudinal ligament limits flexion.
8. The muscle's line of pull is through or close to the center of the frontal axis of trunk flexion and extension, thus making it ineffective in this motion. To be effective in rotation, the muscle's line of pull would have to be horizontal or diagonal. The quadratus lumborum has a vertical line of pull.
9. The erector spinae
10. The right side (same side)
11. The median AA joint is a uniaxial pivot joint, and the 2 lateral AA joints are plane-shaped synovial joints.
12. L4-5 and L5-S1 because the PLL is thinner and more narrow at this level and does not act as an effective barrier between the disc and the spinal cord

13. The occipital condyle glides anteriorly on the superior articular facet of C1.
14. a. Flexion decreases the lumbar lordosis and extension increases the lumbar lordosis.
    b. Increases with flexion and decreases with extension
    c. The annulus compresses anteriorly with flexion and posteriorly with extension.
    d. The nucleus moves posteriorly with flexion and anteriorly with extension.
    e. Increases with flexion and decreases with extension
    f. Decreases with flexion and increases with extension
15. Prevents the dens from slipping posteriorly into the spinal cord

Functional Activity Questions

1. Neck rotation and possibly some hyperextension
2. Neck lateral bending
3. Neck hyperextension
4. Neck flexion
5. Neck hyperextension
6. Trunk rotation to left
7. Trunk rotation to right
8. Trunk lateral bending
9. Trunk flexion
10. Trunk hyperextension
11. Quadratus lumborum performs reverse muscle action to elevate the pelvis.
12. a. Gravity
    b. Spinal extensors are contracting eccentrically to control the rate and degree of flexion being caused by gravity.
13. Left quadratus lumborum contracts concentrically to perform left lateral bending back to the neutral position.

Clinical Exercise Questions

Head and Neck

1. a. Flexion of head on C1
   b. Neck extension
   c. Concentric
   d. Isometric
   e. Neck extensors (splenius capitis, splenius cervicis, erector spinae, interspinales, and transversospinalis)
2. a. Right lateral bending of head and neck
   b. Isometric
   c. Right sternocleidomastoid, right splenius capitis, right splenius cervicis, right scalenes, right erector spinae, and right intertransversarii
3. a. Neck lateral bending to the right
   b. Left neck lateral benders
   c. Right sternocleidomastoid, right scalenes, right splenius capitis and cervicis, right erector spinae, and right intertransversarii
   d. Right lateral benders
   e. Same as answer (c), except on left side
4. Left sternocleidomastoid
5. a. Flexion of head on C1
   b. Concentric
   c. Prevertebral muscles
   d. Neck flexion
   e. Concentric
   f. Sternocleidomastoid (bonus point if you included the longus colli of the prevertebral muscle group)
   g. Isometric
   h. Sternocleidomastoid (another bonus point if you remembered the longus colli)
   i. Neck extension
   j. Eccentric contraction
   k. Sternocleidomastoid and longus colli

Trunk

1. a. Trunk flexion, especially lumbar region
   b. Trunk extensors
   c. Erector spinae, transversospinalis, interspinales
2. a. Trunk flexion
   b. Concentric
   c. Bilateral rectus abdominis, external and internal obliques
3. a. Yes
   b. Flexing
   c. Origin toward insertion
   d. Reverse muscle action
   e. Holding down the feet makes the distal segment more stable and the proximal segment more movable. This allows the hip flexors to flex the hip (and trunk) in a reversal of muscle action.
4. a. Trunk flexion with rotation to the left
   b. Concentric
   c. Both right and left rectus abdominis, right external oblique, and left internal oblique
5. a. Hyperextension
   b. Trunk flexors
   c. Isometrically

Chapter 16 Respiratory System

General Anatomy Questions

1. The sternum, ribs, costal cartilages, and thoracic vertebrae
2. The bodies of the thoracic vertebrae articulate with the heads of the ribs (costovertebral joint), and the transverse processes of the thoracic vertebrae articulate with the tubercles of the ribs (costotransverse joint).
3. The chondrosternal joint is the articulation of the costal cartilage of ribs 1-7 with the sternum.
4. Elevation and depression bringing about inspiration and expiration
5. During inspiration, the ribs elevate and the diaphragm lowers, and during expiration, the ribs depress and the diaphragm muscle elevates.
6. The origin, or more stable attachment, is above the rib cage and in a position to pull the rib cage up.
7. The line of pull does not change from front to back, but the muscle moves 180 degrees around the rib cage, giving the appearance of changing direction from front to back.
8. The origin, or more stable attachment, has a bony attachment, but the insertion attaches to a central tendon. When the muscle is relaxed, it is dome-shaped. When it contracts, the muscle flattens out, allowing more room in the thoracic cavity.
9. You talk only during expiration, when air is moving out through the airway.
10. The accessory muscles of inspiration pull up on the sternum and rib cage while the accessory muscles of expiration pull down.
11. a. Bucket handle movement
    b. Pump handle movement
    c. A bellows
12. The person with a C3 injury will not have an innervated diaphragm; they will need the assistance of a ventilator to breathe. A person with a C5 injury will have a neurologically intact diaphragm and can breathe without mechanical assistance.

Functional Activity Questions

1. Forced inspiration followed by forced expiration
2. Deep inspiration
3. Forced expiration
4. Forced expiration
5. Quiet inspiration and expiration
6. a. The trunk extensors contract to neutralize the trunk flexion force created by the abdominals, allowing the abdominals to pull down on the ribs instead of flexing the trunk.
   b. Reverse muscle action causes the pectoralis minor to lift up on the rib cage assisting in inspiration.
   c. They perform a concentric contraction to produce scapular elevation. This exerts an upward pull on the rib cage via the scapula's connection to the clavicle, assisting in inspiration.
   d. The muscles of scapular elevation stabilize the scapula so the pectoralis minor, in a reverse muscle action, pulls up on the ribs instead of pulling down on the coracoid process.

Clinical Exercise Questions

1. a. Chest breathing
   b. Diaphragmatic breathing
2. Anterior trunk muscles—rectus abdominis, external and internal oblique, and transverse abdominis
3. a. Chest rose during sniffing
   b. Muscles contracted
   c. Sniffing requires deep inspiration. Accessory muscles of inspiration assisted by pulling up the rib cage in a reversal of muscle action. These muscles were the scalenes and sternocleidomastoids.
4. a. Ribcage moves up and out during inspiration.
   b. The pectoralis major is assisting in deep inspiration by pulling up on the ribs.
   c. This is a closed-chain activity.

Chapter 17 Pelvic Girdle

General Anatomy Questions

1. a. Anterior/posterior pelvic tilt
   b. Lateral tilt
   c. Pelvic rotation
2. a. To the left
   b. Right hip hiking
3. The hip joints
4. a. Hip flexion
   b. Hip extension
   c. Hip abduction on the unsupported side and hip adduction on the weight-bearing side

5. a. Right hip medial rotation
   b. Right hip lateral rotation
6. a. Hyperextension
   b. Flexion
   c. Lateral bending to opposite side
7. a. Trunk extensors, hip flexors
   b. Trunk flexors and hip extensors
8. Left leg
9. Decrease
10. Iliolumbar and lumbosacral ligaments

Functional Activity Questions

1. Posterior pelvic tilt
2. Anterior pelvic tilt
3. Posterior pelvic tilt
4. Left hip adducted and right hip abducted
5. a. Hip flexors
   b. Hip extensors
   c. Trunk extensors
   d. Trunk flexors

Clinical Exercise Questions

1. Motions: posterior pelvic tilt, trunk flexion, hip extension
   Muscles: gluteus maximus and trunk flexors
2. Motions: left lateral pelvic tilt; left hip adduction and right hip abduction
   Muscles: right hip abductors (gluteus medius and minimus) and left quadratus lumborum

Chapter 18 Hip Joint

General Anatomy Questions

1. a. Two innominate bones, the sacrum, and the coccyx
   b. The fused bones of the ilium, ischium, and pubis
   c. Acetabulum of the innominate and head of the femur
   d. The ilium, ischium, and pubis
   e. The ischium and pubis
   f. The ilium and ischium
2. With the greater sciatic notch posterior and the body of the pubis anterior, the acetabulum faces laterally. Therefore, if the acetabular opening is facing to the right in this position, it is a right innominate bone.
3. With the femur in the vertical position, the linea aspera and lesser trochanter are posterior, and the head faces medially. Therefore, in this position the head of the right femur faces toward the left.
4. a. Number of axes: 3
   b. Shape of joint: ball and socket
   c. Type of motion allowed: flexion/extension, abduction/adduction, and rotation
5. a. Medial and lateral rotation
   b. Flexion/extension
   c. Abduction/adduction
6. The distal attachment of the iliofemoral ligament; because it splits into two parts, forming an upside-down Y
7. a. Anterior/ hips are in extension
   b. Posterior
   c. Extension
   d. Extensor
8. The acetabulum forms a deep socket holding most of the femoral head, and the joint is surrounded by three very strong ligaments.
9. The line of attachment of the ligaments is a spiral. This arrangement causes the ligaments to become taut as the joint moves into extension and to slacken with flexion, thus limiting hyperextension without impeding flexion.
10. The rectus femoris, sartorius, gracilis, semitendinosus, semimembranosus, biceps femoris (long head), and tensor fascia latae muscles
11. The sartorius muscle is involved in hip flexion, abduction, and lateral rotation; the tensor fasciae latae muscle is involved in flexion and abduction.
12. When you lift your right foot off the floor, the left hip abductors and right trunk extensors contract to keep the right side of the pelvis from dropping. A force couple exists when the hip abductors are pulling down while the trunk extensors are pulling up.
13. Opposite
14. Anterior
15. Hip flexion—soft; hip extension—firm

Functional Activity Questions

1. Hip extension and medial rotation, and maybe some adduction
2. a. Greater hip flexion is required with a low surface.
   b. Medial rotation and adduction may accompany the increased flexion.

3. a. Adduction
   b. Right hip adductors
   c. Closed
4. a. Swing phase includes hip flexion, extension, and hyperextension.
   b. Greater hip flexion than walking
   c. Hip flexion and abduction
   d. Combination of hip hyperextension, abduction, flexion, adduction as you swing your leg over the bike, and may also include some rotation
5. Opposite so the cane can bear body weight and help prevent lateral tilt on the non-weight-bearing side
6. a. Posterior tilt
   b. Anterior tilt with increased lumbar lordosis
7. a. It maintains the pelvis in a posterior tilt.
   b. There is not sufficient length of the hip flexors to complete the range of motion.
   c. Iliopsoas
   d. The anterior hip muscles must be elongated more when the pelvis is in a posterior tilt position versus an anterior tilt position.
8. You may compensate by standing with the lumbar spine in lordosis and the pelvis in anterior tilt or by leaning forward in a slightly flexed hip position.
9. a. The right hip is flexed, adducted, and medially rotated.
   b. The left hip is extended, abducted, and laterally rotated.
10. Hip—closed chain; shoulder—open chain

Clinical Exercise Questions

1. a. Hip hyperextension
   b. Strengthening
   c. Gluteus maximus
2. a. Hip hyperextension
   b. Stretching
   c. Iliopsoas
3. a. Yes. The rectus femoris is being stretched over both joints at the same time.
4. a. Hip abduction
   b. Strengthening
   c. Hip abductors—gluteus medius and gluteus minimus
5. a. Combination of hip abduction and flexion
   b. Strengthening
   c. Tensor fascia lata
6. a. Concentric
   b. Third class
   c. Anterior tilt
   d. Trunk flexors
7. a. No
   b. By having the knee flexed, the hamstrings are already shortened. As the hip goes into more hyperextension, the hamstrings will quickly become actively insufficient.
8. a. Hip abduction and flexion
   b. Stretching
   c. Adductors—pectineus, adductor longus, adductor brevis, adductor magnus
      Extensors (hamstrings)—semimembranosus, semitendinosus, biceps femoris
9. a. Exercise B is more difficult.
   b. With the knees in extension, the resistance arm is much longer than in Exercise A. The force arm remains the same length in both.
   c. Exercise B, because the legs have created a longer lever and therefore exert more torque at the pelvis
10. a. Closed
    b. Hip extension
    c. Concentric
    d. Hip extensors—gluteus maximus and hamstrings
    e. Hip flexor—rectus femoris

Chapter 19 Knee Joint

General Anatomy Questions

1. a. *Number of axes:*
      Knee joint: 1
      Patellofemoral joint: 0
   b. *Shape of joint:*
      Knee joint: hinge
      Patellofemoral joint: irregular
   c. *Type of motion:*
      Knee joint: flexion/extension
      Patellofemoral joint: gliding
2. Knee flexion and extension occur in the sagittal plane around the frontal axis.
3. The Q angle is formed by the intersection of the line between the tibial tuberosity and middle of the patella and the line between the ASIS and the middle of the patella. The greater the angle, the higher the stress on the patellofemoral joint during knee flexion and extension.
4. Femur and tibia

5. Because it initiates knee flexion, moving the knee out of the "locked" position of extension
6. The distal attachments of the sartorius, gracilis, and semitendinosus muscles
7. Weakened knee extension (quadriceps = L2–L4) and no knee flexion (hamstrings = L5–S2)
8. a. Closed kinetic chain
   b. No. This could only happen as a closed-chain action.
   c. The gastrocnemius is pulling origin toward insertion—a reversal of muscle action.
9. Rotary
10. a. Bending
    b. Tensile stress on medial side
    c. Compressive stress on lateral side
11. a. Lateral
    b. Lateral
    c. Medial

Functional Activity Questions

1. a. Hamstring action: hip extension and knee flexion
   b. Hip position (see Fig. 19-25A): extension
   c. Hip position (see Fig. 19-25B): partly flexed
   d. Position of hamstring active insufficiency: hip extension and knee flexion
   e. See Figure 19-25B: hip partly flexed
   f. Keeping the hip in slight flexion keeps some elongation of the hamstrings while they are being shortened at the knee, thus avoiding active insufficiency. Keeping the hip in extension has the hamstrings shortened over the hip while they are shortening over the knee. Thus, active insufficiency will be reached more quickly.
2. a. Hip position in Figure 19-26A = partial hip flexion; the hip position in Figure 19-26B = greater hip flexion.
   b. Vasti muscle
   c. Rectus femoris—hip flexion and knee extension
   d. The one-joint vasti muscles are elongated with knee flexion. Because they do not cross the hip, hip position has no effect on them. The two-joint rectus femoris is elongated in hip extension and knee flexion. Therefore, it is elongated more in position A. In position B, it is already shortened (on slack) at the hip.
   e. If you want to strengthen the rectus femoris, use a more extended hip position (see Fig. 19-26A).
   f. If you want to isolate and strengthen only the vasti muscles, use a more flexed hip position (see Fig. 19-26B), where the rectus femoris is shortened and is not as strong.
3. a. Placing foot onto curb—knee flexion
   b. Moving up onto curb—knee extension
4. a. Preparing to kick—bringing knee into flexion and hip into hyperextension
   b. Rectus femoris is being stretched over both hip and knee.
   c. Point of ball contact—knee extension and hip extension
   d. Rectus femoris is shortening at the knee but is still elongated at the hip.
   e. Follow-through—knee remains in extension, hip going into flexion.
   f. Rectus femoris is shortened over both joints and is becoming actively insufficient.
5. a. Left foot, not right foot, would lead
   b. Hip hiking (pelvic elevation on right side; also called *right trunk lateral bending* in a reversal of muscle action)

Clinical Exercise Questions

1. Slide down:
   a. Knee flexion
   b. Eccentric contraction
   c. Knee extensors (quadriceps)
   d. Closed chain
   Hold position:
   a. Isometric
   b. Knee extensors (quadriceps)
   Return to standing:
   a. Knee extension
   b. Concentric contraction
   c. Knee extensors (quadriceps)
2. a. Hip flexion and knee extension
   b. Stretching of hamstrings, which extend hip and flex knee
   c. Hamstrings consist of semimembranosus, semitendinosus, biceps femoris
3. a. Hip flexion and knee extension
   b. Strengthening
   c. Hip flexors (rectus femoris, iliopsoas, and pectineus) and knee extensors (quadriceps group)
   d. Open chain
4. a. Hip extension and knee flexion
   b. Stretching
   c. Rectus femoris (which does hip flexion and knee extension)
5. Flexion—soft; extension—firm

6. a. Position C is easier to hold, position A is more difficult to hold.
   b. Force is the quadriceps muscle, resistance is the leg and foot, and axis is the knee joint. It is a third-class lever (AFR).
   c. Resistance arm shortens
   d. Force arm remains the same
7. See Figure 19-28
   Straighten knee:
   a. Knee extension
   b. Concentric contraction
   c. Knee extensors (quadriceps)
   d. Closed-chain activity
   Hold position:
   a. Knee extension
   b. Isometric contraction
   c. Knee extensors (quadriceps)
   Bend knee:
   a. Knee flexion
   b. Eccentric contraction
   c. Knee extensors (quadriceps)
8. The clinician can apply greater force just above the ankle than just below the knee because the force lever arm is longer. The axis is the knee joint. The resistance is being applied by the patient in this case. The resistance arm is the distance between the axis and the insertion of the quadriceps muscle, which does not change. The force arm is the distance between the axis and the place on the patient's leg where force is applied. Stated another way, the clinician does not need to apply as much force when using a longer force lever arm as she would with a shorter force lever arm to accomplish the same result.

Chapter 20 Ankle Joint and Foot

General Anatomy Questions

1. a. 1
   b. Hinge
   c. Dorsiflexion, plantar flexion
   d. Tibia and talus (primarily)
2. a. The subtalar joint involves the talus and calcaneus.
   b. The transverse tarsal joint involves the talus and calcaneus with the navicular and cuboid bone.
   c. Inversion and eversion
3. The function of the interosseous membrane, which is located between the tibia and fibula, is to hold the two bones together and to provide a large area for muscle attachment.
4. The deltoid ligament, made up of the tibionavicular, tibiocalcaneal, and posterior tibiotalar ligaments
5. The lateral ligament, made up of the posterior and anterior talofibular and calcaneofibular ligaments
6. The medial and lateral longitudinal arches
7. The medial longitudinal arch is made up of the calcaneus, navicular, cuneiform, and first three metatarsal bones. The lateral longitudinal arch is made up of the calcaneus, cuboid, and fourth and fifth metatarsals.
8. The transverse arch, made up of the cuboid and three cuneiform bones
9. The function of the arches is to provide some shock absorption, adjust to uneven terrain, and propel the body forward.
10. Tibialis posterior, flexor digitorum longus, and flexor hallucis longus muscles
11. Tibialis posterior, tibialis anterior, fibularis longus muscles
12. Fibularis longus and fibularis brevis muscles
13. Fibularis brevis and tertius muscles
14. Tibialis anterior and fibularis longus muscles; together, the fibularis longus and tibialis anterior muscles are sometimes referred to as the stirrup of the foot because the fibularis longus muscle descends the leg laterally before crossing the foot medially to join the tibialis anterior muscle. The tibialis anterior muscle descends the leg medially to meet the fibularis longus muscle, forming a "U," or stirrup.
15. No, the strongest plantar flexors are the gastrocnemius and soleus, which are innervated at the S1–S2 levels. The posterior deep group is innervated at the L5–S1 level primarily.
16. Toe flexion, extension/hyperextension
17. Supination = plantar flexion, inversion, and adduction.
    Pronation = dorsiflexion, eversion, and abduction.

Functional Activity Questions

1. Ankle plantar flexion
2. Ankle plantar flexion
3. Ankle dorsiflexion
4. Ankle plantar flexion
5. Ankle inversion/eversion
6. Ankle dorsiflexion

7. Ankle plantar flexion
8. Ankle inversion prevented by the fibularis muscle group

Clinical Exercise Questions

1. Gastrocnemius:
   a. *Number of joints crossed:* 2
   b. Knee motion: knee flexion
   c. Ankle motion: ankle plantar flexion
   Soleus:
   a. *Number of joints crossed:* 1
   b. Knee motion: no knee motion
   c. Ankle motion: ankle plantar flexion
2. a. Left knee: extension
   Left ankle: dorsiflexion
   b. Left gastrocnemius is stretching
   c. Left soleus is stretching
   d. Gastrocnemius
   e. The gastrocnemius is stretched more because it has to stretch over the combined range of both knee and ankle joints, while the soleus is being stretched over only the ankle joint.
3. a. Left knee: flexion
   Left ankle: dorsiflexion
   b. The left gastrocnemius is slack at the knee.
   c. The left gastrocnemius is stretched at the ankle.
   d. The left soleus is not stretched at the knee because it does not cross the knee.
   e. Yes. The left soleus is stretched at the ankle.
   f. Soleus
   g. The soleus is stretched more because there is more ankle ROM. With the gastrocnemius slack over the knee, more ankle motion is possible, which stretches the soleus more.
4. a. Left knee: extension
   Left ankle: plantar flexion
   b. The left gastrocnemius is elongating.
   c. The left gastrocnemius is shortening.
   d. The left soleus is not acting over the knee.
   e. The left soleus is shortening over the ankle.
   f. The two-joint gastrocnemius is able to elongate over the knee while shortening over the ankle, thus keeping more tension in the muscle through a greater range. The one-joint soleus is shortening over the ankle and will lose tension quickly.
5. a. Inversion
   b. Concentric, then isometric contraction to hold the feet in position
   c. Tibialis anterior and tibialis posterior
6. a. Ankle dorsiflexion, ankle dorsiflexion, ankle plantar flexion
   b. Concentric, isometric, eccentric
   c. Ankle dorsiflexion—tibialis anterior is the prime mover for all three phases.
   d. Open
7. To prevent passive insufficiency of the gastrocnemius from limiting ankle motion

Chapter 21 Posture

General Anatomy Questions

1. Cervical extensors
2. The side view
3. Hip flexors
4. The side
5. Level and not elevated or depressed
6. From the front or back
7. Slightly in front of the lateral malleolus
8. a. Knee—slightly posterior to the patella
   b. Hip—through the greater trochanter
   c. Shoulder—through the tip of the acromion process
   d. Head—through the earlobe

Functional Activity Questions

1. Shoulder girdle protraction
2. Shoulder girdle retraction, maybe some elevation
3. Cervical flexion and possibly some forward head
4. Right shoulder higher
5. The woman's COG shifts anteriorly.
6. Anterior tilt
7. Increased lordosis
8. a. Posterior trunk—lumbar erector spinae and paraspinals become tight.
   b. Anterior trunk—abdominals become stretched.
9. Hip flexors

Clinical Exercise Questions

1. Cervical hyperextension
2. a. Cervical extensors—tighter
   b. Cervical flexors—stretched
3. No. Left side of pelvis is higher.

4. a. Left side muscles—tighter
   b. Right side muscles—stretched
5. a. Left side of disk more compressed
   b. Right side more distracted
   c. Intervertebral foramen—right side opened more
   d. Intervertebral foramen on left made smaller
6. a. Trunk extensors—posterior
   b. Anterior part
7. a. Trunk flexors—anterior
   b. Posterior part

Chapter 22 Gait

General Anatomy Questions

1. a. There are no periods of double support in running, but one period of non-support.
   b. Decreases
   c. Increases
   d. Decreases
   e. Decreases
2. Traditional terminology refers to single points in a time frame, whereas RLA terminology refers to periods within a time frame.
3. Stance phase
4. Period of double support; between heel-off and toe-off of one foot and heel strike and foot flat on the opposite foot
5. During midstance of the stance phase
6. Swing phase
7. Step length lengthens and cadence increases.
8. Walk with feet farther apart to widen the base of support.
9. Heel strike of stance phase and midswing of swing phase
10. Push-off of stance phase
11. Right, right

Functional Activity Questions

1. Shorter step length
   Flatter foot during stance
   Less arm swing
2. Narrower walking base
   Arms more out to side to help maintain balance
3. Wider walking base
   Greater horizontal displacement
4. Increased forward lean
5. Greater vertical displacement
   Greater arm swing
6. Circumducted gait during swing
   Greater horizontal displacement during stance
7. Curvilinear motion

Clinical Exercise Questions

1. a. Ankle—dorsiflexion
   b. Hip—flexion
   c. Pelvis—anterior pelvic tilt
   d. Lumbar spine—lordosis
2. a. Type of contraction: concentric
   Muscle group involved: knee extensors
   b. Type of contraction: eccentric
   Muscle group involved: ankle plantar flexors
   c. Type of contraction: concentric
   Muscle group involved: hip extensors
   d. Type of contraction: isometric
   Muscle group involved: contralateral hip abductors
   e. Type of contraction: eccentric
   Muscle group involved: knee flexors
3. a. Increasing lateral pelvic tilt to involved side
   b. Leaning over the involved (shorter) leg during stance phase
   c. Walking in an equinus gait (shorter leg)
   d. Flexing the knee of the uninvolved (longer) leg
4. Moving the center of gravity toward the weak area decreases the force that gravity exerts on the joint and reduces the demand for muscle contraction.
5. a. Hip extensors and ankle plantar flexors
   b. Closed chain
   c. Reverse muscle action
6. Vaulting gait (on uninvolved side), circumducted gait, abducted gait
7. End of stance phase (heel-off to toe-off) because the hip should be in maximal extension at that point.
8. It shortens because the involved side cannot perform a strong push-off.
9. Hip adductors
10. a. Painful
    b. Non-painful

Index

AA joint. *See* Atlantoaxial (AA) joint
Abdomen, 4, 4f
Abdominal aponeurosis, 247, 253f
Abducens nerve, 71f, 71t
Abducted gait, 394
Abduction, 7, 9f
  ankle and foot, 346, 346f
  fingers, 198, 198f
  hip joint, 298f
  shoulder joint, 146f
  thumb, 196f
  toes, 350f
Abductor digiti minimi muscle, 207f, 210
Abductor pollicis brevis muscle, 206, 207f
Abductor pollicis longus muscle, 202–203, 203f
Abnormal end feel, 31, 32
Abnormal gait, 390–396
AC joint. *See* Acromioclavicular (AC) joint
Acceleration, 104, 382f, 384t, 385t, 387–388, 388f
Accessory expiratory muscles, 275
Accessory inspiratory muscles, 274–275
Accessory motion forces, 33–34
Accessory motion terminology, 32
Accessory nerves, 70
Accommodating resistance, 57
Acetabular labrum, 302
Acetabulum, 300, 300f
Achilles tendon, 334
Achilles tendonitis, 366
Acquired bursae, 26
Acromioclavicular (AC) joint, 127f, 130–131, 131f
Acromioclavicular ligament, 131, 131f
Acromioclavicular separation, 141
Acromion process, 129, 129f, 131f, 147f, 148
Actin filament, 45, 46f
Action-reaction, 105
Active insufficiency, 49, 50f
Active range of motion (AROM), 31
Active tension, 45
Adam's apple, 270
Adaptive lengthening, 51
Adaptive shortening, 51
Adduction, 7, 9f
  ankle and foot, 346, 346f
  fingers, 198, 198f
  hip joint, 298f
  shoulder joint, 146f
  thumb, 196f
  toes, 350f
Adductor brevis muscle, 306, 306f
Adductor hiatus, 303
Adductor longus muscle, 306, 306f
Adductor magnus muscle, 306–307, 306f
Adductor pollicis muscle, 207f, 208
Adductor tubercle, 301, 301f, 327, 327f
Adhesive capsulitis, 147, 159
Afferent impulses, 65
Afferent lymph vessels, 99, 99f
Age-related gait patterns, 390
Agonist, 57
AIIS. *See* Anterior inferior iliac spine (AIIS)
Ala, 284, 284f
Alveolus (alveoli), 270f, 271
Alzheimer's disease, 82
Amphiarthrodial joint, 22
Amphiarthrosis, 23t
Amyotrophic lateral sclerosis, 82
Anastomosis, 97, 97f
Anatomical position, 4, 5f
Anatomical snuffbox, 204, 205f
Anconeus muscle, 171–172, 172f
Aneurysm, 101
Angina, 101
Angion, 98, 99f
Angle of inclination, 313, 315f
Angle of pull, 58, 58f
Angle of ramus, 224
Angle of torsion, 313, 315f
Angular force, 109
Angular motion, 6, 6f
Ankle fracture, 365–366
Ankle fusion, 395, 395f
Ankle joint and foot, 343–348
  anatomical relationships, 360–362
  anterior muscle group, 354t, 357–358
  arches, 351–352
  arthrokinematics, 349, 349f
  bones and landmarks, 344–345
  common ankle pathologies, 364–366
  deep posterior muscle group, 354t, 355–357, 357t
  extensor digitorum longus muscle, 358, 359f
  extensor hallucis longus muscle, 358, 358f
  extrinsic muscles, 353–360
  fibularis brevis muscle, 359–360, 359f
  fibularis longus muscle, 359, 359f
  fibularis tertius muscle, 359f, 360
  flexor digitorum longus muscle, 356, 357f
  flexor hallucis longus muscle, 356, 356f
  functional aspects of foot, 345–346
  gastrocnemius muscle, 354, 354f
  intrinsic muscles, 360, 361t
  joint capsule, 350
  joints and motions, 346–350
  lateral muscle group, 358–360
  ligaments and other structures, 350–353
  metatarsophalangeal (MTP) joints, 350, 350f
  muscle innervation, 361t, 362–364, 365t, 366t
  plantar fascia, 352, 353f
  plantaris muscle, 355, 355f
  soleus muscle, 354–355, 355f
  subtalar and transverse tarsal joints, 349–350
  superficial posterior muscle group, 354–355, 354t
  talocrural joint, 347–348
  tibialis anterior muscle, 357, 358f
  tibialis posterior muscle, 355–356, 356f
  toes, 345, 345f, 350, 350f
  weight-bearing surfaces of foot, 351f
  windlass effect, 353
Ankle sprain, 365
Ankylosing spondylitis, 262
Annular ligament, 168, 168f
Annulus fibrosus, 243, 243f
ANS. *See* Autonomic nervous system (ANS)
Anserine bursa, 331f
Antagonist, 57
Antalgic gait, 396
Anterior, 4, 5f
Anterior arch, 243
Anterior cerebral artery, 96
Anterior communicating artery, 97
Anterior cord syndrome, 81
Anterior cruciate ligament, 329, 329f, 330f
Anterior deep hip muscles, 312f
Anterior deltoid muscle, 150, 150f
Anterior elbow muscles, 175f
Anterior fibular vein, 93
Anterior hand muscles, 211f
Anterior horn, 69, 69f
Anterior inferior iliac spine (AIIS), 299f, 300, 300f
Anterior knee muscles, 331–333, 336f
Anterior longitudinal ligament, 246, 247f
Anterior ramus, 72
Anterior root, 64, 65f, 68f, 69f
Anterior sacroiliac ligament, 285, 285f
Anterior scalene muscle, 249, 249f
Anterior shoulder dislocation, 159
Anterior shoulder girdle muscles, 139f
Anterior shoulder muscles, 156f
Anterior superficial hip muscles, 311f
Anterior superior iliac spine (ASIS), 285f, 288, 288f, 289f, 299f, 300, 300f
Anterior tibial artery, 93, 94f
Anterior tibial vein, 93, 94f
Anterior tibiotalar ligament, 351f
Anterior tilt, 288, 288f
Anterior wrist muscles, 190f
Anteversion, 313, 315f
Antigravity muscles, 373, 373f
AO joint. *See* Atlantooccipital (AO) joint
Aorta, 91–92, 92f, 96f
Aortic arch, 92f, 93f, 96f
Aortic valve, 87
Ape hand, 82, 207
Aponeurosis, 26
Apophyseal joint, 240, 246
Appendicular skeleton, 13, 14t, 15f
Applications. *See* Clinical applications
Arachnoid (arachnoid mater), 67, 67f, 68f
Arches in palm of hand, 200, 201f
Arches of foot, 351–352
Arm, 4, 4f
AROM. *See* Active range of motion (AROM)
Arteries, 88, 91t, 94f, 95f, 96f
Arterioles, 88
Arteriosclerosis, 101

Arthritis, 279
Arthrokinematic motion
  accessory motion forces, 33–34
  accessory motion terminology, 32
  ankle joint and foot, 349, 349f
  concave-convex rule, 35–36
  defined, 32
  elbow joint, 165
  fingers, 198
  hip joint, 298–299
  joint mobilization, 33
  joint surface positions, 36–39
  joint surface shape, 34
  knee joint, 324–325, 324f
  shoulder joint, 146, 147f
  thumb, 197
  types of, 34–35
  wrist joint, 183
Arthrokinematics, 103
Articular cartilage, 22, 22f, 25
Articular disk, 183f, 184, 228, 228f
Articular fossa, 225
Articular process, 242, 245f
Articular system, 21–29
  degrees of freedom, 28
  joint structure, 25–26
  pathological terms, 28
  planes and axes, 26–27
  types of joints, 21–24
Articular tubercle, 225, 226f, 229f
Ascending aorta, 91
ASIS. *See* Anterior superior iliac spine (ASIS)
Assisting mover, 57
Assistive device, 314
Asthma, 278
Ataxic gait, 395
Atherosclerosis, 101
Atlantoaxial (AA) joint, 240, 244, 246f
Atlantooccipital (AO) joint, 240, 244
Atlas, 243, 243f
Atrioventricular (AV) valve, 87, 88
Atrium (atria), 86, 87
Atypical vertebral articulations, 244
Auricular surface, 284, 284f
Autonomic dysreflexia, 81
Autonomic nervous system (ANS), 63, 63f
AV valve. *See* Atrioventricular (AV) valve
Avascular necrosis, 189
Axes, 27, 28f
Axial extension, 241
Axial skeleton, 13, 14t, 15f
Axillary artery, 95, 95f
Axillary border, 147, 147f
Axillary nerve, 75, 76, 76f
Axillary vein, 95f
Axis
  cervical vertebra, 243, 243f
  lever, 113, 113f
Axon, 64, 64f
Axon terminal, 64, 64f

Back, 5
Back knees, 337
Baker's cyst, 337
Balance, stability, and motion, 111–113
Ball-and-socket joint, 24, 25f
Ballet dancers, 373–374, 374f
Basal ganglia, 66
Basic information, 3–11
  descriptive terminology, 4–6
  joint movements, 7–10
  segments of the body, 4
  types of motion, 6–7
Basilar area, 241, 241f
Basilar artery, 96
Basilic vein, 95
Bell-clapper gait, 394, 394f
Bell's palsy, 82
Bench press, 59
Bending, 33, 33f
Biaxial joint, 23t, 24
Biceps femoris muscle, 308, 309, 309f
Biceps muscle, 116f, 118f, 169–170, 169f, 174f
Bicipital groove, 148, 148f
Bicipital ridges, 148
Bicipital tendonitis, 159
Bicuspid valve, 87
Bilateral, 6
Bimalleolar fracture, 366
Biomechanics, 3, 103–123
  defined, 103
  force, 105–107
  inclined plane, 120–121
  laws of motion, 104–105
  lever, 113–118
  mechanics/biomechanics relationship flowchart, 104f
  pulley, 118–119
  simple machines, 113–121
  stability, 109–113
  torque, 107–109
  wheel and axle, 119–120
Bipennate muscle, 44, 44f
Birth canal, 282
Blood clot, 88–89, 101
Blood pressure, 90–91
Blood vessels, 89–90
Body proportions (adult/child), 110f
Body segments, 4
Boggy end feel, 32
Bone, 25
  appendicular skeleton, 14t
  axial skeleton, 14t
  cancellous, 14, 15f
  compact, 14, 15f
  markings, 17, 18t
  normal bone structure, 15f
  organic/inorganic material, 14
  types, 16–17, 16f, 17t
Bone markings, 17, 18t
Bony end feel, 32
Bony landmarks. *See* Landmarks
BOS. *See* Base of support (BOS)
Boutonnière deformity, 212
Bowlegs, 336. *See also* Genu varum
Brachial artery, 95, 95f, 168
Brachial plexus, 74–78
  formation, 74f
Brachial pulse, 168
Brachial vein, 95, 95f
Brachialis muscle, 169, 169f
Brachiocephalic trunk, 92, 92f, 93f, 96f
Brachioradialis muscle, 118f, 170–171, 171f
Brachium, 64
Brain
  blood supply, 96–97, 97f
  brainstem, 66, 66f
  cerebellum, 66, 66f
  cerebrospinal fluid, 67, 67f, 68
  cerebrum, 65–66
  lobes, 65–66, 66f
  midsagittal section, 66f
  skull, 66, 67f
Brain protection, 66–68
Brainstem, 66, 66f
Breathing. *See* Respiratory system
Broken bone, 17. *See also* Fracture
Bronchial tree, 271
Bronchioles, 270f, 271
Bronchitis, 278
Bronchopneumonia, 278
Brown-Séquard syndrome, 81
Brushing hair, 193
Buccinator muscle, 235f
Burner syndrome, 82
Bursa (bursae), 26, 26f, 148–149
Bursitis, 28

C1, C2, ... C7, 68f, 73f, 240f, 240t
C7 (vertebra prominens), 244
Cadence, 381
Calcaneal positions, 347, 347f
Calcaneal tuberosity, 344, 345f
Calcaneal valgus, 347, 347f
Calcaneal varus, 347, 347f
Calcaneus, 328, 328f, 344, 345f, 352f
Calcaneus foot, 364
Calcific tendonitis, 159
Cancellous bone, 14, 15f
Cane, 314
Capillaries, 88
Capitate, 183f, 184f, 197f
Capitulum, 166, 166f
Capsular ligaments, 25
Capsular patterns, 28, 28f
Capsule, 25. *See also* Joint capsule
Capsulitis, 28
Cardiac cycle, 88–89
Cardinal plane, 27
Cardiopulmonary resuscitation (CPR), 86
Cardiovascular system, 85–97
  anastomosis, 97, 97f
  aorta, 91–92, 92f, 96f
  arteries, 91t, 94f, 95f, 96f
  blood flow through the heart, 87–88, 89f
  blood pressure, 90–91
  blood vessels, 89–90
  cardiac cycle, 88–89
  circle of Willis, 96, 97f

common pathologies, 101
heart, 86–89
heart sounds, 88
pulmonary and systemic circulation, 85–86, 86f
pulse, 90, 90f
veins, 91–92t, 94f, 95f, 96
Carpal tunnel, 200f
Carpal tunnel syndrome, 82, 211
Carpals, 196f
Carpometacarpal (CMC) joint
fingers, 197–198, 197f
thumb, 24, 24f, 34, 34f, 195–197
Carrying angle, 165, 165f
Cartilage, 25
Cartilaginous joint, 22, 22f
Cauda equina, 5, 68, 68f
Caudal, 5, 5f
Cell body, 64, 64f
Center of gravity (COG), 27, 27f, 109–110, 110f, 111f, 112f
Central cord syndrome, 81
Central nervous system (CNS), 63, 63f
brain, 65–68
common pathologies, 81–82
spinal cord, 68–70
Cephalad, 5
Cephalic vein, 95, 95f
Cerebellum, 66, 66f, 67f
Cerebral hemispheres, 65
Cerebral hemorrhage, 101
Cerebral palsy, 81
Cerebrospinal fluid, 67, 67f, 68
Cerebrovascular accident, 70, 101
Cerebrum, 65–66, 67f
Cervical curve, 371, 372f
Cervical nerve-vertebra relationship, 72
Cervical nerves, 68f, 70
Cervical plexus, 74, 74f
Cervical protraction, 241
Cervical retraction, 241
Cervical vertebrae, 68f, 73f, 240f, 240t, 245f, 245t
Chest breathing, 277
Chondromalacia patella, 337–338
Chondrosternal joint, 268f, 269
Chuck, 216
Circle of Willis, 96, 97f
Circumducted gait, 394, 394f
Circumduction, 8, 9f, 146f
Classical motion, 31
Clavicle, 129, 129f, 258f
Clavicular fracture, 141
Claw hand, 83, 209
Claw toe, 364
Clinical applications
assistive device, 314
crutch walking, reverse muscle action, 153
elbow flexion strength testing, 171
genu varus/genu valgus, 330
hand, functional position, 217
heel lift, 355
impaired lateral prehension, 218
knee flexion/extension, 326
lifting, 261
osteokinematics & arthrokinematics, 147
paradoxical breathing, 274
piriformis stretch position, 309
plantar fascia and support for arch of foot, 353
posture and latissimus dorsi, 160
posture and pelvic girdle, 292
posture and shoulder girdle, 138
posture and temporomandibular junction (TMJ), 236
pushing and pulling, 173
respiration, biomechanical impediments, 279
sit-ups, 252
spinal stability, compressive forces, 257
straight leg raise (SLR), 309
temporomandibular joint (TMJ), mechanical advantage, 230
text neck, 378
walking/running, compared, 391
wall slide exercise, 335
wrist flexor/extensors, joint positioning, 190
wrist immobilization, 217
wrist joint, lever systems, 191–192
wrist muscles, dual role, 189
Clinical motion analysis, 36, 38t
Close-packed position, 36–37, 38t
Closed-chain exercise equipment, 59
Closed-chain exercises, 59t
Closed fracture, 18
Closed kinetic chain, 58, 58f
Closing the jaw, 228, 229f
CMC joint. *See* Carpometacarpal (CMC) joint
CNS. *See* Central nervous system (CNS)
Coccygeal nerve, 68f, 70
Coccyx, 68f, 284f
Cock-up wrist splint, 217
Cocontraction, 57
COG. *See* Center of gravity (COG)
Collapsed lung, 278
Collateral ligaments, 329
Colles fracture, 189
Column, 64
Common carotid artery, 95, 96f
Common extensor tendon, 185
Common fibular nerve, 78, 78f, 80, 80f, 81f
Common flexor tendon, 185
Common iliac artery, 93, 93f
Common iliac vein, 93, 93f
Common pathologies
ankle joint and foot, 364–366
cardiovascular system, 101
central nervous system (CNS), 81–82
elbow joint, 175–176
hand, 211–212
hip joint, 312–315
knee joint, 336–338
lymphatic system, 101
muscular system, 59
nervous system, 81–83
peripheral nervous system (PNS), 82–83
postural deviations, 375t, 378–379
respiratory system, 278
shoulder girdle, 141
shoulder joint, 159
skeletal system, 17–18
vertebral column, 260–262
wrist joint, 189–190, 211–212
Common tendon, 255f
Compact bone, 14, 15f
Component motions, 32
Compression force, 33, 33f
Compression fracture, 262
Concave-convex rule, 35–36
Concave joint surface, 36, 36f
Concentric contraction, 54, 54f, 55f, 55t, 56t
Concentric exercise, 59t
Conceptual motion analysis, 36, 37t
Concurrent force, 105
Concurrent force system, 105f
Condylar process, 225
Condyle, 18t, 225, 225f
Condyloid joint, 24, 24f, 181–182
Congenital hip dislocation, 312
Congestive heart failure, 101
Congruent, 36
Contractility, 45
Contracture, 51
Contralateral, 6
Conus medullaris, 68, 68f
Convex joint surface, 36
Coracoacromial ligament, 131, 131f
Coracobrachialis muscle, 156, 156f
Coracoclavicular ligament, 131, 131f
Coracohumeral ligament, 148, 149f
Coracoid process, 129, 129f, 131f, 166, 166f
Coronal plane, 27
Coronary arteries, 91
Coronoid process, 167, 167f, 225, 225f
Corpus callosum, 65, 66f
Cortex, 65
Corticospinal tract, 65f, 69, 70f
Costal cartilage, 268, 268f
Costal facet, 244, 268, 269, 269f
Costoclavicular ligament, 130, 130f
Costotransverse joint, 268f, 269
Costovertebral joint, 268f, 269
Counternutation, 283, 283f
Coxa plana, 312
Coxa valga, 313, 315f
Coxa vara, 313, 315f
CPR. *See* Cardiopulmonary resuscitation (CPR)
Cracked bone, 17. *See also* Fracture
Cranial, 5, 5f
Cranial meninges, 66–67, 67f
Cranial nerves, 70, 71–72t, 71f
Crest, 18t
Crest of greater tubercle, 148
Crest of lesser tubercle, 148
Crouch gait, 396
Cruciate ligaments, 329, 329f

Crutch walking, 59, 140, 140f, 153
Cubital fossa, 168
Cubital tunnel, 82
Cubital tunnel syndrome, 82
Cuboid, 344, 345f
Cuneiforms, 344, 345f
Curvilinear motion, 6, 6f
Cylindrical grip, 215, 215f
Cylindrical grip variation, 215, 215f

da Vinci, Leonardo, 110
De Quervain's disease, 212
Deceleration, 382f, 384t, 385t, 388, 388f
Deep, 5
Deep fibular nerve, 80, 81f, 363
Deep infrapatellar bursa, 331f
Deep inspiration, 272, 276t
Deep palm group, 208
Deep palm muscles, 206, 206t
Deep rotator muscles, 307–308, 308f, 308t
Definitions. *See* Terminology
Degenerative arthritis, 28
Degenerative diseases, 82
Degrees of freedom, 28t
Deltoid ligament, 350–351, 351f
Deltoid muscle, 150–151, 150f
Deltoid tuberosity, 148, 148f
Demifacets, 269
Demyelinating diseases, 82
Dendrites, 64, 64f
Dens, 244, 244f
Depression, 269
Dermatomes, 72, 73f
Descending aorta, 92, 93f
Descriptive terminology, 4–6
Designer jeans syndrome, 277
Diagonal line of pull, 58
Diaphragm muscle, 270f, 272–273, 272f
Diaphragmatic breathing, 276–277
Diaphysis, 15, 15f
Diarthrodial joint, 22, 23t
Diarthrosis, 23t
Diastolic pressure, 91
Digastric muscle, 232, 232f, 233, 233f
DIP joint. *See* Distal interphalangeal (DIP) joint
Disk, 22f, 25
Dislocating force, 109
Dislocation, 28
Disorders/diseases. *See* Common pathologies
Distal, 5, 5f
Distal carpal arch, 200, 201f
Distal interphalangeal (DIP) joint, 196f, 198, 350, 350f
Distal phalanges, 196f
Distal radioulnar joint, 164, 164f
Dorsal, 5, 5f
Dorsal columns, 69
Dorsal interossei muscles, 208, 208f, 208t
Dorsal radiocarpal ligament, 184, 184f
Dorsal venous arch, 94f
Dorsalis pedis artery, 93
Dorsiflexion, 7, 8f
  ankle and foot, 346f
  wrist joint, 182f
Double support, 382f, 383
Drainage watersheds, 100, 100f
Drop foot, 393
Dupuytren's contracture, 212
Dura mater, 67, 67f, 68f
Dynamic systems, 3
Dynamics, 103
Dysplasia, 312

Eccentric contraction, 54, 54f, 55t, 56t
Eccentric exercise, 59t
Efferent impulses, 64
Efferent lymph vessels, 99, 99f
Effort, 113
Elastic cartilage, 26
Elastic tubing, 56
Elasticity, 45
Elbow complex, 163
Elbow dislocation, 176
Elbow flexion, 7
Elbow flexion strength testing, 171
Elbow joint, 163–179
  anatomical relationships, 174, 175f
  anconeus muscle, 171–172, 172f
  anterior elbow muscles, 175f
  arthrokinematics, 165
  biceps muscle, 169–170, 169f
  bones and landmarks, 165–167
  brachialis muscle, 169, 169f
  brachioradialis muscle, 170–171, 171f
  carrying angle, 165, 165f
  common elbow pathologies, 175–176
  defined, 163
  end feel, 165
  ligaments and other structures, 167–168
  muscle innervation, 175, 176t
  muscles, 168–174
  posterior elbow muscles, 175f
  prime movers, 176t
  pronator quadratus muscle, 172f, 173
  pronator teres muscle, 172–173, 172f
  supinator muscle, 174, 174f, 176f
  triceps muscle, 171, 172f
Elevation, 257, 269
Ellipsoid joint, 24
Embolism, 101
Eminence, 18t
Emphysema, 278
Empty end feel, 32
End feel, 31–32
  elbow joint, 165
  hip joint, 298, 303
  knee joint, 324
Endosteum, 15, 15f
Epicondyle, 18t
Epidural bleed, 101
Epiglottis, 227f
Epiphyseal plate, 14, 15f
Epiphysis, 14, 15f
Equinus foot, 364
Equinus gait, 392, 393f, 396
Erb's palsy, 82
Erector spinae muscle group, 255–256, 255f
Eversion, 9, 10f, 346, 346f, 349
Excursion, 45, 46f
Exercise equipment, 59
Exercise terminology, 59t
Expiration, 272, 276t
Extensibility, 45
Extension, 7, 8f
  elbow joint, 163, 164f
  fingers, 198f
  hip joint, 298f
  knee joint, 324f, 326
  neck, 241f
  sacroiliac (SI) joint, 283
  shoulder joint, 146f
  thumb, 196f
  toes, 350f
  trunk, 241f
  wrist joint, 182f
Extensor carpi radialis brevis muscle, 187–188, 188f
Extensor carpi radialis longus muscle, 187, 187f
Extensor carpi ulnaris muscle, 188
Extensor digiti minimi muscle, 205–206, 206f
Extensor digitorum longus muscle, 358, 359f
Extensor digitorum muscle, 204, 205f
Extensor expansion ligament, 200, 200f
Extensor hallucis longus muscle, 358, 358f
Extensor hood, 200, 200f
Extensor indicis muscle, 204–205, 205f
Extensor pollicis brevis muscle, 203, 204f
Extensor pollicis longus muscle, 203–204, 204f
Extensor retinaculum ligament, 189, 190f, 200, 200f
External auditory meatus, 226, 226f, 241f
External carotid artery, 96, 96f
External iliac artery, 93, 93f, 94f
External iliac vein, 93, 93f, 94f
External intercostal muscles, 273, 273f
External jugular vein, 96, 96f
External oblique muscle, 251–252, 253f, 277f
External rotation, 9
Extrinsic muscles of ankle and foot, 353–360
Extrinsic muscles of hand, 201–206

FA. *See* Force arm (FA)
Facet, 18t, 240
Facet joint, 240, 243f, 246
Facial nerve, 71f, 71t
False pelvis, 282, 282f
False ribs, 267, 268f
Fascicle, 45, 46f
Fasciculus, 64
Faucet handle, 119–120, 119f, 120f
Femoral artery, 93, 94f
Femoral nerve, 78, 78f, 79, 79f
Femoral triangle, 93, 94f
Femoral vein, 93, 94, 94f
Femur, 301, 327–328, 327f

Festinating gait, 395
Fibrocartilage, 25–26
Fibrous joint, 21, 22f
Fibula, 328, 328f
Fibular collateral ligament, 329
Fibular head, 328f
Fibular nerves, 80, 81f
Fibularis brevis muscle, 359–360, 359f
Fibularis longus muscle, 352f, 359, 359f
Fibularis tertius muscle, 359f, 360
Fifth finger opposition, 197
Filum terminale, 68, 68f
Fingers, 197–199
Firm end feel, 32
First-class lever, 113–114, 114f, 115f
Fixator, 57
Fixed pulley, 118, 119f
Flail chest, 278
Flat back, 261, 371
Flat bones, 16, 16f, 17t
Flexion, 7, 8f
 ankle and foot, 346, 346f
 elbow joint, 163, 164f
 fingers, 198f
 hip joint, 298f
 knee joint, 324f, 326
 neck, 241f
 sacroiliac (SI) joint, 283
 shoulder joint, 146f
 thumb, 196f
 toes, 350f
 trunk, 241f
 wrist joint, 182f
Flexor carpi radialis muscle, 185–186, 186f
Flexor carpi ulnaris muscle, 185, 186f
Flexor digiti minimi muscle, 207f, 210
Flexor digitorum longus muscle, 356, 357f
Flexor digitorum profundus muscle, 202, 202f
Flexor digitorum superficialis muscle, 201–202, 201f, 202f
Flexor hallucis longus muscle, 356, 356f
Flexor pollicis longus muscle, 202, 203f
Flexor retinaculum, 184, 198f, 199, 207f
Floating ribs, 267, 268f
Foot, 4, 4f, 298f. *See also* Ankle joint and foot
Foot drop, 83
Foot flat, 382f, 383t, 384t, 386, 387f
Foot joints, 350
Foot slap, 392
Foramen, 18t
Foramen magnum, 241f, 242
Force, 103, 105–107, 113
Force arm (FA), 113, 113f
Force couple, 107, 107f, 108f, 139, 291f, 293f
Forced expiration, 272, 276t
Forced inspiration, 272, 276t
Forearm, 4, 4f
Forearm pronation, 4, 10f
Forearm supination, 10f
Forefoot, 345f, 346
Forward bend lift, 261
Fossa, 18t
Fracture
 ankle and foot, 365–366
 clavicular, 141
 defined, 17
 hip, 314
 neck and trunk, 262
 scaphoid, 212
 shoulder joint, 159
 supracondylar, 176
 wrist joint, 189
Fractures with dislocation, 262
Free weights, 59
Friction, 104
Front, 5
Frontal axis, 27, 28f
Frontal lobe, 65, 66f
Frontal plane, 27, 27f
Frozen shoulder, 159
Fulcrum, 113
Functional position of hand, 214, 214f, 217
Funny bone, 176
Fused hip, 393
Fusiform muscle, 44, 44f

Gait, 381–398
 abnormal (atypical), 390–396
 age-related gait patterns, 390
 analysis of stance phase, 386–387
 analysis of swing phase, 387–388
 defined, 381
 horizontal displacement, 389
 joint/muscle range-of-motion limitation, 393–395
 key events of gait cycle, 384–385t
 lateral pelvic tilt, 389, 390f
 leg length discrepancy, 396
 muscular weakness/paralysis, 391–393
 neurological involvement, 395–396
 pain, 396
 phases of gait cycle, 382f
 Rancho Los Amigos (RLA) terms vs. traditional terminology, 383–384t
 terminology, 381–383, 383–384t
 Trendelenburg gait, 392
 Trendelenburg sign, 389
 vertical displacement, 388–389, 389f
 walking/running, compared, 391
 width of walking base, 389, 389f
Gait cycle, 381, 382f
Gamekeeper's thumb, 212
Ganglion cyst, 189–190
Gastrocnemius muscle, 334–335, 334f, 354, 354f
Gemellus inferior, 308f, 308t
Gemellus superior, 308f, 308t
Geniohyoid muscle, 232, 232f, 233, 233f
Genitofemoral nerve, 78, 78f
Genu recurvatum, 337
Genu recurvatum gait, 392, 393f
Genu valgum, 330, 336
Genu varum, 330, 336
Glenohumeral joint, 127f. *See also* Shoulder joint
Glenohumeral ligaments, 148, 149f
Glenohumeral subluxation, 159
Glenoid fossa, 129, 129f, 131f, 147, 147f
Glenoid labrum, 147, 147f, 148, 149f
Glide, 34–35, 35f
Gliding motion, 33
Glossopharyngeal nerve, 71f, 71t
Gluteus maximus gait, 391, 392f
Gluteus maximus muscle, 307, 307f
Gluteus medius gait, 392, 392f
Gluteus medius muscle, 309–310, 310f
Gluteus minimus muscle, 310, 310f
Golfer's elbow, 175
Gomphosis, 22, 22f, 23t
Gracilis muscle, 307, 307f, 335
Grasps (grips), 214–217
Gravitation force, 109
Gravity, 109
Gravity-eliminated position, 56
Gray matter, 64, 65f, 68f, 69, 69f
Great saphenous vein, 94, 94f
Great toe, 345, 350f
Greater sciatic foramen, 284, 285f
Greater sciatic notch, 284, 285f, 299f, 300, 300f
Greater trochanter, 301, 301f, 327, 327f
Greater tubercle, 148, 148f
Greater wing, 226, 226f
Greenstick fracture, 189
Groove, 18t
Ground reaction force, 105

Habitual anterior tilt, 292
Habitual posterior tilt, 292
Hair brushing, 193
Hallux rigidus, 364
Hallux valgus, 364
Hamate, 183f, 184f, 197f
Hammer toe, 364
Hamstring curl exercise, 339
Hamstring muscles, 308–309, 309f, 333, 333f
 active insufficiency, 49, 50f
 ascending a step, 49t
 optimal length, 48, 48f
 passive insufficiency, 51, 51f
 strain, 59
 strain (pulled hamstrings), 315
 stretching, 52f
Hamstring strain, 315
Hand, 4, 4f, 197–222
 abductor digiti minimi muscle, 207f, 210
 abductor pollicis brevis muscle, 206, 207f
 abductor pollicis longus muscle, 202–203, 203f
 adductor pollicis muscle, 207f, 208
 anatomical relationships, 210–211
 anatomical snuffbox, 204, 205f
 anterior hand muscles, 211f
 arches, 200, 201f
 bones and landmarks, 199
 common wrist and hand pathologies, 211–212
 deep palm muscles, 206, 206t

dorsal interossei muscles, 208, 208f, 208t
extensor digiti minimi muscle, 205–206, 206f
extensor digitorum muscle, 204, 205f
extensor indicis muscle, 204–205, 205f
extensor pollicis brevis muscle, 203, 204f
extensor pollicis longus muscle, 203–204, 204f
extrinsic muscles, 201–206
fingers, 197–199
flexor digiti minimi muscle, 207f, 210
flexor digitorum profundus muscle, 202, 202f
flexor digitorum superficialis muscle, 201–202, 201f, 202f
flexor pollicis longus muscle, 202, 203f
functional position, 214, 214f, 217
grasps, 214–217
hypothenar muscles, 206, 206t
intrinsic muscles, 206–210
joints, 199t
ligaments and other structures, 199–200
lumbrical muscles, 209–210, 210f
muscle innervation, 213, 213t, 214t
muscles, 201–210
nonprehensile hand functions, 213
opponens digiti minimi muscle, 207f, 210
opponens pollicis muscle, 207, 207f
palmar interossei muscles, 208–209, 209f, 209t
posterior hand muscles, 211f
power grips, 214, 215–216, 215f, 216
precision grips, 215, 215f, 216–217
prehension, 213–214
prime movers, 212t
sensory innervation of hand, 213f, 214
thenar muscles, 206, 206t
thumb, 195–197
Hand function, 213–214
Hand of benediction, 82
Hand sensation, 213f, 214
Hangman's fracture, 262
Hard end feel, 32
Hardening of the arteries, 101
Head
body segment, 4, 4f
bone marking, 18t
Heart
blood flow, 87–88, 88f
chambers, 86–87, 87f
function, 86
location, 86, 86f
valves, 87
Heart attack, 101
Heart chambers, 86–87, 87f
Heart murmur, 101
Heart sounds, 88
Heart valves, 87
Heel, 328
Heel cord, 334
Heel lift, 355
Heel-off, 382f, 383t, 385t, 386, 387f
Heel strike, 382f, 383t, 384t, 386, 387f
Height-body span, 110, 110f
Heimlich maneuver, 271, 271f
Hemiplegic gait, 395, 395f
Hemorrhage, 101
Herniated disk, 262
Hiccups, 278
Hindfoot, 345, 345f
Hinge joint, 23, 23f
Hip flexion, 7
Hip flexion contracture, 393, 394f
Hip flexion exercise, 321
Hip fracture, 314
Hip hiking, 257, 289
Hip joint, 297–321
adductor brevis muscle, 306, 306f
adductor hiatus, 303
adductor longus muscle, 306, 306f
adductor magnus muscle, 306–307, 306f
anatomical relationships, 311–312
arthrokinematics, 298–299
biceps femoris muscle, 308, 309, 309f
bones and landmarks, 299–301
common hip pathologies, 312–315
deep rotator muscles, 307–308, 308f, 308t
end feel, 298, 303
gluteus maximus muscle, 307, 307f
gluteus medius muscle, 309–310, 310f
gluteus minimus muscle, 310, 310f
gracilis muscle, 307, 307f
hamstring muscles, 308–309, 309f
iliopsoas muscle, 304, 304f
joint structure and motions, 297–299
ligaments and other structures, 302–303
muscle innervation, 316, 316t, 317t
muscles, 303–311
pectineus muscle, 305–306, 305f
prime movers, 316t
rectus femoris muscle, 304, 305f
sartorius muscle, 305, 305f
semimembranous muscle, 308–309, 309f
semitendinosus muscle, 308, 309, 309f
tensor fascia lata muscle, 310–311, 311f
Hip joint capsule, 302, 302f
Hip pointer, 315
Hitting with backswing, 264
Holding a baby, 219
Holding a box, 194
Hook grip, 215, 216f
Hook of the hamate, 183
Horizontal abduction, 8, 9f, 146f
Horizontal adduction, 8, 9f
Horizontal displacement, 389
Horizontal plane, 27
Horse's foot, 364
Housemaid's knee, 338
Humeral neck fracture, 159
Humeroradial articulation, 163
Humeroulnar articulation, 163
Humerus, 148, 148f, 166
Hyaline cartilage, 22, 25
Hydrocephalus, 81
Hyoid bone, 227, 227f, 258f
Hyperextension, 7, 8f
hip joint, 298f
neck, 241f
shoulder joint, 146f
toes, 350f
trunk, 241f
wrist joint, 182f
Hyperreflexia, 81
Hyperventilation, 278
Hypoglossal nerve, 71f, 72t
Hypothalamus, 66, 66f, 67f
Hypothenar muscles, 206, 206t

Iliac crest, 284, 285f, 299, 299f
Iliac fossa, 299, 299f
Iliacus, 304f
Iliocostalis cervicis, 255f
Iliocostalis muscle group, 256
Iliocostalis thoracis, 255f
Iliofemoral ligament, 25f, 302, 303f
Iliohypogastric nerve, 78, 78f
Ilioinguinal nerve, 78, 78f
Iliolumbar ligament, 285f, 286, 286f, 287
Iliopsoas muscle, 304, 304f
Iliotibial band, 302, 310, 311f
Iliotibial band syndrome, 314–315
Iliotibial tract, 302
Ilium, 284, 285f, 299–300
Impaired lateral prehension, 218
Impingement syndrome, 159
Inchworm effect, 151
Inclined plane, 120–121
Incomplete spinal cord injury (SCI), 81
Index finger, 197
Inertia, 104
Inferior, 5, 5f
Inferior articular process, 242f, 243f, 245f, 245t
Inferior gluteal nerve, 78, 78f
Inferior lamina, 229f
Inferior pubic ligament, 286, 286f
Inferior pubic ramus, 285f, 287, 299f, 300f
Inferior ramus, 300
Inferior tibiofibular joint, 347, 347f
Inferior trunk, 74
Inferior vena cava, 93, 93f
Infraglenoid tubercle, 166, 166f
Infrahyoid muscles, 233–234, 233f
Infraspinatus muscle, 154, 154f
Infraspinous fossa, 147, 147f
Inguinal ligament, 94f, 253f, 302, 303f
Initial contact, 383t, 384t, 386, 387f
Initial swing, 384t, 385t, 388, 388f
Injuries. *See* Common pathologies
Innervation of muscles. *See* Muscle innervation
Innominate bone, 299, 299f
Insertion, 41, 42f
Inspiration, 272, 276t
Intercarpal joint, 182
Intercellular fluid, 98
Interclavicular ligament, 130, 130f
Intercondylar eminence, 328, 328f
Intercostal muscles, 273–274
Intercostal nerves, 72
Intercostal space, 268
Intermediate group, 208
Internal carotid artery, 96, 96f
Internal iliac artery, 93, 93f

Internal intercostal muscles, 274, 274f
Internal jugular vein, 93f, 96, 96f
Internal oblique muscle, 252, 253f, 277f
Internal rotation, 9
Interneuron, 65, 65f
Interosseous membrane, 168, 168f
Interosseous sacroiliac ligament, 285f, 286
Interphalangeal (IP) joint, 196f, 197, 198, 350, 350f
Interspinal ligament, 246–247, 247f
Interspinales muscles, 257, 257f
Interstitial fluid, 98
Interstitial spaces, 98
Intertransversarii muscles, 257, 257f
Intertrochanteric crest, 301, 301f
Intervertebral disk, 22f, 25, 242
Intervertebral foramen, 68, 242, 243f
Intervertebral joint, 246
Intracapsular ligaments, 329
Intrinsic foot muscles, 360, 361t
Intrinsic hand muscles, 206–210
Inversion, 9, 10f, 346, 346f, 349
IP joint. *See* Interphalangeal (IP) joint
Ipsilateral, 6
Irregular bones, 16, 16f, 17t
Irritability, 45
Ischemia, 101
Ischial body, 285, 285f, 299f, 300, 300f
Ischial ramus, 299f, 300, 300f
Ischial spine, 285, 285f, 299f, 300, 300f
Ischial tuberosity, 285, 285f, 299f, 300, 300f
Ischiofemoral ligament, 302, 303f
Ischium, 285, 285f, 300
Isokinetic contraction, 56, 57, 57t
Isometric contraction, 53, 54f, 55f, 57t
Isotonic contraction, 57, 57t

Jaw, 224
Joint
  defined, 21
  trade-offs, 21
  types, 21–25
Joint approximation, 33
Joint capsule
  ankle joint and foot, 350
  elbow joint, 168, 168f
  function, 25
  hip joint, 25f, 302, 302f
  shoulder joint, 148, 149f
  temporomandibular joint (TMJ), 228
  wrist joint, 184f
Joint classification, 23t
Joint congruency, 36–39
Joint degeneration, 279
Joint distraction, 33
Joint ligaments, 25, 25f
Joint mobilization, 33
Joint motions, 28t
  neck and trunk, 240t–241, 241f
  shoulder girdle, 131–133
  shoulder joint, 145–147
  temporomandibular joint (TMJ), 223–224, 224f
  wrist joint, 182–183
Joint movements, 7–10
  abduction/adduction, 7, 9f
  circumduction, 8, 9f
  extension, 7, 8f
  flexion, 7, 8f
  inversion/eversion, 9, 10f
  protraction/retraction, 9, 10f
  radial/ulnar deviation, 8, 9f
  rotation, 9, 10f
  supination/pronation, 9, 10f
Joint play, 32, 37
Joint rotation motions, 9, 10f
Joint structure, 25–26
Joint surface motion, 32. *See also* Arthrokinematic motion
Joint surface positions, 36–39
Joint surface shape, 34
Jumper's knee, 337

Keystone, 352
Kienböck's disease, 212
Kinematics, 3, 103
Kinesiology, 3
Kinetic chains, 58–59, 59t
Kinetics, 3, 103
Knee extension, 324f, 326
Knee extension exercise, 340
Knee flexion, 324f, 326
Knee flexion contracture, 394
Knee fusion, 394
Knee joint, 323–342
  anatomical relationships, 335
  anterior muscles, 331–333
  arthrokinematics, 324–325, 324f
  bones and landmarks, 325–328
  bursae, 330, 331f, 331t
  common knee pathologies, 336–338
  end feel, 324
  gastrocnemius muscle, 334–335, 334f
  hamstring muscles, 333, 333f
  joint structure and motions, 323–325
  ligaments and other structures, 328–330
  muscle innervation, 335–336, 337t
  muscles, 330–335
  popliteus muscle, 333–334, 334f
  posterior muscles, 333–335
  prime movers, 336t
  Q angle, 325, 327f
  quadriceps muscle group, 331–333
  rectus femoris muscle, 331, 332f
Kneeling stool posture, 377f
Knock knees, 336. *See also* Genu valgum
Kyphosis, 261
Kyphotic curves, 379

L1, L2, ... L5, 68f, 73f, 240f, 240t
Labral tear, 159
Labrum, 26, 26f
Lamina, 242, 242f, 244f
Landmarks
  ankle joint and foot, 344–345
  clavicle, 129
  elbow joint, 165–167
  femur, 301, 327–328
  forearm, 199
  hand, 199
  hip joint, 299–301
  humerus, 148, 166
  ilium, 284, 299–300
  ischium, 285, 300
  knee joint, 325–328
  mandible, 224–225
  maxilla, 227
  metatarsals, 345
  neck and trunk, 241–244
  pelvic girdle, 283–285, 286–287
  pubis, 286–287, 300
  radius, 167
  respiratory system, 267–269
  ribs, 268
  sacrum, 283–284
  scapula, 128–129, 129f, 147–148, 166
  shoulder girdle, 128–130
  shoulder joint, 147–148
  skull, 241–242, 241f
  sphenoid bone, 226–227
  sternum, 130, 268
  tarsal bones, 344, 345f
  temporal bone, 225–226
  temporomandibular joint (TMJ), 224–227
  thoracic vertebra, 268–269
  tibia, 328, 344
  ulna, 166–167
  vertebrae, 242–243
  wrist joint, 183
  zygomatic bone, 227
Laryngopharynx, 270f
Larynx, 270, 270f
Lateral, 4, 5f
Lateral atlantoaxial joint, 244, 246f
Lateral bending, 8, 9f, 240, 241f
Lateral collateral ligament, 167, 168f, 329
Lateral condyle, 301, 301f, 344
Lateral cord, 75
Lateral epicondyle, 166, 166f, 183, 301, 301f
Lateral epicondylitis, 175
Lateral femoral condyle, 327, 327f
Lateral flexion, 8, 240
Lateral hip muscles, 314f
Lateral ligament, 227, 228f, 351, 351f
Lateral lip of bicipital groove, 148
Lateral longitudinal arch, 351f, 352
Lateral malleolus muscle, 119f, 328f, 344
Lateral meniscus, 329f, 330, 330f
Lateral pelvic tilt, 372, 389, 390f
Lateral plantar nerve, 80f
Lateral prehension, 216
  impaired, 218
Lateral pterygoid muscle, 231f, 232, 235f
Lateral pterygoid plate, 226, 226f
Lateral rotation, 9, 10f
  hip joint, 298f
  shoulder joint, 146f
Lateral shoulder girdle muscles, 139f
Lateral supracondylar ridge, 166, 166f, 183
Lateral tibial condyle, 328, 328f
Lateral tilt, 288, 289f
Latissimus dorsi muscle, 152, 152f
Law of acceleration, 104
Law of action-reaction, 105

Law of inertia, 104
Laws of motion, 104–105
Left common carotid artery, 95
Leg, 4, 4f, 298f
Leg advancement, 382
Leg length discrepancy, 396
Legg-Calvé-Perthes disease, 18, 312
Lemniscus, 64
Lengthening contraction, 54
Lesser pelvis, 282
Lesser sciatic notch, 285, 285f, 299f, 300f
Lesser toes, 345, 350f
Lesser trochanter, 301, 301f, 327, 327f
Lesser tubercle, 148, 148f
Levator costarum muscles, 275f
Levator scapula muscle, 136, 136f, 277f
Lever
  classes, 113–117
  components, 113, 113f
  factors which cause change of class, 117–118
  first-class, 113–114, 114f, 115f
  second-class, 114–116
  third-class, 116–117, 116f
Lifting, 261
Ligament, 25
Ligament of Bigelow, 302
Ligamentous-type joint, 21, 22f
Ligamentum flavum, 246, 247f
Ligamentum nuchae, 247, 247f
Line, 18t
Line of gravity (LOG), 110
Line of pull, 57–58, 58f
Linea alba, 26, 248, 253f
Linea aspera, 301, 301f, 327, 327f
Linear force, 105, 106f
Linear motion, 6
Little finger, 197
Little League elbow, 175–176
Loading response, 383t, 384t, 386, 387f
Lobar bronchi, 270
Lobes, 65–66, 66f
LOG. *See* Line of gravity (LOG)
Long bones, 16, 16f, 17t
Long plantar ligament, 352, 352f
Long posterior sacroiliac ligament, 286, 286f
Longissimus capitis, 255f
Longissimus muscle group, 255–256
Longissimus thoracis, 255f
Longitudinal arch, 200, 201f
Longitudinal axis, 27, 28f
Longus capitis, 249f, 250t
Longus colli, 249f, 250t
Loose-packed position, 37, 38f
Lordosis, 261, 287–288, 287f, 372
Lordotic curves, 379
Lou Gehrig's disease, 82
Lower jaw, 224
Lower joint space, 224, 228f, 229f
Lower motor neuron, 69
Lower motor neuron lesion, 70, 70t
Lower respiratory infection (LRI), 278
Lower respiratory tract, 270
Lower trapezius muscle, 135, 135f
Lumbar aponeurosis, 149
Lumbar curve, 371, 372f
Lumbar lordosis, 287–288, 287f, 379
Lumbar nerves, 68f, 70
Lumbar plexus, 78, 78f
Lumbar vertebrae, 68f, 73f, 240f, 240t, 245f, 245t
Lumbosacral angle, 283, 287–288, 287f
Lumbosacral joint, 281, 281f, 287–288
Lumbosacral ligament, 285f, 287
Lumbosacral plexus, 74f, 78–81
Lumbosacral trunk, 78f
Lumbrical grip, 217, 217f
Lumbrical muscles, 209–210, 210f
Lunate, 183f, 184f
Lungs, 270f, 271
Lying posture, 378, 378f
Lymph, 98
Lymph angion, 98, 99f
Lymph capillaries, 98
Lymph glands, 99
Lymph nodes, 98, 100f
Lymph vessels, 98
Lymphatic system, 97–101
  common pathologies, 101
  drainage patterns, 99–100
  filtration and protection, 99
  functions, 98
  lymph collection, 98
  regional lymph nodes and drainage watersheds, 100f
  transport, 98–99
Lymphatic trunks, 100
Lymphedema, 101

Main stem bronchi, 270
Mallet finger, 212
Mallet toe, 364
Mandible, 224–225, 225f, 258f
Mandibular bone (mandible), 224–225, 225f, 258f
Mandibular depression, 224f
Mandibular elevation, 224f
Mandibular fossa, 225, 226f
Mandibular lateral deviation, 224f
Mandibular protrusion, 224f
Mandibular retrusion, 224f
Manipulation, 33
Manual muscle testing, 59
Manubrium, 129f, 130, 268, 268f
Mass, 103
Masseter muscle, 231, 231f, 234f
Mastoid process, 226, 226f, 241f, 242
Maxilla, 226f, 227
Maxillary bone (maxilla), 226f, 227
MCP joint. *See* Metacarpophalangeal (MCP) joint
Meatus, 18t
Mechanical advantage, 118, 119f
Mechanics, 103
Mechanics/biomechanics relationship flowchart, 104f
Medial, 4, 5f
Medial collateral ligament, 167, 168f, 329
Medial condyle, 301, 301f, 344
Medial cord, 75
Medial epicondyle, 166, 166f, 183, 301, 301f, 327, 327f
Medial epicondylitis, 175
Medial femoral condyle, 327, 327f
Medial hip muscles, 312f
Medial lip of bicipital groove, 148
Medial longitudinal arch, 351f, 352
Medial malleolus, 344
Medial meniscus, 330, 330f
Medial plantar nerve, 80f
Medial pterygoid muscle, 231, 231f, 235f
Medial rotation, 9, 10f
  hip joint, 298f
  shoulder joint, 146f
Medial tibial condyle, 328, 328f
Medial tibial stress syndrome, 364
Median atlantoaxial joint, 244, 246f
Median cubital vein, 95, 95f
Median nerve, 75, 76–77, 77f
Mediastinum, 86, 86f, 270f, 271
Medulla oblongata (medulla), 66, 66f, 67f
Medullary canal, 15, 15f
Meninges, 66–67, 67f
Meningocele, 81
Meniscus, 25
Mental spine, 225, 225f
Metacarpals, 196f, 197f
Metacarpophalangeal (MCP) joint
  fingers, 198
  thumb, 196f, 197
Metaphysis, 15, 15f, 16
Metatarsalgia, 364–365
Metatarsals, 344, 345, 345f
Metatarsophalangeal (MTP) joints, 350, 350f
Mid-sagittal plane, 27
Midbrain, 66, 66f, 67f
Midcarpal joint, 181f, 182
Middle cerebral artery, 96
Middle deltoid muscle, 150–151, 150f
Middle finger, 197
Middle phalanges, 196f
Middle scalene muscle, 249, 249f
Middle trapezius muscle, 135, 135f
Middle trunk, 74
Midfoot, 345f, 346
Midhumeral fracture, 159
Midstance, 382f, 383t, 385t, 386, 387f
Midswing, 382f, 384t, 385t, 388, 388f
Mild sprain, 28
Minor pelvis, 282
Miserable malalignment syndrome, 338
Mitral valve, 87
Moderate sprain, 28
Moment arm, 108, 108f, 109f
Moment of force, 107
Mortise, 348
Morton's neuroma, 83, 365
Motion
  balance, stability, and motion, 111–113
  laws of, 104–105
  types of, 6–7
Motor endplate, 64
Motor neuron, 64, 65f
Movable pulley, 118

MTP joints. *See* Metatarsophalangeal (MTP) joints
Multiaxial joint, 24
Multifidus muscles, 256, 256f
Multijoint muscles, 48, 52t
Multipennate muscle, 44, 44f
Multiple sclerosis, 70, 82
Muscle, 41. *See also* Muscles
Muscle attachments, 41–42
Muscle contraction, 53–57
Muscle fascicle, 45, 46f
Muscle fiber, 45, 46f
Muscle fiber anatomy, 46f
Muscle fiber arrangement, 43–44
Muscle innervation
  ankle joint and foot, 361t, 362–364, 365t, 366t
  elbow joint, 175, 176t
  general innervation level of major muscles, 73, 74f
  hand, 213, 213t, 214t
  hip joint, 316, 316t, 317t
  knee joint, 335–336, 337t
  neck and trunk, 260
  respiratory system, 277
  shoulder girdle, 141
  shoulder joint, 158–159, 158t, 159t
  temporomandibular joint (TMJ), 235, 235t
  wrist joint, 191, 191t
Muscle names, 42–43
Muscle paralysis, 82
Muscle spasm, 32
Muscle stretching, 52–53
Muscle-tendon unit, 42f
Muscle tissue, 45
Muscles
  ankle joint and foot, 353–360
  cervical spine, 248–251
  elbow joint, 168–174
  hand, 201–210
  hip joint, 303–311
  insertion/origin, 41, 42f
  knee joint, 330–335
  mouth and hyoid bone, 250t
  names, 42–43
  respiration system, 272–275, 277f
  shoulder girdle, 133–138
  shoulder joint, 150–156
  temporomandibular joint (TMJ), 229–234
  tight, 51
  trunk, 251–258
  weak, 51
  wrist joint, 184–188
Muscular dystrophy, 70, 82
Muscular system, 41–61
  active and passive insufficiency, 49–51
  adaptive shortening and lengthening, 51–52
  common muscle pathologies, 59
  functional characteristics of muscle tissue, 45
  kinetic chains, 58–59, 59t
  length-tension relationship, 45–53
  line of pull, 57–58, 58f
  muscle attachments, 41–42
  muscle contraction, 53–57
  muscle fiber anatomy, 46f
  muscle fiber arrangement, 43–44
  muscle names, 42–43
  optimal length, 47–48
  roles of muscles, 57
  sliding filament theory, 45
  stretching, 52–53
  tendon action of a muscle (tenodesis), 53
Musculocutaneous nerve, 75, 76, 76f
Musculotendinous junction, 41, 42f
Myasthenia gravis, 70, 82
Myelin, 64
Myelin sheath, 64f
Myelomeningocele, 81
Mylohyoid muscle, 232, 232f, 233f
Myocardial infarction, 101
Myofibril, 45, 46f
Myosin filament, 45, 46f

Nasal cavity, 270, 270f
Nasal nares, 270
Nasopharynx, 270f
Natural bursae, 26
Navicular, 344, 345f
Navicular tuberosity, 344, 345f
Neck and trunk, 4, 4f, 239–265
  abdominal aponeurosis, 247
  anatomical relationships, 258–260
  atypical vertebral articulations, 244
  bones and landmarks, 241–244
  cervical/thoracic/lumbar vertebrae, compared, 245f, 245t
  common vertebral column pathologies, 260–262
  erector spinae muscle group, 255–256, 255f
  external oblique muscle, 251–252, 253f
  iliocostalis muscle group, 256
  internal oblique muscle, 252, 253f
  interspinales muscles, 257, 257f
  intertransversarii muscles, 257, 257f
  joint motions, 240t–241, 241f
  joints and ligaments, 244–248
  linea alba, 248
  longissimus muscle group, 255–256
  muscle innervation, 260
  muscles of cervical spine, 248–251
  muscles of mouth and hyoid bone, 250t
  muscles of trunk, 251–258
  posterior trunk muscles, 254–255, 254t
  prevertebral muscles, 249, 249f, 250t
  prime movers, 261t
  quadratus lumborum muscle, 257, 258f
  rectus abdominis muscle, 251, 251f
  scalene muscles, 249, 249f
  spinalis muscle group, 255
  splenius capitis muscle, 250, 251f
  splenius cervicis muscle, 250, 251f
  sternocleidomastoid muscle, 248, 248f
  suboccipital muscles, 249, 250f, 251t
  thoracolumbar fascia, 248
  transverse abdominis muscle, 252, 253f, 254
  transversospinalis muscle group, 256, 256f
  typical vertebral articulations, 244–247
  vertebral curves, 239, 240f, 240t
  vertebral segments, 240t
Nerve cell, 64
Nerve fiber, 64
Nervous system, 63–83
  brain, 65–68
  checks and balances, 63
  common pathologies, 81–83
  congenital defects, 81
  cranial nerves, 70, 71–72t, 71f
  degenerative diseases, 82
  demyelinating diseases, 82
  disorders of muscle and neuromuscular junction, 82
  functional significance of spinal cord level, 72–74
  innervation level of major muscles, 73, 74f
  neuron, 64–65
  overview, 63f
  plexus formation, 74–80
  spinal cord, 68–70
  spinal cord trauma, 81
  spinal nerves, 68f, 70–72
Nervous tissue (neuron), 64–65
Neural arch, 68, 69f, 242, 242f
Neuron, 64–65
Neutral equilibrium, 111, 111f
Neutralizer, 57
Newton's three laws of motion, 104–105
Node of Ranvier, 64, 64f
Non-weight-bearing exercise, 59t
Nonaxial joint, 22–23, 23t
Nonprehensile hand functions, 213
Nonsupport, 383
Normal end feel, 31, 32
Normal resting length, 45
Nose, 270, 270f
Nuchal ligament, 247, 247f
Nuchal line, 241
Nucleus pulposus, 243, 243f
Nursemaid's elbow, 176
Nutation, 283, 283f

Oblique muscle, 43, 44, 44f
Obliquus capitis inferior, 250f, 251t
Obliquus capitis superior, 250f, 251t
Obturator externus, 308f, 308t
Obturator foramen, 299f, 300, 300f
Obturator internus, 308f, 308t
Obturator nerve, 78, 78f, 79–80, 79f
Occipital bone, 241, 241f
Occipital condyles, 241f, 242
Occipital lobe, 65–66, 66f
Occipital protuberance, 241
Occiput, 241, 249f
Occlusion, 101
Oculomotor nerve, 71f, 71t
Odontoid process, 244
Olecranon fossa, 166, 166f
Olecranon process, 166, 167f
Olfactory nerve, 71f, 71t
Omohyoid muscle, 233f, 234
One-joint muscle, 48, 52t
Open-chain exercise equipment, 59

Open-chain exercises, 59t
Open fracture, 18
Open kinetic chain, 59, 59f
Open-packed position, 37
Opening mouth against pressure, 238
Opening the jaw, 228, 229f
Opponens digiti minimi muscle, 207f, 210
Opponens pollicis muscle, 207, 207f
Opposition, 196f, 197
Optic nerve, 71f, 71t
Optimal length, 47–48
Oral cavity, 270, 270f
Oral pharynx, 270f
Origin, 41, 42f
Osgood-Schlatter disease, 18, 337
Osteoarthritis, 28, 314
Osteoclasts, 15
Osteokinematic motion, 31–32
Osteokinematics, 7, 103. *See also* Joint movements
Osteomyelitis, 18
Osteopenia, 18
Osteoporosis, 18
Osteoporotic bone, 18f
Overstretched muscle, 51
Ovoid joint, 34, 34f

Pad-to-pad grip, 216
Pad-to-side grip, 216–217, 217f
"Palm down" position, 9
"Palm up" position, 9
Palmar aponeurosis, 184, 185f
Palmar carpal ligament, 199
Palmar flexion, 7, 8f
Palmar interossei muscles, 208–209, 209f, 209t
Palmar radiocarpal ligament, 184, 184f
Palmaris longus muscle, 186–187, 186f
Paradoxical breathing, 274
Parallel force, 105
Parallel muscle, 43, 44, 44f
Parallelogram method, 105, 106f
Paraplegia, 81
Parasympathetic system, 63, 63f
Parietal lobe, 66, 66f
Parkinsonian gait, 395, 395f
Parkinsonism, 70
Passive insufficiency, 51, 51f
Passive range of motion (PROM), 31
Passive tension, 45, 47f
Patella, 17, 328, 328f, 329f
Patellar surface, 301, 301f, 327f, 328
Patellar tendon, 304, 331
Patellar tendonitis, 337
Patellofemoral angle, 325
Patellofemoral joint, 324, 325f
Patellofemoral pain syndrome, 337
Pathological fracture, 159
Pathological terms, 28
Pathologies. *See* Common pathologies
Pectineal line, 301, 301f, 327f, 328
Pectineus muscle, 305–306, 305f
Pectoralis major muscle, 151–152, 151f, 275, 275f, 277f
Pectoralis minor muscle, 137–138, 138f, 275, 277f
Pedicle, 242, 242f
Peduncle, 64
Peg-in-socket, 22, 22f
Pelvic cavity, 282
Pelvic girdle, 281–294, 299
  bones and landmarks, 283–285, 286–287
  ligaments, 285–286
  lumbosacral joint, 287–288
  male vs. female pelvis, 282, 282f
  muscle control, 291, 291f, 293f
  pelvic rotation, 290, 290f
  pelvic tilt, 288, 288f, 289f
  posture, 292
  pubic symphysis, 286, 286f
  sacroiliac (SI) joint, 283
  structure and function, 281–282
  true/false pelvis, 282
Pelvic girdle motions, 288–290
Pelvic hiking, 289
Pelvic inlet, 282, 282f
Pelvic outlet, 282, 282f
Pelvic rotation, 290, 290f
Pelvic surface, 283, 284
Pelvic tilt, 288, 288f, 289f
Pelvis, 281, 298f, 299. *See also* Pelvic girdle
Periosteum, 16
Peripheral nerve injuries, 70
Peripheral nerves, 75
Peripheral nervous system (PNS), 63, 63f
  common pathologies, 82–83
  cranial nerves, 70, 71–72t, 71f
  functional significance of spinal cord level, 72–74
  plexus formation, 74–80
  spinal nerves, 68f, 70–72
Pes anserine muscle group, 330
Pes cavus, 364
Pes planus, 364
Phalanges
  foot, 345, 345f
  hand, 196f
Pharynx, 270, 270f
Phlebitis, 101
Physiological motion, 31
Pia mater, 67, 67f, 68f
Picking up suitcase, 264
PIIS. *See* Posterior inferior iliac spine (PIIS)
Pincer grip, 216
Pinch grip, 216, 216f
PIP joint. *See* Proximal interphalangeal (PIP) joint
Piriformis muscle, 80f, 308f, 308t
Piriformis stretch position, 309
Pisiform, 181, 183f, 184f
Pituitary gland, 66f
Pivot joint, 24, 24f
Plane of the scapula, 128
Planes of action, 26–27, 27f
Plantar calcaneonavicular ligament, 352
Plantar fascia, 352, 353f
Plantar fasciitis, 366
Plantar flexion, 7, 8f, 346, 346f
Plantaris muscle, 355, 355f
Plantigrade, 364
Plate grip, 217
Platysma muscle, 258, 258f
Pleura, 271
Pleurisy, 278
Plexus, 74–80
  brachial, 74–78, 74f
  cervical, 74, 74f
  defined, 74
  lumbosacral, 74f, 78–81
PLL. *See* Posterior longitudinal ligament (PLL)
Plumb line, 374
Pneumonia, 278
Pneumothorax, 278
PNS. *See* Peripheral nervous system (PNS)
Poliomyelitis, 70
Pons, 66, 66f
Pope's blessing, 82
Popliteal artery, 93, 94f
Popliteal cyst, 337
Popliteal space, 330
Popliteal vein, 94, 94f
Popliteus muscle, 333–334, 334f
Posterior, 4, 5f
Posterior cerebral artery, 97
Posterior column, 65f, 69
Posterior communicating artery, 97
Posterior cruciate ligament, 329, 329f, 330f
Posterior deep hip muscles, 313f
Posterior deltoid muscle, 150f, 151
Posterior elbow muscles, 175f
Posterior fibular vein, 93
Posterior hand muscles, 211f
Posterior horn, 69, 69f
Posterior inferior iliac spine (PIIS), 284, 285f, 299f, 300, 300f
Posterior knee muscles, 333–335
Posterior longitudinal ligament (PLL), 246, 247f
Posterior ramus, 72
Posterior root, 65f, 68f, 69f
Posterior scalene muscle, 249, 249f
Posterior shoulder girdle muscles, 139f
Posterior shoulder muscles, 157f
Posterior superficial hip muscles, 313f
Posterior superior iliac spine (PSIS), 284, 285f, 299f, 300, 300f
Posterior tibial artery, 93, 94f
Posterior tibial vein, 93, 94f
Posterior tibiotalar ligament, 351f
Posterior tilt, 288, 288f
Posterior trunk muscles, 254–255, 254t
Posterior wrist muscles, 190f
Postglenoid tubercle, 225, 226f
Postural sway, 373, 373f
Posture, 371–380
  antigravity muscles, 373, 373f
  common postural deviations, 375t, 378–379
  development of postural curves, 372–374

disk pressures in various positions, 376, 377f
latissimus dorsi, 160
lying down, 378
pelvic girdle, 292
plumb line, 374
postural sway, 373, 373f
respiration, 279
shoulder girdle, 138
sitting, 376-378
standing, 374-376
supine, 378
temporomandibular junction (TMJ), 236
vertebral alignment, 371-374
Power grips, 214, 215-216, 215f, 216
Practical applications. *See* Clinical applications
Precision grips, 215, 215f, 216-217
Precision prehension, 215
Prehension, 213-214
Prepatellar bursa, 331f
Prepatellar bursitis, 338
Pressure epiphysis, 15, 16f
Preswing, 384t, 385t, 387, 387f
Prevertebral muscles, 249, 249f, 250t
Primary curve, 372, 372f
Prime mover, 57
Prime movers
elbow joint, 176t
hand, 212t
hip joint, 316t
knee joint, 336t
neck and trunk, 261t
shoulder girdle, 138t
shoulder joint, 158t
temporomandibular joint (TMJ), 235t
wrist joint, 190t
Pringles potato chips, 195, 196f
PROM. *See* Passive range of motion (PROM)
Pronation, 9, 10f
ankle and foot, 346
elbow joint, 163, 164f
Pronator quadratus muscle, 172f, 173
Pronator teres muscle, 172-173, 172f
Prone, 5-6
Propulsion phase, 386
Protraction, 9, 10f
Proximal, 5, 5f
Proximal carpal arch, 200, 201f
Proximal interphalangeal (PIP) joint, 196f, 198, 350, 350f
Proximal phalanges, 196f
Proximal radioulnar joint, 164, 164f
PSIS. *See* Posterior superior iliac spine (PSIS)
Psoas major, 304f
Pterygoid muscles, 231, 231f, 232, 235f
Pubic body, 285f, 286, 299f, 300, 300f
Pubic symphysis, 286, 286f, 288f
Pubic tubercle, 285f, 287, 299f, 300, 300f
Pubis, 285f, 286-287
Pubofemoral ligament, 25f, 303f
Pulled elbow, 176
Pulled hamstring, 315
Pulley, 118-119
Pulmonary circuit, 85, 86f
Pulmonary valve, 87
Pulmonic valve, 87
Pulse, 90, 90f
Pump-handle effect, 269
Push-off, 386
Push-pull activity, 173

Q angle, 325, 327f
Quadratus femoris muscle, 308f, 308t
Quadratus lumborum muscle, 257, 258f, 275, 277f
Quadriceps muscle, 109, 109f
Quadriceps muscle group, 331-333
Quadriceps "setting" exercises, 54
Quadriceps tendon, 330f
Quadriplegia, 81
Quiet expiration, 272, 276t
Quiet inspiration, 272, 276t

RA. *See* Resistance arm (RA)
Radial artery, 95, 95f
Radial collateral ligament, 183f, 184, 184f
Radial deviation, 8, 9f, 182f, 183f
Radial nerve, 75, 76, 77f
Radial nerve injury, 159
Radial notch, 167, 167f
Radial tuberosity, 167, 167f
Radial vein, 95
Radiocarpal joint, 181, 181f
Radioulnar joint, 164, 164f
Radius, 167, 167f, 176f
Ramus, 225, 225f
Rancho Los Amigos (RLA) terms, 383-384t
Range of motion (ROM), 31
Rectilinear motion, 6, 6f
Rectus abdominis muscle, 251, 251f, 275, 277f
Rectus capitis anterior, 249f, 250t
Rectus capitis lateralis, 249f, 250t
Rectus capitis posterior major, 250f, 251t
Rectus capitis posterior minor, 250f, 251t
Rectus femoris muscle, 49t, 304, 305f, 331, 332f
Reposition, 196f, 197
Resistance, 113
Resistance arm (RA), 113, 113f
Resistance training machine, 59
Respiratory system, 267-280
accessory expiratory muscles, 275
accessory inspiratory muscles, 274-275
anatomical relationships, 275-276
biomechanical impediments to respiration, 279
bones and landmarks, 267-269
common respiratory conditions/ pathologies, 278
diaphragm muscle, 272-273, 272f
diaphragmatic versus chest breathing, 276-277
Heimlich maneuver, 271, 271f
intercostal muscles, 273-274
joints of the thorax, 269
mechanics of respiration, 271
movements of thorax, 269-270
muscle innervation, 277
muscles of respiration, 272-275, 277f
paradoxical breathing, 274
phases of respiration, 272, 276t
structures of respiration, 270-271
thoracic cage, 267, 268f
Valsalva's maneuver, 277-278
Resting position, 37
Resultant force, 105-107, 107f
Retraction, 9, 10f
Retroversion, 314, 315f
Reverse Colles fracture, 189
Reverse muscle action, 42, 139-141
Rhomboid muscles, 136-137, 137f, 277f
Rhomboidal muscle, 44
Rib, 268
Rib cage, 267
Rib dislocation, 278
Rib separation, 278
Right common carotid artery, 95
Right lateral bending, 8
Right lymphatic duct, 100, 100f
Right neck rotation, 9, 10f
Ring finger, 197
RLA terms. *See* Rancho Los Amigos (RLA) terms
Rocking horse gait, 392
Roll, 34, 34f
ROM. *See* Range of motion (ROM)
Rotary force, 33-34, 34f
Rotary motion, 6
Rotation, 9, 10f
neck and trunk, 240, 241f
pelvic girdle, 290, 290f
Rotator cuff, 149, 149f
Rotator cuff muscles, 155
Rotatores muscles, 256, 256f
Rowing machine, 59
Running/walking, compared, 391
Ruptured Achilles tendon, 366

S1, S2, ... S5, 68f, 73f, 240t
Sacral curve, 371, 372f
Sacral extension, 283
Sacral flexion, 283
Sacral nerves, 68f, 70
Sacral plexus, 78, 78f
Sacral promontory, 282f, 283, 284f
Sacral vertebrae, 68f, 73f, 240f, 240t
Sacroiliac (SI) joint, 281, 281f, 283
Sacrospinalis muscle group, 255
Sacrospinous ligament, 285f, 286, 286f
Sacrotuberous ligament, 285f, 286, 286f
Sacrum, 283-284, 284f
Saddle joint, 24, 24f
Saddle-shaped joint, 34
Sagittal axis, 27, 28f
Sagittal plane, 26-27, 27f
"Sally Likes To Push The Toy Car Hard," 191
Saltwater taffy, 45
Sarcomere, 45, 46f

Sartorius muscle, 305, 305f, 335
Saturday night palsy, 82
SC joint. *See* Sternoclavicular (SC) joint
Scalar, 103
Scalar terms, 103
Scalene muscles, 249, 249f, 277f
Scaphoid, 183f, 184f
Scaphoid fracture, 189, 212
Scaption, 146, 146f
Scapula, 128–129, 129f, 147, 147f, 166
Scapular abduction, 132
Scapular adduction, 132
Scapular depression, 132
Scapular downward rotation, 132
Scapular elevation, 132
Scapular motion, 132, 132f
Scapular protraction, 132
Scapular retraction, 132
Scapular tilt, 132, 132f
Scapular upward rotation, 132
Scapular winging, 82, 132, 133f
Scapulohumeral rhythm, 133
Scapulothoracic articulation, 127–128, 127f, 131
SCI. *See* Spinal cord injury (SCI)
Sciatic nerve, 78, 78f, 80, 80f
Sciatica, 83, 261
Scissors gait, 395–396, 396f
Scoliosis, 261, 279, 372, 373, 379
Screw-home mechanism, 324, 325f
Second-class lever, 114–116
Segments of the body, 4
Self-stretch at forearm, 179
Sellar joint, 34, 34f
Semilunar notch, 167
Semilunar (SL) valve, 87, 88
Semimembranosus bursa, 331f
Semimembranosus muscle, 308–309, 309f, 333
Semispinalis muscles, 256, 256f
Semitendinosus muscle, 308, 309, 309f, 333, 333f
Sensory innervation of hand, 213f, 214
Sensory neuron, 65, 65f
Sentinel node, 99
Serratus anterior muscle, 43, 43f, 137, 137f
Serratus posterior inferior muscle, 276, 276f
Serratus posterior superior muscle, 276, 276f
Sesamoid bones, 17, 17t
Severe sprain, 28
Shearing force, 33, 33f
Shin splints, 364
Short bones, 16, 16f, 17t
Short plantar ligament, 352, 352f
Short posterior sacroiliac ligament, 286, 286f
Shortening contraction, 54, 55f
Shoulder abduction, 9f
Shoulder adduction, 9f
Shoulder complex, 127
Shoulder girdle, 127–143. *See also* Shoulder joint
  acromioclavicular (AC) joint, 130–131, 131f
  anatomical relationships, 138–139
  anterior shoulder girdle muscles, 139f
  bones and landmarks, 128–130
  common pathologies, 141
  crutch walking, 140, 140f
  force couples, 139
  joint motions, 131–133
  lateral shoulder girdle muscles, 139f
  levator scapula muscle, 136, 136f
  muscle innervation, 141
  pectoralis minor muscle, 137–138, 138f
  posterior shoulder girdle muscles, 139f
  prime movers, 138t
  reverse muscle action, 139–141
  rhomboid muscles, 136–137, 137f
  scapulohumeral rhythm, 133
  scapulothoracic articulation, 131
  serratus anterior muscle, 137, 137f
  sternoclavicular (SC) joint, 130, 130f
  terminology, 127–128
  trapezius muscle, 134–136
Shoulder horizontal abduction, 9f
Shoulder horizontal adduction, 9f
Shoulder joint, 128, 145–162. *See also* Shoulder girdle
  anatomical relationships, 156–157
  anterior shoulder muscles, 156f
  arthrokinematic motion, 146, 147f
  bones and landmarks, 147–148
  common shoulder pathologies, 159
  coracobrachialis muscle, 156, 156f
  deltoid muscle, 150–151, 150f
  glenohumeral movement, 157–158
  infraspinatus muscle, 154, 154f
  joint motions, 145–147
  latissimus dorsi muscle, 152, 152f
  ligaments and other structures, 148–150
  muscle innervation, 158–159, 158t, 159t
  pectoralis major muscle, 151–152, 151f
  posterior shoulder muscles, 157f
  prime mover actions, 158t
  subscapularis muscle, 155–156, 155f
  supraspinatus muscle, 153–154, 154f
  teres major muscle, 153, 153f
  teres minor muscle, 154–155, 154f
Shoulder joint capsule, 148, 149f
Shoulder subluxation, 28
SI joint. *See* Sacroiliac (SI) joint
Side bending, 240
Side-to-side grip, 217, 217f
Simple machines, 113–121
Single-joint muscle, 48, 52t
Single-leg support, 382, 382f
Single support, 382f, 383
Sinus, 18t
SIT muscles, 155
Sit-ups, 248, 252
SITS muscles, 155
Sitting posture, 376–378
Skeletal system, 13–19
  bone. *See* Bone
  common skeletal pathologies, 17–18
  functions of the skeleton, 13
  types of skeletons, 13, 14t, 15f
Skier's thumb, 212
Skull, 66, 67f, 241–242, 241f
SL valve. *See* Semilunar (SL) valve
Slide, 34
Sliding board transfer, 162
Sliding filament theory, 45
Slipped capital femoral epiphysis, 18, 313
Slouched posture, 377f
Small saphenous vein, 94, 94f
Smith's fracture, 189
Soft end feel, 32
Soft tissue approximation, 32
Soleus muscle, 354–355, 355f
Sphenomandibular ligament, 227, 228f
Spherical grip, 215, 216f
Sphygmomanometer, 90
Spin, 35, 35f
Spina bifida, 81
Spina bifida occulta, 81
Spinal accessory nerve, 71f, 72t
Spinal column, 239
Spinal cord, 68–70
Spinal cord injury (SCI), 70, 81
Spinal cord trauma, 81–82
Spinal meninges, 66–67, 67f
Spinal nerves, 68f, 70–72
Spinal osteoarthritis, 261
Spinal stability, compressive forces, 257
Spinal stenosis, 262
Spinalis cervicis, 255f
Spinalis muscle group, 255
Spinalis thoracis, 255f
Spine, 18t
Spinous process, 242, 242f, 244f, 245f, 245t
Spiral groove, 166
Splenius capitis muscle, 250, 251f
Splenius cervicis muscle, 250, 251f
Spondylolisthesis, 262
Spondylolysis, 262
Spondylosis, 261
Sprain
  ankle, 365
  defined, 28
  severity, 28
  wrist, 190
Spring block, 32
Spring ligament, 351f, 352, 352f
Squat lift, 261
Stability
  balance, stability, and motion, 111–113
  base of support (BOS), 110, 111f, 112f
  center of gravity (COG), 109–110, 110f, 111f, 112f
  line of gravity (LOG), 110
  states of equilibrium, 110–111, 111f
Stabilizer, 57
Stabilizing force, 109
Stable equilibrium, 110–111, 111f
Stair stepper, 59
Stance phase, 382, 382f, 383t–384t, 386–387
Standing posture, 374–376
Standing with one foot on telephone book, 294
State of equilibrium, 109, 110–111, 111f
Statics, 103
Stationary bicycle, 59
Stenosing tenosynovitis, 212
Step, 381
Step length, 381, 382f

Steppage gait, 393, 393f, 395
Sternoclavicular (SC) joint, 127f, 130, 130f
Sternoclavicular ligament, 130, 130f
Sternocleidomastoid muscle, 43, 43f, 248, 248f, 258, 258f, 277f
Sternohyoid muscle, 233–234, 233f
Sternothyroid muscle, 233f, 234
Sternum, 129, 129f, 130, 258f, 268, 268f
Stinger syndrome, 82
Stirrup of foot, 359
Stitch, 278
Straight leg raise (SLR), 309
Strain
  defined, 28
  hamstring muscles, 59
  severity, 28
Strap muscle, 44, 44f
Stretching the muscles, 52–53
Stride, 381
Stride length, 381, 382f
Stroke, 101
Student's bursa, 26
Stylohyoid ligament, 227f, 228
Stylohyoid muscle, 232, 232f, 233, 233f
Styloid process, 167, 167f, 183, 183f, 226, 226f
Stylomandibular ligament, 227, 228f
Subacromial bursa, 149
Subarachnoid space, 67, 67f
Subclavian artery, 94–95, 95f, 96f
Subclavian vein, 95, 95f, 96f
Subdeltoid bursa, 148–149
Subdural bleed, 101
Subluxation, 28
Subluxing of biceps tendon, 159
Suboccipital muscles, 249, 250f, 251t
Subscapular fossa, 147, 147f
Subscapularis muscle, 155–156, 155f
Subtalar joint, 349, 349f
Superficial, 5
Superficial fibular nerve, 80, 81f, 363
Superficial infrapatellar bursa, 331f
Superior, 5, 5f
Superior articular process, 242f, 243f, 245f, 245t, 284, 284f
Superior gluteal nerve, 78, 78f
Superior lamina, 229f
Superior pubic ligament, 286, 286f
Superior pubic ramus, 285f, 286, 299f, 300f
Superior ramus, 300
Superior tibiofibular joint, 347, 347f
Superior trunk, 74
Superior vena cava, 93f, 96f
Supination, 4, 9, 10f
  ankle and foot, 346
  elbow joint, 163, 164f
Supinator muscle, 174, 174f, 176f
Supine, 5
Supine posture, 378
Supracondylar fracture, 176
Supraglenoid tubercle, 166, 166f
Suprahyoid muscles, 232–233, 233f
Suprapatellar bursa, 331f
Supraspinal ligament, 246, 247f
Supraspinatus muscle, 153–154, 154f
Supraspinous fossa, 147, 147f
Sustentaculum tali, 344, 345f, 351f
Suture-type joint, 21, 22f
Swan neck deformity, 212
Sway back, 371
Swimmer's shoulder, 159
Swing phase, 382, 382f, 384t, 387–388
Sympathetic system, 63, 63f
Symphysis pubis, 281, 281f, 282f, 300
Synapse, 64, 65f
Synarthrosis, 21, 22f, 23t
Syndesmosis, 21, 22f, 23t
Synergist, 57
Synovial fluid, 25
Synovial joint, 22, 22f
Synovial membrane, 22f, 25
Synovitis, 28
Systemic circuit, 86, 86f
Systolic pressure, 90–91

T1, T2, ... T12, 68f, 73f, 240f, 240t
Tabletop position, 209
Talocalcaneal joint, 349
Talocrural joint, 347–348
Talotibial joint, 347
Talus, 344, 345f, 352f
Tarsal bones, 344, 345f
Temporal bone, 225–226, 241f, 242
Temporal fossa, 226f, 227
Temporal lobe, 66, 66f
Temporal process, 226f, 227
Temporalis muscle, 230, 231f, 234f
Temporomandibular dysfunction (TMD), 236
Temporomandibular joint (TMJ), 223–238
  anatomical relationships, 234–235
  bones and landmarks, 224–227
  closing the jaw, 228, 229f
  digastric muscle, 232, 232f, 233, 233f
  geniohyoid muscle, 232, 232f, 233, 233f
  infrahyoid muscles, 233–234, 233f
  joint motions, 223–224, 224f
  lateral pterygoid muscle, 231f, 232, 235f
  ligaments and other structures, 227–228
  location, 223
  masseter muscle, 231, 231f, 234f
  mechanical advantage, 230
  mechanics of movement, 228, 229f
  medial pterygoid muscle, 231, 231f, 235f
  muscle innervation, 235, 235t
  muscles, 229–234
  mylohyoid muscle, 232, 232f, 233f
  omohyoid muscle, 233f, 234
  opening the jaw, 228, 229f
  postural influences, 236
  prime movers, 235t
  sternohyoid muscle, 233–234, 233f
  sternothyroid muscle, 233f, 234
  stylohyoid muscle, 232, 232f, 233, 233f
  suprahyoid muscles, 232–233, 233f
  temporalis muscle, 230, 231f, 234f
  thyrohyoid muscle, 233f, 234
  TMJ dysfunction, 236
Temporomandibular ligament, 227
Tendon, 26, 26f, 41, 42f
Tendon action of a muscle (tenodesis), 53
Tendon position of anterior wrist muscles, 188f
Tendon sheath, 26
Tendonitis, 28, 59
Tennis backswing, 263
Tennis elbow, 175
Tennis forehand swing, 318
Tenodesis, 53, 54f
Tenon, 348
Tenoperiosteal junction, 41, 42f
Tenosynovitis, 28, 212
Tension, 45
Tensor fascia lata muscle, 310–311, 311f, 335
Teres major muscle, 153, 153f
Teres minor muscle, 154–155, 154f
Terminal nerves
  brachial plexus, 75, 76–78
  lumbosacral plexus, 79–81
Terminal stance, 383t, 385t, 386, 387f
Terminal swing, 384t, 385t, 388, 388f
Terminology
  accessory arthrokinematic motions, 32
  ankle and foot, 346–347
  descriptive terms, 4–6
  exercise terms, 59t
  gait, 381–383, 383–384t
  pathological terms, 28
  scalar terms, 103
  shoulder, 127–128
Terrible triad, 338
Text neck, 378
Thalamus, 66, 66f
Thenar muscles, 206, 206t
Thigh, 4, 4f, 298f
Third-class lever, 116–117, 116f
Thoracic cage, 267, 268f
Thoracic curve, 371, 372f
Thoracic duct, 100, 100f
Thoracic nerves, 68f, 70, 72
Thoracic outlet, 95, 101, 261
Thoracic outlet syndrome, 82, 101, 260–261
Thoracic vertebrae, 68f, 73f, 240f, 240t, 245f, 245t
Thoracolumbar fascia, 149, 157f, 248, 253f
Thorax, 4, 4f, 267
Three-jaw chuck, 216
Thrombophlebitis, 101
Thrombosis, 101
Thumb, 195–197
Thyrohyoid muscle, 233f, 234
Thyroid cartilage, 227, 227f
Tibia, 301, 302f, 328, 328f, 344
Tibial collateral ligament, 329
Tibial nerve, 78, 78f, 80, 80f, 362
Tibial plateau, 328, 328f
Tibial tuberosity, 301, 302f, 328, 328f
Tibialis anterior muscle, 357, 358f
Tibialis posterior muscle, 355–356, 356f
Tibiocalcaneal ligament, 351f
Tibionavicular ligament, 351f
Tight muscle, 51
Tip position, 82
Tip-to-tip grip, 216
TMD. *See* Temporomandibular dysfunction (TMD)

TMJ. *See* Temporomandibular joint (TMJ)
Toe-off, 382f, 384t, 385t, 386–387, 387f
Toes, 345, 345f, 350, 350f
Tone, 45
Torn rotator cuff, 159
Torque, 104, 107–109
Torque arm, 108
Torsional force, 33–34, 34f
Torticollis, 261
Trabeculae, 14
Trachea, 227f, 270, 270f
Tract, 64
Traction epiphysis, 15, 16f
Traction force, 33, 33f
Translatory motion, 6
Transverse abdominis muscle, 252, 253f, 254, 277f
Transverse arch, 352, 352f
Transverse carpal ligament, 198f, 199
Transverse foramen, 243f, 244, 244f
Transverse ligament, 243f, 244, 330f
Transverse plane, 27, 27f
Transverse process, 242, 242f, 245f, 245t
Transverse spinal muscle group, 256
Transverse tarsal joint, 349, 349f
Transversospinalis muscle group, 256, 256f
Trapezium, 183f, 184f, 197f
Trapezius muscle, 43, 43f, 134–136
Trapezoid, 183f, 184f, 197f
Treadmill, 59
Trendelenburg gait, 310, 392
Trendelenburg sign, 389
Triangular muscle, 44, 44f
Triaxial joint, 23t, 24
Triceps muscle, 171, 172f
Triceps surae contracture, 394
Triceps surae group, 393
Tricuspid valve, 87
Trigger finger, 212
Trigger points, 59
Trimalleolar fracture, 366
Triplanar, 346, 348
Triple arthrodesis, 366, 395
Tripod grip, 216f
Triquetrum, 183f
Trochanter, 18t
Trochanteric bursitis, 315
Trochanteric fossa, 301, 301f
Trochlea, 166, 166f
Trochlear nerve, 71f, 71t
Trochlear notch, 167, 167f
True pelvis, 282, 282f
True ribs, 267, 268f
Trunk, *See* Neck and trunk
Trunk left lateral bending, 9f
Trunk right lateral bending, 9f
Tubercle, 18t
Tuberosity, 18t
Tuberosity of Navicular, 344, 345f
Tunica adventitia, 88
Tunica intima, 88
Tunica media, 88
Turf toe, 365
Twisted neck, 261
Twisting motion, 33
Typical vertebral articulations, 244–247

Ulna, 164f, 166–167, 176f
Ulnar artery, 95, 95f
Ulnar collateral ligament, 183f, 184, 184f
Ulnar deviation, 8, 9f, 182f, 183f
Ulnar drift, 212
Ulnar nerve, 75, 77, 78f
Ulnar nerve compression, 176
Ulnar tuberosity, 167, 167f
Ulnar vein, 95
Uniaxial, 23–24, 23t
Unipennate muscle, 44, 44f
Unstable equilibrium, 111, 111f
Unstable fracture, 262
Upper extremity closed-chain activities, 59
Upper joint space, 224, 228f, 229f
Upper motor neuron, 69
Upper motor neuron lesion, 70, 70t
Upper respiratory infection (URI), 278
Upper respiratory tract, 270
Upper trapezius muscle, 43f, 134–135, 134f, 277f

Vagus nerve, 71f, 72t
Valsalva's maneuver, 277–278
Varicose veins, 101
Vastus intermedialis muscle, 331, 332f, 333
Vastus lateralis muscle, 331, 332, 332f
Vastus medialis muscle, 331, 332–333, 332f
Vaulting gait, 394, 394f
Vector, 103
Vector force, 105
Vector quantity, 105
Veins, 88, 91–92t, 94f, 95f, 96
Velcro strap (on shoe), 118
Velocity, 103
Ventral, 4, 5f
Ventricles, 67, 86, 87, 87f
Venules, 88
Vertebra, 69f
Vertebra prominens, 244
Vertebral alignment, 371–374
Vertebral arch, 242
Vertebral artery, 96, 96f
Vertebral column, 239, 240, 240f
Vertebral curves, 239, 240f, 240t
Vertebral foramen, 68, 69f, 242, 242f, 245f, 245t
Vertebral notches, 242, 245f, 245t
Vertebral segments, 240t
Vertebral vein, 96, 96f
Vertical axis, 27, 28f
Vertical displacement, 388–389, 389f
Vestibulocochlear nerve, 71f, 71t
Voice box, 270
Volkmann's ischemic contracture, 176

Waddling gait, 393, 393f
Walking, 381. *See also* Gait
Walking base width, 389, 389f
Walking gait cycle, 391
Walking pneumonia, 278
Wall slide exercise, 335
Water on the brain, 81
Watersheds, 100, 100f
Weak muscle, 51
Weight acceptance, 382, 382f
Weight-bearing exercise, 59t
Wheel and axle, 119–120
Wheelbarrow, 114
Wheelchair accessibility, 120
Wheelchair pushing, 59
Wheelchair ramp, 120–121, 121f
Whiplash, 262
White matter, 64, 65f, 68f, 69, 69f
Width of walking base, 389, 389f
Windlass effect, 353
Windpipe, 270
Winging of the scapula, 132, 133f
Wire spring, 45
Wrist drop, 82
Wrist immobilization, 217
Wrist joint, 181–194. *See also* Hand
  anatomical relationships, 188–189, 190f
  anterior wrist muscles, 190f
  arthrokinematic motion, 183
  bones and landmarks, 183
  common wrist pathologies, 189–190
  dual role of wrist muscles, 189
  extensor carpi radialis brevis muscle, 187–188, 188f
  extensor carpi radialis longus muscle, 187, 187f
  extensor carpi ulnaris muscle, 188
  flexor carpi radialis muscle, 185–186, 186f
  flexor carpi ulnaris muscle, 185, 186f
  joint motions, 182–183
  ligaments and other structures, 184
  muscle innervation, 191, 191t
  muscles, 184–188
  osteokinematic motion, 182
  palmaris longus muscle, 186–187, 186f
  posterior wrist muscles, 190f
  prime movers, 190t
  tendon position of anterior wrist muscles, 188f
  terminology, 182t
Wrist radial deviation, 9f
Wrist sprain, 190
Wrist ulnar deviation, 9f
Wry neck, 261

Xiphoid process, 129f, 130, 268, 268f

Y ligament, 302

Z-line, 45, 46f
Zygapophyseal joint, 246
Zygomatic arch, 226f, 227
Zygomatic bone, 226f, 227
Zygomatic process, 226, 226f